IMMUNOLOGY

9th edition

IMMUNOLOGY

David Male, BA, MA, PhD

Professor of Biology
Department of Life Sciences
The Open University
Milton Keynes, United Kingdom

R. Stokes Peebles, Jr., MD

Elizabeth and John Murray Professor of Medicine
Division of Allergy, Pulmonary, and Critical Care Medicine
Vanderbilt University School of Medicine
Nashville, Tennessee, United States

Victoria Male, BA, MA, PhD

Sir Henry Dale Fellow
Department of Metabolism
Digestion and Reproduction
Imperial College London
London, United Kingdom

For additional online content visit StudentConsult.com

ELSEVIER

ISBN: 978-0-7020-7844-6
International ISBN: 978-0-7020-7845-3

Content Strategist: Alexandra Mortimer
Content Development Specialist: Trinity Hutton
Senior Project Manager: Karthikeyan Murthy
Design: Ryan Cook
Art Buyer: Anitha Rajarathnam
Marketing Manager: Melissa Darling

Printed in Poland

Last digit is the print number: 9 8 7 6 5 4 3 2 1

Working together
to grow libraries in
developing countries

www.elsevier.com • www.bookaid.org

CONTENTS

v

PREFACE TO THE 9TH EDITION

This is the first edition of *Immunology* that has not included two of our original editors, Ivan Roitt and Jonathan Brostoff. We would like to pay tribute to their foresight in developing this text, which was originally planned as a slide atlas of immunology. They have steered the book through its eight previous editions, during which time the subject has advanced beyond all recognition. In 1985 when the first edition was published, the structure and function of antibodies were well known and MHC molecules had just been described, but how T cells became activated was still a matter of conjecture and debate.

Nowadays, antibodies have become key therapeutic agents, not just for immunological conditions, but particularly for treatment of cancer and the targeting of therapeutic agents. Cytokine-based treatments for many diseases are following closely behind. Hence, the subject of immunology impinges on diverse areas of clinical practice, as well as providing tools and important theoretical concepts for many of the biological sciences.

For this edition, and with two new editors, we have made a major reorganisation in the first half of the book, with innate immunity and cell-mediated immunity introduced first. This rearrangement responds to our improved understanding of these areas of immunology, and it also presents material in a more logical chronological order, since innate immune reactions and lymphocyte activation precede antibody production.

Despite these changes we have maintained the overall balance of the text with the first two sections describing how the immune system works. Section three is concerned with immune responses against pathogens—the primary function of the immune system—and the final three sections deal with aspects of clinical immunology, including autoimmune disease, immunodeficiency, transplantation, tumour immunology and hypersensitivity. All chapters have been fully updated with many new diagrams.

We have followed the style of the 8th edition by including two levels of detail in the text. The printed text includes those elements that we consider essential for understanding basic and clinical immunology; the online version includes additional information at appropriate points (indicated by a symbol in the margin), for readers who want to delve deeper. The critical thinking sections that follow each chapter require an understanding of the material presented and the implications in a laboratory or clinical setting—they may be used as the basis of class discussion. Another important teaching tool is the summaries which distil the key points of each chapter and are a solid basis for revision for exams.

The contributors to this edition include many experts in different fields of immunology, with seven new contributors who have brought their own expertise to individual chapters. We also greatly appreciate the hard work of colleagues at Elsevier, particularly Trinity Hutton, Alex Mortimer and Karthikeyan Murthy.

Immunology bridges basic science and medicine and encompasses genetics, cell biology and molecular biology. Advances in biotechnology in the last 10 years have driven forward antibody-based therapies. In the next 10 years we anticipate that understanding of genetic diversity in the immune system will lead to advances in personalised medicine, while gene therapies are becoming available to correct primary immunodeficiencies. For the past century, immunology has fascinated and inspired some of the greatest scientific thinkers and Nobel prize winners. Most recently the prize for Medicine or Physiology was awarded to James Allison and Tasuko Honjo for advances in cancer immunotherapy. We wish our readers well in their study of immunology, a subject that continues to excite and surprise us, and which underpins many areas of medicine and biomedical science.

David Male
R. Stokes Peebles, Jr.
Victoria Male
2019

CONTRIBUTORS

The editors would like to acknowledge and offer grateful thanks for the input of all previous editions' contributors, without whom this new edition would not have been possible.

Gregory J. Bancroft, BSc Hons, PhD
Professor
Department of Infection Biology
Faculty of Infectious and Tropical Diseases
London School of Hygiene & Tropical
    Medicine
London, United Kingdom

David Bending, BA, MA, PhD
Institute of Immunology and
    Immunotherapy
University of Birmingham
Birmingham, United Kingdom

Persephone Borrow, BA, MA, PhD
Professor of Viral Immunology
Nuffield Department of Clinical Medicine
University of Oxford
Oxford, United Kingdom

Colin Casimir, BSc, PhD
Department of Natural Sciences
Middlesex University
London, United Kingdom

Daniel Cook, MD, PhD
Resident Physician
Department of Internal Medicine
Vanderbilt University Medical Center
Nashville, Tennessee, United States

David P. D'Cruz, MD, FRCP
Consultant Rheumatologist
The Louise Coote Lupus Unit
Guy's and St Thomas' Hospitals
London, United Kingdom

Daniel Dulek, MD
Assistant Professor
Department of Pediatric Infectious Diseases
Vanderbilt University Medical Center
Nashville, Tennessee, United States

**Hakimeh Ebrahimi-Nik, Doctorate of
    Veterinary Medicine, PhD**
Postdoctoral Fellow
Department of Immunology
UConn Health
Farmington, Connecticut, United States

**Andrew George, MBE, MA, PhD, DSc,
    FRCPath, FHEA, FRSA, FRSB**
Emeritus Professor
Brunel University London
Uxbridge, United Kingdom

David Isenberg, MD, FRCP, FAMS
Professor
The Centre for Rheumatology Research,
    Department of Medicine
University College London
London, United Kingdom

**Roy Jefferis, BSc, PhD, FRSC, CChem,
    MRCP, FRCPath, DSc**
Emeritus Professor
Institute of Immunology & Immunotherapy
University of Birmingham
Birmingham, United Kingdom

Thomas Kamradt, Dr. med.
Professor
Department of Immunology
University Hospital Jena
Jena, Germany

Yasmin Khan, MD
Assistant Professor of Pediatrics
Department of Pediatric Allergy,
    Immunology, and Pulmonary Medicine
Vanderbilt University Medical Center
Nashville, Tennessee, United States

**Peter Maldwyn Lydyard, BSc, MSc, PhD,
    FRCPath**
Emeritus Professor
University College London
Visiting Professor
University of Westminster
London, United Kingdom

Arti Mahto, BSc, MBBCh, MRCP, PhD
Department of Rheumatology
University College Hospital,
London, United Kingdom

David Male, BA, MA, PhD
Professor of Biology
Department of Life Sciences
The Open University
Milton Keynes, United Kingdom

Victoria Male, BA, MA, PhD
Sir Henry Dale Fellow
Department of Metabolism
Digestion and Reproduction
Imperial College London
London, United Kingdom

Luisa Martinez-Pomares, BSc, PhD
Associate Professor
School of Life Sciences
University of Nottingham
Nottingham, United Kingdom

**Bryan Paul Morgan, BSc, MBBCh, PhD,
    FRCPath, MRCP**
Professor of Immunology
School of Medicine
Cardiff University
Cardiff, United Kingdom

Luigi D. Notarangelo, MD
Chief
Laboratory of Clinical Immunology
    and Microbiology
National Institute of Allergy and
    Infectious Diseases, National
    Institutes of Health
Bethesda, Maryland, United States

R. Stokes Peebles, Jr., MD
Elizabeth and John Murray
    Professor of Medicine
Division of Allergy, Pulmonary,
    and Critical Care Medicine
Vanderbilt University School of Medicine
Nashville, Tennessee, United States

**Thomas A.E. Platts-Mills, MD,
    PhD, FRS**
Head, Asthma and Allergic Disease Center
Department of Medicine
University of Virginia
Charlottesville, Virginia, United States

Richard John Pleass, BSc, MSc, PhD
Professor
Department of Parasitology
Liverpool School of Tropical Medicine
Liverpool, Merseyside, United Kingdom

Nina Porakishvili, BSc, MSc, PhD
School of Life Sciences
University of Westminster
London, United Kingdom

Theo Rispens, PhD
Department of Immunopathology
Sanquin Research, Amsterdam
Amsterdam, Netherlands

Pramod K. Srivastava, PhD, MD
Professor of Immunology and Medicine
Director, Carole and Ray Neag
    Comprehensive Cancer Center and
    Department of Immunology
University of Connecticut School of Medicine
Farmington, Connecticut, United States

Gestur Vidarsson, BSc, MSc, PhD
Head of Laboratory
Department of Experimental
    Immunohematology/Immunoglobulin
    Research Laboratory
Sanquin Research
Amsterdam, Netherlands

Introduction to the Immune System

SUMMARY

- **The immune system has evolved to protect us from pathogens.** Intracellular pathogens infect individual cells (e.g. viruses), whereas extracellular pathogens divide outside cells in blood, tissues or the body cavities (e.g. many bacteria and parasites). These two kinds of pathogen require fundamentally different immune responses.

- **Phagocytes and lymphocytes are key mediators of immunity.** Phagocytes internalize pathogens and degrade them. Lymphocytes (B and T cells) have receptors that recognize specific molecular components of pathogens and have specialized functions. B cells make antibodies (effective against extracellular pathogens), cytotoxic T lymphocytes (CTLs) kill virally infected cells and helper T cells coordinate the immune response by direct cell–cell interactions and the release of cytokines.

- **Inflammation is a response to tissue damage.** It allows antibodies, complement system molecules and leukocytes to enter the tissue at the site of infection, resulting in phagocytosis and destruction of the pathogens. Lymphocytes are also required to recognize and to destroy infected cells in the tissues.

- **Specificity and memory are two essential features of adaptive immune responses.** As a result, the adaptive arm of the immune system (B and T lymphocytes) mounts a more effective response on second and subsequent encounters with a particular antigen. Non-adaptive (innate) immune responses (mediated, for example, by complement and phagocytes) do not alter on repeated exposure to an infectious agent.

- **Antigens are molecules that are recognized by receptors on B cells and T cells.** B cells usually recognize intact antigen molecules, whereas T cells recognize antigen fragments displayed on the surface of the body's own cells.

- **An immune response occurs in two phases – antigen recognition and antigen eradication.** In the first phase, clonal selection involves recognition of antigen by particular clones of lymphocytes, leading to expansion of specific clones of T and B cells and differentiation to effector and memory cells. In the effector phase, these lymphocytes coordinate an immune response, which eliminates the source of the antigen.

- **Vaccination depends on the specificity and memory of adaptive immunity.** Vaccination is based on the key elements of adaptive immunity, namely specificity and memory. Memory cells allow the immune system to mount a much stronger and more rapid response on a second encounter with antigen.

- **The immune system may fail (immunopathology).** This can be a result of immunodeficiency, hypersensitivity or dysregulation leading to autoimmune diseases.

- **Normal immune reactions can be inconvenient in modern medicine**, for example blood transfusion reactions and graft rejection.

The immune system is fundamental to survival, as it protects the body from **pathogens**: viruses, bacteria and parasites that cause disease. To do so, it has evolved a powerful collection of defence mechanisms to recognize and protect against potential invaders that would otherwise take advantage of the rich source of nutrients provided by the vertebrate host. At the same time it must differentiate between the individual's own cells and those of harmful invading organisms while not attacking the beneficial commensal flora that inhabit the gut, skin and other tissues.

This chapter provides an overview of the complex network of processes that form the immune system of higher vertebrates:

- It illustrates how the components of the immune system fit together to allow students to grasp the big picture before delving into the material in more depth in subsequent chapters.

- It introduces the basic elements of the immune system and of immune responses, which are mediated principally by white blood cells or **leukocytes** (from the Greek for white cell) and are detailed in Chapters 2–13.

Over many millions of years, different types of immune defence, appropriate to the infecting pathogens, have evolved in different groups of organisms. In this book, we concentrate on the immune systems of mammals, especially humans. Because mammals are warm-blooded and long-lived, their immune systems have evolved particularly sophisticated systems for recognizing and destroying pathogens.

Many of the immune defences that have evolved in other vertebrates (e.g. reptiles, amphibians) and other phyla (e.g. sponges, worms, insects) are also present in some form in mammals. Consequently the mammalian immune system consists of multi-layered, interlocking defence mechanisms that incorporate both ancient and recently evolved elements.

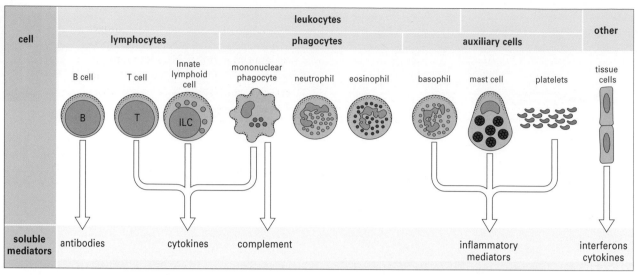

Fig. 1.1 Components of the immune system The principal cells of the immune system and the mediators they produce are shown. Neutrophils, eosinophils and basophils are collectively known as polymorphonuclear granulocytes (see Chapter 2). B cells and T cells have highly specific receptors for foreign material (antigens), whereas innate lymphoid cells (ILCs) do not have the specific receptors. Cytotoxic describes the function of different cells, including cytotoxic T lymphocytes (CTLs), natural killer (NK) cells (a type of ILC) and eosinophils. Complement is made primarily by the liver, although there is some synthesis by mononuclear phagocytes. Note that each cell produces and secretes only a particular set of cytokines or inflammatory mediators.

CELLS AND SOLUBLE MEDIATORS OF THE IMMUNE SYSTEM

Cells of the Immune System

Immune responses are mediated by a variety of cells and the soluble molecules that these cells secrete (Fig. 1.1). Although the leukocytes are central to all immune responses, other cells in the tissues also participate by signalling to the lymphocytes and responding to the cytokines (soluble intercellular signalling molecules) released by T cells and macrophages.

Phagocytes internalize antigens and pathogens and break them down. The most important long-lived phagocytic cells belong to the **mononuclear phagocyte** lineage (see Chapter 5). These cells are all derived from bone marrow stem cells and their function is to engulf particles, including infectious agents, internalize them and destroy them (Fig. 1.2). To do so, mononuclear phagocytes have surface receptors that allow them to recognize and bind to a wide variety of microbial

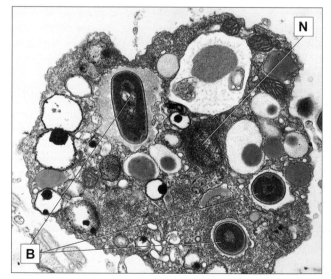

Fig. 1.3 Phagocytes internalize and kill invading organisms Electron micrograph of a phagocyte from a tunicate (sea squirt) that has endocytosed three bacteria *(B)*. *N*, Nucleus. (Courtesy Dr AF Rowley.)

macromolecules. They can then internalize and kill the microorganism (Fig. 1.3). The process of **phagocytosis** describes the internalization (endocytosis) of large particles or microbes. The primitive responses of phagocytes are highly effective and people with genetic defects in phagocytic cells often succumb to infections in infancy.

To intercept pathogens, mononuclear phagocytes are strategically placed where they will encounter them. For example, the Kupffer cells of the liver line the sinusoids along which blood flows, while the synovial A cells line the synovial cavity (Fig. 1.4).

Leukocytes of the mononuclear phagocyte lineage are called **monocytes**. These cells migrate from the blood into the tissues, where they develop into tissue **macrophages**.

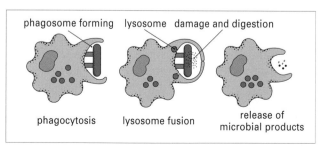

Fig. 1.2 Phagocytosis Phagocytes attach to microorganisms using cell surface receptors for microbial products or via adapter molecules. Pseudopods extend around the microorganism and fuse to form a phagosome. Killing mechanisms are activated and lysosomes fuse with the phagosomes, releasing digestive enzymes that break down the microbe. Undigested microbial products may be released to the outside.

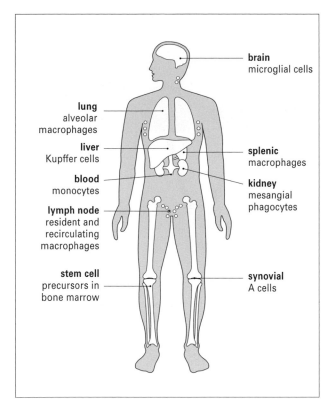

lung
alveolar
macrophages

liver
Kupffer cells

blood
monocytes

lymph node
resident and
recirculating
macrophages

stem cell
precursors in
bone marrow

brain
microglial cells

splenic
macrophages

kidney
mesangial
phagocytes

synovial
A cells

Fig. 1.4 Cells of the mononuclear phagocyte lineage Many organs contain cells belonging to the mononuclear phagocyte lineage. These cells are derived from blood monocytes and ultimately from stem cells in the bone marrow.

Polymorphonuclear neutrophils (often just called **neutrophils** or **PMNs**) are another important group of phagocytes. Neutrophils constitute the majority of the blood leukocytes and develop from the same early precursors as monocytes and macrophages. Like monocytes, neutrophils migrate into tissues, particularly at sites of inflammation. However, neutrophils are short-lived cells that phagocytose material, destroy it and then die within a few days.

B cells and T cells are responsible for the specific recognition of antigens. Adaptive immune responses are mediated by a specialized group of leukocytes, the **lymphocytes**, which include T and B lymphocytes (T cells and B cells) that specifically recognize foreign material or **antigens**. All lymphocytes are derived from bone marrow stem cells, but T cells then develop in the thymus, while B cells develop in the bone marrow (in adult mammals).

These two classes of lymphocytes carry out very different protective functions:
- **B cells** are responsible for the production of antibodies that act against extracellular pathogens.
- **T cells** are mainly concerned with cellular immune responses to intracellular pathogens, such as viruses. They also regulate the responses of B cells and the overall immune response.

B cells express specific antigen receptors on their cell surface during their development and, when mature, secrete soluble **immunoglobulin** molecules (also known as antibodies) into the extracellular fluids. The B cell's receptor for antigen (BCR) is in fact a cell-surface form of its secreted antibody. Each

B cell is genetically programmed to express a surface receptor which is specific for a particular antigen. If a B cell binds to its specific antigen and receives appropriate signals from T cells, it will multiply and differentiate into **plasma cells**, which produce large amounts of the secreted antibody (see Chapter 10).

Secreted antibody molecules are large glycoproteins found in the blood and tissue fluids. Because secreted antibody molecules are a soluble version of the original receptor molecule (BCR), they bind to the same antigen that initially activated the B cells. Antibodies are an essential component of an immune response and, when bound to their cognate antigens, they help phagocytes to take up antigens, a process called **opsonization** (from the Latin, opsono, 'to prepare food').

There are several different types of T cell, and they have a variety of functions (Fig 1.5):
- TH1 cells (type-1 T helpers) interact with mononuclear phagocytes and help them destroy intracellular pathogens.
- TH2 cells (type-2 T helpers) interact with B cells and help them to divide, differentiate and make antibodies.
- TH17 cells are defined according to a cytokine they produce (IL-17) and are involved in defence against microbes, particularly in mucosal tissues.
- Regulatory T cells, or Tregs, help to control the development of immune responses and limit reactions against self tissues.
- CTLs (cytotoxic T lymphocytes), also called Tc cells (cytotoxic T cells), are responsible for the destruction of host cells that have become infected by viruses or other intracellular pathogens.

In every case, the T cells recognize antigens present on the surface of other cells using a specific receptor, the **T cell antigen receptor (TCR)** (see Chapter 6), which is quite distinct from, but related in structure to, the antigen receptor on B cells (BCR) (see Chapter 9). T cells generate their effects either by releasing soluble proteins, called **cytokines**, which signal to other cells, or by direct cell–cell interactions.

Cytotoxic cells recognize and destroy other cells that have become infected. Several cell types have the capacity to kill other cells should they become infected. Cytotoxic cells include CTLs, natural killer (NK) cells and eosinophils (see Chapter 8). Of these, the CTL is especially important, but other cell types may be active against particular types of infection.

All of these cell types damage their different targets by releasing the contents of their intracellular granules close to them. Cytokines secreted by the cytotoxic cells, but not stored in granules, contribute to the damage.

NK cells have the capacity to recognize the surface changes that occur on a variety of tumour cells and virally infected cells. They use a different recognition system to the CTLs and are one member of the population of innate lymphoid cells **(ILCs)**. Some NK cells are larger and more granular than T cells and were previously referred to as **large granular lymphocytes (LGLs).**

Eosinophils are a specialized group of leukocytes that have the ability to engage and damage large extracellular parasites, such as schistosomes.

Auxiliary cells control inflammation. The main purpose of inflammation is to attract leukocytes and the soluble mediators

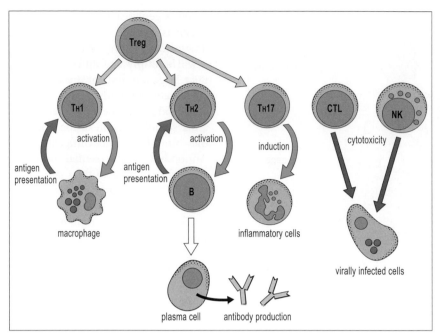

Fig. 1.5 Functions of different types of lymphocyte Macrophages present antigen to T$_H$1 cells, which then activate the macrophages to destroy phagocytosed pathogens. B cells present antigen to T$_H$2 cells, which activate the B cells, causing them to divide and differentiate into antibody-secreting plasma cells. T$_H$17 cells help to protect mucosal surfaces by attracting and activating other leukocytes. Cytotoxic T lymphocytes *(CTL)* and natural killer cells *(NK)* recognize and destroy virally infected cells. Regulatory T cells *(Treg)* modulate activity of other T-cell populations.

of immunity towards a site of infection. Inflammation is mediated by a variety of other cells, including basophils, mast cells and platelets.

Basophils and **mast cells** have granules that contain a variety of mediators, which induce inflammation in surrounding tissues and are released when the cells are triggered. Basophils and mast cells can also synthesize and secrete a number of mediators that control the development of immune reactions. Mast cells lie close to blood vessels in most tissues and some of their mediators act on cells in the vessel walls. Basophils are functionally similar to mast cells, but are mobile, circulating cells.

Platelets are small cellular fragments that are essential in blood clotting, but they can also be activated during immune responses to release mediators of inflammation.

Soluble Mediators of Immunity

A wide variety of molecules are involved in the development of immune responses, including antibodies, opsonins and complement system molecules. The serum concentration of a number of these proteins increases rapidly during acute infection and they are therefore called **acute phase proteins**.

One example of an acute phase protein is **C-reactive protein (CRP)**, so-called because of its ability to bind to the C protein of pneumococci; it promotes the uptake of pneumococci by phagocytes. Molecules such as CRP that promote phagocytosis are said to act as **opsonins**. There are a number of these evolutionarily ancient molecules in mammals and they recognize conserved structures on the surface of pathogens called **pathogen-associated molecular patterns (PAMPs)** (see Chapter 3). Another important group of molecules that can act as opsonins are components of the complement system (see Chapter 4).

Complement proteins mediate phagocytosis, control inflammation and interact with antibodies in immune defence. The complement system, a key component of innate immunity, is a group of about 20 serum proteins whose overall function is to promote inflammation (Fig. 1.6) and clearance of microbes and damaged cells. The components interact with each other and with other elements of the immune system. For example, a number of microorganisms spontaneously activate the complement system, via the so-called '**alternative pathway**', which is an innate immune defence. This results in the microorganism being opsonized (i.e. coated by complement molecules, leading to its uptake by phagocytes). The complement system can also be activated by antibodies bound to the pathogen via the '**classical pathway**' or by mannose binding lectin bound to the pathogen surface via the '**lectin pathway**'.

Complement activation is a cascade reaction, where one component acts enzymatically on the next component in the cascade to generate an enzyme, which mediates the following step in the reaction sequence, and so on. (The blood clotting system also works as an enzyme cascade.)

Activation of the complement system generates protein molecules or peptide fragments, which have the following effects:

- opsonization of microorganisms for uptake by phagocytes and eventual intracellular killing;
- attraction of phagocytes to sites of infection (chemotaxis);
- increased blood flow to the site of activation and increased permeability of capillaries to plasma molecules;
- damage to plasma membranes on cells, Gram-negative bacteria, enveloped viruses, or other organisms that have caused complement activation;
- release of inflammatory mediators from mast cells.

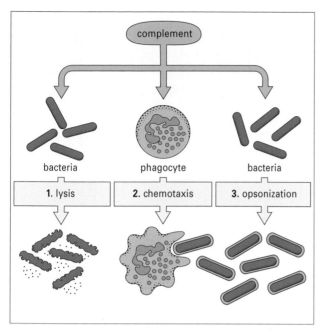

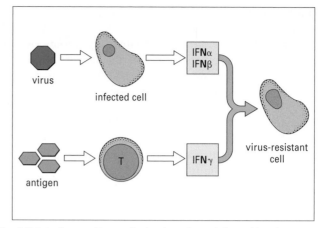

Fig. 1.7 Interferons Host cells that have been infected by virus secrete interferon-α *(IFNα)* and/or interferon-β *(IFNβ)*. TH1 cells secrete interferon-γ *(IFNγ)* after activation by antigens. IFNs act on other host cells to induce resistance to viral infection. IFNγ has many other effects.

Fig. 1.6 Functions of complement Components of the complement system can lyse many bacterial species *(1)*. Complement fragments released in this reaction attract phagocytes to the site of the reaction *(2)*. Complement components opsonize the bacteria for phagocytosis *(3)*. In addition to the responses shown here, activation of the complement system increases blood flow and vascular permeability at the site of activation. Activated components can also induce the release of inflammatory mediators from mast cells.

Cytokines signal between lymphocytes, phagocytes and other cells of the body. **Cytokine** is the general term for a large group of secreted molecules involved in signalling between cells during immune responses. All cytokines are proteins or glycoproteins. The different cytokines fall into a number of categories and the principal subgroups of cytokines are outlined below.

Interferons (IFNs) are cytokines that are particularly important in limiting the spread of certain viral infections: one group of interferons (IFNα and IFNβ or type-1 interferons) is produced by cells that have become infected by a virus; another type, IFNγ, is released by activated TH1 cells.

IFNs induce a state of antiviral resistance in uninfected cells (Fig. 1.7). They are produced very early in infection and are important in delaying the spread of a virus until the adaptive immune response has developed.

The **interleukins (ILs)** are a large group of cytokines produced mainly by T cells, although some are also produced by mononuclear phagocytes or by tissue cells. They have a variety of functions. Many interleukins cause other cells to divide and to differentiate.

Colony stimulating factors (CSFs) are primarily involved in directing the division and differentiation of bone marrow stem cells and the precursors of blood leukocytes. The CSFs partially control how many leukocytes of each type are released from the bone marrow. Some CSFs also promote subsequent differentiation of cells. For example, macrophage CSF (M-CSF, also known as CSF1) promotes the development of monocytes in bone marrow and macrophages in tissues.

Chemokines are a large group of chemotactic cytokines that direct the movement of leukocytes around the body, from the blood stream into the tissues and to the appropriate location within each tissue. Some chemokines also activate cells to carry out particular functions.

Tumour necrosis factors, TNFα and TNFβ, have a variety of functions but are particularly important in promoting inflammation and cytotoxic reactions.

Transforming growth factors (e.g. TGFβ) are important in controlling cell division and tissue repair.

Each set of cells releases a particular blend of cytokines, depending on the type of cell and whether, and how, it has been activated. For example:
* TH1 cells release one set of cytokines, which promote activation of mononuclear phagocytes to deal with pathogens they have phagocytosed;
* TH2 cells release a different set of cytokines, which activate B cells;
* TH17 cells release cytokines that control inflammatory responses.

Some cytokines may be produced by all T cells and some just by a specific subset.

Equally important is the expression of cytokine receptors. Only a cell that has the appropriate receptors can respond to a particular cytokine. For example, the receptors for interferons are present on all nucleated cells in the body, whereas other receptors are much more restricted in their distribution. In general, cytokine receptors are specific for their own individual cytokine, but this is not always so. In particular, many chemokine receptors respond to several different chemokines.

INFLAMMATION

Tissue damage caused by physical agents (e.g. trauma or radiation) or by pathogens results in the tissue response of **inflammation**, which has three principal components:
* increased blood supply to the infected area;
* increased capillary permeability as a result of retraction of the endothelial cells lining the vessels, permitting larger molecules than usual to escape from the capillaries;

- migration of leukocytes from the venules into the surrounding tissues: in the earliest stages of inflammation, neutrophils are particularly prevalent, but in later stages monocytes and lymphocytes also migrate towards the site of infection or damage. Inflammation allows the body's immune defences to concentrate at a site of infection or cell damage.

Leukocytes enter inflamed tissue by crossing venular endothelium. The process of leukocyte migration is controlled by **chemokines** (a particular class of cytokines) on the surface of venular endothelium in inflamed tissues. Chemokines activate the circulating leukocytes, causing them to bind to the endothelium and initiate migration across the endothelium (Fig. 1.8).

Once in the tissues, the leukocytes migrate towards the site of infection by a process of chemical attraction known as **chemotaxis**. For example, phagocytes will actively migrate up concentration gradients of certain (chemotactic) molecules.

A particularly active chemotactic molecule is **C5a**, which is a fragment of one of the complement components (Fig. 1.9) that attracts both neutrophils and monocytes. When purified C5a is applied to the base of a blister in vivo, neutrophils can be seen sticking to the endothelium of nearby venules shortly afterwards. The cells then squeeze between the endothelial cells and move through the basement membrane of the microvessels to reach the tissues. This process is described more fully in Chapter 3.

IMMUNE RESPONSES TO PATHOGENS

Effective immune responses vary depending on the pathogen. The primary function of the immune system is to prevent entry of and/or to eliminate infectious agents and minimize the damage they cause, ensuring that most infections in normal individuals are short-lived and leave little permanent damage. Pathogens, however, come in many different forms, with various modes of transmission and reproductive cycles, and the immune system has therefore evolved different ways of responding to each of them.

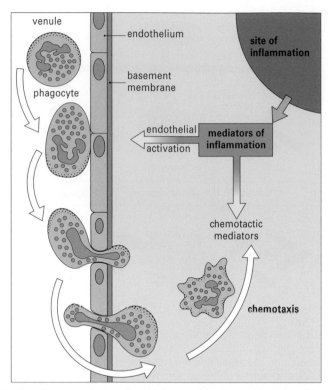

Fig. 1.9 Chemotaxis At a site of inflammation, tissue damage and complement activation cause the release of chemotactic peptides (e.g. chemokines and C5a), which diffuse to the adjoining venules and signal to circulating phagocytes. Activated cells migrate across the vessel wall and move up a concentration gradient of chemotactic molecules towards the site of inflammation.

The exterior defences of the body (Fig. 1.10) present an effective barrier to most organisms. Very few infectious agents can penetrate intact skin. In contrast, many infectious agents gain access to the body across the epithelia of the gastrointestinal or urogenital tracts; others, such as the virus responsible for the common cold, infect the respiratory epithelium of nasopharynx and lung; a small number of infectious agents infect the

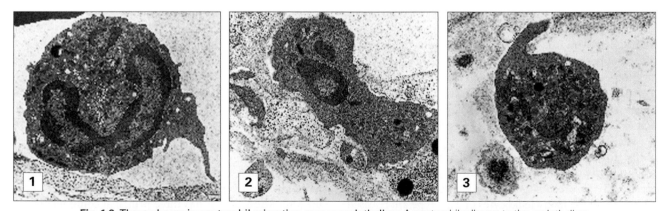

Fig. 1.8 Three phases in neutrophil migration across endothelium A neutrophil adheres to the endothelium in a venule (**1**). It extends its pseudopodium between the endothelial cells and migrates towards the basement membrane (**2**). After the neutrophil has crossed into the tissue, the endothelium reseals behind (**3**). The entire process is referred to as diapedesis. (Courtesy Dr I Jovis.)

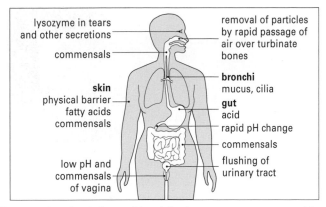

Fig. 1.10 Exterior defences Most infectious agents are prevented from entering the body by physical and biochemical barriers. The body tolerates a number of commensal organisms, which compete effectively with many potential pathogens.

body only if they enter the blood directly (e.g. malaria and sleeping sickness).

Once inside the body, the site of the infection and the nature of the pathogen largely determine which type of immune response will be induced, most importantly (Fig. 1.11) whether the pathogen is:

- an **intracellular pathogen** (i.e. invades the host cells to divide and reproduce); or
- an **extracellular pathogen** (i.e. does not invade the host cells).

Many bacteria and larger parasites live in tissues, body fluids or other extracellular spaces, and are susceptible to the multitude of immune defences, such as **antibodies** and **complement** that are present in these areas. Because these components are present in the tissue fluids of the body (the "humours" of ancient medicine), they have been classically referred to as **humoral immunity**.

Many organisms (e.g. viruses, some bacteria, some parasites) evade these formidable defences by being intracellular pathogens and replicating within host cells. To clear these infections, the immune system has developed ways to recognize and to

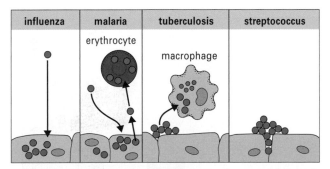

Fig. 1.11 Intracellular and extracellular pathogens All infectious agents spread to infect new cells by passing through the body fluids or tissues. Many are intracellular pathogens and must infect cells of the body to divide and reproduce (e.g. viruses such as influenza viruses and malaria, which has two separate phases of division, either in cells of the liver or in erythrocytes). The mycobacteria that cause tuberculosis can divide outside cells or within macrophages. Some bacteria (e.g. streptococci, which produce sore throats and wound infections) generally divide outside cells and are therefore extracellular pathogens.

destroy infected cells. This is largely the function of **cell-mediated immunity**.

Intracellular pathogens cannot, however, wholly evade the extracellular defences because they must reach their host cells by moving through the blood and tissue fluids. As a result, they are susceptible to humoral immunity during this portion of their life cycle.

Any immune response involves recognition of the pathogen or other foreign material and then a reaction to eliminate it.

Innate immune responses are the same on each encounter with an antigen. Broadly speaking, immune responses fall into two categories: those that become more powerful following repeated encounters with the same antigen (**adaptive immune responses**) and those that do not become more powerful following repeated encounters with the same antigen (**innate immune responses**).

Innate immune responses (see Chapters 3–5) can be thought of as simple, though remarkably effective, systems present in all animals that are the first line of defence against pathogens and allow a rapid response to invasion.

Innate immune response systems range from external barriers (skin, mucous membranes, cilia, secretions and tissue fluids containing anti-microbial agents; see Fig. 1.10) to sophisticated receptors capable of recognizing broad classes of pathogenic organisms, for example:

- innate immune receptors on leukocytes recognize PAMPs;
- intracellular receptors in many cells recognize nucleic acids characteristic of viral replication;
- some plasma proteins bind to bacterial and fungal cell walls and opsonize them;
- the complement system includes components that can be specifically activated by bacterial surface molecules.

Receptors and proteins that recognize PAMPs are broadly referred to as **pattern recognition receptors (PRRs)**. It takes several days for adaptive immune responses to develop and the innate immune responses limit pathogen spread during this critical period. The innate defences are also closely interlinked with adaptive responses.

Adaptive immune responses display specificity and memory. In contrast to the innate immune response, which recognizes common molecular patterns (such as PAMPs), the adaptive immune system takes a highly discriminatory approach, with a very large repertoire of specific antigen receptors that can recognize virtually any component of a foreign invader (see Chapters 6, 9 and 10). This use of highly specific antigen receptor molecules provides the following advantages:

- pathogens that lack stereotypical patterns (which might avoid recognition by the innate immune system) can be recognized;
- responses can be highly specific for a given pathogen;
- the **specificity** of the response allows the generation of **immunological memory**: related to its use of highly individual antigen receptors, the adaptive immune system has the capacity to remember a pathogen.

These features underlie the phenomenon of specific immunity (e.g. diseases such as measles and diphtheria induce adaptive immune responses that generate life-long immunity).

Specific immunity can, very often, be induced by artificial means, allowing the development of vaccines (see Chapter 17).

ANTIGEN RECOGNITION

Originally the term **antigen** was used for any molecule that induced B cells to produce a specific antibody (*anti*body *gener*ator). This term is now more widely used to indicate molecules that are specifically recognized by antigen receptors of either B cells or T cells.

Antigens, defined broadly, are molecules that initiate adaptive immune responses (e.g. components of pathogenic organisms), although purists may prefer the term **immunogen** in this context.

Antigens are not just components of foreign substances such as pathogens. A large variety of 'self' molecules can also act as antigens, provoking autoimmune responses that can be highly damaging and even lethal (see Chapter 20).

Antigens initiate and direct adaptive immune responses. The immune system has evolved to recognize antigens, destroy them and eliminate the source of their production – when an antigen is eliminated, immune responses switch off.

Both T-cell receptors and immunoglobulin molecules (antibodies) bind to their cognate antigens with a high degree of specificity. These two types of receptor molecules have striking structural relationships and are closely related evolutionarily, but they bind to very different types of antigens and carry out quite different biological functions.

Functions of Antibodies

Antibody specifically binds to antigen. Soluble antibodies are a group of serum molecules closely related to and derived from the antigen receptors on B cells. All antibodies have the same basic Y-shaped structure, with two regions (variable regions) at the tips of the Y that bind to antigen. The stem of the Y is referred to as the constant region and is not involved in antigen binding (see Chapter 10).

The two variable regions contain identical antigen-binding sites that, in general, are specific for only one type of antigen. The amino acid sequences of the variable regions of different antibodies vary greatly between antibodies produced by different clones of B cells. As a B cell develops, a process of somatic gene-recombination affects the antibody gene loci so that each clone of B cells produces antibody with a different specificity (binding site). The antibody molecules in the body, derived from millions of B cells, therefore provide an extremely large repertoire of antigen-binding sites. The way in which this great diversity of antibody variable regions is generated is explained in Chapter 9.

Each antibody binds to a restricted part of the antigen called an epitope. Pathogens typically have many different antigens on their surface. Each antibody binds to an **epitope**, which is

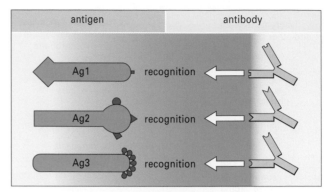

Fig. 1.12 Antigens and epitopes Antibodies recognize molecular shapes (epitopes) on the surface of antigens. Each antigen (*Ag1, Ag2, Ag3*) may have several epitopes recognized by different antibodies. Some antigens have repeated epitopes (e.g. Ag3).

a restricted part of the antigen. A particular antigen can have several different epitopes or repeated epitopes (Fig. 1.12). Antibodies are specific for the epitopes rather than the whole antigen molecule. In some cases, the same epitope may be present on different antigens and an antibody that binds to that epitope will recognize both antigens. This is referred to as **cross-reactivity**.

Fc regions of antibodies act as adapters to link phagocytes to pathogens. The constant region of the antibody (the Fc region) can bind to Fc receptors on phagocytes, so acting as an adapter between the phagocyte and the pathogen (Fig. 1.13). Consequently, if an antibody binds to a pathogen, it can link to a phagocyte and promote phagocytosis, i.e. opsonization. This process is an important example of collaboration between the innate and adaptive immune responses.

Other molecules (such as activated complement proteins) can also enhance phagocytosis when bound to microbial surfaces. Binding and phagocytosis are most effective when more than one type of adapter molecule (**opsonin**) is present (Fig. 1.14). Note that antibody can act as an adapter in many

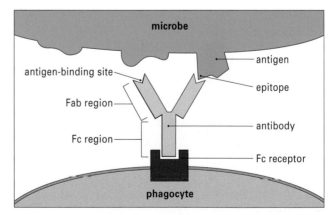

Fig. 1.13 An antibody acts as an adapter linking a microbe to a phagocyte The antibody binds to a region of an antigen (an epitope) on the microbe surface, using one of its antigen-binding sites. These sites are in the Fab regions of the antibody. The stem of the antibody, the Fc region, can attach to receptors on the surface of the phagocytes.

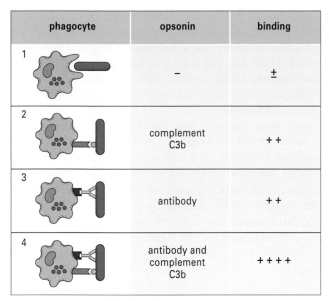

phagocyte	opsonin	binding
1	–	±
2	complement C3b	+ +
3	antibody	+ +
4	antibody and complement C3b	+ + + +

Fig. 1.14 Opsonization Phagocytes have some intrinsic ability to bind to bacteria and other microorganisms via their pattern recognition receptors (**1**). Binding is much enhanced if the bacteria have been opsonized by complement C3b (**2**) or antibody (**3**), each of which cross-links the bacteria to receptors on the phagocyte. Antibody can also activate complement, and if antibody and C3b both opsonize the bacteria, binding is further enhanced (**4**).

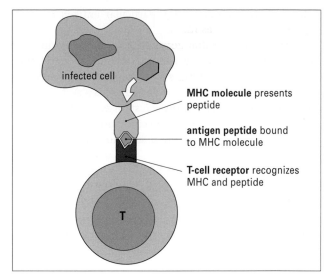

Fig. 1.15 T-cell recognition of antigen Major histocompatibility complex *(MHC)* molecules transport peptides to the surface of an infected cell where they are presented to T cells, which may recognize the MHC–peptide combination. If a cell is infected, MHC molecules present peptides derived from the pathogen and the cell's own proteins.

other circumstances, not just phagocytosis. For example, antibodies bound to parasitic worms allow them to be recognized by eosinophils. Another type of antibody binds to receptors on mast cells and allows them to recognize soluble antigens (see Chapter 10).

Peptides from intracellular pathogens are displayed on the surface of infected cells. Antibodies are present only in extracellular spaces, including blood, lymph and tissue fluids, and they can usually only target extracellular pathogens. Intracellular pathogens (such as viruses) can escape antibody-mediated responses once they are safely located within a host cell. The adaptive immune system has therefore evolved a specific method of displaying portions of virtually all cell proteins on the surface of each nucleated cell in the body so that they can be recognized by T cells.

For example, a cell infected with a virus will present fragments of viral proteins (peptides) on its surface that are recognizable by T cells. The antigenic peptides are transported to the cell surface and presented to the T cells by **MHC molecules** (a group of molecules encoded within the major histocompatibility complex, see Chapter 6). T cells use their antigen-specific receptors (TCRs) to recognize the antigenic peptide–MHC molecule complex (Fig. 1.15). If an infected cell (target) is recognized by a cytotoxic T cell (CTL), the T cell can signal to the target cell to induce apoptosis (programmed cell death). The process by which MHC molecules facilitate recognition of antigenic peptides is one component of a wider process called **antigen presentation** (see Chapter 7).

ANTIGEN PRESENTATION

Virtually all cells of the body can present antigen to CTLs, but there is a more limited group of specialized **antigen-presenting cells (APCs)** which process and present antigens to helper T cells. Several different types of leukocyte can act as APCs, including dendritic cells, macrophages and B cells. All of these cells internalize antigens from the extracellular space by phagocytosis or endocytosis. These APCs then display antigenic peptide–MHC complexes on the cell surface and they express co-stimulatory molecules that are essential for initiating immune responses. Activation of a TH cell requires both the signal from antigenic peptide–MHC and co-stimulation. Co-stimulatory signals are upregulated by the presence of pathogens, which can be detected by the engagement of innate immune receptors that recognize PAMPs.

Most immune responses to infectious organisms are made up of a variety of innate and adaptive components. In the earliest stages of infection, innate responses predominate; later the lymphocytes start to generate adaptive immune responses. After recovery from infection, immunological memory remains within the population of lymphocytes, which can then mount a more effective and rapid response if there is re-infection with the same pathogen at a later date.

The two major phases of any immune response are antigen recognition and a reaction to eliminate the antigen.

Antigen activates specific clones of lymphocytes. In adaptive immune responses, lymphocytes are responsible for immune recognition, which is achieved by clonal selection. Each lymphocyte is genetically programmed to produce one specific antigen receptor (BCR or TCR) capable of recognizing just one particular antigen. However, the immune system as a whole can specifically recognize many thousands of antigens and the lymphocytes that recognize any particular antigen are only a tiny proportion of the total.

How then is an adequate immune response to an infectious agent generated? The answer is that, when an antigen binds to the few lymphocytes that can recognize it, they are induced to proliferate rapidly. Within a few days there is a sufficient number to mount an adequate immune response. In other words, the antigen selects and activates the specific clones to which it binds (Fig. 1.16), a process called **clonal selection**. This operates for both B cells and T cells.

How can the immune system know which specific antibodies will be needed during an individual's lifetime? It does not know. The immune system generates antibodies (and T-cell receptors) that can recognize an enormous range of antigens even before it encounters them. Many of these specificities, which are generated more or less at random, will never be called upon to protect the individual against infection.

What is the advantage of generating billions of lymphocytes that do not recognize any known infectious agent? Many pathogens mutate their surface antigens. Indeed the immune system provides selective pressure for the evolution of new strains of pathogen with altered antigens. If the immune system could not recognize new variants of pathogens, it would not be able to make an effective immune response. By having a wide range of antigen receptors, at least some of the lymphocytes will be able to recognize any pathogen that enters the body.

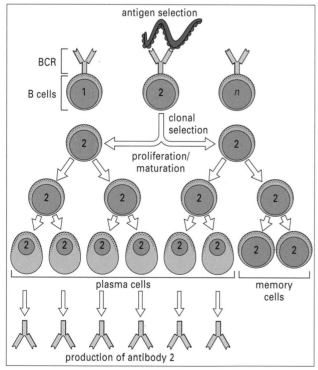

Fig. 1.16 B-cell clonal selection Each B cell expresses just one variant cell surface antibody (i.e. with specificity for a single particular antigen), which it uses as its antigen receptor (BCR). Antigens bind only to B cells with the specific BCR (number 2 in this example), driving these cells to divide and to differentiate into plasma cells and memory cells, all with the same specificity as the original B cell. Thus an antigen selects just the clones of B cells that can react against it.

Lymphocytes that have been stimulated, by binding to their specific antigen, take the first steps towards cell division. They express new receptors that allow them to respond to cytokines from other cells and will usually go through a number of cycles of division before differentiating into mature cells, again under the influence of cytokines. They may also start to produce sets of cytokines themselves.

Even when the infection has been overcome, some of the newly produced lymphocytes remain, available for re-stimulation if the antigen is ever encountered again. These cells are called **memory cells**, because they are generated by past encounters with particular antigens. Memory is partly the result of the expansion of the responding population of lymphocytes in the first immune response and partly because these cells are more easily activated on subsequent encounters with the antigen. Memory cells confer lasting immunity to a particular pathogen.

ANTIGEN ELIMINATION

There are numerous ways in which the immune system can destroy pathogens, each being suited to a given type of infection at a particular stage of its life cycle. These defence mechanisms are often referred to as **effector systems**.

Antibodies can directly neutralize some pathogens. In one of the simplest effector systems, antibodies can combat certain pathogens just by binding to them. For example, antibody to the outer coat proteins of some rhinoviruses (which cause colds) can prevent the viral particles from binding to and infecting host cells.

Phagocytes kill pathogens in endosomes. More often, antibodies activate complement or act as opsonins to promote ingestion by phagocytes (see Fig. 1.14). Phagocytes that have bound to an opsonized microbe engulf it by extending pseudopodia around it. These fuse and the microorganism is internalized (endocytosed) in a phagosome. Phagocytes have several ways of dealing with internalized microbes in phagosomes. For example:

- Macrophages reduce molecular oxygen to form microbicidal reactive oxygen and nitrogen intermediates (ROIs and RNIs), which are secreted into the phagosome.
- Macrophages pump H⁺ ions into the phagosome to lower the pH.
- Neutrophil granules contain anti-microbial peptides called defensins, which fuse with the phagosome.
- Neutrophils contain lactoferrin, which chelates iron and prevents some bacteria from obtaining this vital nutrient.

Once a pathogen has been killed, lysosomes fuse with the phagosome, pouring enzymes into the resulting phagolysosome, to digest the contents.

Cytotoxic cells kill infected target cells. Cytotoxic reactions are usually directed against whole cells, i.e. targets that are too large for phagocytosis.

The target cell may be recognized by:

- specific antibody bound to the cell surface;
- cytotoxic T cells using their specific TCRs;
- NK cells using immunoglobulin-like and lectin-like receptors.

In cytotoxic reactions, the attacking cells direct their granules towards the target cell (in contrast to phagocytosis where the contents are directed into the phagosome). As a result, granules are discharged into the extracellular space close to the target cell.

The granules of CTLs and NK cells contain molecules called **perforins**, which can punch holes in the outer membrane of the target. (In a similar way, antibody bound to the surface of a target cell can direct complement to make holes in the cell's plasma membrane.) Some cytotoxic cells can signal to the target cell to initiate programmed cell death (apoptosis). These processes must be closely regulated as the release of toxic molecules into the extracellular space could cause collateral damage to nearby cells.

Termination of immune responses limits damage to host tissues.

Although it is important to initiate immune responses quickly, it is also critical to terminate them appropriately once the threat has ended. To clear the offending pathogen, immune responses often involve millions of activated lymphocytes and activation of huge numbers of phagocytes. These responses, if left unchecked, can also damage host tissues. A number of mechanisms are employed to dampen or to terminate immune responses. One is a passive process, i.e. simple clearance of antigen should lead to a diminution of immune responses; in the absence of antigen, lymphocytes that recognize the antigen will not be stimulated to divide and to differentiate.

Antigen elimination can be a slow process, however, therefore the immune system also employs a variety of active mechanisms to downregulate responses (see Chapter 12).

Immune responses to extracellular and intracellular pathogens.

In dealing with extracellular pathogens, the immune system aims to destroy the pathogen itself and to neutralize its products.

In dealing with intracellular pathogens, the immune system has two options:

- T cells can destroy the infected cell (i.e. cytotoxicity); or
- T cells can activate the infected cell to deal with the pathogen itself (e.g. helper T cells release cytokines, which activate macrophages to destroy the organisms they have internalized).

Because many pathogens have both intracellular and extracellular phases of infection, different mechanisms are usually effective at different times. For example, the polio virus travels from the gut through the blood stream to infect nerve cells in the spinal cord. Antibodies are particularly effective at blocking the early phase of infection while the virus is in the blood stream, but to clear an established infection CTLs must kill any cell that has become infected.

Consequently, antibodies are important in limiting the spread of infection and preventing reinfection with the same virus, while CTLs are essential to deal with infected cells

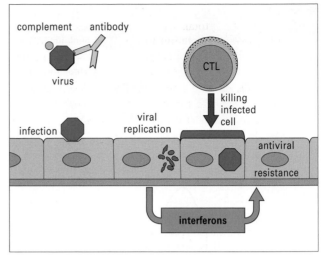

Fig. 1.17 Reaction to extracellular and intracellular pathogens Different immunological systems are effective against different types of infection, here illustrated as a virus infection. Antibodies and complement can block the extracellular phase of the life cycle and promote phagocytosis of the virus. Interferons produced by infected cells signal to uninfected cells to induce a state of antiviral resistance. Viruses can multiply only within living cells; cytotoxic T lymphocytes (CTLs) recognize and destroy the infected cells.

(Fig. 1.17). These factors play an important part in the development of effective vaccines.

VACCINATION

The study of immunology has had its most successful application in vaccination (see Chapter 17), which is based on the key elements of adaptive immunity, namely specificity and memory. Memory cells allow the immune system to mount a much stronger response on a second encounter with antigen. Compared with the primary response, the secondary response is:

- faster to appear;
- more effective.

The aim in vaccine development is to alter a pathogen or its toxins in such a way that they become innocuous without losing antigenicity. This is possible because antibodies and T cells recognize particular parts of antigens (the epitopes) and not the whole organism or toxin.

Take, for example, vaccination against tetanus. The tetanus bacterium produces a toxin that acts on receptors to cause tetanic contractions of muscle. The toxin can be modified by formalin treatment so that it retains its epitopes but loses its toxicity. The resulting molecule (known as a toxoid) is used as a vaccine (Fig. 1.18).

Whole infectious agents, such as the poliovirus, can be attenuated so they retain their antigenicity but lose their pathogenicity.

IMMUNOPATHOLOGY

Strong evolutionary pressure from infectious microbes has led to the development of the immune system in its present form.

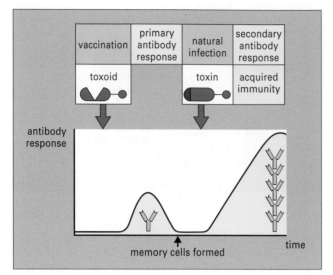

Fig. 1.18 Principle of vaccination Chemical modification of tetanus toxin produces a toxoid, which has lost its toxicity but retains many of its epitopes. A primary antibody response to these epitopes is produced after vaccination with the toxoid. If a natural infection occurs, the toxin re-stimulates memory B cells, which produce a faster and more intense secondary response against that epitope, neutralizing the toxin.

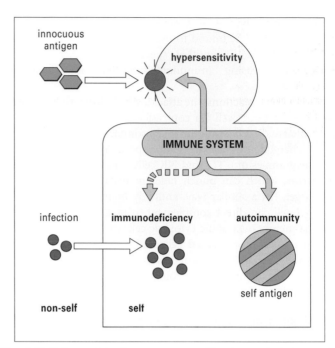

Fig. 1.19 Failure of the immune system The three principal ways in which the immune system can fail result in hypersensitivity (an overactive immune response to an antigen), immunodeficiency (an ineffective immune response to an infection) and autoimmunity (the immune system reacts against the body's own tissues).

Deficiencies in any part of the system leave the individual exposed to a greater risk of infection, but other parts of the system may partly compensate for such deficiencies. However, there are occasions when the immune system is itself a cause of disease or other undesirable consequences.

In essence, the immune system can fail in one of three ways (Fig. 1.19), resulting in autoimmunity, immunodeficiency or hypersensitivity.

Inappropriate Reaction to Self Antigens – Autoimmunity

Normally the immune system recognizes all foreign antigens and reacts against them, while recognizing the body's own tissues as self and making no reaction against them. The mechanisms by which this discrimination between self and non-self is established are described in Chapter 11.

When the immune system reacts against self components, the result is an **autoimmune disease** (see Chapter 20), for example rheumatoid arthritis or pernicious anaemia.

Ineffective Immune Response – Immunodeficiency

If any elements of the immune system are defective, the individual may not be able to fight infections adequately, resulting in **immunodeficiency**. Some immunodeficiency conditions:
- are hereditary and start to manifest shortly after birth; they are primary immunodeficiencies (see Chapter 18);

- develop later in life, for example the acquired immune deficiency syndrome (AIDS) and are referred to as secondary immunodeficiencies (see Chapter 19).

Overactive Immune Response – Hypersensitivity

Sometimes immune reactions are out of all proportion to the damage that may be caused by a pathogen. The immune system may also mount a reaction to a harmless antigen, such as a food molecule. Such immune reactions (**hypersensitivity**) may cause more damage than the pathogen or antigen (see Chapters 23–26). For example, molecules on the surface of pollen grains are recognized as antigens by particular individuals, leading to the symptoms of hay fever or asthma.

NORMAL BUT INCONVENIENT IMMUNE REACTIONS

The most important examples of normal immune reactions that are inconvenient in the context of modern medicine are:
- blood transfusion reactions (see Chapter 24);
- graft rejection (see Chapter 21).

In these cases it is necessary to match the donor and recipient tissues carefully so that the immune system of the recipient does not attack the donated blood or graft tissue.

CRITICAL THINKING: SPECIFICITY AND MEMORY IN VACCINATION

See Critical thinking: Explanations, section 1

The recommended schedules for vaccination against different diseases are strikingly different. Two examples are given in the table. For tetanus, the vaccine is a modified form of the toxin released by the tetanus bacterium. The vaccine for influenza is either an attenuated non-pathogenic variant of the virus, given intranasally, or a killed preparation of virus, given intradermally. Both vaccines induce antibodies that are specific for the inducing antigen.

1. Why is it necessary to vaccinate against tetanus only every 10 years when antibodies against the toxoid disappear from the circulation within a year?
2. Why is the vaccine against tetanus always effective, whereas the vaccine against influenza protects on some occasions but not others?
3. Why is tetanus recommended for everyone and influenza for only a restricted group of at-risk individuals, even though influenza is a much more common disease than tetanus?

Schedules for Vaccination Against Tetanus and Influenza A

Pathogen	Type of vaccine	Recommended for	Vaccination	Effectiveness (%)
Tetanus	Toxoid	Everyone	Every 10 years	100
Influenza A	Attenuated virus	Health workers and older people	Annually	Variable, 0–90

2

Cells, Tissues and Organs of the Immune System

SUMMARY

- **Most cells of the immune system** derive from haematopoietic stem cells. The primary lymphoid organs in mammals are the thymus and bone marrow, where lymphocyte differentiation occurs.
- **Phagocytic cells** are found in the circulation as monocytes and granulocytes. Monocytes differentiate into macrophages that reside in tissues (e.g. Kupffer cells in the liver). Neutrophils are short-lived phagocytes present in high numbers in the blood and at sites of acute inflammation.
- **Eosinophils, basophils, mast cells and platelets, together with cytokines and complement,** take part in the inflammatory response.
- **Innate lymphoid cells** are of two kinds: those that produce cytokines in response to micro-environmental signals and the cytotoxic NK cells that recognize and kill virus-infected cells and certain tumour cells by inducing apoptosis.
- **Antigen-presenting cells** link the innate and adaptive immune systems and are required by T cells to enable them to respond to antigens.
- **Lymphocytes** are phenotypically, functionally and morphologically heterogeneous.
- **B lymphocytes and T lymphocytes express specific antigen receptors** called the B-cell receptor (BCR) and T-cell receptor (TCR), respectively.

- **There are three major subpopulations of T cells that have helper, cytotoxic and regulatory activities (TH, Tc and Treg).**
- **B cells can differentiate into antibody-secreting plasma cells and memory cells.**
- **T cells developing in the thymus** are subject to positive and negative selection processes.
- **Mammalian B cells develop mainly in the fetal liver and from birth onwards in the bone marrow.** This process continues throughout life. B cells also undergo a negative selection process at the site of B-cell generation.
- **Lymphocytes** migrate to, and function in, the secondary lymphoid organs and tissues.
- **Secondary lymphoid organs and tissue protect different body sites**: the spleen responds to blood-borne organisms; the lymph nodes respond to lymph-borne antigens; and the mucosa-associated lymphoid tissue (**MALT**) protects the mucosal surfaces.
- **Most lymphocytes recirculate around the body:** there is continuous lymphocyte traffic from the blood stream into lymphoid tissues and back again into the blood via the thoracic duct and right lymphatic duct.

CELLS OF THE IMMUNE SYSTEM

There is great heterogeneity in the cells of the immune system, most of which originate from haematopoietic stem cells in the fetal liver and in the postnatal bone marrow – mainly in the vertebrae, sternum, ribs, femur and tibia (Fig. 2.1). This morphological heterogeneity reflects the fact that cells of the immune system are called on to provide a wide variety of functions including:

- phagocytosis,
- antigen presentation,
- lysis of virus-infected cells and
- secretion of specific antibodies.

In general, cells of the immune system can be divided into two broad functional categories, which work together to provide innate immunity and the adaptive immune response. Innate immunity represents an ancient defence system that has evolved to recognize conserved patterns characteristic of a variety of pathogens and often serves as the first line of defence. Adaptive immunity, a more recent evolutionary development, recognizes novel molecules produced by pathogens by virtue of a large repertoire of specific antigen receptors.

Cells of the innate immune system include mononuclear phagocytes, granulocytes, mast cells, and innate lymphoid cells. Phagocytic cells of the innate immune system belong to the myeloid lineage and include:

- the monocytes: circulating blood cells;
- the macrophages: differentiated from monocytes and residing in various tissues;
- the **polymorphonuclear granulocytes** (polymorphonuclear neutrophils (PMNs), basophils, and eosinophils): circulating blood cells.

All phagocytic cells are mainly involved in defence against extracellular microbes.

Innate lymphoid cells are mainly involved in the defence against intracellular microbes and virus-infected cells.

Mast cells and platelets are pivotal in inducing and maintaining inflammation.

Microbes express various cell surface and intracellular molecules called pathogen-associated molecular patterns (PAMPs). Cells of the innate system recognize microbes through their receptors for PAMPs called pattern recognition receptors (PRRs). PRRs have broad specificity and a non-clonal distribution, features that distinguish them from the specific antigen receptors of the adaptive immune system.

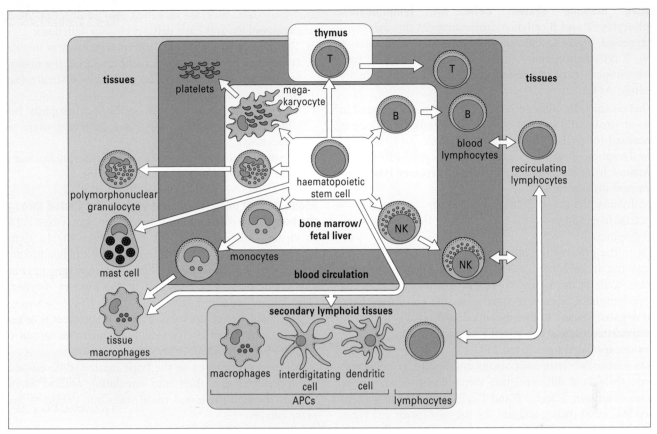

Fig. 2.1 Origin of cells of the immune system All cells shown here arise from the haematopoietic stem cell. Platelets (cellular fragments produced by megakaryocytes) are released into the circulation. Polymorphonuclear granulocytes and monocytes pass from the circulation into the tissues. Mast cells are identifiable in all tissues. B cells mature in the fetal liver and bone marrow in mammals, whereas T cells mature in the thymus. The origin of the large granular lymphocytes with natural killer *(NK)* activity is probably the bone marrow. Lymphocytes recirculate through secondary lymphoid tissues. Interdigitating cells and dendritic cells act as antigen-presenting cells *(APCs)* in secondary lymphoid tissues.

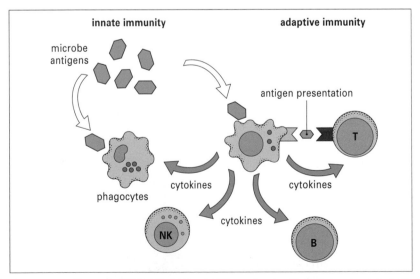

Fig. 2.2 Antigen-presenting cells (APCs) Specialized APCs are involved in both innate and adaptive immunity to bacteria and viruses by the production of cytokines and by presentation of processed antigens to T cells.

Antigen-presenting cells (APCs) link the innate and adaptive immune systems. A specialized group of cells termed antigen-presenting cells (APCs) link the innate and adaptive immune systems by taking up and processing antigens so that they can be recognized by T cells and by producing cytokines. APCs enhance innate immune cell function and they are essential for activation of T cells (Fig. 2.2).

Adaptive immune system cells are lymphocytes. Lymphocytes (T and B cells) recognize antigens through clonally expressed, highly specific antigen receptors (see Chapters 6 and 9). T cells are produced in the thymus (see Fig. 2.1) and require antigen to be processed and presented to them by specialized APCs.

Whereas the cells of the innate immune system are found in the blood stream and in most organs of the body, lymphocytes are localized to specialized organs and tissues.

The lymphoid organs where the lymphocytes differentiate and mature from stem cells are called the **primary lymphoid organs** and include:
- the thymus: the site of T cell development;
- the fetal liver and postnatal bone marrow: the sites of B-cell development.

It is in the primary lymphoid organs that the lymphocytes undergo the antigen-independent part of their differentiation program. Cells of the T- and B-cell lineages migrate from the primary lymphoid organs to function in the **secondary lymphoid organs**. These can be subdivided into:
- encapsulated organs: the spleen and lymph nodes;
- non-encapsulated tissues, e.g. MALT.

In the secondary lymphoid organs and tissues, lymphocytes undergo their final differentiation steps, which occur in the presence of antigen. Effector B and T cells generated in the secondary lymphoid tissues account for the two major cell types participating in adaptive immune responses of humoral and cellular immunity, respectively.

As the cells of the immune system develop, they acquire molecules that are important for their function. These specific functional molecules are referred to as **lineage markers** because they identify the cell lineage. For example:
- myeloid cells: polymorphs and monocytes; and
- lymphoid cells: T and B cells.

Other marker molecules include those involved in regulating cell differentiation (maturation, development), proliferation and function and those involved in regulating the number of cells participating in the immune response.

MYELOID CELLS

Mononuclear phagocytes and polymorphonuclear granulocytes are the two major phagocyte lineages. Phagocytes are found both in the circulation and in tissues; they belong to two major lineages that differentiate from myeloid precursors:
- mononuclear phagocytes: monocytes/macrophages; and
- polymorphonuclear granulocytes.

The mononuclear phagocytes consist of circulating cells (the monocytes) and macrophages that differentiate from monocytes and reside in a variety of organs (e.g. spleen, liver, lungs, kidneys) where they display distinctive morphological features and perform diverse functions.

The other family of phagocytes, polymorphonuclear granulocytes, have a lobed, irregularly shaped (polymorphic) nucleus. On the basis of how their cytoplasmic granules stain with acidic and basic dyes, they are classified into neutrophils, basophils and eosinophils, and have distinct effector functions:
- The neutrophils, also called polymorphonuclear neutrophils (PMNs), are most numerous and constitute the majority of leukocytes (white blood cells) in the blood stream (around 60%–70% in adults).
- The primary actions of eosinophils and basophils, both of which can function as phagocytes, involve granule release (exocytosis).

The mononuclear phagocytes and polymorphonuclear granulocytes develop from a common precursor.

Mononuclear phagocytes are widely distributed throughout the body. Cells of the mononuclear phagocytic system are found in virtually all organs of the body where the local microenvironment determines their morphology and functional characteristics, e.g. in the lung as alveolar macrophages, in kidney as glomerular mesangial cells and in the liver as Kupffer cells (Fig. 2.3 and see Fig. 1.4).

The main role of the mononuclear phagocytes is to remove particulate matter of foreign origin (e.g. microbes) or self-origin (e.g. aged erythrocytes).

Myeloid progenitors in the bone marrow differentiate into pro-monocytes and then into circulating monocytes, which migrate through the blood vessel walls into organs to become macrophages.

The human blood monocyte:
- is large (10–18 μm in diameter) relative to the lymphocyte;
- has a horseshoe-shaped nucleus;
- contains primary azurophilic (blue-staining) granules; and
- possesses ruffled membranes, a well-developed Golgi complex, and many intracytoplasmic lysosomes (Fig. 2.4).

The lysosomes contain peroxidase and several acid hydrolases, which are important for killing phagocytosed microorganisms. Monocytes/macrophages actively phagocytose microorganisms (mostly bacteria and fungi) and the body's own aged and dead cells, or even tumour cells.

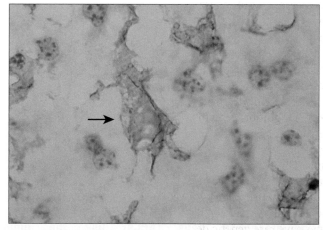

Fig. 2.3 Kupffer cells Kupffer cells in the normal mouse liver stain strongly positive with antibody to F4/80 *(arrow)*. Sinusoidal endothelial cells and hepatocytes are F4/80-negative. (Courtesy Professor S Gordon and Dr DA Hume.)

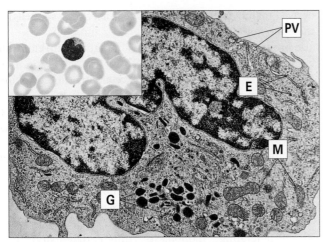

Fig. 2.4 Morphology of the monocyte Ultrastructure of a monocyte showing the horseshoe-shaped nucleus, pinocytotic vesicles *(PV)*, lysosomal granules *(G)*, mitochondria *(M)*, and isolated rough endoplasmic reticulum cisternae *(E)*. × 8000. *Inset*: Light microscope image of a monocyte from the blood. × 1200. (Courtesy Dr B Nichols.)

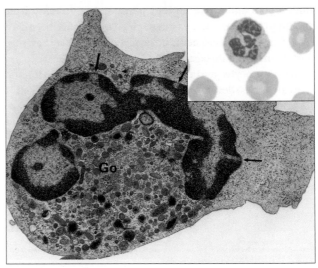

Fig. 2.5 Morphology of the neutrophil At the ultrastructural level, the azurophilic (primary) granules are larger than the secondary (specific) granules with a strongly electron-dense matrix; the majority of granules are specific granules and contain a variety of toxic materials to kill microbes. A pseudopod *(to the right)* is devoid of granules. *Arrows* indicate nuclear pores. *Go*, Golgi region. *Inset*: A mature neutrophil in a blood smear showing a multi-lobed nucleus. × 1500. (Reprinted from Shiland, BJ, Medical Assistant: Urinary, Blood, Lymphatic and Immune Systems with Laboratory Procedures—Module E, Second Edition, Copyright Elsevier Inc. 2015.)

Microbial adherence occurs through pattern recognition receptors (see Chapters 3 and 5), followed by phagocytosis. Coating microbes with complement components and/or antibodies (opsonization) enhances phagocytosis by monocytes/macrophages and is mediated by specialized complement receptors and antibody receptors expressed by the phagocytic cells (see Chapters 4 and 10). Several subsets of macrophages have now been described associated with different markers, cytokine profiles and functions.

There are three different types of polymorphonuclear granulocyte.

The polymorphonuclear granulocytes (often referred to as **polymorphs** or **granulocytes**) consist mainly of neutrophils (PMNs):

- They are released from the bone marrow at a rate of around 7 million per minute.
- They are short-lived (2–3 days) relative to monocytes/macrophages, which may live for months or years.

Like monocytes, PMNs adhere to endothelial cells lining the blood vessels and squeeze between the endothelial cells to leave the circulation (see Fig. 1.8) and reach the site of infection in tissues. This process is known as **diapedesis**. Adhesion is mediated by receptors on the granulocytes and ligands on the endothelial cells and is promoted by chemo-attractant cytokines (chemokines; see Chapter 3).

Like monocytes/macrophages, granulocytes also have pattern recognition receptors and PMNs play an important role in acute inflammation (usually synergizing with antibodies and complement) in providing protection against microorganisms. Their predominant role is phagocytosis and destruction of pathogens.

The importance of granulocytes is evident from the observation of individuals who have a reduced number of white cells or who have rare genetic defects that prevent polymorph extravasation in response to chemotactic stimuli (see Chapter 18). These individuals have a markedly increased susceptibility to bacterial and fungal infection.

Neutrophils comprise over 95% of the circulating granulocytes.

Neutrophils have a characteristic multi-lobed nucleus and are 10–20 μm in diameter (Fig. 2.5). Chemotactic agents attracting neutrophils to the site of infection include:

- protein fragments released when complement is activated (e.g. C5a);
- factors derived from the fibrinolytic and kinin systems;
- the products of other leukocytes and platelets; and
- the products of certain bacteria (see Chapter 3).

Neutrophils have a large arsenal of enzymes and antimicrobial proteins stored in two main types of granule:

- the primary (azurophilic) granules are lysosomes containing acid hydrolases, myeloperoxidase, and muramidase (lysozyme); they also contain the antimicrobial proteins including defensins, serprocidins, cathelicidins and bacterial permeability inducing (BPI) protein; and
- the secondary granules (specific to neutrophils) contain lactoferrin and lysozyme (see Fig. 2.5).

During phagocytosis the lysosomes containing the antimicrobial proteins fuse with vacuoles containing ingested microbes (termed **phagosomes**) to become **phagolysosomes** where the killing takes place.

Neutrophils can also release granules and cytotoxic substances extracellularly when they are activated by immune complexes (antibodies bound to their specific antigen molecules) through their Fc receptors. This is an important example of collaboration between the innate and adaptive immune systems and may be an important pathogenic mechanism in immune complex diseases (type III hypersensitivity, see Chapter 25).

Granulocytes and mononuclear phagocytes develop from a common precursor. Studies in which colonies have been grown in vitro from individual stems cells have shown that the progenitor of the myeloid lineage (CFU-GEMM) can give rise to granulocytes, monocytes and megakaryocytes (Fig. 2.6). Monocytes and neutrophils develop from a common precursor cell, the CFU-granulocyte macrophage cells (CFU-GMs). **Myelopoiesis** (the development of myeloid cells) commences in the liver of the human fetus at about 6 weeks of gestation.

CFU-GEMMs mature under the influence of colony-stimulating factors (CSFs) and several interleukins. These factors, which are relevant for the positive regulation of haematopoiesis, are:

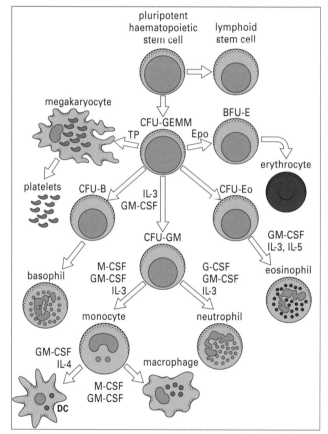

Fig. 2.6 Development of granulocytes and monocytes Pluripotent haematopoietic stem cells generate colony-forming units *(CFUs)* that can give rise to granulocytes, erythrocytes, monocytes and megakaryocytes *(CFU-GEMMs)*. CFU-GEMMs therefore have the potential to give rise to all blood cells except lymphocytes. IL-3 and granulocyte–macrophage colony-stimulating factor *(GM-CSF)* are required to induce the CFU-GEMM stem cell to enter one of five pathways (i.e. to give rise to megakaryocytes, erythrocytes via burst-forming units, basophils, neutrophils or eosinophils). IL-3 and GM-CSF are also required during further differentiation of the granulocytes and monocytes. Eosinophil *(Eo)* differentiation from CFU-Eo is promoted by IL-5. Neutrophils and monocytes are derived from the CFU-GM through the effects of G-CSF and M-CSF, respectively. Both GM-CSF and M-CSF and other cytokines (including IL-1, IL-4 and IL-6) promote the differentiation of monocytes into macrophages. Thrombopoietin *(TP)* promotes the growth of megakaryocytes. *BFU-E*, Erythrocytic burst-forming unit; *DC*, dendritic cell; *Epo*, erythropoietin; *G*, granulocyte; *M*, monocyte.

- derived mainly from stromal cells (connective tissue cells) in the bone marrow;
- also produced by mature forms of differentiated myeloid and lymphoid cells.

Bone marrow stromal cells, stromal cell matrix and cytokines form the micro-environment to support stem cell differentiation into individual cell lineages. Stromal cells produce an extracellular matrix, which is very important in establishing cell–cell interactions and enhancing stem cell differentiation. The major components of the matrix are proteoglycans, fibronectin, collagen, laminin, haemonectin and thrombospondin.

Other cytokines, such as transforming growth factor-β (TGFβ) may downregulate haematopoiesis. CFU-GMs taking the monocyte pathway give rise initially to proliferating monoblasts. Proliferating monoblasts differentiate into promonocytes and finally into mature circulating monocytes, which serve as a replacement pool for the tissue-resident macrophages (e.g. lung macrophages).

Monocytes express CD14 and significant levels of MHC class II molecules. The non-differentiated haematopoietic stem cell marker CD34, like other early markers in this lineage, is lost in mature neutrophils and mononuclear phagocytes. Other markers may be lost as differentiation occurs along one pathway, but retained in the other. For example, the common precursor of monocytes and neutrophils, the CFU-GM cell, expresses **major histocompatibility complex (MHC) class II molecules**, but only monocytes continue to express significant levels of this marker.

Mononuclear phagocytes and granulocytes display different functional molecules. Mononuclear phagocytes express CD14, which is part of the receptor complex for the lipopolysaccharide of Gram-negative bacteria. In addition, they acquire many of the same surface molecules as mature or activated neutrophils (e.g. the adhesion molecules CD11a and CD11b and Fc receptors, which recognize the constant regions of antibodies such as CD64 and CD32 – FcγRI and FcγRII, respectively).

Neutrophils express adhesion molecules and receptors involved in phagocytosis. CFU-GMs go through several differentiation stages to become neutrophils. As the CFU-GM cell differentiates along the neutrophil pathway, several distinct morphological stages are distinguished. Myeloblasts develop into promyelocytes and myelocytes, which mature and are released into the circulation as neutrophils.

The one-way differentiation of the CFU-GM into mature neutrophils is the result of acquiring specific receptors for growth and differentiation factors at progressive stages of development. Surface differentiation markers disappear or are expressed on the cells as they develop into granulocytes. For example, MHC class II molecules are expressed on the CFU-GM, but not on mature neutrophils.

Other surface molecules acquired during the differentiation process include:
- adhesion molecules (e.g. the leukocyte integrins see Table 3.w1); and
- receptors involved in phagocytosis, including complement and antibody Fc receptors.

Neutrophils constitutively express FcγRIII and FcγRII, and FcγRI is induced on activation.

It is difficult to assess the functional activity of different developmental stages of granulocytes, but it seems likely that the full functional potential is realized only when the cells are mature.

To become active in the presence of opsonins, neutrophils must interact directly with microorganisms and/or with cytokines generated by a response to antigen. This limitation could reduce neutrophil activity in early life.

Activation of neutrophils by cytokines and chemokines is also a prerequisite for their migration into tissues (see Chapter 3).

EOSINOPHILS, BASOPHILS AND MAST CELLS IN INFLAMMATION

Eosinophils play a role in immunity to parasitic worms.
Eosinophils comprise 2%–5% of blood leukocytes in healthy, non-allergic individuals. Human blood eosinophils usually have a bi-lobed nucleus and many cytoplasmic granules, which stain with acidic dyes such as eosin (Fig. 2.7). Although not their primary function, eosinophils appear to be capable of phagocytosing and killing ingested microorganisms.

The granules in mature eosinophils are membrane-bound organelles with crystalloid cores that differ in electron density from the surrounding matrix. The crystalloid core contains the **major basic protein (MBP)**, which:

- is a potent toxin for helminths;
- induces histamine release from mast cells;
- activates neutrophils and platelets; and

- provokes bronchospasm, a symptom of allergic asthma.

Other proteins with similar effects are found in the granule matrix, for example:
- eosinophil cationic protein (ECP); and
- eosinophil-derived neurotoxin (EDN).

Release of the granules on eosinophil activation is the only way eosinophils can kill large pathogens (e.g. schistosomula), which cannot be phagocytosed. Eosinophils are therefore thought to play a specialized role in immunity to parasitic worms using this mechanism (see Fig. 16.11).

Basophils and mast cells play a role in immunity against parasites.
Basophils are found in very small numbers in the circulation and account for less than 0.2% of leukocytes (Fig. 2.8).

The mast cell (Fig. 2.9), which is present in tissue and not in the circulation, is indistinguishable from the basophil in a number of its characteristics but displays some distinctive morphological features (Table 2.w1). Their shared functions may indicate a convergent differentiation pathway.

The stimulus for mast cell or basophil degranulation is often an **allergen** (i.e. an antigen causing an allergic reaction). To be effective, an allergen must cross-link IgE molecules bound to the surface of the mast cell or basophil via its high-affinity Fc receptors for IgE (FcεRI). Degranulation of a basophil or mast cell results in all contents of the granules being released very rapidly. This occurs by intracytoplasmic fusion of the granules, followed by discharge of their contents (Fig. 2.10).

Mediators such as histamine, released by degranulation, cause the adverse symptoms of allergy but, on the positive side, also play a role in immunity against parasites by enhancing acute inflammation.

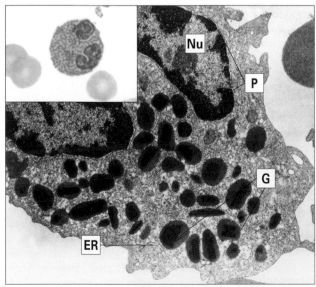

Fig. 2.7 Morphology of the eosinophil The ultrastructure of a mature eosinophil shows granules *(G)* with central crystalloids. × 17 500. *ER*, Endoplasmic reticulum; *Nu*, nucleus; *P*, nuclear pores. *Inset*. A mature eosinophil in a blood smear is shown with a bi-lobed nucleus and eosinophilic granules. × 1000. (Reprinted from Shiland, BJ, Medical Assistant: Urinary, Blood, Lymphatic and Immune Systems with Laboratory Procedures—Module E, Second Edition, Copyright Elsevier Inc. 2015.)

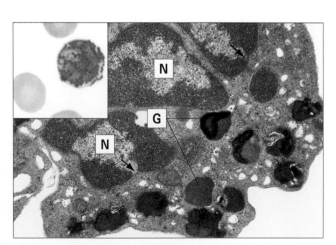

Fig. 2.8 Morphology of the basophil Morphology of the basophil: ultrastructural analysis shows a segmented nucleus *(N)* and the large cytoplasmic granules *(G). Arrows* indicate nuclear pores. × 11 000. *Inset*. This blood smear shows a typical basophil with its deep violet-blue granules. × 1000. (Reprinted from Shiland, BJ, Medical Assistant: Urinary, Blood, Lymphatic and Immune Systems with Laboratory Procedures—Module E, Second Edition, Copyright Elsevier Inc. 2015.)

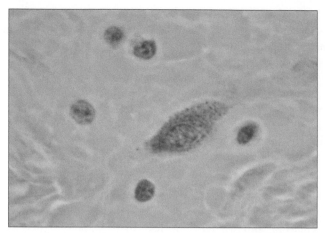

Fig. 2.9 Histological appearance of human connective tissue mast cells This micrograph of a mast cell shows dark blue cytoplasm with purple granules. Alcian blue and safranin stain. × 600. (Courtesy Dr TS Orr.)

Adipocytes produce inflammatory cytokines. Over the last 10 years it has become clear that adipocytes are players in immune reactions. Although adipose tissue was thought to be solely involved in energy storage and release, the metabolic and immunological functions of preadipocytes and adipocytes have emerged. They are potent producers of pro-inflammatory cytokines (e.g. IL-6 and TNFα) and chemokines, regulating monocyte/macrophage function and they produce other molecules associated with the innate immune system, such as the C1q-related superfamily (see Chapter 4). Finally, preadipocytes and adipocytes express a broad spectrum of functional Toll-like receptors and can convert into macrophage-like cells and express MHC molecules. They are thought to play an important role in the inflammation that occurs in type 2 diabetes.

ANTIGEN-PRESENTING CELLS

APCs are a heterogeneous population of leukocytes that are important in innate immunity (see Fig. 2.2) and play a pivotal role in activating T helper (TH) cells. In this regard, APCs are seen as a critical interface between the innate and adaptive immune systems. There are **professional APCs** (dendritic cells, macrophages and B cells) constitutively expressing MHC class II and co-stimulatory molecules, and **non-professional APCs,** which express MHC class II and co-stimulatory molecules for short periods of time throughout sustained inflammatory responses. This group comprises fibroblasts, glial cells, pancreatic β cells, thymic epithelial cells, thyroid epithelial cells and vascular endothelial cells.

Both macrophages and B cells are rich in membrane MHC class II molecules, especially after activation, and are thus able to process and to present specific antigens to (activated) T cells (see Chapter 7).

Somatic cells other than immune cells do not normally express class II MHC molecules, but cytokines such as IFNγ and tumour necrosis factor-α (TNFα) can induce the expression of class II molecules on some cell types and thus allow them to present antigen (non-professional APCs). This induction of inappropriate class II expression might contribute to the pathogenesis of autoimmune diseases and to prolonged inflammation (see Chapter 20).

Dendritic cells are derived from several different lineages. Functionally, dendritic cells (DC) are divided into those that both process and present foreign protein antigens to T cells – 'classical' dendritic cells (DCs) – and a separate type that passively presents foreign antigen in the form of immune complexes to B cells in lymphoid follicles – **follicular dendritic cells** (FDCs; Fig. 2.11).

Most DCs derive from one of two precursors:
- a myeloid progenitor (DC1) that gives rise to myeloid DCs, otherwise called bone-marrow derived or **bm-DCs**; and
- a lymphoid progenitor (DC2) that develops into plasmacytoid DCs (**pDCs**).

A summary of the main properties of myeloid and plasmacytoid dendritic cells is shown in Table 2.1.

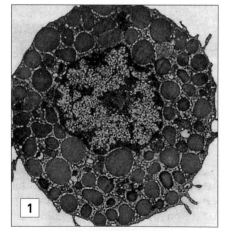
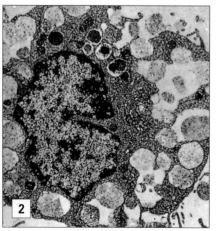

Fig. 2.10 Electron micrograph of rat mast cells Rat peritoneal mast cells show electron-dense granules (**1**). Vacuolation with exocytosis of the granule contents has occurred after incubation with anti-IgE (**2**). Transmission electron micrographs. × 2700. (Courtesy Dr D Lawson.)

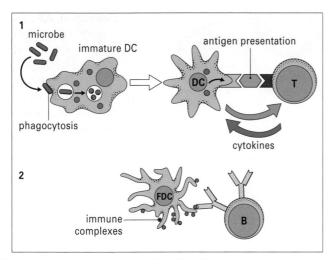

Fig. 2.11 Antigen-presenting cells (APCs) There are two main types of dendritic cells *(DC)*: classic DC and follicular dendritic cells *(FDCs)*. (**1**) Immature DCs are derived from bone marrow and interact mainly with T cells. They are highly phagocytic, take up microbes, process the foreign microbial antigens into small peptides and become mature APCs carrying the processed antigen (a peptide) on their surface with specialized MHC molecules. Specific T cells recognize the displayed peptide in a complex with MHC and, in the presence of cytokines produced by the mature DC, proliferate and also produce cytokines. (**2**) FDCs are not bone marrow derived and interact with B cells. In the B-cell follicles of lymphoid organs and tissues they bind small immune complexes. Antigen contained within the complex is presented to specific B cells in the lymphoid follicles.

TABLE 2.1 Myeloid and Plasmacytoid Dendritic Cells

	Myeloid DCs	Plasmacytoid DCs
Origin of precursor	Myeloid (DC1)	Lymphoid (DC2)
Localization	Diffuse – epidermis, mucosae, thymus and T-cell areas of secondary lymphoid organs and tissues	Restricted to T-cell areas of secondary lymphoid organs and tissues
Myeloid markers	Many	None
Characteristic cytokines produced	Mainly IL-8, IL-12	Mainly type I interferons (on challenge with enveloped viruses)

DC, Dendritic cell.
There are two main types of dendritic cells defined by their origin. They have differences in their localization, markers and cytokine production.

Myeloid DCs can also be divided into at least three types: Langerhans cells (LCs), dermal or interstitial DCs (DDC-IDCs) and blood monocyte-derived DCs (moDCs).

Different populations of DCs can be identified by their surface markers. Myeloid DCs, but not pDCs express CD1a and CD208, and DDC-IDC and moDC also express CD11b.

Langerhans cells have so-called Birbeck granules containing langerin. It appears that various populations of myeloid DCs may represent different stages in their maturation and migration in the body (see later).

BM-DCs express various receptors that are involved in antigen uptake:

- C-type lectin receptors, e.g. macrophage mannose receptor (MMR) family;
- Fc receptors for IgG, IgE;
- receptors for heat shock protein–peptide complexes;
- receptors for apoptotic bodies;
- 'scavenger' receptors – for sugars, lipid, etc.; and
- Toll-like receptors (TLRs).

Before DCs take up antigen (become loaded) they are called immature DCs and express various markers characteristic for this resting stage, the most important being chemokine receptors CCR1, CCR5 and CCR6. DCs are attracted to the infection site by chemokines through these receptors (see Chapter 3).

Mature DCs loaded with antigen downregulate expression of CCR1, 5, 6 and upregulate CCR7. This encourages their migration into peripheral lymphatics, where CCR7 interacts with secondary lymphoid tissue chemokine SLC (CCL21) expressed on vascular endothelium (see Fig. 3.15).

DCs are found primarily in the skin, lymph nodes and spleen, and within or underneath most mucosal epithelia. They are also present in the thymus, where they present self-antigens to developing T cells.

Langerhans cells and interdigitating dendritic cells are rich in MHC class II molecules. Langerhans cells in the epidermis and in other squamous epithelia migrate via the afferent lymphatics into the paracortex of the draining lymph nodes (Fig. 2.12). Here, they interact with T cells and are termed interdigitating cells (IDCs, Fig. 2.13). These DCs are rich in class II MHC molecules, which are important for presenting antigen to helper T cells.

BM-DCs are also present within the germinal centres (GCs) of secondary lymphoid follicles (i.e. they are the MHC class II molecule-positive germinal centre DCs (GCDCs)). In contrast to FDCs, they are migrating cells, which on arrival in the GC interact with germinal centre T cells and are involved in B-cell development (see Chapter 9).

The thymus is of crucial importance in the development and maturation of T cells. In thymus there are cortical DCs and IDCs, which are especially abundant in the medulla. They participate in two important stages in T-cell maturation/differentiation in thymus positive and negative selection, respectively (see later).

FDCs lack class II MHC molecules and are found in B cell areas. Unlike the APCs that actively process and present protein antigens to T cells, FDCs have a passive role in presenting antigen in the form of immune complexes to B cells. They are therefore found in the primary and secondary follicles of the B-cell areas of secondary lymphoid tissues. They are a non-migratory population of cells and form a stable

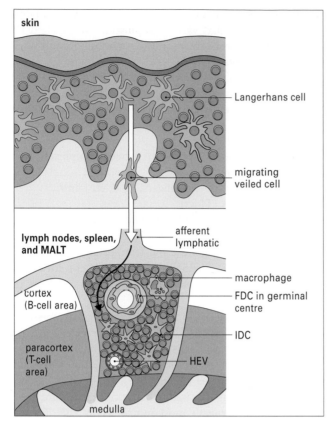

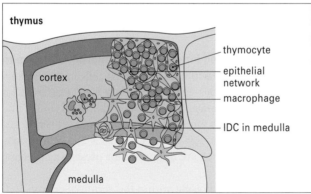

Fig. 2.12 Migration of antigen-presenting cells (APCs) into lymphoid tissues Bone marrow-derived dendritic cells (DCs) are found especially in lymphoid tissues, in the skin and in mucosa. DCs in the form of Langerhans cells are found in the epidermis and in mucosa and are characterized by special (tennis racquet-shaped) Birbeck granules. Langerhans cells are rich in MHC class II molecules and carry processed antigens. They migrate via the afferent lymphatics (where they appear as veiled cells) into the paracortex of the draining lymph nodes. Here they make contact with T cells. These interdigitating dendritic cells (IDCs), localized in the T-cell areas of the lymph node, present antigen to T helper cells. The antigen is exposed to B cells on the follicular dendritic cells (FDCs) in the germinal centres of B-cell follicles. Some macrophages located in the outer cortex and marginal sinus may also act as APCs. In the thymus, APCs occur as IDCs in the medulla. HEV, High endothelial venule; MALT, mucosa-associated lymphoid tissue.

network by establishing strong intercellular connections via desmosomes.

FDCs lack class II MHC molecules, but bind antigen via complement receptors (CD21 and CD35), which attach to

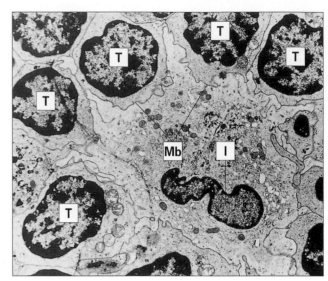

Fig. 2.13 Ultrastructure of an Interdigitating dendritic cell In the T-cell area of a lymph node, intimate contacts are made by antigen-presenting cells with the membranes of the surrounding T cells. The cytoplasm contains a well-developed endosomal system and does not have Birbeck granules. × 2000. *I*, IDC nucleus; *Mb*, IDC membrane; *T*, T-cell nucleus. (Courtesy Dr BH Balfour.)

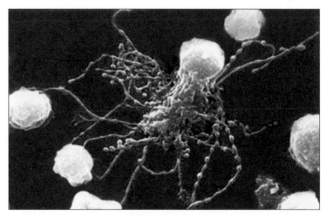

Fig. 2.14 Follicular dendritic cell An isolated follicular dendritic cell (FDC) from the lymph node of an immunized mouse 24 hours after injection of antigen. The FDC is of intermediate maturity with smooth filiform dendrites typical of young FDCs, and beaded dendrites, which bind immune complexes (iccosomes) in mature FDCs. The adjacent small white cells are lymphocytes. (Electron micrograph kindly provided by Dr Andras Szakal, Isolated follicular dendritic cells: cytochemical antigen localization, Nomarski, SEM and TEM morphology. J.Immunology 1985;134: 1349–1359. Reproduced by permission of the Journal of Immunology.)

complement associated with immune complexes (iccosomes; Fig. 2.14). They also express Fc receptors. The FDCs produce chemokines that are important in B cells homing to the follicular areas in lymphoid tissues. They are not bone-marrow derived but are of mesenchymal origin.

LYMPHOCYTES

Lymphocytes are phenotypically and functionally heterogeneous. Large numbers of lymphocytes are produced daily in the primary or central lymphoid organs (i.e. thymus and postnatal bone marrow). Some migrate via the circulation into the secondary lymphoid tissues (i.e. spleen, lymph nodes and MALT).

The average human adult has about 2×10^{12} lymphoid cells and lymphoid tissue as a whole represents about 2% of total body weight. Lymphoid cells account for about 20% of the leukocytes in the adult circulation.

Many mature lymphoid cells are long-lived and persist as memory cells for many years.

Lymphocytes are morphologically heterogeneous. In a conventional blood smear, lymphocytes vary in size (from 6 to 10 μm in diameter) and morphology.

Differences are seen in:
- nuclear to cytoplasmic (N:C) ratio;
- nuclear shape; and
- the presence or absence of azurophilic granules.

Two distinct morphological types of lymphocyte are seen in the circulation as determined by light microscopy and a haematological stain such as Giemsa (Fig. 2.15):
- The first type is relatively small, is typically agranular and has a high nuclear to cytoplasmic (N:C) ratio (see Fig. 2.15(1)).
- The second type is larger, has a lower N:C ratio, contains cytoplasmic azurophilic granules and is known as the large granular lymphocyte (LGL).

LGLs should not be confused with granulocytes, monocytes, or their precursors, which also contain azurophilic granules.

Most T cells express the αβ T-cell receptor (see later) and, when resting, can show either of the above morphological patterns.

Most T$_H$ cells (approximately 95%) and a proportion (approximately 50%) of cytotoxic T cells (T$_C$ or CTL) have the morphology shown in Figure 2.15(1).

The LGL morphological pattern displayed in Figure 2.15(2) is shown by less than 5% of T$_H$ cells and by about 30%–50% of T$_C$ cells. These cells display LGL morphology with primary lysosomes dispersed in the cytoplasm and a well-developed Golgi apparatus, as shown in Figure 2.15(3).

Most B cells, when resting, have a morphology similar to that seen in Figure 2.15(1).

Lymphocytes express characteristic surface and cytoplasmic markers. Lymphocytes (and other leukocytes) express a large number of different functionally important molecules mostly on their surfaces but also in their cytoplasm, which can be used to distinguish (mark) cell subsets. Many of these cell markers can be identified by specific monoclonal antibodies (mAb) and can be used to distinguish T cells from B cells (Table 2.2).

Lymphocytes express a variety of cell surface molecules that belong to different families, which have probably evolved from a few ancestral genes. These families of molecules are shared with other leukocytes and are distinguished by their structure. The major families include:
- the immunoglobulin superfamily;
- the integrin family;
- selectins; and
- proteoglycans.

Marker molecules allow lymphocytes to communicate with their environment. The major function of these families of molecules is to allow lymphocytes to communicate with their environment. They are extremely important in cell trafficking, adhesion and activation. Markers expressed by lymphocytes can often be detected on cells of other lineages.

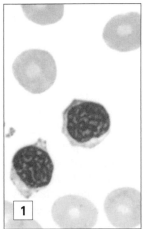
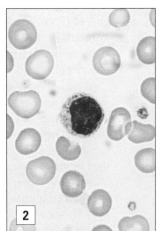
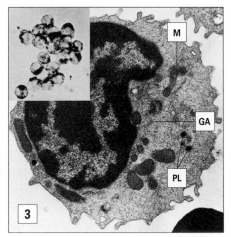

Fig. 2.15 Morphological heterogeneity of lymphocytes Lymphocyte morphology. (**1**) The small lymphocyte has no granules, a round nucleus and a high N:C ratio. (**2**) The large granular lymphocyte (LGL) has a lower N:C ratio, indented nucleus and azurophilic granules in the cytoplasm. Giemsa stain. (**3**) Ultrastructure of the LGL shows characteristic electron-dense peroxidase-negative granules (primary lysosomes, *PL*), scattered throughout the cytoplasm, with some close to the Golgi apparatus *(GA)* and many mitochondria *(M)*. × 10 000. (Reprinted from Shiland, BJ, *Medical Assistant: Urinary, Blood, Lymphatic and Immune Systems with Laboratory Procedures—Module E, Second Edition*, Copyright Elsevier Inc. 2015.)

TABLE 2.2	Main Distinguishing Markers of T and B Cells	
CD number	T cells	B cells
antigen receptor	TCR – (αβ or γδ)	immunoglobulin (Ig)
CD1	–	+
CD3	+ (part of the TCR complex)	–
CD4	+ (subset)	–
CD8	+ (subset)	–
CD19	–	+
CD20	–	+
CD23	+ (subset)	+
CD40	–	+
CD79a	–	+ (part of the BCR complex)
CD79b	–	+ (part of the BCR complex)

BCR, B-cell receptor; *TCR*, T-cell receptor.

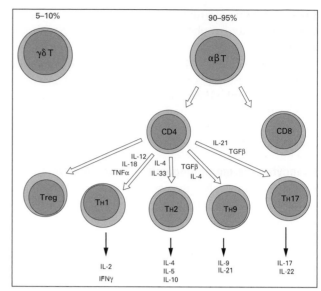

Fig. 2.16 Naïve T-cell subsets In the thymus, naïve T cells develop as two distinct populations of cells, based on the composition of their T-cell receptor (TCR); 90%–95% have an α/β TCR and 5%–10% a γ/δ TCR. αβ T cells diverge into CD4⁺ or CD8⁺ cells through the ability of their TCR to interact, respectively, with MHC class II (CD4⁺) or class I (CD8⁺) molecules. CD4⁺ and CD8⁺ αβT cells have very distinct effector functions. About 5% of CD4⁺ cells are so-called natural regulatory cells *(Tregs)*. CD4 subpopulations differentiate in response to the cytokines indicated and the differentiated cells go on to produce distinct sets of cytokines.

T cells can be distinguished by their different antigen receptors. The definitive T-cell lineage marker is the TCR. The two defined types of TCR are:

- a heterodimer of two disulfide-linked polypeptides (α and β); and
- a structurally similar heterodimer consisting of γ and δ polypeptides.

Both receptors are associated with a set of five polypeptides (the CD3 complex) and together form the TCR complex (TCR–CD3 complex; see Chapter 6).

Approximately 90%–95% of blood T cells in humans are αβ T cells and the remaining 5%–10% are γδ T cells.

There are three major subpopulations of αβ T cells.

- Tн cells that express the CD4 marker (CD4⁺ T cells) and mainly help or induce immune responses, divided into two main subsets (Tн1 and Tн2).
- Tregs that express the CD4 marker (CD4⁺ T cells) and regulate immune responses.
- Tc cells that express the CD8 marker (CD8⁺ T cells) – also called CTLs.

CD4⁺ T cells recognize their specific antigens in association with MHC class II molecules, whereas CD8⁺ T cells recognize antigens in association with MHC class I molecules (see Chapter 7). Thus, the presence of CD4 or CD8 limits (restricts) the type of cell with which the T cell can interact.

A small proportion of αβ T cells express neither CD4 nor CD8; these double negative T cells might have a regulatory function. Most circulating γδ cells are double negative.

Tн subsets are distinguished by their cytokine profiles. CD4⁺ Tн cells can be further divided into functional subsets on the basis of the spectrum of the cytokines they produce. They initially develop from Tн0 naive (antigen inexperienced) precursor cells (Fig. 2.16):

- Tн1 cells develop in response to IL-12, IL-18 and IFNγ and secrete IL-2 and IFNγ.

- Tн2 cells develop in response to IL-4 and IL-33 and produce IL-4, IL-5, IL-6 and IL-10.

Tн1 cells mediate several functions associated with cytotoxicity and local inflammatory reactions. They help cytotoxic T-cell precursors develop into effector cells to kill virally infected target cells and to activate macrophages infected with intracellular pathogens (e.g. *Mycobacteria* and *Chlamydia*), enhancing intracellular killing of the pathogens by the production of IFNγ. Consequently, they are important for combating intracellular pathogens, including viruses, bacteria and parasites. Some Tн1 cells also help B cells to produce different classes of antibodies.

Tн17 cells are similar to the Tн1 subset but their development from Tн0 cells is dependent on TGFβ and IL-21. Their induction by TGFβ suggests that they are related to the regulatory T-cell subsets. They produce both IL-17 and IL-22 and play an important role in maintaining the integrity of mucosal epithelia and thus in protection against microbial entry into the body.

Another subset of T cells, Tн9, can be produced from Tн0 cells by a combination of IL-4 and TGFβ. They, in turn, can produce IL-9 and IL-21 cytokines. The suggested function of Tн9 cells is to carry out immune responses to intestinal worms. In addition, they are implicated in autoimmune and allergic reactions and in immunosurveillance of melanoma.

Tн2 cells are effective at stimulating B cells to proliferate and to produce antibodies of some IgG subclasses and especially IgE and therefore function primarily to protect against free-living, extracellular microorganisms (humoral immunity).

Several CD4$^+$ regulatory T-cell populations have been described as being capable of suppressing T-cell responses (see later).

γδ T Cells and NKT Cells

γδ T cells maintain epithelial integrity, kill stressed cells and contribute to antimicrobial immunity. γδT cells display LGL characteristics (see Fig. 2.15) and some have a dendritic morphology in lymphoid tissues (Fig. 2.17). They have a broad specificity for recognition of unconventional antigens such as heat shock proteins, phospholipids and phosphoproteins. Unlike αβ T cells, they do not generally recognize antigens in association with classical MHC class I and II molecules. γδT cells express several of the Toll-like receptor families either spontaneously or after activation and most express CD16.

Human γδ T cells have been divided into three main populations based on the expression of their δ chain.

- γδ T cells expressing Vδ1 chains are prominent in the intra-epithelial layer of mucosal surfaces in the skin, lung and gut. Here, as the majority of the intra-epithelial T cells, they are involved in the maintenance of epithelial tissue integrity when facing damage, infection or responding to stressed or neoplastic epithelial cells. They produce IL-17 and some IL-10, but little or no IL-2, IL-4 or IFN γ. Vδ1 cells are also present as a minor population in the peripheral blood.
- The second population using Vδ2 chains represent the majority of circulating γδ T lymphocytes (50%–90%) in healthy human adults. Vδ2 chain pairing is mainly with Vγ9 (also termed Vγ2) and is thought to recognize conformational changes in the butyrophilin molecule (a widely expressed member of the Ig supergene family) and may represent a mechanism to identify infected or transformed cells. Interestingly, Vδ2 T cells have been reported to act as professional APCs on activation acquiring co-stimulatory molecules, MHC class II, CD80 and CD86.

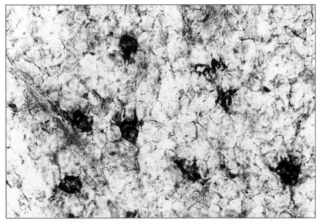

Fig. 2.17 Dendritic morphology of γδ T cells in the tonsil The γδ T-cell population is predominantly localized in the interfollicular T-cell-dependent zones. Note the dendritic morphology of the cells. Anti-γδ T-cell monoclonal antibody and immunoperoxidase. × 900. (Courtesy Dr A Favre, from Arancia G, Malorni W, Iosi F, et al. Morphological features of cloned lymphocytes expressing gamma/delta T cell receptors. Eur J Immunol 1991;21:173, with permission.)

- The third population is Vδ3 T cells, which make up about 0.2% of circulating T cells. They express CD56, CD161, HLA-DR and NKG2D but not NKG2A or NKG2C and although poorly represented in the blood, they are rich in the liver and in patients with leukaemias and some chronic viral infections.

γδ T cells show some long-term memory characteristics even though they are generally regarded, like NKT cells, as being part of innate immunity.

iNKT cells recognize glycolipid antigens. NKT cells have T-cell markers and also some NK-cell markers (see later): they express CD3 and have a unique αβ TCR (expressing an invariant Vα and Vβ11, hence called invariant NKT cells (iNKT cells). Human iNKT cells are infrequent in the blood, being between 0.01% and 1% of the peripheral mononuclear cells. iNKT cells recognize glycolipid antigens presented by CD1d molecules (see Fig. 7.11), but not conventional MHC molecules. iNKT cells are therefore thought to act as an interface between the innate and adaptive systems by initiating T-cell responses to non-peptide antigens.

NKT cells are also thought to regulate immune responses (especially dendritic cell function) through the production of cytokines (e.g. IL-4, IL-10 and IFNγ) in response to antigens.

B cells recognize antigen using the B cell receptor complex. About 5%–15% of the circulating lymphoid pool are B cells, which are defined by the presence of **surface immunoglobulin**, transmembrane molecules, which are constitutively produced and inserted into the B-cell membrane, where they act as specific antigen receptors.

Most human B cells in peripheral blood express two immunoglobulin isotypes on their surface: IgM and IgD (see Chapter 9).

On any B cell, the antigen-binding sites of these IgM and IgD isotypes are identical.

Fewer than 10% of the B cells in the circulation express IgG, IgA, or IgE, but B cells expressing IgG, IgA or IgE are present in larger numbers in specific locations of the body (e.g. IgA-bearing cells in the intestinal mucosa).

Immunoglobulin associated with other accessory molecules on the B-cell surface forms the **B cell antigen receptor complex (BCR)**. These accessory molecules consist of disulfide-bonded heterodimers of Igα (CD79a) and Igβ (CD79b).

The heterodimers interact with the transmembrane segments of the immunoglobulin receptor (see Fig. 10.1), and, like the separate molecular components of the TCR/CD3 complex (see Fig. 6.17), are involved in cellular activation. Intracellular domains of CD79a/b have immunoreceptor tyrosine-based activation motifs (ITAMs). BCR interaction with specific antigen triggers ITAM phosphorylation and this initiates a downstream cascade of intracellular events, leading to the activation-related changes in gene expression.

Other B-cell markers include MHC class II antigens and complement and Fc receptors. Most B cells carry MHC class II antigens, which are important for co-operative (cognate) interactions with T cells (see Fig. 7.3).

Complement receptors for C3b (CD35) and C3d (CD21) are commonly found on B cells and are associated with activation and, together with chemokine receptors, possibly homing of the cells in the peripheral lymphoid organs and tissues. CD19/CD21 interactions with complement, associated with antigen, play a role in antigen-induced B-cell activation via the antigen-binding antibody receptor.

Fc receptors for exogenous IgG (FcγRII, CD32) are also present on B cells and play a role in negative signalling to the B cell (see Fig. 10.15). CD19 and CD20 are the main markers currently used to identify human B cells. Other human B-cell markers are CD22 and CD72–CD78.

Murine B cells also express CD72 (Lyb-2) and B220, a high molecular weight (220 kDa) isoform of CD45 (Lyb-5).

CD40 is an important molecule on B cells and is involved in cognate interactions between T and B cells (see Fig. 9.10) with T cells expressing CD40 ligand (CD40L). Activated B cells upregulate expression of B7.1 (CD80) and B7.2 (CD86) molecules that interact with their CD28 expressed by T cells. This provides a co-stimulatory signal for T/B cognate interactions.

CD5⁺ B-1 cells and marginal zone B Cells produce natural antibodies.

Many of the first B cells that appear during ontogeny express CD5, a marker originally found on T cells. These cells (termed B-1 cells) are found predominantly in the peritoneal cavity in mice and there is some evidence for a separate differentiation pathway from conventional B cells (termed **B-2 cells**).

CD5⁺ B-1 cells express their immunoglobulins from unmutated germline genes (see Chapter 9) and produce mostly IgM, but also some IgG and IgA. These so-called natural antibodies are of low avidity, but, unusually, they are polyreactive and are found at high concentration in the adult serum. CD5⁺ B-1 cells:

- respond well to TI (T-independent) antigens (i.e. antigens that can directly stimulate B cells without T cell help);
- may be involved in antigen processing and antigen presentation to T cells; and
- probably play a role in both tolerance and antibody responses.

Functions proposed for natural antibodies include:
- the first line of defence against microorganisms;
- clearance of damaged self components; and
- regulatory interactions within the immune system.

Characteristically, natural antibodies react against auto-antigens including:
- DNA;
- Fc of IgG;
- phospholipids; and
- cytoskeletal components.

CD5 is expressed by B-2 cells when they are activated appropriately and there is therefore some controversy about whether CD5 represents an activation antigen on B cells. Current theories therefore support the notion for two different kinds of CD5⁺ B cells.

A ligand for CD5 is CD72 and there is some suggestion that it self-associates and can bind directly to IL6. However, the exact function of CD5 on human B cells is currently unclear but is highly likely to be involved in the regulation of B-cell activation.

Marginal zone B cells are thought to protect against polysaccharide antigens.

Much has been learned about **marginal zone B cells** over the past few years. These cells accumulate slowly in the marginal zone of the spleen – a process that takes between 1 and 2 years in humans.

Like B-1 cells, marginal zone B cells respond to thymus-independent antigens and they are thought to be our main protection against polysaccharide antigens. They also produce natural antibodies and, together with B-1 cells, have recently been termed innate-like B cells.

B cells can differentiate into antibody-secreting plasma cells.

Following B-cell activation, many B-cell blasts mature into **antibody-forming cells** (AFCs), which progress in vivo to terminally differentiated **plasma cells**, and a subset of B cells remains in the periphery as long-lived memory B cells.

Some B-cell blasts do not develop rough endoplasmic reticulum cisternae. These cells are found in germinal centres and are named **follicle centre cells** or **centrocytes**.

Under light microscopy, the cytoplasm of the plasma cells is basophilic because of the large amount of RNA being used for antibody synthesis in the rough endoplasmic reticulum. At the ultra-structural level, the rough endoplasmic reticulum can often be seen in parallel arrays (Fig. 2.18).

Plasma cells are infrequent in the blood, comprising less than 0.1% of circulating lymphocytes. They are normally restricted to the secondary lymphoid organs and tissues, but are also abundant in the bone marrow. Since their sole function is to produce immunoglobulins, plasma cells have few surface receptors and do not respond to antigens. Unlike resting B cells or memory B cells, plasma cells do not express surface BCR or MHC class II.

Antibodies produced by a single plasma cell are of one specificity (idiotype) and immunoglobulin class (isotype and allotype; see Chapter 10).

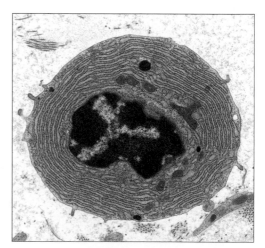

Fig. 2.18 Plasma cell, transmission electron micrograph (TEM) This section has revealed the cell's large central nucleus. Surrounding this is large amounts of rough endoplasmic reticulum thin lines. Plasma cells, which are found in the blood and lymph, are mature B lymphocytes (white blood cells) that produce and secrete antibodies during an immune response. Magnification x6000 when printed at 10 centimetres wide. (© Steve Gschmeissner/Science Photo Library.)

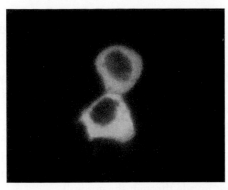

Fig. 2.19 Immunofluorescent staining of intracytoplasmic immuno-globulin in plasma cells Fixed human plasma cells, treated with fluores-ceinated anti-human-IgM *(green)* antibody and rhodaminated anti-human-IgG *(red)* antibody, show extensive intracytoplasmic staining. As the distinct staining of the two cells shows, plasma cells normally produce only one class or subclass (isotype) of antibody. × 1500.

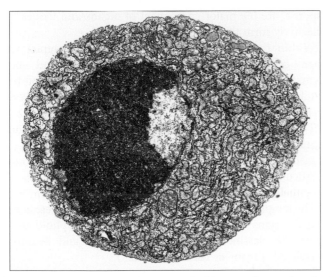

Fig. 2.20 Plasma cell death by apoptosis Plasma cells are short-lived and die by apoptosis (cell suicide). Note the nuclear chromatin changes, which are characteristic of apoptosis. × 5000.

Immunoglobulins can be visualized in the plasma cell cytoplasm by staining with fluorochrome-labelled specific antibodies (Fig. 2.19).

Many plasma cells have a short life span, surviving for a few days and dying by apoptosis (Fig. 2.20). However, there is a subset of plasma cells with a long life span (months) in the bone marrow that might be important in giving rise to sustained antibody responses.

INNATE LYMPHOID CELLS (ILC)

ILCs are lymphocytes that do not express rearranged antigen receptors. ILCs are a heterogeneous population of non-T and non-B lymphoid cells that carry out many of the functions of conventional T cells and play an important first-line

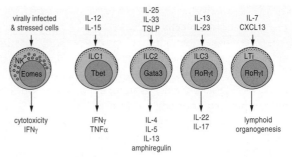

Fig. 2.21 Innate lymphoid cells Innate lymphoid cells are subdivided into five categories according to cytokines required to induce their differentiation *(top)*, the transcription factors that are required to induce their differentiation and the cytokines they produce. *NK*, Natural killer cells.

role in defence against pathogens, wound healing and maintenance of epithelial integrity. Unlike T and B cells, they do not have rearranged antigen receptors and are therefore not able to recognize specific antigens.

Five groups of ILC are defined by lineage and functional traits. The classification of the ILCs is still under development but there appear to be five distinct groups based on the transcription factors required for their development and functional traits (Fig. 2.21)

Four of these groups can be considered as innate equivalents to T cells. Natural killer (NK) cells, like CD8$^+$ T cells, are cytotoxic. ILC1, ILC2 and ILC3 are sometimes called helper ILCs and show similar cytokine and transcriptional factor profiles to the CD4 T-cell lineage as innate counterparts to TH1, TH2 and TH17 cells, respectively. The final group of ILCs are lymphoid tissue inducer (LTi) cells, which are important for the organogenesis of secondary lymphoid tissues (see Fig 2.21).

NK cells kill virally infected and cancerous cells. NK cells are very important cytotoxic cells in innate immunity. They account for up to 15% of blood lymphocytes, are derived from the bone marrow and morphologically have the appearance of large granular lymphocytes (see Fig. 2.15). The function of NK cells is to recognize and to kill virally infected cells (Fig. 2.22) and certain tumour cells by mechanisms described in Chapter 8.

NK cells are identified by their expression of CD56 and CD16. In humans, NK cells are most often identified by the absence of the T-cell receptor component CD3 and the expression of CD56 (NCAM), a homophilic adhesion molecule of the immunoglobulin superfamily. CD16 (FcγRIII) is another marker that may be used to identify NK cells, although about 10% of human NK cells do not express this molecule and are thought to represent immature NK cells.

CD16 is involved in the activation pathways of NK cells by antibody-coated targets and is also expressed by neutrophils, some macrophages and γδ T cells. However, on neutrophils,

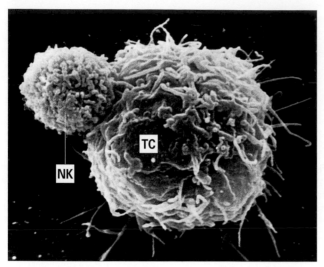

Fig. 2.22 NK cell attached to a target A natural killer *(NK)* cell attached to a target cell *(TC)* × 4500. (Courtesy Drs G Arancia and W Malorni, Rome.)

CD16 is linked to the surface membrane by a glycoinositol phospholipid (GPI) linkage, whereas NK cells, some macrophages and γδ T cells express the transmembrane form of the molecule.

In mice, NK cells do not express CD56 and have historically been defined by their expression of the activating NK cell receptors NK1.1 or NKp46. However, the recent discovery that some helper ILCs also express these molecules means that this definition is now treated with some caution.

Resting NK cells in both species express the β chain of the IL-2 receptor and the signal transducing common γ chain of IL-2 and other cytokine receptors (see Fig. 7.16). Therefore, direct stimulation with IL-2 activates NK cells.

Helper ILCs polarize the immune response by producing cytokines. ILC1, ILC2 and ILC3 are ubiquitous but are most often found at protective barriers in tissues associated with gastrointestinal, bronchial tracts and skin. Many of the ILCs are found in higher numbers during neonatal development than in adult life. There is some evidence that ILC2 and ILC3 subsets can change into ILC1 in the appropriate cytokine micro-environment.

The phenotypic definition of most helper ILC subsets has not yet been fully agreed upon. One complicating factor is that the phenotype of these cells varies between species and even between organs in the same species. One definition that is currently widely used is expression of IL-7Rα (CD127) in the absence of lineage markers that define other immune cell subsets (for example, CD3 and CD19).

One key role of the helper ILCs is to sense changes in the environment through their intracellular and extracellular cytokine receptors and to produce cytokines in response (see Chapter 7). For example, ILC1 are activated by IL-12 released from macrophages following ingestion of pathogens; in turn, they produce IFNγ and TNFα, both polarizing the immune response to an anti-viral state. Expression of NKp44 and NKp46 by ILC1 and ICL3 cells also allows sensing of stressed cells (see Chapter 8), which stimulates the production of cytokines.

ILC2 and ILC3 help to maintain epithelial integrity. Another important role of ILC2 and ILC3 at barrier sites is to maintain epithelial integrity. ILC2 produce a member of the epidermal growth factor family, Amphiregulin (Areg), which promotes the division of epidermal cells. The cytokine IL-22, which is produced by ILC3, also acts to promote epidermal cell division. Mice lacking ILC3 are particularly susceptible to infection by bacteria that invade through the gut wall.

There is also evidence that in certain circumstances ILC2 and ILC3 can act as antigen-presenting cells, but the importance of this is not yet fully understood.

LYMPHOCYTE DEVELOPMENT

Lymphocytes, the effector cells of the adaptive immune response, are the major component of organs and tissues that collectively form the lymphoid system.

Within the lymphoid organs, lymphocytes interact with other cell types of both haematopoietic and non-haematopoietic origin that are important for lymphocyte maturation, selection, function and disposal of terminally differentiated cells.

These other cell types are termed accessory cells and include:
* antigen-presenting cells;
* macrophages;
* reticular cells; and
* epithelial cells.

The lymphoid system is arranged into either discrete encapsulated organs or accumulations of diffuse lymphoid tissue, which are classified into primary (central) and secondary (peripheral) organs or tissues (Fig. 2.23).

In essence, lymphocytes:
* are produced, mature and are selected in primary lymphoid organs; and
* exert their effector functions in the secondary lymphoid organs and tissues.

Tertiary lymphoid tissues are anatomical sites that under normal conditions contain sparse lymphocytes, if any, but may be selectively populated by these cells in pathological conditions (e.g. skin, synovium, lungs).

Lymphoid stem cells develop and mature within primary lymphoid organs. In the primary lymphoid organs, lymphocytes (B and T cells) differentiate from lymphoid stem cells, proliferate, are selected and mature into functional cells.

In mammals, T cells mature in the thymus and B cells mature in the fetal liver and postnatal bone marrow. Birds have a specialized site of B-cell generation, the bursa of Fabricius.

In the primary lymphoid organs:
* lymphocytes acquire their repertoire of specific antigen receptors to cope with the antigenic challenges that individuals encounter during their lifetime;

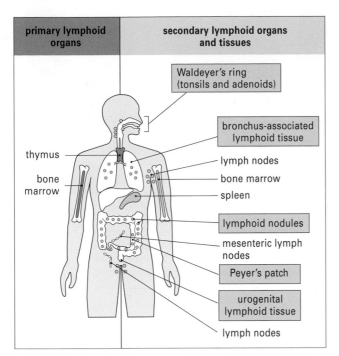

Fig. 2.23 **Major lymphoid organs and tissues** Thymus and bone marrow are the primary (central) lymphoid organs. They are the sites of maturation for T and B cells, respectively. Cellular and humoral immune responses occur in the secondary (peripheral) lymphoid organs and tissues. Secondary lymphoid organs can be classified according to the body regions they defend. The spleen responds predominantly to blood-borne antigens. Lymph nodes mount immune responses to antigens circulating in the lymph, entering through the skin (subcutaneous lymph nodes) or through mucosal surfaces (visceral lymph nodes). Tonsils, Peyer's patches and other mucosa-associated lymphoid tissue (MALT) *(blue boxes)* react to antigens that have entered via the surface mucosal barriers. Note that the bone marrow is both a primary and a secondary lymphoid organ because it gives rise to B and NK cells, but it is also the site of B-cell terminal differentiation (long-lived plasma cells).

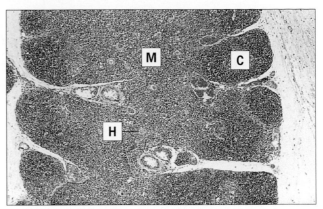

Fig. 2.24 **Thymus section showing the lobular organization** This section shows the two main areas of the thymus lobule: an outer cortex of immature cells *(C)* and an inner medulla of more mature cells *(M)*. Hassall's corpuscles *(H)* are found in the medulla. H&E stain. × 25. (Courtesy Dr A Stevens and Professor J Lowe.)

- cells with receptors for **auto-antigens** are mostly eliminated; and
- in the thymus, T cells learn to recognize appropriate **self MHC molecules**.

There is evidence that some lymphocyte development might occur outside primary lymphoid organs.

T cells develop in the thymus. The thymus in mammals is a bi-lobed organ in the thoracic cavity overlying the heart and major blood vessels. Each lobe is organized into lobules separated from each other by connective tissue trabeculae.

Within each lobule, the lymphoid cells (thymocytes) are arranged into:

- an outer tightly packed cortex, which contains the majority of relatively immature proliferating thymocytes; and
- an inner medulla containing more mature cells, implying a differentiation gradient from cortex to medulla (Fig. 2.24).

The main blood vessels that regulate cell traffic in the thymus are high endothelial venules (HEVs) at the corticomedullary junction of thymic lobules. Through these veins, the T-cell

progenitors formed in the fetal liver and bone marrow enter the **epithelial anlage** and migrate towards the cortex.

In the cortex of the thymus, the T-cell progenitors undergo proliferation and then differentiate into mature T cells as they migrate from the cortex to the medulla.

A network of epithelial cells throughout the lobules plays a role in the differentiation and selection processes involved in thymocyte development.

The mature T cells probably leave the thymus through the same venules, at the corticomedullary junction from which the T-cell progenitors entered (Fig. 2.25).

Three types of thymic epithelial cell have important roles in T-cell production. At least three types of epithelial cell can be distinguished in the thymic lobules according to distribution, structure, function and phenotype:

- The epithelial nurse cells are in the outer cortex.
- The cortical thymic epithelial cells (TECs) form an epithelial network.
- The medullary TECs are mostly organized into clusters (Fig. 2.26).

These three types of epithelial cell have different roles for thymocyte proliferation, maturation and selection:

- **Nurse cells** in the outer cortex sustain the proliferation of progenitor T cells, mainly through cytokine production (e.g. IL-7).
- **Cortical TECs** are responsible for the positive selection of maturing thymocytes, allowing survival of cells that recognize MHC class I and II molecules with associated peptides via TCRs of intermediate affinity.
- **Medullary TECs** display a large variety of organ-specific self peptides through transcription factors such as AIRE (autoimmune regulator).

Hassall's corpuscles (see Fig. 2.24) are found in the thymic medulla. Their function is unknown, but they appear to contain degenerating epithelial cells rich in high molecular weight cytokeratins.

The mammalian thymus involutes with age (Fig. 2.27). In humans, atrophy begins at puberty and continues throughout

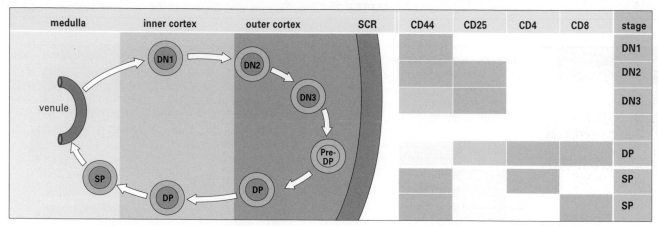

medulla	inner cortex	outer cortex	SCR	CD44	CD25	CD4	CD8	stage
								DN1
								DN2
								DN3
								DP
								SP
								SP

Fig. 2.25 Cell migration to and within the thymus T-cell progenitors enter the thymic lobule through postcapillary venules (PCVs) at the corticomedullary junction. These cells are double negative 1 *(DN1)* for CD4 and CD8 expression but are also CD25⁻, but CD44⁺. They move progressively towards the outer cortex and differentiate into *DN2* (CD25⁺, CD44⁺) and *DN3* cells (CD25⁺, CD44^{lo}). Thymocytes accumulate in the subcapsular region where they actively proliferate and differentiate into double positive (*DP*; CD4⁺, CD8⁺) cells. DP thymocytes reverse their polarity and move towards the medulla. In the course of this migration, thymocytes are selected and as single positive (*SP*; CD4⁺ or CD8⁺) cells ultimately leave the thymus, presumably via high endothelial venules at the corticomedullary junction.

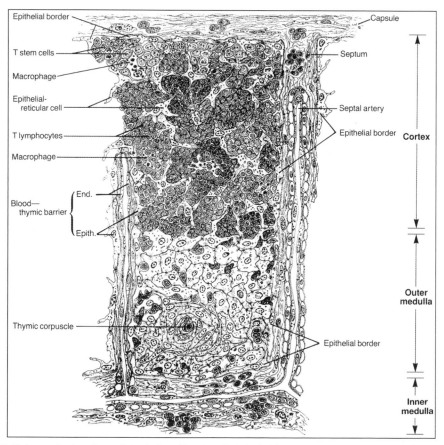

Fig. 2.26 Schematic drawing of a portion of a thymic lobule The cortex is heavily infiltrated with lymphocytes that stretch the epithelioreticular cells and their desmosomal connections. The proportion of epithelioreticular cells is greater in the medulla than in the cortex. A thymic corpuscle is seen in the medulla. The capsule and trabeculae are rich in collagenous fibers and contain blood vessels, plasmocytes, granulocytes, and lymphocytes. A border of flattened epithelial cells surrounds the cortex and outer medulla. (Reprinted from Mcmillan D, Harris R, An Atlas of Comparative Vertebrate Histology, Copyright Elsevier Inc., 2018.)

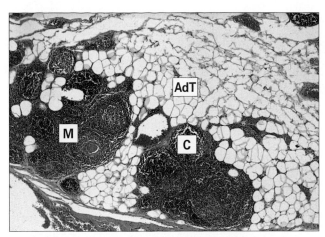

Fig. 2.27 Atrophic adult thymus There is an involution of the thymus with replacement by adipose tissue *(AdT)*. The cortex *(C)* is largely reduced and the less cellular medulla *(M)* is still apparent. (Courtesy Dr A Stevens and Professor J Lowe.)

life. Thymic involution begins within the cortex and this region may disappear completely, whereas medullary remnants persist.

Cortical atrophy is related to a sensitivity of the cortical thymocytes to corticosteroid and all conditions associated with an acute increase in corticosteroids (e.g. pregnancy and stress) promote thymic atrophy.

It is conceivable that T-cell generation within the thymus continues into adult life, albeit at a low rate. Evidence for de novo T-cell production in the thymus (recent thymic emigrants) has been shown in humans over the age of 76 years.

Stem cell migration to the thymus initiates T-cell development. The thymus develops from the endoderm of the third pharyngeal pouch as an epithelial rudiment that becomes seeded with blood-borne stem cells. Relatively few stem cells appear to be needed to give rise to the enormous repertoire of mature T cells with diverse antigen receptor specificities. From experimental studies, migration of stem cells into the thymus is not a random process but results from chemotactic signals periodically emitted from the thymic rudiment. β_2-Microglobulin, a component of the MHC class I molecule, is one such putative chemo-attractant.

In birds, stem cells enter the thymus in two or possibly three waves, but it is not clear whether there are such waves in mammals.

Once in the thymus, the stem cells begin to differentiate into thymic lymphocytes, under the influence of the epithelial micro-environment.

Whether or not the stem cells are pre-T cells (i.e. cells committed to becoming T cells before they arrive in the thymus) is controversial. Although the stem cells express CD7, substantial evidence exists that they are in fact multipotent. Granulocytes, APCs, NK cells, B cells and myeloid cells have all been generated in vitro from haematopoietic precursors isolated from the thymus. This suggests that the prethymic bone marrow-derived cell entering the thymic rudiment is multipotent.

Notch1 receptor has proved to be essential for T-cell development, and is involved in T- versus B-cell fate determination through interaction with thymic epithelial cells expressing

Notch ligands. At this level, Notch1 acts as a lineage specifier. Notch1-deficient bone marrow progenitors migrate from the bone marrow to the thymus but can no longer develop towards the T-cell lineage. Since these progenitors are still at least bipotential they develop into B cells instead.

Epithelial cells, macrophages and bone marrow-derived IDCs, molecules rich in MHC class II, are important for the differentiation of T cells from this multipotent stem cell. For example, specialized epithelial cells in the peripheral areas of the cortex (the thymic nurse cells, see earlier) contain thymocytes within pockets in their cytoplasm. The nurse cells support lymphocyte proliferation by producing the cytokine IL-7.

The subcapsular region of the thymus is the only site where thymocyte proliferation occurs. Thymocytes develop into large, actively proliferating, self-renewing lymphoblasts, which generate the thymocyte population.

There are many more developing lymphocytes (85%–90%) in the thymic cortex than in the medulla and studies of function and cell surface markers have indicated that cortical thymocytes are less mature than medullary thymocytes. This reflects the fact that cortical cells migrate to, and mature in, the medulla.

Most mature T cells leave the thymus via HEVs at the corticomedullary junction, though other routes of exit may exist, including lymphatic vessels.

T cells change their phenotype during maturation. As with the development of granulocytes and monocytes, differentiation markers of functional significance appear or are lost during the progression from stem cell to mature T cell.

Analyses of genes encoding αβ and γδ TCRs and other studies examining changes in surface membrane antigens suggest that there are multiple pathways of T-cell differentiation in the thymus. It is not known whether these pathways are distinct, but it seems more likely that they diverge from a common pathway.

Only a small proportion (<1%) of mature T lymphocytes express the γδ TCR. Most thymocytes differentiate into αβ TCR cells, which account for the majority (>95%) of T lymphocytes in secondary lymphoid tissues and in the circulation.

Phenotypic analyses have shown sequential changes in surface membrane antigens during T-cell maturation (Fig. 2.w8). The phenotypic variations can be simplified into a three-stage model.

Stage I thymocytes are CD4⁻, CD8⁻. There are two phases of stage I (early) thymocytes. In the first phase, the TCR genes are in the germline configuration and the cells:

- express CD44 and CD25; and
- are CD4⁻, CD8⁻ (i.e. double negative cells).

In this first phase, cells entering the thymus via the HEVs in the corticomedullary junction express CD44, which allows them to migrate towards the outermost cortex, the zone of thymocyte proliferation. These cells are not fully committed to the T-cell lineage, because outside the thymic environment they can give rise to other haematopoietic lineages. Surface expression of CD44 is downregulated once the cells are in the external cortex.

In the second phase the cells:
- become CD44$^-$;
- are CD25$^+$;
- remain double negative for CD4 and CD8;
- rearrange the β chain of the TCR;
- express cytoplasmic but not surface TCR-associated CD3;
- are irreversibly committed to become T cells with continuous expression of Notch1; and
- continue to express CD7 with CD2 and CD5.

Proliferation markers such as the transferrin receptor (CD71) and CD38 (a marker common to all early haematopoietic precursors) are also expressed at this stage.

Stage II thymocytes become CD4$^+$ and CD8$^+$.

Stage II (intermediate or common) thymocyte cells account for around 80% of thymocytes in the fully developed thymus. Characteristically they:
- are CD1$^+$, CD44$^-$, CD25$^-$; and
- become CD4$^+$, CD8$^+$ (double positives).

Genes encoding the TCR α chain are rearranged in these intermediate thymocytes; both chains of the αβ TCR are expressed at low density on the cell surface in association with polypeptides of the CD3/antigen receptor complex.

Stage III thymocytes become either CD4$^+$ or CD8$^+$.

Stage III (mature) thymocytes show major phenotypic changes:
- loss of CD1;
- cell surface CD3 associated with the αβ TCR expressed at a higher density; and
- the distinction of two subsets of cells expressing either CD4 or CD8 (i.e. single positives).

Most stage III thymocytes:
- lack CD38 and the transferrin receptor; and
- are virtually indistinguishable from mature, circulating T cells.

All stage III cells re-express the receptor CD44, which is thought to be involved in migration and homing to peripheral lymphoid tissues. L-selectin (CD62L) is also expressed at this time.

The T cell receptor is generated during development in the thymus.

TCR gene recombination takes place within the subcapsular and outer cortex of the thymus, where there is active cell proliferation. Through a random assortment of different gene segments, a large number of different TCRs are made and thymocytes that fail to make a functional receptor die. The TCRs associate with peptides of the CD3 complex, which transduces activating signals to the cell (see Chapter 6).

Positive and negative selection of developing T cells takes place in the thymus.

The processes involved in the education of T cells are shown in Figure 2.28, and self-tolerance is discussed fully in Chapter 11. Positive selection ensures only TCRs with an intermediate affinity for self MHC develop further.

T cells:
- recognize antigenic peptides only when presented by self MHC molecules on APCs; and
- show dual recognition of both the antigenic peptides and the polymorphic part of the MHC molecules.

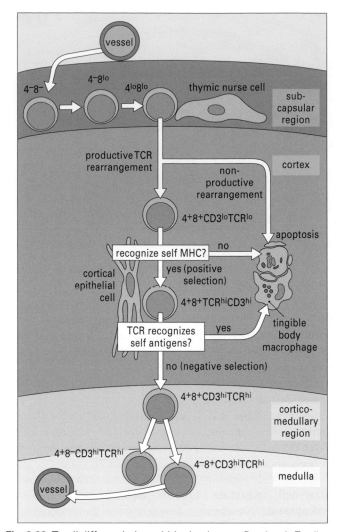

Fig. 2.28 T-cell differentiation within the thymus Pre-thymic T cells are attracted to and enter the thymic rudiment at the corticomedullary junction. They reach the subcapsular region where they proliferate as large lymphoblasts, which give rise to a pool of cells entering the differentiation pathway. Many of these cells are associated with epithelial thymic nurse cells. Cells in this region first acquire CD8 and then CD4 at low density. They also rearrange their T-cell receptor *(TCR)* genes and may express the products of these genes at low density on the cell surface. Maturing cells move deeper into the cortex and adhere to cortical epithelial cells. These epithelial cells are elongated and branched, and thus provide a large surface area for contact with thymocytes. The TCRs on the thymocytes are exposed to epithelial major histocompatibility complex *(MHC)* molecules through these contacts. This leads to positive selection. Those cells that are not selected undergo apoptosis and are phagocytosed by macrophages. There is an increased expression of CD3, TCR, CD4 and CD8 during thymocyte migration from the subcapsular region to the deeper cortex. Those TCRs with self reactivity are now deleted through contact with auto-antigens presented by medullary thymic epithelial cells, interdigitating cells and macrophages at the corticomedullary junction, a process called negative selection. After this stage, cells expressing either CD4 or CD8 appear and exit to the periphery via specialized vessels at the corticomedullary junction.

Positive selection (the first stage of **thymic education**) ensures that only those TCRs with an intermediate affinity for self MHC are allowed to develop further. There is evidence that positive selection is mediated by TECs acting as APCs.

T cells displaying very high or very low receptor affinities for self MHC undergo apoptosis and die in the cortex. Apoptosis is a pre-programmed suicide, achieved by activating endogenous nucleases that cause DNA fragmentation.

T cells with TCRs that have intermediate affinities are rescued from apoptosis, survive and continue along their pathway of maturation. A possible exception is provided by some T cells equipped with γδ receptors, which (like B cells) recognize native antigenic conformations with no need for APCs.

Negative selection ensures that only T cells that fail to recognize self antigen proceed in their development. Some of the positively selected T cells may have TCRs that recognize self components other than self MHC. These cells are deleted by a negative selection process, which occurs:

- in the deeper cortex;
- at the corticomedullary junction; and
- in the medulla.

T cells interact with antigen presented by interdigitating cells, macrophages and medullary TECs. Medullary TECs are particularly important for negative selection because they produce peptides for virtually all tissue antigens in the body, genes for these being activated by the AIRE transcription factor (auto-immune regulator).

Only T cells that fail to recognize self-antigen are allowed to proceed in their development. The rest undergo apoptosis and are destroyed. These, and all the other apoptotic cells generated in the thymus, are phagocytosed by (tingible body) macrophages (see Fig. 2.41) in the deep cortex.

T cells at this stage of maturation (CD4$^+$ CD8$^+$ TCR^{lo}) go on to express TCR at high density and lose either CD4 or CD8 to become single positive mature T cells.

The separate subsets of CD4$^+$ and CD8$^+$ cells possess specialized homing receptors (e.g. CD44) and exit to the T-cell areas of the peripheral (secondary) lymphoid tissues where they function as mature helper and cytotoxic T cells, respectively.

Less than 5% of thymocytes leave the thymus as mature T cells. The rest die as the result of:

- selection processes; or
- failure to undergo productive rearrangements of antigen receptor genes.

Adhesion of maturing thymocytes to epithelial and accessory cells is crucial for T-cell development. Adhesion of maturing thymocytes to epithelial and other accessory cells is mediated by the interaction of complementary adhesion molecules, such as:

- CD2 with LFA-3 (CD58); and
- LFA-1 (CD11a/CD18) with ICAM-1 (CD54).

These interactions induce the production of the cytokines IL-1, IL-3, IL-6, IL-7 and GM-CSF, which are required for T-cell proliferation and maturation in the thymus.

Early thymocytes also express receptors for IL-2, which together with IL-7 sustains cell proliferation.

Negative selection may also occur outside the thymus in peripheral lymphoid tissues. Not all self-reactive T cells are eliminated during intra-thymic development, probably because not all self antigens can be presented in the thymus. The thymic epithelial barrier that surrounds blood vessels may also limit access of some circulating antigens.

Given the survival of some self-reacting T cells, a separate mechanism is required to prevent them attacking the body. Experiments with transgenic mice have suggested that peripheral inactivation of self-reactive T cells (**peripheral tolerance**, see Chapter 11) could occur via several mechanisms:

- downregulation of the TCR and CD8 (in cytotoxic cells) so that the cells are unable to interact with target auto-antigens;
- **anergy**, because of the lack of crucial co-stimulatory signals provided by the target cells, followed by induction of apoptosis after interaction with auto-antigen;
- Tregs.

Regulatory T cells are involved in peripheral tolerance. Tregs have been the subject of intensive research over the past few years, especially in the areas of autoimmunity and vaccine development.

The general consensus is that there are two main types of Tregs: naturally occurring and inducible following activation by specific antigen.

Naturally occurring Tregs:

- constitutively express CD25 (the α chain of the receptor for IL-2);
- constitute about 5%–10% of the peripheral CD4$^+$ T cells;
- express the unique transcription factor FoxP3;
- constitutively express the marker CTLA-4 (CD152);
- do not proliferate in response to antigenic challenge; and
- are thought to produce their suppressive effects through cell contact (e.g. with APCs, T$_H$1 or T$_H$2 cells).

Antigen-induced Tregs:

- also express CD25;
- can develop from CD25$^-$, CD4$^+$ T cells; and
- are believed to exert their suppressive effects through IL-10.

There is some evidence for extrathymic development of T cells. The vast majority of T cells require a functioning thymus for differentiation, but small numbers of cells carrying T-cell markers that are often oligoclonal in nature have been found in athymic (nude) mice. Although the possibility that these mice possess thymic remnants cannot be ruled out, there is accumulating evidence to suggest that bone marrow precursors can home to mucosal epithelia and mature without the need for a thymus to form functional T cells with γδ TCRs and probably also T cells with αβ TCRs.

The importance of extrathymic development in animals that are euthymic (i.e. that have a normal thymus) is at present unclear.

B CELLS

B cells develop mainly in the fetal liver and bone marrow. In humans, the liver is the primary site for haematopoiesis, but in adults this function moves to the bone marrow.

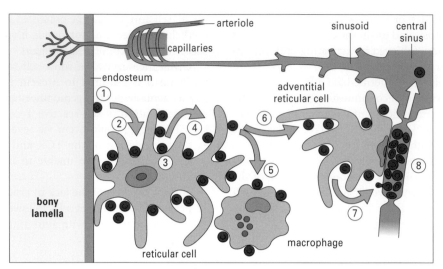

Fig. 2.29 Schematic organization of B-cell development in the bone marrow The earliest B-cell progenitors are found close to the endosteum *(1)* where they interact with stromal reticular cells *(2)*. The stromal reticular cells prompt precursor B-cell proliferation and maturation *(3 and 4)*. During these processes, selection occurs, which implies B-cell apoptosis and phagocytosis of apoptotic cells by macrophages *(5)*. B cells that have survived selection mature further and interact with adventitial reticular cells *(6)*, which may facilitate their ingress *(7)* into bone marrow sinusoids *(8)* and finally the central venous sinuses, from which they enter the general circulation. In this model, maturation and selection events follow a gradient from the periphery of the bone marrow tissue contained in the bony spaces towards the centre.

B-cell progenitors in bone marrow are seen adjacent to the endosteum of the bone lamellae (Fig. 2.29). Each B-cell progenitor, at the stage of immunoglobulin gene rearrangement, may produce up to 64 progeny. The progeny migrate towards the centre of each cavity of the spongy bone and reach the lumen of a venous sinusoid (Fig. 2.30). B cells mature in close association with **stromal reticular cells**, which are found both adjacent to the endosteum and in close association with the central sinus, where they are termed **adventitial reticular cells**.

Where the B cells differentiate, the reticular cells have mixed phenotypic features with some similarities to fibroblasts, endothelial cells and myofibroblasts. The reticular cells produce type IV collagen, laminin and the smooth muscle form of actin. Experiments in vitro have shown that reticular cells sustain B-cell differentiation, possibly by producing the cytokine IL-7.

Adventitial reticular cells may be important for the release of mature B cells into the central sinus.

B cells are subject to selection processes. Most B cells (>75%) maturing in the bone marrow do not reach the circulation but (like thymocytes) undergo a process of programmed cell death (apoptosis) and are phagocytosed by bone marrow macrophages.

B cell–stromal cell interactions enhance the survival of developing B cells and mediate a form of selection that rescues a minority of B cells with productive rearrangements of their immunoglobulin genes from programmed cell death.

Many self-reactive B cells are also eliminated through negative selection in the bone marrow.

From kinetic data, it is estimated that about 5×10^7 murine B cells are produced each day. As the mouse spleen contains approximately 7.5×10^7 B cells, a large proportion of B cells

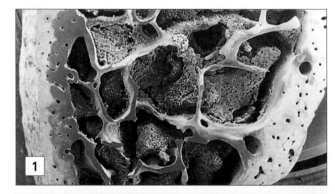

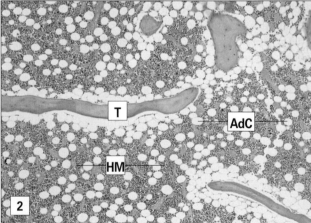

Fig. 2.30 Bone marrow. (1) Low-power scanning electron micrograph showing the architecture of bone and its relationship to bone marrow. Within the cavities of spongy bone between the bony trabeculae, B-cell lymphopoiesis takes place, with maturation occurring in a radial direction towards the centre (from the endosteum to the central venous sinus). **(2)** The biopsy shows haematopoietic bone marrow *(HM)* in the spaces between the bony trabeculae (lamellae) *(T)*. Some of the space is also occupied by adipocytes *(AdC)*. (Courtesy Dr A Stevens and Professor J Lowe.)

must die, probably at the pre-B cell stage, because of non-productive rearrangements of receptor genes or if they express self-reactive antibodies and are not rescued.

Immunoglobulins are the definitive B-cell lineage markers.

Lymphoid stem cells expressing terminal deoxynucleotidyl transferase (TdT) proliferate, differentiate and undergo immunoglobulin gene rearrangements to emerge as pre-B cells (see Chapter 9). A sequence of immunoglobulin gene rearrangements and phenotypic changes takes place during B-cell ontogeny, similar to that described above for T cells.

Heavy-chain gene rearrangements occur in B-cell progenitors and represent the earliest indication of B-lineage commitment. This is followed by light-chain gene rearrangements, which occur at later pre-B cell stages.

Once a B cell has synthesized light chains, it becomes committed to the antigen-binding specificity of its surface IgM (sIgM) antigen receptor.

One B cell can therefore make only one specific antibody – a central tenet of the **clonal selection theory** for antibody production.

Surface immunoglobulin-associated molecules Igα and Igβ (CD79a and b) are present by the pre-B cell stage of development.

B cells migrate to and function in the secondary lymphoid tissues.

Early B-cell immigrants into fetal lymph nodes (17 weeks in humans) are surface IgM⁺ and are B-1 cells. CD5⁺ B-cell precursors are found in the fetal omentum.

Some CD5⁺ B cells are also found in the marginal zone of the spleen and mantle zone of secondary follicles in adult lymph nodes (see Fig. 2.39).

Following antigenic stimulation, mature B cells can develop into memory cells or antibody-forming cells (AFCs).

LYMPHOID ORGANS

The generation of lymphocytes in primary lymphoid organs is followed by their migration into peripheral secondary tissues, which include:

- well-organized encapsulated organs, the spleen and lymph nodes (systemic lymphoid organs); and
- non-encapsulated accumulations of lymphoid tissue.

Lymphoid tissue found in association with mucosal surfaces is called mucosa-associated lymphoid tissue (MALT).

Lymphoid organs and tissues protect different body sites.

The systemic lymphoid organs and the mucosal system have different functions in immunity:

- The spleen is responsive to blood-borne antigens and patients who have had their spleen removed are much more susceptible to pathogens that reach the blood stream.
- The lymph nodes protect the body from antigens that come from skin or from internal surfaces and are transported via the lymphatic vessels.
- The MALT protects mucosal surfaces.

Responses to antigens encountered via the spleen and lymph nodes result in the secretion of antibodies into the circulation and local cell-mediated responses.

Being the major port of entry into the body for pathogens, the MALT is the site of first encounter (priming) of immune cells with antigens entering via mucosal surfaces and lymphoid tissues and are associated with surfaces lining:

- the intestinal tract – gut-associated lymphoid tissue (GALT);
- the respiratory tract – bronchus-associated lymphoid tissue (BALT); and
- the genitourinary tract.

The major effector mechanism at mucosal surfaces is secretory IgA antibody (sIgA), which is actively transported via the mucosal epithelial cells to the lumen of the tracts.

The spleen is made up of white pulp, red pulp and a marginal zone.

The spleen lies at the upper left quadrant of the abdomen, behind the stomach and close to the diaphragm. The adult spleen is around 13×8 cm and weighs approximately 180–250 g.

The outer layer of the spleen consists of a capsule of collagenous bundles of fibres, which enter the parenchyma of the organ as short trabeculae. These, together with a reticular framework, support two main types of splenic tissue: the white pulp and the red pulp.

A third compartment, the **marginal zone**, is located at the outer limit of the white pulp.

The white pulp consists of lymphoid tissue.

The white pulp of the spleen consists of lymphoid tissue, the bulk of which is arranged around a central arteriole to form the peri-arteriolar lymphoid sheaths (PALS; Fig. 2.31). PALS are composed of T- and B-cell areas:

- the T cells are found around the central arteriole;
- the B cells may be organized into either primary unstimulated follicles (aggregates of virgin B cells) or secondary

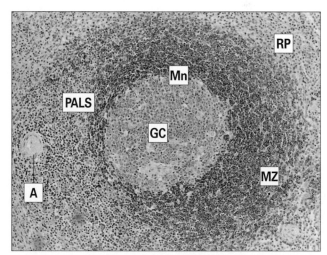

Fig. 2.31 White pulp of the spleen Spleen section showing a white pulp lymphoid aggregate. A secondary lymphoid follicle, with germinal centre *(GC)* and mantle *(Mn)*, is surrounded by the marginal zone *(MZ)* and red pulp *(RP)*. Adjacent to the follicle, an arteriole *(A)* is surrounded by the peri-arteriolar lymphoid sheath *(PALS)* consisting mainly of T cells. Note that the marginal zone is present only at one side of the secondary follicle. (Courtesy Professor I MacLennan.)

stimulated follicles (which possess a germinal centre with memory cells).

The germinal centres also contain FDCs and phagocytic macrophages. Macrophages and the FDCs present antigen to B cells in the spleen.

B cells and other lymphocytes are free to leave and enter the PALS via branches of the central arterioles, which enter a system of blood vessels in the marginal zone (see later). Some lymphocytes, especially maturing plasmablasts, can pass across the marginal zone via bridges into the red pulp.

The red pulp consists of venous sinuses and cellular cords. The venous sinuses and cellular cords of the red pulp contain:

- resident macrophages;
- erythrocytes;
- platelets;
- granulocytes;
- lymphocytes; and
- numerous plasma cells.

In addition to immunological functions, the spleen serves as a reservoir for platelets, erythrocytes and granulocytes. Aged platelets and erythrocytes are destroyed in the red pulp in a process referred to as haemocatheresis.

The functions of the spleen are made possible by its vascular organization (Fig. 2.32). Central arteries surrounded by PALS end with arterial capillaries, which open freely into the red pulp cords. Circulating cells can therefore reach these cords and become trapped. Aged platelets and erythrocytes are recognized and phagocytosed by macrophages.

Blood cells that are not ingested and destroyed can re-enter the blood circulation by squeezing through holes in the discontinuous endothelial wall of the venous sinuses, through which plasma flows freely.

The marginal zone contains B cells, macrophages and dendritic cells. The marginal zone surrounds the white pulp and exhibits two major features:

- a characteristic vascular organization; and
- unique subsets of resident cells (B cells, macrophages and dendritic cells).

The blood vessels of the marginal zone form a system of communicating sinuses, which receive blood from branches of the central artery (see Fig. 2.32).

Most of the blood from the marginal sinuses enters the red pulp cords and then drains into the venous sinuses, but a small proportion passes directly into the venous sinuses to form a closed circulation.

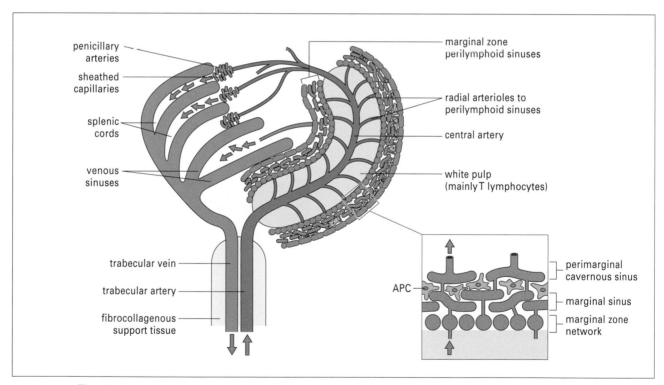

Fig. 2.32 Vascular organization of the spleen The splenic artery branches to form trabecular arteries, which give rise to central arteries surrounded by peri-arteriolar lymphoid sheaths (PALS), which are the T-cell areas of the white pulp. Leaving the PALS, the central arteries continue as penicillar arteries and sheathed capillaries, which open in the splenic cords of the red pulp. From the red pulp (where haemocatheresis takes place) the blood percolates through the wall of the venous sinuses. The central arterioles surrounded by PALS give collateral branches that reach a series of sinuses in the marginal zone. Most of the blood from the marginal sinuses enters the red pulp cords and then drains into the venous sinuses, but a proportion passes directly into the sinuses to form a closed circulation. *APC*, Antigen-presenting cells. (Courtesy Dr A Stevens and Professor J Lowe.)

Cells residing in the marginal zone are:

- various types of APC – metallophilic macrophages, marginal zone macrophages, dendritic cells;
- a subset of B cells with distinctive phenotype and function – they express high levels of IgM and low or absent IgD and, in humans, are long-lived recirculating cells; and
- some B-1 cells.

Lymph nodes filter antigens from the interstitial tissue fluid and lymph. The lymph nodes form part of a network that filters antigens from the interstitial tissue fluid and lymph during its passage from most of the body to the thoracic duct and the right side of the thorax, upper arm and right side of the head and neck into the right lymphatic duct (Fig. 2.33).

Lymph nodes frequently occur at the branches of the lymphatic vessels. Clusters of lymph nodes are strategically placed in areas that drain various superficial and deep regions of the body, such as:

- neck;
- axillae;
- groin;
- mediastinum; and
- abdominal cavity.

Lymph nodes protect the skin (superficial subcutaneous nodes) and mucosal surfaces of the respiratory, digestive and genitourinary tracts (visceral or deep nodes).

Human lymph nodes are 2–10 mm in diameter, are round or kidney shaped and have an indentation called the hilus where blood vessels enter and leave the node.

Lymph arrives at the lymph node via several afferent lymphatic vessels and leaves the node through a single efferent lymphatic vessel at the hilus.

Lymph nodes consist of B and T cell areas and a medulla. A typical lymph node is surrounded by a collagenous capsule. Radial trabeculae, together with reticular fibres, support the various cellular components. The lymph node consists of:

- a B-cell area (**cortex**);
- a T-cell area (**paracortex**); and
- a central **medulla**, consisting of cellular cords containing T cells, B cells, abundant plasma cells and macrophages (Figs 2.34–2.36).

The paracortex contains many APCs (interdigitating cells), which express high levels of MHC class II surface molecules. These are cells migrating from the skin (Langerhans cells) or from mucosae (dendritic cells), which transport processed antigens into the lymph nodes from the external and internal surfaces of the body (Fig. 2.37). The bulk of the lymphoid tissue is found in the cortex and paracortex.

The paracortex contains specialized postcapillary vessels – **high endothelial venules (HEVs)** – which allow the traffic of lymphocytes out of the circulation into the lymph node (see the section on lymphocyte recirculation later).

The medulla is organized into cords separated by lymph (medullary) sinuses, which drain into a terminal sinus – the origin of the efferent lymphatic vessel (see Fig. 2.36).

Scavenger phagocytic cells are arranged along the lymph sinuses, especially in the medulla. As the lymph passes across the nodes from the afferent to the efferent lymphatic vessels,

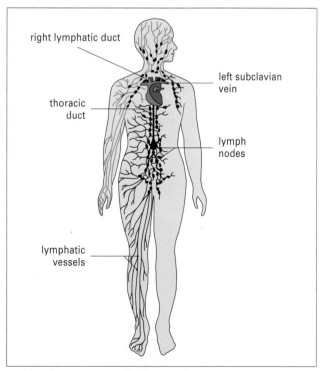

Fig. 2.33 The lymphatic system Lymph nodes are found at junctions of lymphatic vessels and form a network that drains and filters interstitial fluid from the tissue spaces. They are either subcutaneous or visceral, the latter draining the deep tissues and internal organs of the body. The lymph eventually reaches the thoracic duct or right lymphatic duct, which open into the left and right subclavian veins, respectively, and thus back into the circulation.

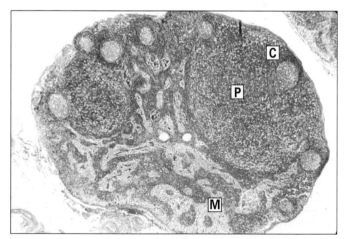

Fig. 2.34 Lymph node section The lymph node is surrounded by a connective tissue capsule and is organized into three main areas: the cortex (C), which is the B-cell area; the paracortex (P), which is the T-cell area; and the medulla (M), which contains cords of lymphoid tissue (T-cell and B-cell areas rich in plasma cells and macrophages). H&E stain. × 10. (Reprinted from Arber, DA, et al., Hematopathology, Second Edition, Copyright Elsevier Inc., 2017.)

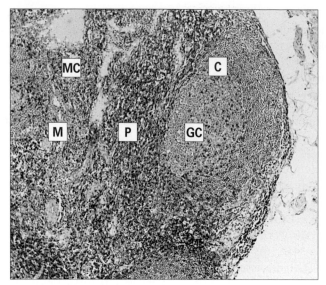

Fig. 2.35 Histological structure of the lymph node Cortex *(C)*, paracortex *(P)* and medulla *(M)* are shown. The section has been stained to show the localization of T cells. They are most abundant in the paracortex, but a few are found in the germinal centre *(GC)* of the secondary lymphoid follicle, in the cortex and in the medullary cords *(MC)*. (Courtesy Dr A Stevens and Professor J Lowe.)

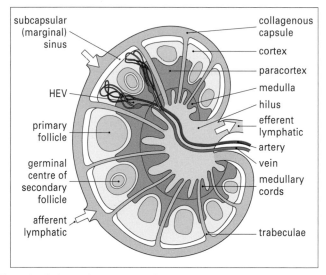

Fig. 2.36 Schematic structure of the lymph node Beneath the collagenous capsule is the subcapsular sinus, which is lined by endothelial and phagocytic cells. Lymphocytes and antigens from surrounding tissue spaces or adjacent nodes pass into the sinus via the afferent lymphatics. The cortex is mainly a B-cell area. B cells are organized into primary or, more commonly, secondary follicles, i.e. with a germinal centre. The paracortex contains mainly T cells. Each lymph node has its own arterial and venous supply. Lymphocytes enter the node from the circulation through the highly specialized high endothelial venules *(HEVs)* in the paracortex. The medulla contains both T and B cells in addition to most of the lymph node plasma cells organized into cords of lymphoid tissue. Lymphocytes leave the node through the efferent lymphatic vessel.

particulate antigens are removed by the phagocytic cells and transported into the lymphoid tissue of the lymph node.

The cortex contains aggregates of B cells in the form of primary or secondary follicles.

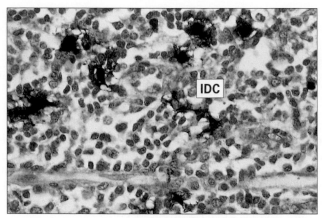

Fig. 2.37 Interdigitating cells in the lymph node paracortex Interdigitating dendritic cells *(IDC;* stained dark brown) form contacts with each other and with paracortical T cells. (Courtesy Dr A Stevens and Professor J Lowe.)

B cells are also found in the subcapsular region, adjacent to the marginal sinus. It is possible that these cells are similar to the splenic marginal zone B cells that intercept incoming pathogens primarily by mounting a rapid, IgM-based, T-independent response.

T cells are found mainly in the paracortex. Therefore, if an area of skin or mucosa is challenged by a T-dependent antigen, the lymph nodes draining that particular area show active T-cell proliferation in the paracortex.

Further evidence for this localization of T cells in the paracortex comes from patients with congenital thymic aplasia (DiGeorge's syndrome), who have fewer T cells in the paracortex than normal. A similar feature is found in neonatally thymectomized or congenitally athymic (nude) mice or rats.

Secondary follicles are made up of a germinal centre and a mantle zone. Germinal centres in secondary follicles are seen in antigen-stimulated lymph nodes. These are similar to the germinal centres seen in the B-cell areas of the splenic white pulp and of MALT.

Germinal centres are surrounded by a mantle zone of lymphocytes (Fig. 2.38). Mantle zone B cells (Fig. 2.39) co-express

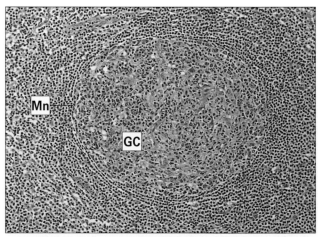

Fig. 2.38 Structure of the secondary follicle A large germinal centre *(GC)* is surrounded by the mantle zone *(Mn)*.

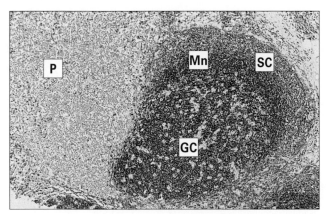

Fig. 2.39 Distribution of B cells in the lymph node cortex Immunohistochemical staining of B cells for surface immunoglobulin shows that they are concentrated largely in the secondary follicle, germinal centre *(GC)*, mantle zone *(Mn)* and between the capsule and the follicle – the subcapsular zone *(SC)*. A few B cells are seen in the paracortex *(P)*, which contains mainly T cells.

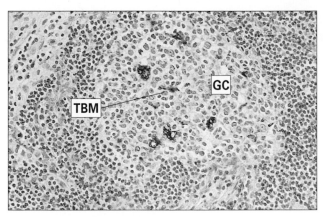

Fig. 2.41 Germinal centre macrophages Immunostaining for cathepsin D shows several macrophages localized in the germinal centre *(GC)* of a secondary follicle. These macrophages, which phagocytose apoptotic B cells, are called tingible body macrophages *(TBM)*. (Courtesy Dr A Stevens and Professor J Lowe.)

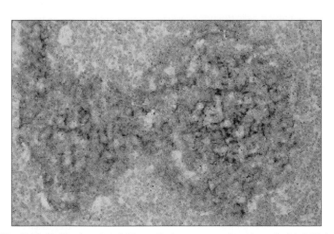

Fig. 2.40 Follicular dendritic cells in a secondary lymphoid follicle This lymph node follicle is stained by immunohistochemistry to demonstrate follicular dendritic cells.

surface IgM, IgD, and CD44. This is taken as evidence that they are naive, actively recirculating B cells.

In most secondary follicles, the thickened mantle zone or corona is oriented towards the capsule of the node. Secondary follicles contain:
- FDCs (Fig. 2.40);
- some macrophages (Fig. 2.41); and
- a few follicular Tн cells.

All the cells in the secondary follicle together with specialized marginal sinus macrophages, appear to play a role in generating B-cell responses and, in particular, in the development of B-cell memory.

In the germinal centres B cells proliferate, are selected and differentiate into memory cells or plasma cell precursors.

The germinal centre consists of a dark zone and a light zone:
- the dark zone is the site where one or a few B cells enter the primary lymphoid follicle and undergo active proliferation

leading to clonal expansion – these B cells are termed **centroblasts**. Their immunoglobulin genes undergo a process of **somatic hypermutation**, which leads to the generation of cells with a wide range of affinities for antigen;
- in the light zone, B cells (**centrocytes**) encounter the antigen on the surface of FDCs (see Fig. 2.14) and only those cells with higher affinity for antigen survive.

Cells with mutated antibody receptors of lower affinity die by apoptosis and are phagocytosed by germinal centre macrophages.

Selected centrocytes interact with germinal centre CD4+ Tн cells and their BCRs undergo **class switching** (i.e. replacement of their originally expressed immunoglobulin heavy-chain constant region genes by another class, for instance IgM to IgG or IgA, see Chapter 9).

The selected germinal centre B cells differentiate into **memory B cells** or **plasma cell** precursors and leave the germinal centre (Fig. 2.42).

MALT includes all lymphoid tissues associated with mucosa.

Aggregates of encapsulated and non-encapsulated lymphoid tissue are found especially in the lamina propria and submucosal areas of the gastrointestinal, respiratory and genitourinary tracts (see Fig. 2.23).

The tonsils contain a considerable amount of lymphoid tissue, often with large secondary follicles and intervening T-cell zones with HEVs. The three main kinds of tonsil that constitute Waldeyer's tonsillar ring are:
- palatine tonsil;
- pharyngeal tonsil (called adenoids when diseased); and
- lingual tonsil (Fig. 2.43).

Aggregates of lymphoid tissue are also seen lining the bronchi and along the genitourinary tract.

The digestive, respiratory and genitourinary mucosae contain dendritic cells for the uptake, processing and transport of antigens to the draining lymph nodes.

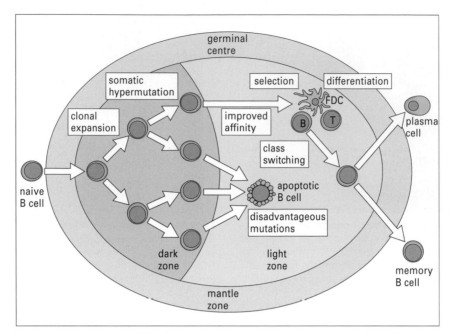

Fig. 2.42 Structure and function of the germinal centre One or a few B cells (founder cells) in the dark zone proliferate actively. This proliferation leads to clonal expansion and is accompanied by somatic hypermutation of the immunoglobulin V region genes. B cells with the same specificity, but different affinity, are therefore generated. In the light zone, B cells with disadvantageous mutations or with low affinity undergo apoptosis and are phagocytosed by macrophages. This process is also called affinity maturation. Cells with appropriate affinity encounter the antigen on the surface of the follicular dendritic cells *(FDCs)* and, with the help of CD4+ T cells, undergo class switching, leaving the follicle as memory B cells or plasma cells precursors.

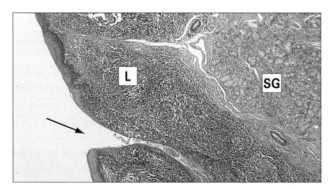

Fig. 2.43 Structure of the lingual tonsil The lingual tonsil, situated in the posterior one-third of the tongue, consists of accumulations of lymphoid tissue *(L)* with large secondary follicles associated with a mucosa that forms deep cleft-like invaginations *(arrow)*. Mucus-containing salivary glands *(SG)* are seen around the tonsil. These are common features of all types of tonsil. (Courtesy Dr A Stevens and Professor J Lowe.)

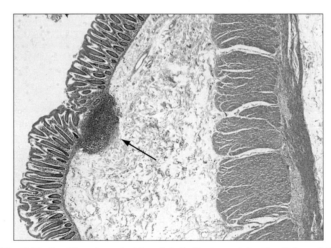

Fig. 2.44 A solitary lymphoid nodule in the large intestine This nodule is localized in the mucosa and submucosa of the intestinal wall *(arrow)*. (Courtesy Dr A Stevens and Professor J Lowe.)

Lymphoid tissues seen in the lamina propria of the gastrointestinal wall often extend into the submucosa and are found as either:
- solitary nodules (Fig. 2.44); or
- aggregated nodules such as in the appendix (Fig. 2.45).

Follicle-associated epithelium is specialized to transport pathogens into the lymphoid tissue. Peyer's patches are found in the lower ileum. The intestinal epithelium overlying Peyer's patches (follicle-associated epithelium, FAE) and other mucosa-associated lymphoid aggregates (e.g. the tonsils) is specialized to allow the transport of antigens into the lymphoid tissue. This particular function is carried out by epithelial cells termed

M cells, which are scattered among other epithelial cells and so-called because they have numerous microfolds on their luminal surface.

M cells contain deep invaginations in their basolateral plasma membrane, which form pockets containing B and T lymphocytes, dendritic cells and macrophages (Fig. 2.46). Antigens and microorganisms are transcytosed into the pocket and to the organized mucosal lymphoid tissue under the epithelium (Fig. 2.47) and taken up by the dendritic cells.

M cells are not exclusive to Peyer's patches but are also found in epithelia associated with lymphoid cell accumulations at antigen sampling areas in other mucosal sites.

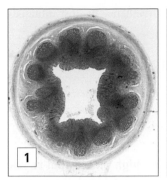
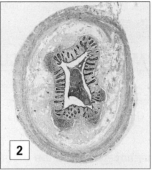

Fig. 2.45 Lymphoid nodules in the human appendix (1) Appendix of a 10-year-old child showing large lymphoid nodules extending into the submucosa. **(2)** Appendix from a 36-year-old man. Note the dramatic reduction of lymphoid tissue, with the virtual disappearance of lymphoid follicles. This illustrates the atrophy of lymphoid tissues during ageing, which is not limited to the appendix. (Courtesy Dr A Stevens and Professor J Lowe.)

The dome area of Peyer's patches and the subepithelial regions of tonsils harbour B cells that display a phenotype and function similar to that seen for the splenic marginal zone B cells.

A major defence at mucosal surfaces is IgA, which is secreted across the mucosal epithelium and is resistant to enzymes in the gut (see Fig. 10.7). B cells producing IgA are found at high levels in gut and MALT and these B cells also selectively migrate to these tissues.

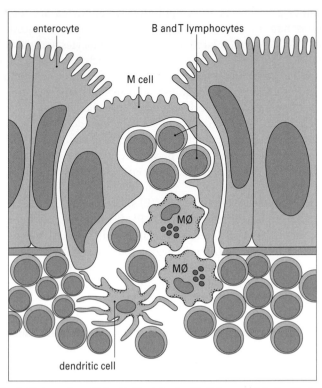

Fig. 2.46 Location of M cells The intestinal follicle-associated epithelium contains M cells. Note the lymphocytes and occasional macrophages *(MØ)* in the pocket formed by invagination of the basolateral membrane of the M cell. Antigens endocytosed by the M cell are passed via this pocket into the subepithelial tissues (not shown).

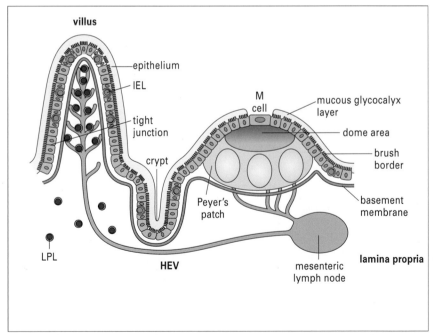

Fig. 2.47 Mucosal lymphoid tissue Peyer's patches, as well as tonsils and other lymphoid areas of mucosa-associated lymphoid tissues, are sites of lymphocyte priming by antigens, which are internalized by M cells in the follicle-associated epithelium. The subepithelial region, the dome, is rich in antigen-presenting cells and also contains a subset of B cells similar to those found in the splenic marginal zone. Lymphoid follicles and intervening T-dependent zones are localized under the dome region. Lymphocytes primed by antigens in these sites of the gut mucosa migrate to the mesenteric lymph nodes and then to the intestinal villi, where they are found both in the lamina propria *(LPL)* and within the surface epithelium *(IEL)*. *HEV*, High endothelial venules.

Lamina propria and intra-epithelial lymphocytes are found in mucosa. In addition to organized lymphoid tissue forming the MALT system, a large number of lymphocytes and plasma cells are found in the mucosa of the stomach, small and large intestine, upper and lower respiratory airways and several other organs. Lymphocytes are found both in the connective tissue of the lamina propria and within the epithelial layer:

- Lamina propria lymphocytes (LPLs) are predominantly activated T cells, but numerous activated B cells and plasma cells are also detected. These plasma cells secrete mainly IgA, which is transported across the epithelial cells and released into the lumen.
- Intra-epithelial lymphocytes (IELs) are mostly T cells. The population is different from the LPLs because it includes a high proportion of $\gamma\delta$ T cells (10%–40%) and CD8$^+$ cells (70%).

Most LPL and IEL T cells belong to the CD45RO$^+$ subset of memory cells. They respond poorly to stimulation with antibodies to the TCR (CD3) but may be triggered via other activation pathways (e.g. via CD2 or CD28).

IELs express an integrin (αE/β_7), which is found on other lymphocytes, only after they have been activated. E-cadherin on epithelial cells is the ligand for αE/β_7 and binding of αE/β_7 to E-cadherin may be important in the homing and retention of αE/β_7-expressing lymphocytes in the intestinal epithelium. IELs release cytokines, including IFNγ and IL-5; one function

suggested for IELs is immune surveillance against mutated or virus-infected host cells.

LYMPHOCYTE RECIRCULATION

Once in the secondary tissues, the lymphocytes do not simply remain there; many move from one lymphoid organ to another via the blood and lymph (Fig. 2.48).

Lymphocytes leave the blood via high endothelial venules. Although some lymphocytes leave the blood through non-specialized venules, the main exit route in mammals is through a specialized section known as HEVs (Figs 2.49 and 2.50). In the lymph nodes, the HEVs are mainly in the paracortex, with fewer in the cortex and none in the medulla.

Some lymphocytes, primarily T cells, arrive from the drainage area of the node through the afferent lymphatics, not via HEVs, which is the main route by which antigen enters the nodes.

Besides lymph nodes, HEVs are also found in MALT and in the thymus (see Fig. 2.26).

HEVs express a distinctive set of chemokines that signal lymphocytes to migrate into the lymphoid tissue and a specialized set of adhesion molecules that allow the cells to attach to the endothelial cells as they migrate.

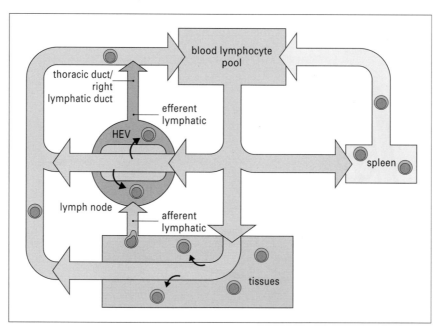

Fig 2.48 Patterns of lymphocyte traffic Lymphocytes move through the circulation and enter the lymph nodes and mucosa-associated lymphoid tissues (MALT) via the specialized endothelial cells of the postcapillary venules (i.e. high endothelial venules (*HEVs*)). They leave the lymph nodes and MALT through the efferent lymphatic vessels and pass through other nodes, finally entering the thoracic duct and right lymphatic duct, which empty into the circulation at the left and right subclavian veins, respectively (in humans). Lymphocytes enter the white pulp areas of the spleen in the marginal zones, pass into the sinusoids of the red pulp and leave via the splenic vein.

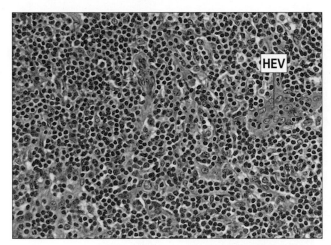

Fig. 2.49 Lymph node paracortex showing high endothelial venules *(HEVs).* Lymphocytes leave the circulation through HEVs to enter the node. H&E. × 200. (Courtesy Dr A Stevens and Professor J Lowe.)

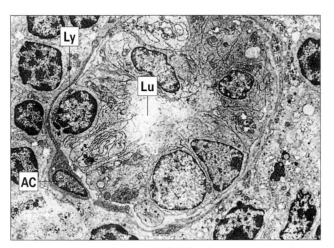

Fig. 2.50 High endothelial venule *(HEV)* **in the paracortex of a lymph node.** The electron micrograph shows a lymphocyte *(Ly),* transiting from the lumen *(Lu)* close to the basal lamina of an HEV. The HEV is partly surrounded by an adventitial cell *(AC).* × 1600.

HEVs are permanent features of secondary lymphoid tissues but can also develop from normal endothelium at sites of chronic inflammatory reactions (e.g. in the skin and in the synovium). This, in turn, may direct specific T-cell subsets to the area where HEVs have formed.

The movement of lymphocytes across endothelium is controlled by adhesion molecules and chemokines (see Chapters 3 and 13). For example:

- The adhesion molecule MadCAM-1 is expressed on endothelial cells in intestinal tissues.
- VCAM-1 is present on endothelial cells in the lung and skin.

Homing molecules on lymphocytes selectively direct lymphocytes to particular organs by interaction with these adhesion molecules (see Chapter 3). In the case of the intestine, a critical role is played by α_4/β_7-integrins, which mediate adherence of lymphocytes to HEVs of Peyer's patches that express MadCAM-1.

Lymphocyte trafficking exposes antigen to a large number of lymphocytes.

- Lymphoid cells within lymph nodes return to the circulation by way of the efferent lymphatics, which pass via the thoracic duct (left subclavian vein) or right lymphatic duct (right subclavian vein).
- About 1%–2% of the lymphocyte pool recirculates each hour. Overall, this process allows a large number of antigen-specific lymphocytes to come into contact with their specific antigen in the peripheral lymphoid organs.

Under normal conditions there is continuous lymphocyte traffic through the lymph nodes, but when antigens enter the lymph nodes of an animal already sensitized to that antigen there is a temporary shutdown in the traffic, which lasts for approximately 24 hours. Thus, antigen-specific lymphocytes are preferentially retained in the lymph nodes draining the source of antigen. In particular, blast cells do not recirculate but appear to remain in one site.

Antigen stimulation at one mucosal area elicits an antibody response largely restricted to MALT. One reason for considering MALT as a system distinct from the systemic lymphoid organs is that mucosa-associated lymphoid cells mainly recirculate within the mucosal lymphoid system. Thus, lymphoid cells stimulated in Peyer's patches pass via regional lymph nodes to the blood stream and then back into the intestinal lamina propria (Fig. 2.51 and see Fig. 2.47).

Specific recirculation is made possible because the lymphoid cells expressing homing molecules attach to adhesion molecules that are specifically expressed on endothelial cells of the mucosal venules but are absent from lymph node HEVs (see earlier).

Thus, antigen stimulation at one mucosal area elicits an antibody response largely, but not exclusively, at other mucosal tissue sites.

The microbiome modulates lymphocyte development. We have described the different kinds of cells present at mucosal surfaces. Over the last 10 years, it has become clear that the microbiome (sum total of the different bacterial species living in/on the body, but especially in the intestine) plays a role in the development of our immune system.

The products of these early colonizing bacteria act on the intestinal epithelial cells and local innate lymphocytes to maintain defence and to regulate immune homeostasis. These bacterial products promote anti-peptide production and IgA secretion and regulate the overall balance between effector and regulatory T cells throughout life. The composition of the microbiome varies from individual to individual, but there are common genera and species. Recent data suggest that composition of the microbiome and therefore their products are more common in patients with different diseases than in control individuals. There are many ongoing studies aimed at identifying the roles of the microbiome in different disease states.

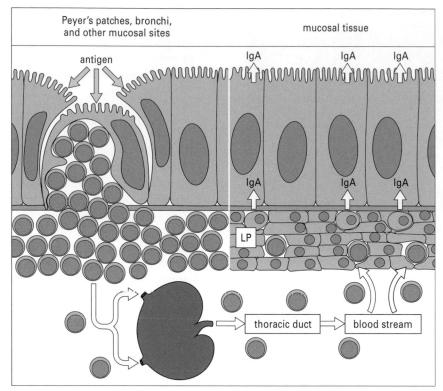

Fig. 2.51 Lymphocyte circulation within the mucosal lymphoid system. Lymphoid cells that are stimulated by antigen in Peyer's patches (or another mucosal site) migrate via the regional lymph nodes and thoracic duct into the blood stream and hence to the lamina propria *(LP)* of the gut or other mucosal surfaces, which might be close to or distant from the site of priming. Thus lymphocytes stimulated at one mucosal surface may become distributed selectively throughout the mucosa-associated lymphoid tissue (MALT) system. This is mediated through specific adhesion molecules on the lymphocytes and mucosal high endothelial venules (HEV).

CRITICAL THINKING: DEVELOPMENT OF THE IMMUNE SYSTEM

See Critical thinking: Explanations, section 2

Immunodeficiencies can tell us a lot about the way the immune system normally functions. Mice that congenitally lack a thymus (and have an associated gene defect that produces hairlessness), termed nude mice, are often used in research.

1. What effect would you expect this defect to have on numbers and types of lymphocytes in the blood? How would this affect the structure of the lymph nodes? What effect would this have on the ability of the mice to fight infections?

Occasionally adult patients develop a tumour in the thymus (thymoma) and it is necessary to remove the thymus gland completely.

2. What effect would you expect adult thymectomy to have on the ability of such patients to fight infections?

With the development of modern techniques in molecular biology, it is possible to produce animals that completely lack individual genes. Such animals are called gene knockouts. Sometimes these knockouts can have quite surprising effects on development and sometimes only minor effects. Others, such as the immunodeficiencies, are very informative. Based on the information provided in this chapter, which effects would you expect the following knockouts to have on the development of leukocytes and/or lymphoid organs?

3. RAG-1? (*RAG-1* and *RAG-2* genes are involved in the recombination processes that generate antigen receptors on B and T cells)
4. Interleukin-7?
5. The β_7-integrin chain?

FURTHER READING

Belkaid Y, Hand T. Role of the microbiota in immunity and inflammation. Cell 2014;157:12–141.

Delves P, Martin SJ, Burton DR, Roitt IM. Roitt's Essential Immunology, 13th edn. Wiley-Blackwell; 2017.

Liston A, ed. Regulatory T cells in health and disease. In: Progress in Molecular Biology and Translational Science. Vol 136. Academic Press; 2015.

Lydyard PM, Whelan A, Fanger MW. Instant Notes in Immunology, 3rd edn. London: Garland Science/Bios Scientific Publishing; 2011.

Mestecky J, Russell MW, Cheroutre H, Strober W, Kelsall BL, Lambrecht BN, eds. Mucosal Immunology, 4th edn. Academic Press; 2015.

Murphy K, Janeway S, Weaver C. Immunobiology, 9th edn. Garland Science; 2016.

Punt J, Stranford S, Jones P, Owen JA. Kuby Immunology, 8th edn. WH Freeman: New York; 2018.

Playfair JHL, Chain BM. Immunology at a Glance, 10th edn, Wiley-Blackwell; 2012.

Zhang L-J, Gallo RL. Antimicrobial peptides, Current Biology, 2016;26: R14–R19.

Van de Broek T, Borghans JAM, Van Wijk F. A Full Spectrum of Human Naïve T cells, Nature Rev Immunol., 2018;18:363–373.

3

Mechanisms of Innate Immunity

SUMMARY

- **Innate immune responses do not depend on immune recognition by B cells or T cells but have co-evolved with and are functionally integrated with the adaptive elements of the immune system.**
- **The body's responses to damage include inflammation, phagocytosis, clearance of debris and pathogens, and remodelling and regeneration of tissues** Inflammation is a response that brings leukocytes and plasma molecules to sites of infection or tissue damage.
- **The phased arrival of leukocytes in inflammation depends on chemokines and adhesion molecules expressed on the endothelium.** Adhesion molecules fall into families that are structurally related. They include the cell-adhesion molecules (CAMs) of the immunoglobulin supergene family which interact with leukocyte integrins, and the selectins which interact with carbohydrate ligands. Chemokines are a large group of signalling molecules that initiate chemotaxis and/or cellular activation. Most chemokines act on more than one receptor, and most receptors respond to more than one chemokine.
- **Plasma enzyme systems modulate inflammation and tissue remodelling.** The kinin system and mediators from mast cells including histamine contribute to the enhanced blood supply and increased vascular permeability at sites of inflammation.

- **Collectins, ficolins and pentraxins** belong to families of proteins present in serum and tissue fluids, which can act as opsonins, either directly or by activating the complement system.
- **Pathogen-associated molecular patterns (PAMPs) are biological macromolecules that can be recognized by pattern recognition receptors (PRRs)**
- **PRRs** include cell-surface scavenger receptors and lectin-like receptors on macrophages, which allow them to directly bind to pathogens and cell debris.
- **Toll-like receptors (TLRs) are a family of PRRs that recognize molecules of bacteria, viruses and fungi.** They are present on many cell types, and can activate macrophages, using signalling systems that are closely related to those used by inflammatory cytokines tumour necrosis factor-α (TNFα) and interleukin-1 (IL-1).
- **Intracellular PRRs recognize products of intracellular pathogens.** The receptors may be located in the cytoplasm or endosomes. Nod family receptors recognize bacterial products, while the RLR receptors and ALRs recognize nucleic acid products of viral replication.

INNATE IMMUNE RESPONSES

The immune system deals with pathogens by means of a great variety of different types of immune response, but these can be broadly divided into:

- adaptive responses; and
- innate immunity.

The adaptive immune responses depend on the recognition of antigen by lymphocytes, a cell type that has evolved relatively recently – lymphocytes are present in all vertebrates, but not invertebrates, although lymphocyte-like cells are present in closely related phyla, including the tunicates and echinoderms (Fig. 3.1).

Before the evolution of lymphocytes, and the emergence of specific antigen receptors (antibodies and the TCR), different types of immune defence were already present in precursor organisms. For example, the antimicrobial peptides (defensins) present in neutrophil granules and encoded in the germline, are also present in invertebrates. Many of these primordial defence systems have been retained in vertebrates and have continued to evolve and diversify alongside the adaptive immune system. Hence, in present-day mammals we see an integrated immune system in which innate and adaptive immune defences work in concert.

In reality it is quite artificial to try to segregate adaptive and innate immune responses. For example, a macrophage:

- displays the very primitive immune defence of phagocytosis; but also
- expresses major histocompatibility complex (MHC) molecules and acts as an antigen-presenting cell, a function that makes sense only in relation to the evolution of T cells.

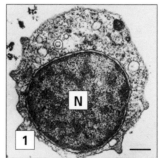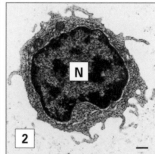

Fig. 3.1 Electron micrographs of lymphocyte-like cells Electron micrographs of lymphocyte-like cells from the tunicate *Ciona intestinalis* (**1**), and from a fish, the blenny, *Blennius pholis* (**2**). Note the similar morphology – both cells have a large nucleus (N) and a thin rim of undifferentiated cytoplasm. Scale bar 0.5 μm. (Courtesy Dr AF Rowley from Endeavour 1989:13;72–77. Copyright 1989 with permission from Elsevier.)

We can identify some of the ancient innate immune defence systems because related systems are seen in distant phyla. For example, the family of **Toll-like receptors (TLRs)** (see Table 3.2) were first identified in insects. We can therefore infer that the distant ancestor of mammals and insects had a receptor molecule of this type that probably recognized microbial components.

Having stated how the functional distinction between adaptive and immune systems is essentially artificial, this chapter outlines some of the immune defences that do not depend on antigen recognition by lymphocytes.

INFLAMMATION – A RESPONSE TO TISSUE DAMAGE

The body's response to tissue damage depends on what caused the damage, its location, and severity. In many cases damage can be caused by physical means, and does not involve infection or an adaptive immune response. However, if an infection is present, the body's innate systems for limiting damage and repairing tissues work in concert with the adaptive immune responses. The overall process involves a number of overlapping stages, which typically take place over a number of days or weeks. These may include some or all of the following:

- stopping bleeding;
- acute inflammation;
- killing of pathogens, neutralizing toxins and limiting pathogen spread;
- phagocytosis of debris, pathogens and dead cells;
- proliferation and mobilization of fibroblasts or other tissue cells to contain an infection and/or repair damage;
- removal or dissolution of blood clots and remodelling of the components of the extracellular matrix;
- regeneration of cells of the tissue and re-establishing normal structure and function.

Inflammation brings leukocytes to sites of infection or tissue damage. Many immune responses lead to the complete elimination of a pathogen (sterile immunity), followed by resolution of the damage, disappearance of leukocytes from the tissue and full regeneration of tissue function – the response in such cases is referred to as **acute inflammation**. In some cases an infection is not cleared completely. Most pathogenic organisms have developed systems to deflect the immune responses that would eliminate them. In this case the body often tries to contain the infection or minimize the damage it causes; nevertheless, the persistent antigenic stimulus and the cytotoxic effects of the pathogen itself lead to ongoing **chronic inflammation**.

The cells seen in acute and chronic inflammation are quite different, and reflect the phased arrival of different populations of leukocytes into a site of infection (Fig. 3.2). Consequently:

- sites of acute inflammation tend to have higher numbers of neutrophils and activated helper T cells, particularly TH1 and TH17 cells; whereas
- sites of chronic inflammation have a higher proportion of macrophages, cytotoxic T cells and B cells.

The phased arrival of different populations of leukocytes at a site of inflammation is dependent on **chemokines** (chemotactic cytokines) expressed on the endothelium. These chemokines activate distinct leukocyte populations, causing them to migrate into the tissue.

The cell types seen in sites of damage and the capacity of the tissue for repair and regeneration also depend greatly on the tissue involved. For example, in the brain the capacity for cell regeneration is very limited, so in chronic inflammatory diseases such as multiple sclerosis, the area of damage often becomes occupied by scar tissue formed primarily by a specialized CNS cell type, the astrocyte. In contrast, the liver has a high capacity for regeneration, and can replace hepatocytes lost through infection, cytotoxic damage or by immune reactions. Nevertheless, chronic tissue damage can still result in fibrosis. How inflammation develops

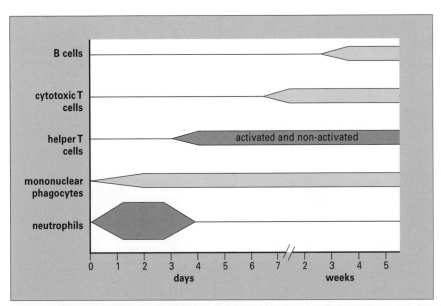

Fig. 3.2 The phased arrival of different populations of leukocytes into a site of infection Leukocytes enter sites of infection in phases controlled primarily by the release of chemokines from that tissue, and the expression of chemokine receptors on different populations of leukocytes.

in a tissue depends on the type of infection, the tissue involved and the immune status of the individual.

Cytokines control the movement of leukocytes into tissues.

Tissue damage leads to the release of a number of inflammatory cytokines, either from:

- cells within the tissue, including resident mononuclear phagocytes; or
- leukocytes that have migrated into the tissue.

The cytokines **tumour necrosis factor-α** (TNFα), interleukin-1 (IL-1) and interferon-γ (IFNγ) are particularly important in this respect. TNFα is produced primarily by macrophages and other mononuclear phagocytes and has many functions in the development of inflammation and the activation of other leukocytes (Fig. 3.3). Notably, TNFα induces the adhesion molecules and chemokines on the endothelium, which are required for the accumulation of leukocytes. TNFα and the related cytokines, **lymphotoxins**, act on a family of receptors causing the activation of the transcription factor **NF-κB** (Fig. 3.4), which has been described as a master-switch of the immune system. NF-κB is, in fact, a group of related transcription factors, which can also be activated by TLRs and IL-1. The activation of vascular endothelium by TNFα or IL-1 causes chemokine production and adhesion molecules to be expressed on the endothelial surface.

Once an immune reaction has developed in tissue, leukocytes generate their own cytokines (e.g. IFNγ is produced by active TH1 cells), which also activate the endothelium and promote further leukocyte migration. The chemokines that are produced at the site depend on the type of immune response that is occurring within the tissue, and this in turn affects which leukocytes migrate into the tissue. This partly explains why different patterns of leukocyte migration and inflammation are seen in different diseases.

Leukocytes migrate across the endothelium of microvessels.

The mechanisms that control leukocyte migration into inflamed tissues have been carefully studied because of their biological and medical importance. These mechanisms are also applicable in principle to the cell movement that occurs between lymphoid tissues during development and normal life.

The routes that leukocytes take as they move around the body are determined by interactions between circulating cells and the endothelium of blood vessels. Leukocyte migration is controlled by signalling molecules, which are expressed on the surface of the endothelium, and occurs principally in venules (Fig. 3.5).

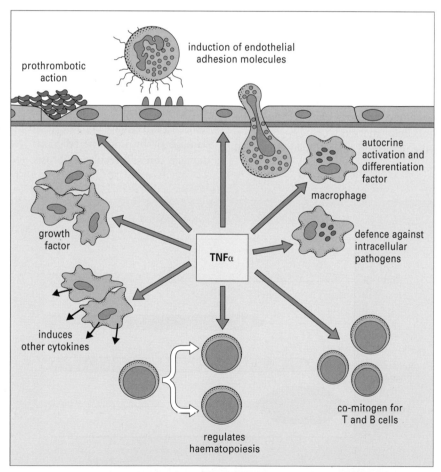

Fig. 3.3 Tumour necrosis factor-α (TNFα) is a cytokine with many functions TNFα has several functions in inflammation. It is prothrombotic and promotes leukocyte adhesion and migration *(top)*. It has an important role in the regulation of macrophage activation and immune responses in tissues *(centre)*, and it also modulates haematopoiesis and lymphocyte development *(bottom)*.

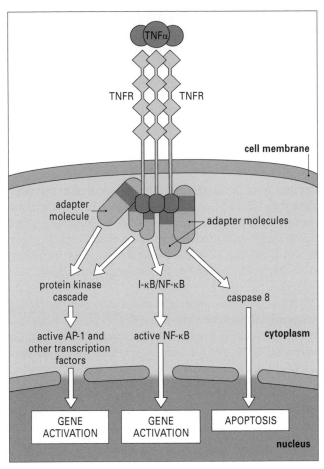

Fig. 3.4 Intracellular signalling pathways induced by tumour necrosis factor-α (TNFα) TNFα induces the trimerization of the TNF receptor *(TNFR)*, which causes adapter molecules to be recruited to the receptor complex. One pathway leads to the activation of caspase 8 and apoptosis. Other pathways lead to the activation of transcription factors AP-1 and NF-κB, which activate many genes involved in adaptive and innate immune responses.

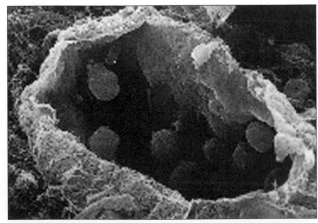

Fig. 3.5 Leukocytes adhering to the wall of a venule Scanning electron micrograph showing leukocytes adhering to the wall of a venule in inflamed tissue. ×16,000. (Courtesy Professor MJ Karnovsky.)

There are three reasons for this:
- the signalling molecules and adhesion molecules that control migration are selectively expressed in venules;
- the haemodynamic shear force in the venules is relatively low, and this allows time for leukocytes to receive signals from the endothelium and allows adhesion molecules on the two cell types to interact effectively; and
- the endothelial surface charge is lower in venules (Fig. 3.6).

Although the patterns of leukocyte migration are complex, the basic mechanism appears to be universal. The initial interactions are set out in a three-step model (Fig. 3.7).

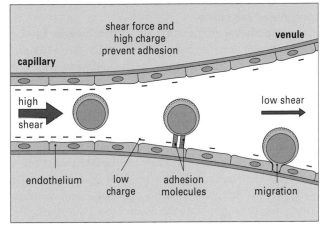

Fig. 3.6 Leukocyte migration across endothelium Leukocytes circulating through a vascular bed may interact with venular endothelium via sets of surface adhesion molecules. In the venules, haemodynamic shear is low, surface charge on the endothelium is low and adhesion molecules are selectively expressed.

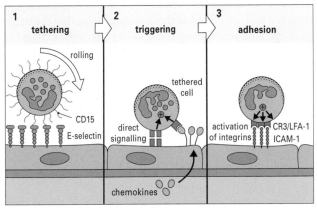

Fig. 3.7 Three-step model of leukocyte adhesion The three-step model of leukocyte adhesion and activation is illustrated by a neutrophil, though different sets of adhesion molecules would be used by other leukocytes in different situations. (**1**) Tethering – the neutrophil is slowed in the circulation by interactions between E-selectin and carbohydrate groups on CD15, causing it to roll along the endothelial surface. (**2**) Triggering – the neutrophil can now receive signals from chemokines bound to the endothelial surface or by direct signalling from endothelial surface molecules. The longer a cell rolls along the endothelium, the longer it has to receive sufficient signal to trigger migration. (**3**) Adhesion – the triggering upregulates integrins *CR3* and *LFA-1* ($\alpha_M\beta_2$- and $\alpha_L\beta_2$-integrin) so that they bind to *ICAM-1* induced on the endothelium by inflammatory cytokines. *ICAM-1*, Intercellular adhesion molecule-1; *LFA-1*, leukocyte-functional-antigen-1.

- Step 1: leukocytes are slowed as they pass through a venule and roll on the surface of the endothelium before being halted – this is mediated primarily by adhesion molecules called **selectins** interacting with carbohydrates on glycoproteins.
- Step 2: the slowed leukocytes now have the opportunity to respond to signalling molecules held at the endothelial surface – particularly important are the **chemokines**, which activate populations of leukocytes expressing the appropriate chemokine receptors.
- Step 3: activation upregulates the affinity of the leukocytes' **integrins**, which now engage the cellular adhesion molecules on the endothelium to cause firm adhesion and initiate a programme of migration.

Transendothelial migration is an active process involving both leukocytes and endothelial cells (Fig. 3.8). Generally, leukocytes migrate through the junctions between cells, but in specialized tissues such as the brain and thymus, where the endothelium is connected by continuous tight junctions, lymphocytes migrate across the endothelium in vacuoles, near the intercellular junctions, which do not break apart.

Migrating cells extend pseudopods down to the basement membrane and move beneath the endothelium using new sets of adhesion molecules. Enzymes are now released that digest the collagen and other components of the basement membrane, allowing cells to migrate into the tissue. Once there, the cells can respond to new sets of chemotactic stimuli, which allow them to position themselves appropriately in the tissue.

Leukocyte traffic into tissues is determined by adhesion molecules and signalling molecules. Intercellular adhesion molecules are membrane-bound proteins that allow one cell to interact with another. Often these molecules traverse the membrane and are linked to the cytoskeleton so that the migrating cell can gain traction against another cell or the extracellular matrix, thus allowing cell movement.

In many cases, a particular adhesion molecule can bind to more than one ligand, using different binding sites. Although the binding affinity of individual adhesion molecules to their ligands is usually low, clustering of the molecules in patches on the cell surface means that the avidity of the interaction can be high.

Cells can modulate their interactions with other cell types by increasing the numbers of adhesion molecules on the surface or altering their affinity and avidity. They can alter the level of expression of adhesion molecules in two ways:

- many cells retain large intracellular stores of these molecules in vesicles, which can be directed to the cell surface within minutes following cellular activation;
- alternatively, new molecules can be synthesized and transported to the cell surface, a process that usually takes several hours.

Selectins bind to carbohydrates to slow the circulating leukocytes. Selectins are involved in the first step of transendothelial migration. The selectins are E-selectin and P-selectin, which are expressed predominantly on endothelium and platelets, and L-selectin, which is expressed on naive lymphocytes and is involved in traffic to secondary lymphoid tissues (Fig. 3.9).

Selectins are transmembrane molecules; their extracellular N-terminal domain has lectin-like properties (i.e. it binds to carbohydrate residues), hence the name selectins. When tissue is damaged, TNFα or IL-1 induces synthesis and expression of E-selectin on endothelium. P-selectin acts similarly to E-selectin,

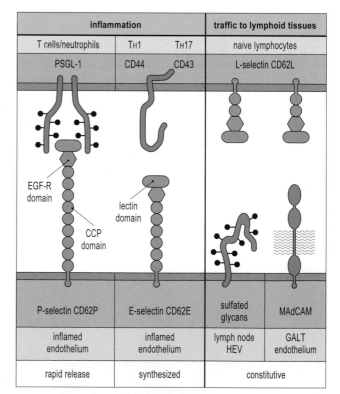

inflammation			traffic to lymphoid tissues
T cells/neutrophils	TH1	TH17	naive lymphocytes
PSGL-1	CD44	CD43	L-selectin CD62L
P-selectin CD62P	E-selectin CD62E	sulfated glycans	MAdCAM
inflamed endothelium	inflamed endothelium	lymph node HEV	GALT endothelium
rapid release	synthesized	constitutive	

Fig. 3.9 Selectins The structures of the three selectins are shown. They have terminal lectin domains, which bind to carbohydrates on the cells listed. The EGF-R domain is homologous to a segment in the epidermal growth factor receptor. The CCP domains are homologous to domains found in complement control proteins, such as factor H. E-selectin and P-selectin are expressed on endothelium at sites of inflammation – P-selectin is released from stores in vesicles, whereas E-selectin is induced by inflammatory cytokines. L-selectin is a ligand for glycosylated molecules on high endothelial venules (*HEV*) in peripheral lymph node or in gut-associated lymphoid tissue.

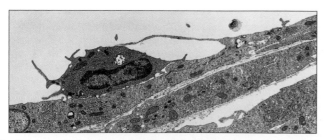

Fig. 3.8 Lymphocyte migration Electron micrograph showing a lymphocyte adhering to brain endothelium close to the inter-endothelial cell junction in an animal with experimental allergic encephalomyelitis. Adhesion precedes transendothelial migration into inflammatory sites. (Courtesy Dr C Hawkins.)

but is held ready-made in storage granules of the endothelium (Weibel–Palade bodies) and released to the cell surface if the endothelium becomes activated or damaged. Both E-selectin and P-selectin can slow circulating platelets or leukocytes by binding to a tetrasaccharide, sialyl Lewis-X (sLeX), which is constitutively expressed on monocytes and neutrophils and is induced on antigen-activated T cells. sLeX was originally identified as a cell-surface structure by immunostaining – CD15 and this carbohydrate group may be linked to different proteoglycans and glycolipids on different cell types.

On leukocytes, the sLeX group may be associated with:
- P-selectin glycoprotein ligand (PSGL-1), which also binds to E-selectin. It is a heavily glycosylated transmembrane molecule that can bind to the cytoskeleton via adapter proteins, allowing intracellular signalling. Lymphocyte subpopulations express different variants of PSGL-1, which contributes to selective migration of those populations – TH1 cells, TH17 cells and neutrophils interact strongly with endothelium via this ligand.
- Leukosialin (CD43), which is the principal ligand on TH17 cells for E-selectin.
- CD44, which is a widely expressed adhesion molecule that binds hyaluronic acid. It is expressed in a number of variants with different glycosylation patterns, one of which is present on T cells and neutrophils and which acts as a ligand for E-selectin.
- E-selectin ligand (ESL), which is an adhesion molecule found on murine (but not human) neutrophils.

When selectins bind to their ligands the circulating cells are slowed within the venules. Video pictures of cell migration show that the cells stagger along the endothelium. During this time the leukocytes have the opportunity of receiving migration signals from the endothelium. This is a process of signal integration – the more time the cell spends in the venule, the longer it has to receive sufficient signals to activate migration. If a leukocyte is not activated it detaches from the endothelium and returns to the venous circulation. A leukocyte may therefore circulate many times before it finds an appropriate place to migrate into the tissues.

Chemokines and other chemotactic molecules trigger the tethered leukocytes. The chemokines are a group of at least 50 small cytokines involved in cell migration, activation, and chemotaxis. They determine which cells will cross the endothelium and where they will move within the tissue. Most chemokines have two binding sites:
- one for their specific receptors; and
- a second for carbohydrate groups on proteoglycans (such as heparan sulfate), which allows them to attach to the extracellular matrix or to the luminal surface of endothelium (blood side), ready to trigger any tethered leukocytes (Fig. 3.10).

The chemokines may be produced by the endothelium itself, and this varies according to the distinct types of endothelium present in each tissue. In addition, chemokines produced by cells in the tissues can be transported to the luminal side of the endothelium, by the process of transcytosis. Immune reactions or events occurring within the tissue can therefore induce the release of chemokines, which signal the inward migration of populations of leukocytes. Once they have crossed the endothelium, chemokines bound to extracellular matrix can form gradients for chemotactic movement through the tissue.

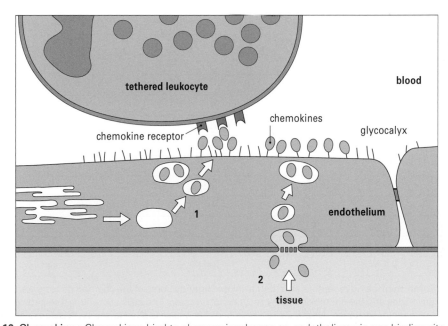

Fig. 3.10 Chemokines Chemokines bind to glycosaminoglycans on endothelium via one binding site while a second site interacts with chemokine receptors expressed on the surface of the leukocyte. Chemokines may be synthesized by the endothelial cell and stored in vesicles (Weibel–Palade bodies) to be released to the luminal surface (blood side) following activation (**1**). Alternatively, chemokines may be produced by cells in the tissues and transported across the endothelium (**2**). Cells in the tissue can therefore signal either directly or indirectly to circulating leukocytes.

Chemokines fall into four different families, based on the spacing of conserved cysteine (C) residues in a characteristic motif sequence. For example:

- α-Chemokines have a CXC structure, where 'X' is any amino acid residue.
- β-Chemokines have a CC structure, where the cysteines are directly linked.
- Fractalkine (CX3CL1), with three intervening residues, is produced as a cell-surface adhesion molecule, involved in limiting cell activation.
- Lymphotactins (XCL1) have a single cysteine residue in the motif.

Chemokines, receptors have promiscuous binding properties. All chemokines act via receptors that have seven transmembrane segments (**7tm receptors**) linked to GTP-binding proteins (**G-proteins**), which cause cell activation. There are also three non-signalling, scavenger receptors, which bind and clear chemokines, thereby helping to maintain chemotactic gradients.

Most chemokines act on more than one receptor, and most receptors will respond to several chemokines. Because of this complexity, it is easiest to understand what chemokines do by considering their receptors:

- the receptors for the CXC chemokines are called CXCR1, CXCR2, and so on,
- the receptors for the CC chemokines are called CCR1, CCR2, etc.

Originally most chemokines had a descriptive name and an acronym such as macrophage chemotactic protein-1 (MCP-1). The current nomenclature describes them according to their type: hence MCP-1 is CCL2, meaning that it is a **ligand** for the CC family of chemokine receptors (Fig. 3.11).

The chemokine receptors are selectively expressed on particular populations of leukocytes and this determines which cells can respond to signals coming from the tissues. The profile of

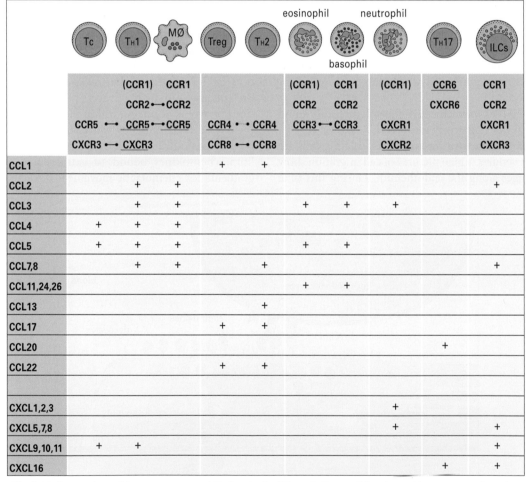

Fig. 3.11 Some chemokine receptors and their principal ligands Some of the chemokine receptors found on particular leukocytes and the chemokines they respond to are listed. The cells are grouped according the principal types of effector response. Note that TH1 cells and mononuclear phagocytes both express chemokine receptor CCR5, which allows them to respond to chemokine CCL3, whereas eosinophils and basophils express CCR3, which allows them to respond to CCL11. This allows selective recruitment of sets of leukocytes into areas with particular types of immune/inflammatory response. Both groups of cells express chemokine receptors CCR1 and CCR2, which allow responses to macrophage chemotactic proteins (CCL2, CCL7, CCL8 and CCL13). Neutrophils express chemokine receptors CXCR1 and CXCR2, which allow them to respond to CXCL8 (IL-8), CXCL1 and CXCL2.

chemokine receptors on a cell depends on its type and state of differentiation. For example:

- all T cells express CCR1;
- eosinophils and basophils express CCR3; and
- TH1 cells and cytotoxic T cells preferentially express CCR5 and CXCR3. After activation in lymph nodes, the levels of CXCR3 on a T cell increase, so that it becomes more responsive for the IFNγ-inducible chemokines CXCL9, CXCL10 and CXCL11, which activate CXCR3. As a consequence, antigen-activated lymphocytes are more readily triggered to enter sites of inflammation where these chemokines are expressed.

Cells change their chemokine receptor profiles as they move between tissues. For example naive regulatory T cells express CCR9, which allows them to home to the gut-associated lymphoid tissue. Later, the expression of CCR9 is reduced and CXCR3 and CCR2 increased, which switches them to migrate to peripheral tissues.

Other molecules are also chemotactic for neutrophils and macrophages. Several other molecules are chemotactic for neutrophils and macrophages, both of which have an f.Met-Leu-Phe (f.MLP) receptor. This receptor binds to peptides blocked at the N-terminus by formylated methionine – prokaryotes (i.e. bacteria) initiate all protein translation with this amino acid, whereas eukaryotes do not. Hence this is a specific receptor for a pathogen-associated molecular pattern (PAMP).

Neutrophils and macrophages also have receptors for:

- C5a, which is a fragment of a complement component generated at sites of inflammation following complement activation; and
- LTB4 (leukotriene-B4), a product of arachidonic acid, which is generated at sites of inflammation, particularly by macrophages and mast cells.

In addition, molecules generated by the blood clotting system, notably fibrin peptide B and thrombin, attract phagocytes, though many molecules such as these only act indirectly by inducing chemokines.

The first leukocytes to arrive at a site of inflammation, if activated, are able to release chemokines that attract other cells. For example, CXCL8 (originally identified as IL-8) released by activated monocytes can induce neutrophil and basophil chemotaxis. Similarly, macrophage activation leads to release of LTB4, attracting more monocytes.

All of these chemotactic molecules act via 7tm receptors which activate trimeric G-proteins.

Integrins on the leukocytes bind to cell-adhesion molecules on the endothelium. Activation of leukocytes via their chemokine receptors initiates the next stage of migration.

Leukocytes and many other cells in the body interact with other cells and components of the extracellular matrix using a group of adhesion molecules called integrins.

In the third step of leukocyte migration (see Fig. 3.7), the leukocytes use their integrins to bind firmly to cell-adhesion molecules (CAMs) on the endothelium. Leukocyte activation promotes this step in the following three ways:

- it can cause integrins to be released from intracellular stores;
- it can cause clustering of integrins on the cell surface into high-avidity patches; and
- most importantly, the cell activation induced by the chemokines causes the integrins to become associated with the cytoskeleton and can switch them into a high-affinity form (Fig. 3.12) – this is referred to as 'inside-out signalling' because activation inside the cell causes a change in the position and affinity of the extracellular portion of the integrin.

Normally, the binding affinity of integrins for the CAMs on the endothelium is relatively weak, but when sufficient interactions take place, the cells adhere firmly.

Many of the CAMs on the endothelium belong to the immunoglobulin superfamily. Some of them (e.g. intercellular adhesion molecule (ICAM)-1 and vascular cell-adhesion molecule-1 (VCAM-1)) are induced on endothelium at sites of inflammation by inflammatory cytokines while others (e.g. ICAM-2) are constitutively expressed and not inducible (Fig. 3.13). Specific integrins bind to particular CAMs (Fig. 3.14), and since integrins vary between leukocytes and CAMs vary between endothelium in different tissues, the adhesion step also affects which leukocytes will enter the tissue.

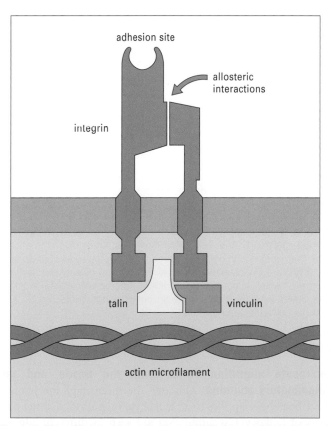

Fig. 3.12 The affinity of integrins is controlled by inside-out signalling Activation of the cell causes a change in the position of the two chains of the integrin, which become linked to the cytoskeleton via the adapter molecules vinculin and talin. The association produces an allosteric change in the extracellular portion of the molecule, causing the binding site to open and allowing the integrin to attach to its ligand.

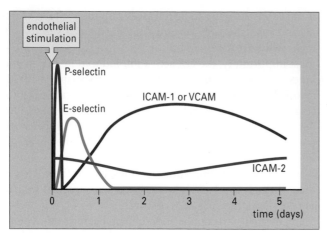

Fig. 3.13 Expression and induction of endothelial adhesion molecules The graph shows the time course of induction of different endothelial molecules on human umbilical vein endothelium in vitro following stimulation by tumour necrosis factor-α. *ICAM*, Intercellular adhesion molecule; *VCAM*, vascular cell-adhesion molecule.

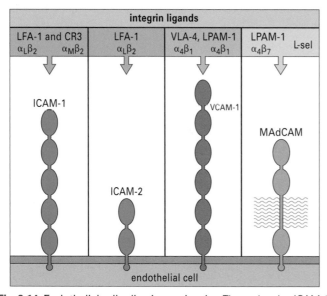

Fig. 3.14 Endothelial cell-adhesion molecules The molecules ICAM-1, ICAM-2, VCAM-1 and MAdCAM are illustrated diagrammatically with their immunoglobulin-like domains. Their integrin ligands (see Fig. 3.w1) are listed above. MAdCAM also has a heavily glycosylated segment, which binds L-selectin. *ICAM*, Intercellular adhesion molecule; *MAdCAM*, mucosal addressin cell-adhesion molecule; *VCAM*, vascular cell-adhesion molecule.

Leukocyte migration varies with the tissue and the inflammatory stimulus. Although the three-stage mechanism described above applies to all leukocyte migration, distinct patterns of leukocyte accumulation are seen in different sites of inflammation, depending on:

- the state of activation of the lymphocytes or phagocytes – the expression of adhesion molecules and their functional affinity vary depending on the type of cell and whether it has been activated by antigen, cytokines or cellular interactions. For

example, activation of T cells induces both the chemokine receptor CXCR3 and the adhesion molecule LFA-1 ($α_Lβ_2$-integrin), which therefore promotes migration of activated T cells into inflamed tissues.

- the types of adhesion molecule expressed by the vascular endothelium, which is related to its anatomical site and whether it has been activated by cytokines. For example, ICAM-1 is expressed at higher levels on brain endothelium than VCAM-1, whereas they are equally expressed on skin endothelium.
- the particular chemotactic molecules and cytokines present; receptors vary between leukocyte populations so that particular chemotactic agents act selectively.

Different chemokines cause different types of leukocyte to accumulate. In the second step of migration, neutrophils are triggered by chemokines such as CXCL8 synthesized by cells in the tissue, or by the endothelium itself. CXCL8 acts on two different chemokine receptors – CXCR1 and CXCR2 (see Fig. 3.11) – to initiate neutrophil migration.

In some tissues different sets of chemokines cause the local accumulation of other groups of leukocytes. For example:

- in the bronchi of individuals with asthma, CCL11 (eotaxin) is released, which causes the accumulation of eosinophils – CCL11 acts on CCR3, which is also present on basophils, so by releasing one chemokine, the tissue can signal to two different kinds of cell to migrate into the tissue and this particular set of cells is characteristic of the cellular infiltrates in asthma;
- in sites of chronic inflammation, the chemokines CXCL10 and CCL2 are released by endothelium in response to IFNγ and TNFα – CXCL10 acts on activated TH1 cells (via CXCR3), while CCL2 acts on macrophages (via CCR2); consequently, macrophages and TH1 cells tend to accumulate at sites of chronic inflammation.

Preventing leukocyte adhesion can be used therapeutically. The importance of leukocyte adhesion has been pinpointed in a group of patients who have leukocyte adhesion deficiency (LAD) syndrome due to the absence of all $β_2$-integrins; they suffer from severe infections. The mechanism was confirmed by studies using antibodies to CR3 ($α_Mβ_2$-integrin) in experimental animals, which inhibit phagocyte migration into tissues.

A number of antibodies against adhesion molecules are now used therapeutically to treat inflammatory diseases. For example, antibodies against VLA-4 ($α_4β_1$-integrin, the ligand for VCAM-1) are used to treat patients with multiple sclerosis, where the aim is to limit the migration of active T cells into the CNS.

LEUKOCYTE MIGRATION TO LYMPHOID TISSUES

Migration of leukocytes into lymphoid tissues is also controlled by chemokines and adhesion molecules on the endothelium. High endothelial venules (HEV, see Fig. 2.50) are present in lymph nodes and gut-associated lymphoid tissues. Up to 25% of lymphocytes that enter a lymph node via the blood may be diverted across the HEV. In contrast, only a tiny proportion of those circulating through other tissues will cross the regular venular endothelium at each transit. HEVs are therefore particularly important in controlling lymphocyte recirculation. Normally they are only present in the secondary lymphoid tissues, but they may be induced at sites of chronic inflammation – referred to as tertiary lymphoid tissue.

In addition to their peculiar shape, HEV cells express distinct sets of heavily glycosylated sulfated adhesion molecules, which bind to circulating T cells and direct them to the lymphoid tissue.

The HEVs in different lymphoid tissues have different sets of adhesion molecules. In particular, there are separate molecules controlling migration to:
- Peyer's patches;
- mucosal lymph nodes; and
- other lymph nodes.

These molecules were previously called vascular addressins, and their expression on different HEVs partly explains how lymphocytes relocalize to their own lymphoid tissue.

Naive lymphocytes express L-selectin, which contributes to their attachment to carbohydrate ligands on HEVs in mucosal and peripheral lymph nodes. Once they have stopped on the HEV, migrating lymphocytes may use the integrin $\alpha_4\beta_7$ (LPAM-1, see Fig. 3.14) to bind to MAdCAM on the HEV of mucosal lymph nodes or Peyer's patches.

Because the expression of $\alpha_4\beta_7$ allows migration to mucosal lymphoid tissue, whereas $\alpha_4\beta_1$ allows attachment to VCAM-1 on activated endothelium or fibronectin in tissues, expression of one or other of these molecules can alternately be used by naive lymphocytes migrating to mucosal lymphoid tissue or by activated T cells migrating to inflammatory sites.

Chemokines are important in controlling cell traffic to lymphoid tissues.
Chemokines are also important in controlling cell traffic to lymphoid tissues. Naive T cells express CXCR4 and CCR7, which allows them to respond to chemokines expressed in lymphoid tissues. Initially, they recognize CCL21 on the endothelium and, subsequently, CCL19 produced by dendritic cells, which directs them to the appropriate T-cell areas of the lymph node where dendritic cells can present antigen to them.

Once T cells have been activated, they lose CXCR4 and CCR7, but gain new chemokine receptors (see Fig. 3.11), which allow them to respond to chemokines produced at sites of inflammation.

Naive B cells express CCR7 and CXCR5, a receptor for CXCL13, which is required for localization to lymphoid follicles within the lymph nodes. A subset of T cells, which are required to help B-cell differentiation, also express CXCR5, causing them to co-localize with B cells in lymphoid follicles. Cells moving into lymphoid tissue therefore respond sequentially to signals on the endothelium and signals from the different areas within the tissue (Fig. 3.15).

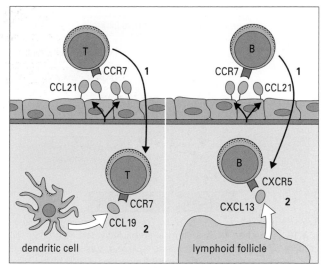

Fig. 3.15 Chemokines and cell migration into lymphoid tissue Cell migration occurs in stages. Naive T cells express CCR7, which allows them to respond to CCL21 expressed by secondary lymphoid tissues (1). Once the cells have migrated across the endothelium, the same receptor can respond to signals from CCL19 produced by dendritic cells (2), which promotes interactions with the T cells in the paracortex (T-cell area) of the lymph node. B cells also express CCR7 and use similar mechanisms to migrate into the lymphoid tissues (1). However, they also express CXCR5, which allows them to respond to CXCL13, a chemokine produced in lymphoid follicles (2); B cells are therefore directed to the B-cell areas of the node. Mice lacking CXCR5 do not develop normal lymphoid follicles.

MEDIATORS OF INFLAMMATION

Increased vascular permeability is another important component of inflammation. However, whereas cell migration occurs across venules, serum exudation occurs primarily across capillaries where blood pressure is higher and the vessel wall is thinnest. This event is controlled in two ways:
- blood supply to the area increases;
- there is an increase in capillary permeability caused by retraction of the endothelial cells and increased vesicular transport across the endothelium – this permits larger molecules to traverse the endothelium than would ordinarily be capable of doing so, and allows antibody and molecules of the plasma enzyme systems to reach the inflammatory site.

The four major plasma enzyme systems that have an important role in haemostasis and control of inflammation are the:
- clotting system;
- fibrinolytic (plasmin) system;
- kinin system; and
- complement system (see Chapter 4).

The kinin system generates powerful vasoactive mediators.
The kinin system generates the mediators bradykinin and lysyl-bradykinin (kallidin). Bradykinin is a very powerful vasoactive nonapeptide that causes:
- venular dilation due to release of nitric oxide (NO);
- increased vascular permeability; and
- smooth muscle contraction.

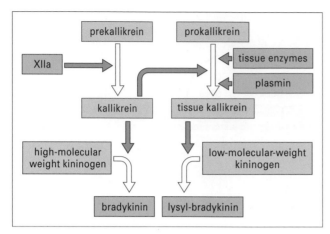

Fig. 3.16 Activation of the kinin system Activated Hageman factor (XIIa) acts on prekallikrein to generate kallikrein, which in turn releases bradykinin from high-molecular-weight kininogen (HMWK). Prekallikrein and HMWK circulate together in a complex. Various enzymes activate prokallikrein to tissue kallikrein, which releases lysyl-bradykinin from low-molecular-weight kininogen. Bradykinin and lysyl-bradykinin are both extremely powerful vasodilators.

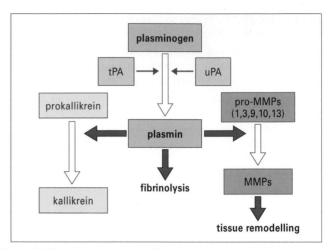

Fig. 3.17 The plasmin system Plasmin is generated by the enzymatic activity of plasminogen activators. *MMPs* are matrix metalloproteinases that can degrade collagen and other matrix components, to promote tissue remodelling. *tPA*, Tissue plasminogen activator produced by vascular endothelium; *uPA*, urokinase plasminogen activator, present in plasma and extracellular matrix.

Bradykinin is generated following the activation of Hageman factor (XII) of the blood clotting system, whereas tissue kallikrein is generated following activation of the plasmin system or by enzymes released from damaged tissues (Fig. 3.16).

The plasmin system is important in tissue remodelling and regeneration. The plasmin system can be activated by a soluble or a tissue-derived plasminogen activator, which leads to the enzymatic conversion of plasminogen into plasmin. Plasmin itself was originally identified by its ability to dissolve fibrin but it has several other activities: in particular it activates some matrix metalloproteases (MMPs), enzymes that are required for the breakdown and remodelling of collagen (Fig. 3.17). Additionally, it can promote angiogenesis (the formation of new blood vessels) by causing the release of cytokines that induce proliferation and migration of endothelial cells.

Mast cells, basophils and platelets release a variety of inflammatory mediators. Auxiliary cells, including mast cells, basophils and platelets, are also very important in the initiation and development of acute inflammation. They act as sources of the vasoactive mediators histamine and 5-hydroxytryptamine (serotonin), which produce vasodilation and increased vascular permeability.

Many of the proinflammatory effects of C3a and C5a result from their ability to trigger mast cell granule release, because they can be blocked by antihistamines. Mast cells and basophils are also a route by which the adaptive immune system can trigger inflammation – IgE sensitizes these cells by binding to their IgE receptors and the cells can then be activated by antigen. They are an important source of slow-reacting inflammatory mediators, including the leukotrienes and prostaglandins, which contribute to a delayed component of acute inflammation and are synthesized and act some hours after pre-formed mediators (e.g. histamine) which are released immediately after mast cell activation.

Table 3.1 lists the principal mediators of acute inflammation. The interaction of the immune system with complement and other inflammatory systems is shown in Figure 3.18.

Platelets may be activated by:

- immune complexes; or
- platelet-activating factor (PAF) from neutrophils, basophils, and macrophages.

Activated platelets release mediators which are important in type II and type III hypersensitivity reactions (see Chapters 24 and 25).

Pain is associated with mediators released from damaged or activated cells. The substances released from damaged cells, mast cells, and basophils are also important in producing the sensation of pain. PAF, histamine, serotonin, prostaglandins and leukotrienes act on C-fibres which are responsible for the poorly localized, dull-aching pain associated with inflammation. Substance-P released from activated nerve fibres further contributes to the feeling of pain. Various types of mechanical and physical damage can also lead to the release of these mediators from the tissue cells, resulting in pain.

Lymphocytes and monocytes release mediators that control the accumulation and activation of other cells. Once lymphocytes and monocytes have arrived at a site of infection or inflammation, they can also release mediators, which control the later accumulation and activation of other cells. For example:

- activated macrophages release the chemokine CCL3 and leukotriene-B4, both of which are chemotactic and encourage further monocyte migration;

TABLE 3.1 Inflammatory Mediators

Mediator	Main source	Actions
Histamine	Mast cells, basophils	Increased vascular permeability, smooth muscle contraction, chemokinesis
5-Hydroxytryptamine (5HT (serotonin))	Platelets, mast cells (rodent)	Increased vascular permeability, smooth muscle contraction
Platelet-activating factor (PAF)	Basophils, neutrophils, macrophages	Mediator release from platelets, increased vascular permeability, smooth muscle contraction, neutrophil activation
IL-8 (CXCL8)	Mast cells, endothelium, monocytes and lymphocytes	Polymorph and monocyte localization
C3a	Complement C3	Mast cell degranulation, smooth muscle contraction
C5a	Complement C5	Mast cell degranulation, neutrophil and macrophage chemotaxis, neutrophil activation, smooth muscle contraction, increased capillary permeability
Bradykinin	Kinin system (kininogen)	Vasodilation, smooth muscle contraction, increased capillary permeability, pain
Fibrinopeptides and fibrin breakdown products	Clotting system	Increased vascular permeability, neutrophil and macrophage chemotaxis
Prostaglandin E$_2$ (PGE$_2$)	Cyclo-oxygenase pathway, mast cells	Vasodilation, potentiates increased vascular permeability produced by histamine and bradykinin
Leukotriene-B$_4$ (LTB$_4$)	Lipoxygenase pathway, mast cells	Neutrophil chemotaxis, synergizes with PGE$_2$ in increasing vascular permeability
Leukotriene-D$_4$ (LTD$_4$)	Lipoxygenase pathway	Smooth muscle contraction, increasing vascular permeability

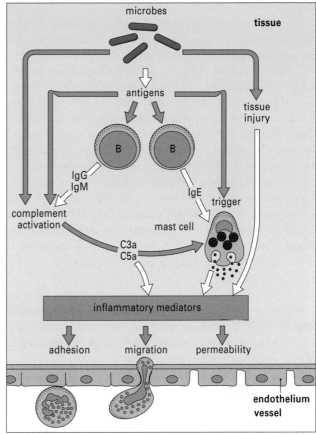

Fig. 3.18 The immune system in acute inflammation The adaptive immune system modulates inflammatory processes via the complement system. Antigens (e.g. from microorganisms) stimulate B cells to produce antibodies including IgE, which binds to mast cells, while IgG and IgM activate complement. Complement can also be activated directly via the alternative pathway (see Table 4.1). When triggered by antigen, sensitized mast cells release their granule-associated mediators and eicosanoids (products of arachidonic acid metabolism, including prostaglandins and leukotrienes). In association with complement (which can also trigger mast cells via C3a and C5a), the mediators induce local inflammation, facilitating the arrival of leukocytes and more plasma enzyme system molecules.

In recurrent inflammatory reactions and in chronic inflammation the patterns of cell migration are different from those seen in an acute response. We now know that the patterns of inflammatory cytokines and chemokines vary over the course of an inflammatory reaction and this can be related to the successive waves of migration of different types of leukocyte into the inflamed tissue (see Fig. 3.2).

Chronic inflammation is characteristic of sites of persistent infection and occurs in autoimmune reactions where the antigen cannot ultimately be eradicated (see Chapter 20).

PATHOGEN-ASSOCIATED MOLECULAR PATTERNS

Before the evolutionary development of B cells and T cells, organisms still needed to recognize and react against microbial

- lymphocytes can modulate later lymphocyte traffic by the release of chemokines and inflammatory cytokines, particularly IFNγ, which induces production of interferon-inducible chemokines CXCL9 and CXCL10.

pathogens. Hence, a variety of soluble molecules and cell surface receptors evolved which were capable of recognizing distinctive molecular structures on pathogens. Such structures are called **pathogen-associated molecular patterns (PAMPs)** and the proteins which recognize them are **pattern recognition receptors (PRRs)**. Typical examples of PAMPs are carbohydrates, lipoproteins and lipopolysaccharide components of bacterial and fungal cell walls, whereas some of the PRRs recognize the distinctive nucleic acids (e.g. dsRNA) formed during viral replication. Such molecules are integral to the function of the pathogen, so they cannot easily be modified to escape immune recognition.

Strictly speaking, many of these molecules are found on non-pathogenic organisms, so some authors prefer to call them **microbe-associated molecular patterns (MAMPs)**, and distinguish them from products of damaged cells, **damage-associated molecular patterns (DAMPs)**, also known as **alarmins**; one example is HMGB1, a nuclear protein released by necrotic, but not apoptotic cells.

Many of the PRRs that evolved in invertebrates have been retained in vertebrates and work alongside the adaptive immune system to recognize pathogens. However, the importance of different PRRs often differs between different species of mammals.

There are three main types of PRR:
- secreted molecules, present in serum and body fluids;
- receptors, present on the cell surface and on endocytic vesicles; and
- intracytoplasmic recognition molecules.

Each type of PRR can scan for PAMPs in a different environment – extracellular, intravesicular or intracytoplasmic. The intracytoplasmic recognition molecules are particularly important for macrophage-mediated recognition of internalized pathogens (see Chapter 5).

The functions of the secreted molecules and the cell surface receptors are explained below. They are divided into families according to structure.

Some of the secreted molecules are **acute phase proteins** (i.e. they are present in the blood and their levels increase during infection). Indeed the first of these molecules to be recognized was C-reactive protein, which can increase by more than 1000-fold in serum, during infection or inflammation. This protein, which recognizes dead cells and some types of bacteria, has been used as a clinical marker of inflammation for more than 75 years.

PRRs allow phagocytes to recognize pathogens. In many cases, the innate recognition mechanisms allow phagocytes to bind and internalize the pathogens and this is often associated with activation of the phagocytes, which enhances their microbicidal activity.

The binding of the pathogen to the phagocyte can be direct or indirect:
- direct recognition involves the surface receptors on the phagocyte directly recognizing surface molecules on the pathogen;
- indirect recognition involves the deposition of serum-derived molecules onto the pathogen surface and their subsequent binding to receptors on the phagocyte (i.e. the process of opsonization) (Fig. 3.19).

Opsonins come from a number of different families of proteins and include pentraxins, collectins, and ficolins. Some of them act directly as adapters for phagocytic cells, for example by binding to the C1q receptor; others activate the complement alternative or lectin pathways.

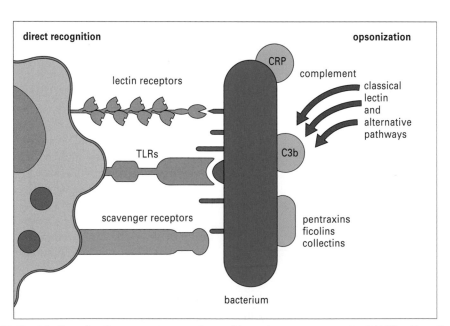

Fig. 3.19 The binding of pathogens to macrophages Macrophages can recognize PAMPs either directly or following opsonization with serum molecules.

Phagocytes have receptors that recognize pathogens directly. Even in the absence of opsonins, phagocytes have a number of receptors that allow them to recognize PAMPs. These include:

- scavenger receptors;
- carbohydrate receptors;
- TLRs.

The scavenger receptors and carbohydrate receptors are primarily expressed on mononuclear phagocytes, and are described more fully in Chapter 5.

Toll-like receptors activate phagocytes. The transmembrane protein Toll was first identified in the fruit fly *Drosophila* as a molecule required during embryogenesis. It was also noted that mutants lacking Toll were highly susceptible to infections with fungi and Gram-positive bacteria, suggesting that the molecule might be involved in immune defence. Subsequently, a series of TLRs was identified in mammals that had very similar intracellular portions to the receptor in the flies.

The intracellular signalling pathways activated by the TLRs and the receptor for IL-1 are very similar and lead to activation of the transcription factor NF-κB.

The family of TLRs include 10 different receptors in humans, many of which are capable of recognizing different microbial components (Table 3.2). All of the TLRs are present on phagocytic cells, and some are also expressed on dendritic cells, mast cells and B cells. Indeed, most tissues of the body express at least one TLR.

Expression of many of the TLRs is increased by inflammatory cytokines (e.g. TNFα, IFNγ) and elevated expression is seen in conditions such as inflammatory bowel disease. The functional importance of the TLRs has been demonstrated in mouse strains lacking individual receptors. Depending on the TLR involved, such animals fail to secrete inflammatory cytokines in response to pathogens and the microbicidal activity of phagocytes is not stimulated. These results show that the TLRs are primarily important in activating phagocytes in addition to any role they may have in endocytosis. Occasionally, humans are deficient in individual TLRs. For example, TLR3 deficiency is associated with susceptibility to herpes simplex, and a variant of TLR7 is associated with higher viral load and disease progression in HIV infection.

The TLRs make an important link between the innate and adaptive immune systems because their activation leads to the expression of co-stimulatory molecules on the phagocytes, which convert them into effective antigen-presenting cells. The binding of microbial components to the TLRs effectively acts as a danger signal to increase the microbicidal activity of the phagocytes and allows them to activate T cells.

TABLE 3.2 Toll-Like Receptors

Receptor	Location	Ligand	Pathogen
TLR1	Cell surface	Lipopeptides	Gram-negative bacteria Mycobacteria
TLR1/TLR2	Cell surface	Tri-acyl lipoprotein	Bacteria
TLR2	Cell surface	Lipoteichoic acid Lipoarabinomannan Zymosan Glycoinositol-phospholipids	Gram-positive bacteria Mycobacteria Fungi *Trypanosoma cruzi*
TLR2/TLR6	Cell surface	Di-acyl lipoprotein	Bacteria
TLR3	Endosome or cell surface	dsRNA	Viruses
TLR4	Cell surface	LPS	Gram-negative bacteria
TLR5	Cell surface	Flagellin	Bacteria
TLR6	Cell surface	Di-acyl lipopeptides	Mycobacteria
TLR7	Endosome	ssRNA	Viruses
TLR8	Endosome	ssRNA	Viruses
TLR9	Endosome	Unmethylated CpG DNA	Bacteria

Toll-like receptors recognize a variety of PAMPs. Gene duplication of the TLR precursor and divergence of function has led to a family of molecules capable of recognizing different types of pathogen. (In humans there is an additional receptor (TLR10) which limits NF-κB activation, although its ligand is not yet identified.)

CRITICAL THINKING: THE ROLE OF ADHESION MOLECULES IN T-CELL MIGRATION

See Critical thinking: Explanations, section 6

An experiment has been carried out to determine which CAMs mediate the migration of antigen-activated T cells across brain endothelium using a monolayer of endothelium overlaid with lymphocytes in vitro. The endothelium is either unstimulated or has been stimulated for 24 hours before the experiment with IL-1. In some cases, the co-cultures were treated with blocking antibodies to different adhesion molecules. The results shown in the following table indicate the percentage of T cells that migrate across the endothelium in a 2-hour period.

| Blocking antibody | PERCENTAGE OF T CELLS MIGRATING IN 2 HOURS | |
	Unstimulated endothelium	IL-1-stimulated endothelium
None	18	48
Anti-ICAM-1	3	16
Anti-VCAM-1	19	28
anti-$\alpha_L\beta_2$-integrin (LFA-1)	2	14
anti-$\alpha_4\beta_1$integrin (VLA-4)	17	32

1. Why does treatment of the endothelium with IL-1 cause an increase in the percentage of migrating cells in the absence of any blocking antibody?
2. Why does it require 24 hours of treatment with IL-1 to enhance the migration (1 hour of treatment does not produce this effect)?
3. Which adhesion molecules are important in mediating T-cell migration across unstimulated endothelium?
4. Which adhesion molecules are important in mediating T-cell migration across IL-1-activated endothelium?

FURTHER READING

Bottazzi B, Doni A, Garlanda C, Mantovani A. An integrated view of humoral innate immunity: pentraxins as the paradigm. Annu Rev Immunol 2010;28:157–183.

Griffith JW, Sokol CL, Luster AD. Chemokines and chemokine receptors: positioning cells for host defense and immunity. Annu Rev Immunol 2014;32:659–702.

Hofman Z, de Maat S, Hack CE, Maas C. Bradykinin: inflammatory product of the coagulation system. Clin Rev Allergy Immunol 2016;51:152–161.

Hynes RO. Integrins: bidirectional allosteric signaling machines. Cell 2002;110:673–687.

Klune JR, Dhupar R, Cardinal J, Billiar TR, Tsung A. HMGB1: endogenous danger signaling. Mol Med 2008;14:476–484.

Kumar H, Kawai T, Akira S. Pathogen recognition by the innate immune system. Int Rev Immunol 2011;30:16–34.

Rubaker SW, Bonhham KS, Zanoni I, Kagan JC. Innate immune pattern recognition: a cell biological perspective. Annu Rev Immunol 2015;33:257–290.

Selsted ME, Ouelette AJ. Mammalian defensins in the antimicrobial immune response. Nat Immunol 2005;6:551–557.

Shattil SJ, Kim C, Ginsberg MH. The final steps of integrin activation: the end game. Nat Rev Mol Cell Biol 2010;11:288–300.

Zarbock A, Ley K, McEver RP, Hidalgo A. Leukocyte ligands for endothelial selectins: specialized glycoconjugates that mediate rolling and signaling under flow. Blood 2011;118:3743–6751.

4

Complement

SUMMARY

- **Complement is central to the development of inflammatory reactions** and forms one of the major immune defence systems of the body. The complement system serves as one of the links between the innate and adaptive arms of the immune system.
- **Complement activation pathways have evolved to label pathogens for elimination.** The classical pathway links to the adaptive immune system through antibody. The alternative and lectin pathways provide antibody-independent innate immunity and the alternative pathway is linked to and amplifies the classical and lectin pathways.
- **The complement system is carefully controlled to protect the body from excessive or inappropriate inflammatory responses**. C1 inhibitor controls the classical and lectin pathways. C3 and C5 convertase activity are controlled by plasma and membrane proteins mediating decay and enzymatic degradation. Membrane attack is inhibited on host cells by CD59.
- **The membrane attack pathway results in the formation of a lytic transmembrane pore**. Regulation of the membrane attack pathway by CD59 reduces the risk of bystander damage to adjacent host cells.

- **Many cells express one or more membrane receptors for complement products.** Receptors for fragments of C3 are widely distributed on different leukocyte populations. Receptors for C1q are present on phagocytes, mast cells and platelets. C5 fragment receptors are present on many cell types. The plasma complement regulator factor H binds cell and non-cell surfaces.
- **Complement has a variety of functions.** Its principal functions include opsonization, chemotaxis and cell activation, lysis of target cells and priming of the adaptive immune response.
- **Complement deficiencies illustrate the homeostatic roles of complement.** Classical pathway deficiencies result in tissue inflammation. Deficiencies of mannan-binding lectin (MBL) are associated with infections in infants and those who are immunosuppressed. Alternative pathway and C3 deficiencies are associated with bacterial infections. Terminal pathway deficiencies predispose to Gram-negative bacterial infections. C1 inhibitor deficiency leads to hereditary angioedema. Deficiencies in alternative pathway regulators produce a secondary loss of C3.

COMPLEMENT AND INFLAMMATION

The complement system was discovered at the end of the 19th century as a heat-labile component of serum that augmented (or complemented) its bactericidal properties.

Complement is now known to comprise some 16 plasma proteins, together constituting nearly 10% of the total serum proteins, and forming one of the major immune defence systems of the body (Fig. 4.1). In addition to acting as a key component of the innate immune system, complement also interfaces with and enhances adaptive immune responses. More than a dozen regulatory proteins are present in plasma and on cells to control complement. The functions of the complement system include:

- triggering and amplification of inflammatory reactions;
- attraction of phagocytes by chemotaxis;
- clearance of immune complexes, apoptotic cells and other debris;
- cellular activation for microbial killing;
- direct microbial killing; and
- contributing to the efficient development of antibody responses.

In evolutionary terms the complement system is ancient and antedates the development of the adaptive immune system: even starfish and worms have a functional complement system.

The importance of complement in immune defence is readily apparent in individuals who lack particular components – for example, children who lack the central component **C3** are subject to frequent and severe bacterial infections.

Like most elements of the immune system, when over-activated or activated in the wrong place, the complement system can cause harm.

Complement is involved in the pathology of many diseases, provoking a search for therapies that control complement activation.

COMPLEMENT ACTIVATION PATHWAYS

One major function of complement is to label pathogens and other foreign or toxic bodies for elimination from the host. The complement activation pathways have evolved to serve this purpose and the multiple ways in which activation can be triggered, together with intrinsic amplification mechanisms, ensure efficient recognition and clearance.

Moreover, there are several different ways to activate the complement system, providing a large degree of flexibility and some redundancy, in response (Fig. 4.2).

The first activation pathway to be discovered, now termed the **classical pathway**, is initiated by antibodies bound to the surface of the target. Although an efficient means of activation, it requires an adaptive immune response: that is, the host must have previously encountered the target microorganism in order for an antibody response to be generated.

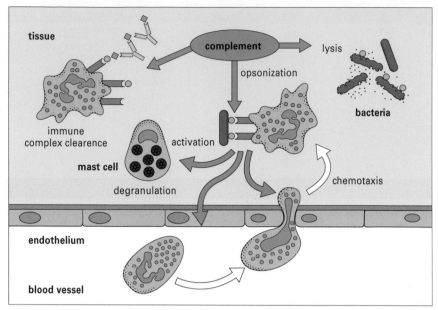

Fig. 4.1 Role of complement in inflammation Complement has a central role in inflammation, causing chemotaxis of phagocytes, activation of mast cells and phagocytes, opsonization and lysis of pathogens and clearance of immune complexes.

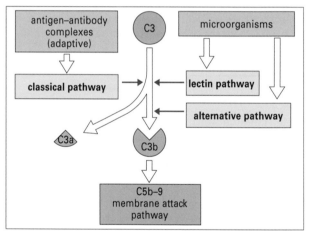

Fig. 4.2 Complement activation pathways Each of the activation pathways generates a C3 convertase, which converts C3 to C3b, the central event of the complement system. C3b in turn activates the terminal lytic membrane attack pathway. The first stage in the classical pathway is the binding of antigen to antibody. The alternative pathway does not require antibody and is initiated by the covalent binding of C3b to hydroxyl and amine groups on the surface of various microorganisms. The lectin pathway is also triggered by microorganisms in the absence of antibody, with sugar residues on the pathogen surface providing the binding sites. The alternative and lectin pathways provide antibody-independent innate immunity, whereas the classical pathway represents a more recently evolved link to the adaptive immune system.

The **alternative pathway**, described in the 1950s, provides an antibody-independent mechanism for complement activation on pathogen surfaces. More importantly, the alternative pathway is an amplification loop that drives activation regardless of the initiating pathway.

The **lectin pathway**, the most recently described of the activation pathways, also bypasses antibody to enable efficient activation on pathogens.

All three pathways – classical, alternative and lectin pathways:

- involve the activation of C3, which is the most abundant and most important of the complement proteins;
- comprise a proteolytic cascade in which complexes of complement proteins create enzymes that cleave other complement proteins in an ordered manner to create new enzymes, thereby amplifying and perpetuating the activation cascade.

Thus, a small initial stimulus can rapidly generate a large effect. Table 4.1 summarizes how each of the pathways is activated.

All activation pathways converge on a common **terminal pathway** – a non-enzymatic system for causing membrane disruption and lytic killing of pathogens.

The immune defence and pathological effects of complement activation are mediated by the fragments and complexes generated during activation:

- the small chemotactic and pro-inflammatory fragments **C3a** and **C5a**;
- the large opsonic fragments **C3b** and **C4b**; and
- the lytic **membrane attack complex (MAC)**.

The details of complement activation, the nomenclature and the ways in which the pathways are controlled are shown in Figure 4.3.

The classical pathway links to the adaptive immune system.

The classical pathway is activated by antibody bound to antigen and requires Ca^{2+}. Only surface-bound IgG and IgM antibodies can activate complement and they do so via the classical pathway. Surface binding is the key:

- IgM is the most efficient activator, but unbound IgM in plasma does not activate complement – surface binding causes a shape change in the IgM molecule from planar to a staple form in which binding sites for C1 are exposed.

TABLE 4.1 Summary of the Activators of the Classical, Lectin and Alternative Pathways

| | Immunoglobulins | MICROORGANISMS | | | |
		Viruses	Bacteria	Other	Other
Classical pathway	Immune complexes containing IgM, IgG1, IgG2 or IgG3	HIV and other retroviruses, vesicular stomatitis virus		*Mycoplasma* spp.	Polyanions, especially when bound to cations PO_4^{3-} (DNA, lipid A, cardiolipin) SO_4^{2-} (dextran sulfate, heparin, chondroitin sulfate)
Lectin pathway		HIV and other retroviruses	Many Gram-positive and Gram-negative organisms		Arrays of terminal mannose groups acetylated sugars
Alternative pathway	Immune complexes containing IgG, IgA or IgE (less efficient than the classical pathway)	Some virus-infected cells (e.g. by Epstein–Barr virus)	Many Gram-positive and Gram-negative organisms	Trypanosomes, *Leishmania* spp., many fungi	Dextran sulfate, heterologous erythrocytes, complex carbohydrates (e.g. zymosan)

- Among IgG subclasses, IgG1 and IgG3 are strong complement activators, whereas IgG4 does not activate because it is unable to bind the first component of the classical pathway – binding of C1 requires a hexameric surface assembly of IgG molecules that mimics bound IgM.

The first component of the pathway, **C1**, is a complex molecule comprising a large, 6-headed recognition unit termed **C1q** and two molecules each of **C1r** and **C1s**, the enzymatic units of the complex (Fig. 4.4). Assembly of the C1 complex is Ca^{2+}-dependent and the classical pathway is therefore inactive if Ca^{2+} ions are absent.

C1 activation occurs only when several of the head groups of C1q are bound to antibody. C1q in the C1 complex binds through its globular head groups to the Fc regions of the immobilized antibody. A single surface-bound IgM can bind multiple head groups and activate C1, but for IgG effective C1q binding depends on the formation of a hexameric IgG complex on the surface. Binding causes changes in shape of C1q that trigger autocatalytic activation of the enzymatic unit C1r. Activated C1r then cleaves an adjacent C1s at a single site in the protein to activate it.

Since C1 activation occurs only when hexameric arrays of IgG are formed on the surface to engage most or all of the six head groups of C1q, only surfaces that are densely coated with IgG antibody will trigger the process. This limitation reduces the risk of inappropriate activation on host tissues.

C1s enzyme cleaves C4 and C2. The C1s enzyme has two substrates – C4 and C2 – which are the next two proteins in the classical pathway sequence. (Note that the apparent lack of logic in numerical order is because complement components were named chronologically, according to the order of their discovery, rather than according to their position in the reaction.) C1s cleaves the abundant plasma protein **C4** at a single site in the molecule:

- releasing a small fragment, **C4a**; and
- exposing a labile thioester group in the large fragment **C4b**.

Through the highly reactive thioester, C4b becomes covalently linked to the activating surface (Fig. 4.5).

Surface-bound C4b binds the next component, **C2**, in an Mg^{2+}-dependent complex and presents it for cleavage by C1s in an adjacent C1 complex:

- the fragment **C2b** is released; and
- **C2a** remains associated with C4b on the surface.

C4b2a is the classical pathway C3 convertase. The complex of C4b and C2a (termed C4b2a – the classical pathway C3 convertase) is the next activation enzyme. C2a in the C4b2a complex cleaves C3, the most abundant of the complement proteins:

- releasing a small fragment, **C3a**; and
- exposing a labile thioester group in the large fragment **C3b**.

As described above for C4b, C3b covalently binds the activating surface via its thioester group.

C4b2a3b is the classical pathway C5 convertase. Where there is strong activation, some of the C3b formed will bind directly to C4b2a, thus forming the trimolecular complex C4b2a3b (the classical pathway C5 convertase). C3b in the complex can bind **C5** and present it for cleavage by C2a:

- a small fragment, **C5a**, is released; and
- the large fragment, **C5b**, remains associated with the C4b2a3b complex.

Cleavage of C5 is the final enzymatic step in the complement activation pathways.

The ability of C4b and C3b to bind surfaces is fundamental to complement function. C3 and C4 are homologous molecules that contain an unusual structural feature – an internal thioester bond between a glutamine and a cysteine residue that, in the intact molecule, is buried within the protein.

When either C3 or C4 is cleaved by the convertase enzyme, a conformational change takes place that exposes the internal thioester bond in C3b and C4b, making it very unstable and highly susceptible to attack by nucleophiles such as hydroxyl groups (-OH) and amine groups ($-NH_2$), present in proteins and carbohydrates on membranes and other surfaces. This reaction creates a covalent bond between the complement fragment

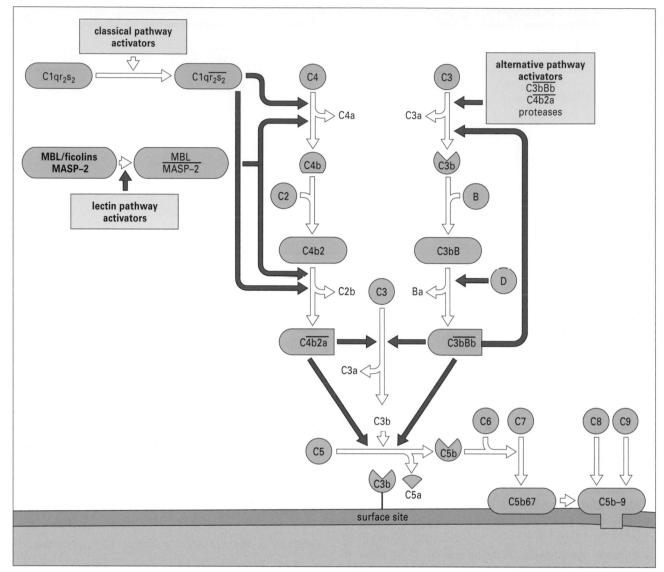

Fig. 4.3 Overview of the complement activation pathways The proteins of the classical and alternative pathways are assigned numbers (e.g. C1, C2). Many of these are zymogens (i.e. pro-enzymes that require proteolytic cleavage to become active). The cleavage products of complement proteins are distinguished from parent molecules by suffix letters (e.g. C3a, C3b). The proteins of the alternative pathway are called factors and are identified by single letters (e.g. factor B, which may be abbreviated to FB or just B). Components are shown in *green*, conversion steps as *white arrows*, and activation/cleavage steps as *red arrows*. The classical pathway is activated by the cleavage of C1r and C1s following association of C1qr$_2$s$_2$ with classical pathway activators (see Table 4.1), including immune complexes. Activated C1s cleaves C4 and C2 to form the classical pathway C3 convertase C4b2a. Cleavage of C4 and C2 can also be effected via MASP-2 of the lectin pathway, which is associated with mannan-binding lectin (MBL) or ficolin. The alternative pathway is activated by the cleavage of C3 to C3b, which associates with factor B and is cleaved by factor D to generate the alternative pathway C3 convertase C4b2a. The initial activation of C3 happens to some extent spontaneously, but this step can also be mediated by classical or alternative pathway C3 convertases or a number of other serum or microbial proteases. Note that C3b generated in the alternative pathway can bind more factor B and generate a positive feedback loop to amplify activation on the surface. Note also that the activation pathways are functionally and structurally analogous and the diagram emphasizes these similarities. For example, C3 and C4 are homologous, as are C2 and factor B. MASP-2 is homologous to C1r and C1s. Either the classical or alternative pathway C3 convertases may associate with C3b bound on a cell surface to form C5 convertases, C4b2a3b or C3bBbC3b, which split C5. The larger fragment C5b associates with C6 and C7, which can then bind to plasma membranes. The complex of C5b67 assembles C8 and multiple molecules of C9 to form a membrane attack complex (MAC), C5b–9.

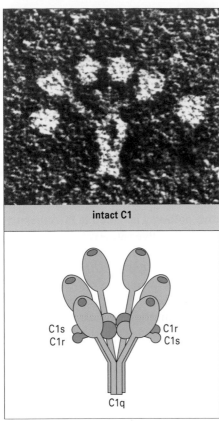

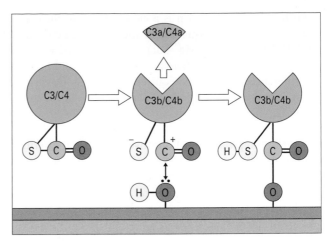

Fig. 4.5 **Activation of the thioester bond in C3 and C4** The α chain of C3 contains a thioester bond formed between a cysteine and a glutamine residue, with the elimination of ammonia. Following cleavage of C3 into C3a and C3b, the bond becomes unstable and susceptible to nucleophilic attack by electrons on -OH and -NH_2 groups, allowing the C3b to form covalent bonds with proteins and carbohydrates – the active group decays rapidly by hydrolysis if such a bond does not form. C4 also contains an identical thioester bond, which becomes activated similarly when C4 is split into C4a and C4b.

Fig. 4.4 **Structure of C1** Electron micrograph *(upper panel)* of a human C1q molecule demonstrates six subunits. Each subunit contains three polypeptide chains, giving 18 in the whole molecule. The receptors for the Fc regions of IgG and IgM are in the globular heads. The connecting stalks contain regions of triple helix and the central core region contains collagen-like triple helix. The *lower panel* shows a model of intact C1 with two C1r and two C1s pro-enzymes positioned within the ring. The catalytic heads of C1r and C1s are closely apposed and conformational change induced in C1q following binding to complexed immunoglobulin causes mutual activation/cleavage of each C1r unit followed by cleavage of the two C1s units. The cohesion of the entire complex is dependent on Ca^{2+}. (Electron micrograph, reproduced courtesy Dr N Hughes-Jones.)

and the surface ligand, locking C3b and C4b onto the surface (see Fig. 4.5).

The exposed thioester remains reactive for only a few milliseconds because it is also highly susceptible to hydrolysis. This lability restricts the surface binding of C3b and C4b to the immediate vicinity of the activating enzyme and prevents damage to surrounding structures.

The alternative and lectin pathways provide antibody-independent innate immunity.

The lectin pathway is activated by microbial carbohydrates.

The lectin pathway differs from the classical pathway only in the initial recognition and activation steps. Indeed, it can be argued that the lectin pathway should not be considered a separate pathway, but rather a route for classical pathway activation that bypasses the need for antibody.

The C1 complex is replaced by a structurally similar multi-molecular complex, comprising a C1q-like pattern recognition lectin, either **MBL**, **collectin-11** or one of the family of **ficolins**,

and several **MBL-associated serine proteases (MASPs)**. MASP-2 provides enzymatic activity. As in the classical pathway, assembly of this initiating complex is Ca^{2+}-dependent.

C1q, MBL and collectin-11 are members of the collectin family of proteins characterized by globular head regions with binding activities and long collagenous tail regions with diverse roles (see Fig. 3.w2). Ficolins are structurally similar, but the head regions comprise fibrinogen-like domains that bind acetyl groups in carbohydrate and other ligands.

MBL binds the simple carbohydrates mannose and *N*-acetyl glucosamine, while ficolins bind acetylated sugars and other molecules. These ligands are abundant in the cell walls of diverse pathogens, including bacteria, yeast, fungi, and viruses, making them targets for lectin pathway activation. Collection 11 ligands are poorly defined, although binding to fucosylated structures on damaged cells has been demonstrated. Binding induces shape changes in MBL, collectin-11 and the ficolins that in turn induce autocatalytic activation of the associated MASP-2. Activated MASP-2 then cleaves C4 and C2 to continue activation exactly as in the classical pathway.

The lectin pathway is not the only means of activating the classical pathway in the absence of antibody. Apoptotic cells, released DNA, mitochondria and other products of cell damage can directly bind C1q, triggering complement activation and aiding the clearance of the dead and dying tissue.

Alternative pathway activation is accelerated by microbial surfaces and requires Mg^{2+}.
The alternative pathway of complement activation also provides antibody-independent activation of complement on pathogen surfaces. This pathway is in a constant state of low-level activation (termed 'tickover').

C3 is hydrolysed at a slow rate in plasma and the product, **C3 (H_2O)**, although incapable of binding surfaces, shares many of the properties of C3b, including the capacity to bind a plasma protein **factor B (FB)**, which is a close relative of the classical pathway protein C2. Formation of the complex between C3b (or C3(H_2O)) and FB is Mg^{2+}-dependent, and the alternative pathway is therefore inactive in the absence of Mg^{2+} ions. (The differences in the ion requirements of the classical and alternative pathway are exploited in laboratory tests for complement activity.)

The C3bBb complex is the C3 convertase of the alternative pathway. Once bound to C3(H_2O) (in the fluid phase) or C3b (primarily on surfaces), FB becomes a substrate for an intrinsically active plasma enzyme termed **factor D (FD)**. FD cuts FB in the C3bB (or C3(H_2O)) complex:

- releasing a fragment, **Ba**; and
- while the residual portion, **Bb**, becomes an active protease.

The **C3bBb** complex is the C3 cleaving enzyme (C3 convertase) of the alternative pathway. C3b generated by this convertase can be fed back into the pathway to create more C3 convertases, thus forming a positive feedback amplification loop (Fig. 4.6). Activation may occur in plasma or, more efficiently, on surfaces.

Amplification of activation, regardless of initiating trigger, is a key role of the alternative pathway. Indeed, it is more accurate to consider it as an amplification loop rather than a separate pathway. Alternative pathway amplification, together with the 'always on' tickover activation, provides an efficient means of pathogen surveillance; just a few C3b molecules deposited on a pathogen surface will trigger amplification, leading to dense C3b coating of the surface, facilitating phagocytic clearance.

Specific features of host cell surfaces, including their surface carbohydrates and the presence of complement regulators (see later), act to protect the host cell from alternative pathway amplification and risk of being destroyed; such surfaces are termed non-activating.

On an activating surface such as a bacterial membrane, amplification will occur unimpeded and the surface will rapidly become coated with C3b (see Fig. 4.6). In a manner analogous to that seen in the classical pathway, C3b molecules binding to the C3 convertase will change the substrate specificity of the complex, creating a C5 cleaving enzyme, **C3bBbC3b**.

Cleavage of C5 is the last proteolytic step in the alternative pathway and the C5b fragment remains associated with the convertase.

The alternative pathway is linked to the classical and lectin pathways. The alternative pathway is inexorably linked to the classical and lectin pathways in that C3b generated through the classical pathway will feed into the alternative pathway to amplify activation. It therefore does not matter whether the initial C3b is generated by the classical, lectin, or alternative pathway – the amplification loop can ratchet up the reactions if they take place in the absence of regulation on an activator surface.

COMPLEMENT PROTECTION SYSTEMS

Control of the complement system is required to prevent the consumption of components through unregulated amplification and to protect the host. Complement activation poses a potential threat to host cells, because it could lead to cell opsonization or even lysis. To defend against this threat, a family of regulators

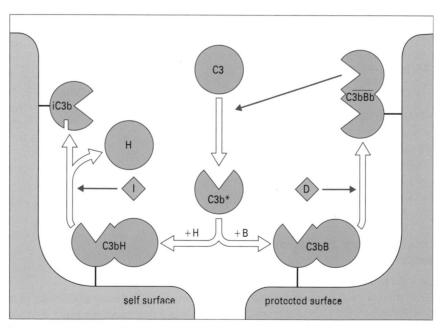

Fig. 4.6 Regulation of the amplification loop Alternative pathway activation depends on the presence of activator surfaces. C3b bound to an activator surface recruits factor B, which is cleaved by factor D to produce the alternative pathway C3 convertase C3bBb, which drives the amplification loop, by cleaving more C3. However, on self surfaces the binding of factor H is favoured and C3b is inactivated by factor I. Thus the binding of factor B or factor H controls the development of the alternative pathway reactions. In addition, proteins such as membrane cofactor protein and decay accelerating factor also limit complement activation on self cell membranes (see Fig. 4.7).

has evolved alongside the complement system to prevent uncontrolled activation and to protect cells from attack.

C1 inhibitor controls the classical and lectin pathways. In the activation pathways, the regulators target the enzymes that drive amplification:

- Activated C1 is controlled by a plasma serine protease inhibitor **(serpin)** termed **C1 inhibitor (C1inh)**, which removes C1r and C1s from the complex, switching off classical pathway activation.
- C1inh also regulates the lectin pathway in a similar manner, removing the MASP-2 enzyme from the MBL, collectin-11 or ficolin recognition unit to switch off activation.

C3 and C5 convertase activity is controlled by decay and enzymatic degradation. The C3 and C5 convertase enzymes are heavily policed with plasma and cell membrane inhibitors to control activation. In the plasma:

- **factor H (FH)** and a truncated form of FH, **factor H-like 1 (FHL-1),** disrupt the convertase enzymes of the alternative pathway;
- **C4 binding protein (C4bp)** performs the same task in the classical pathway.

On membranes, two proteins, **membrane cofactor protein (MCP)** and **decay accelerating factor (DAF)**, collaborate to disrupt the convertases of both pathways (Fig. 4.7).

The regulators of the C3 and C5 convertases are structurally related molecules that have arisen by gene duplication in evolution. These duplicated genes are tightly linked in a cluster on chromosome 1, termed the **regulators of complement activation (RCA) locus**. This locus also encodes several of the complement receptors (see later) and a set of five FH-related proteins, FHR-1 to FHR-5. The FHR proteins do not function as complement regulators but provide a further degree of control of surface activation by competing with FH for surface binding sites.

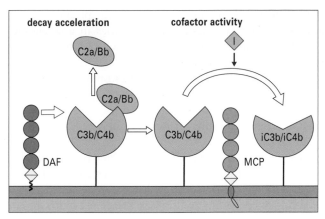

Fig. 4.7 Regulation of C3 convertases Decay accelerating factor *(DAF)* binds the enzyme complex, displacing the enzymatically active component (C2a or Bb). Membrane cofactor protein *(MCP)* binds the C3b/C4b unit released after decay and acts as a cofactor for factor *I* (FI) cleavage of C3b or C4b, resulting in the irreversible inactivation of the convertase.

Control of the convertases is mediated in two complementary ways.

Decay Acceleration. The convertase complexes described above are labile, with a propensity to dissociate within a few minutes of creation. This natural decay is an important part of complement regulation. The regulators FH, FHL-1 and C4bp from the fluid phase and DAF (CD46) on cell membranes bind the convertase complex and markedly accelerate decay, displacing:

- C2a from the classical pathway convertases (C4bp and DAF); and
- Bb from the alternative pathway enzymes (FH. FHL-1 and DAF) (Table 4.2).

Cofactor Activity. **Factor I (FI)** is a fluid-phase enzyme that, in the presence of an appropriate cofactor, can cleave and irreversibly inactivate C4b and C3b (see Table 4.2). MCP (CD46) is a cofactor for FI cleavage of both C4b and C3b, whereas:

- C4bp specifically catalyses cleavage of C4b; and
- FH and FHL-1 specifically catalyse cleavage of C3b.

TABLE 4.2 C3 and C5 Convertase Regulators

The five proteins listed are widely distributed and control aspects of C3b and C4b dissociation or breakdown. Each of these proteins contains a number of short consensus repeat (SCR) domains. They act either by enhancing the dissociation of C3 and C5 convertases or by acting as cofactors for the action of factor I on C3b or C4b

	Number of SCR domains	DISSOCIATION OF C3 AND C5 CONVERTASES		COFACTOR FOR FACTOR I ON		
		Classical pathway	Alternative pathway	C4b	C3b	Localization
C4b binding protein (C4bp)	52 or 56 in 7or 8 chains	+	–	+	–	Plasma
Factor H (fH)	20	–	+	–	+	Plasma
Decay accelerating factor (DAF) (CD55)	4	+	+	–	–	On most cells, including blood cells, endothelia, and epithelia
Membrane cofactor protein (MCP) (CD46)	4	–	–	+	+	On most cells, including blood cells (but not erythrocytes), endothelia, and epithelia
Complement receptor 1 (CR1) (CD35)	30	+	+	+	+	Erythrocytes, B cells, follicular dendritic cells, macrophages

It is interesting to note that, whereas the plasma regulators contain both decay and cofactor activities in a single molecule, the two membrane regulators each contain only one activity.

Efficient regulation of the convertases on membranes therefore requires the concerted action of:
- DAF to dissociate the complex; and
- MCP to irreversibly inactivate it by catalysing cleavage of the central component.

The alternative pathway also has a unique positive regulator, **properdin**, which stabilizes the C3 convertase and markedly increases its life span. Recent evidence has suggested an additional role of properdin as a surface-associated nidus for alternative pathway activation.

Complement receptor 1 (CR1; CD35) is often included in the list of membrane regulators of C3 convertase activity and, indeed, CR1 is a powerful regulator with both decay accelerating and cofactor activities in both pathways. Nevertheless, it is excluded from the above discussion because CR1 is primarily a receptor for complement-coated particles and does not have a role in protecting the host cell.

THE MEMBRANE ATTACK PATHWAY

Activation of the pathway results in the formation of a transmembrane pore. The **terminal or membrane attack pathway** involves a distinctive set of events whereby a group of five globular plasma proteins associate with one another and, in the process, acquire membrane-binding and pore-forming capacity to form a transmembrane pore, the membrane attack complex (MAC) (Fig. 4.8). Cleavage of C5 creates the nidus for MAC assembly to begin. While still attached to the convertase enzyme, C5b binds first **C6** then **C7** from the plasma. Conformational changes occurring during assembly of this trimolecular **C5b67** complex:
- cause release from the convertase; and
- expose a labile hydrophobic site in C5b67.

The complex can stably associate with a membrane through the labile hydrophobic site, although the process is inefficient and most of the C5b67 formed is inactivated in the fluid phase.

Membrane-bound C5b67 recruits **C8** from the plasma and, finally, multiple copies of **C9** are incorporated in the complex to form the MAC.

The latter stages of assembly are accompanied by major conformational changes in the components with globular hydrophilic plasma proteins unfolding to reveal amphipathic regions that penetrate into and through the lipid bilayer.

The fully formed MAC creates a rigid pore in the membrane, the walls of which are formed from multiple copies of C9 arranged like barrel staves around a central cavity.

The MAC is clearly visible in electron microscopic images of complement-lysed cells as doughnut-shaped protein-lined pores, first observed by Humphrey and Dourmashkin 45 years ago (see Fig. 4.8). The pore has an inner diameter approaching 10 nm:

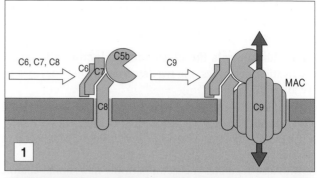

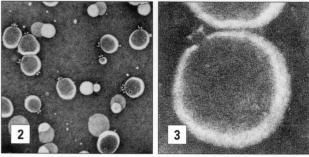

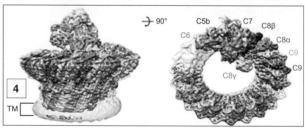

Fig. 4.8 The membrane attack pathway (1) C5b, while still attached to the C5 convertase, binds C6 and C7 from the fluid phase. The trimolecular C5b–7 complex dissociates from the convertase and binds the target cell membrane. Binding of C8 and multiple copies of C9 generates a rigid protein-lined transmembrane channel, the membrane attack complex *(MAC)*. **(2 and 3)** Electron micrographs of the MAC. The complex consists of a cylindrical pore in which the walls of the cylinder, formed by C9, traverse the cell membrane. In these micrographs, the human C5b–9 complex has been incorporated into a lecithin liposomal membrane. (Courtesy Professor J Tranum-Jensen and Dr S Bhakdi.) **(4)** Structure of the MAC pore. The image shows the MAC structure derived from cryo-electron microscopy. (Courtesy Dr Doryen Bubeck.)

- allowing the free flow of solutes and electrolytes across the cell membrane; and
- causing the cell to swell and sometimes burst because of the high internal osmotic pressure.

Recently, high-resolution electron microscopy has revealed the MAC structure in exquisite detail. The MAC pore comprises 22 staves, one each from C6, C7, C8α and C8β, with 18 copies of C9. Surprisingly, the pore is not fixed and rigid; rather, it has a flexible split-washer structure that probably allows the pore size to change.

Metabolically inert targets such as aged erythrocytes are readily lysed by even a small number of MAC lesions, whereas viable nucleated cells resist killing through a combination of ion pump activities and recovery processes that remove MAC lesions and plug membrane leaks.

Even in the absence of cell killing, MAC lesions may severely compromise cell function or cause cell activation.

Regulation of the membrane attack pathway reduces the risk of 'bystander' damage to adjacent cells.

Although regulation in the activation pathways is the major way in which complement is controlled, there are further failsafe mechanisms to protect self cells from MAC damage and lysis.

First, the membrane-binding site in C5b67 is labile. If the complex does not encounter a membrane within a fraction of a second after release from the convertase, the site is lost through:
* hydrolysis; or
* binding of one of the fluid-phase regulators of the terminal pathway – **S protein** (also termed **vitronectin**) or **clusterin** – both of which are multifunctional plasma proteins with diverse roles in homeostasis.

C8, an essential component of the MAC, also behaves as a regulator in that binding of C8 to C5b–7 in the fluid phase blocks the membrane-binding site and prevents MAC formation.

The net effect of all these plasma controls is to limit MAC deposition to membranes in the immediate vicinity of the site of complement activation, hence reducing risk of bystander damage to adjacent cells.

CD59 protects host cells from complement-mediated damage.

Complexes that do bind are further regulated on host cells by **CD59**, a membrane protein that locks into the MAC as it assembles and inhibits recruitment of C9, thereby preventing pore formation (Fig. 4.9). CD59 is a small, highly glycosylated, broadly expressed, glycolipid-anchored protein that is structurally unrelated to the complement regulators described above.

The importance of CD59 in protecting host cells from complement damage is well illustrated in the haemolytic disorder paroxysmal nocturnal haemoglobinuria (PNH), in which erythrocytes and other circulating cells are unable to make glycolipid anchors and as a consequence lack CD59 (and also DAF). The tickover complement activation that routinely occurs on all plasma-exposed cells without much consequence is then sufficient in the absence of CD59 to cause chronic haemolysis and haemolytic crises.

MEMBRANE RECEPTORS FOR COMPLEMENT PRODUCTS

Receptors for fragments of C3 are widely distributed on different leukocyte populations.

Many cells express one or more membrane receptors for complement products (Table 4.3). An understanding of the receptors is essential because the majority of the effects of complement are mediated through these molecules. The best characterized of the complement receptors are those binding fragments of C3.

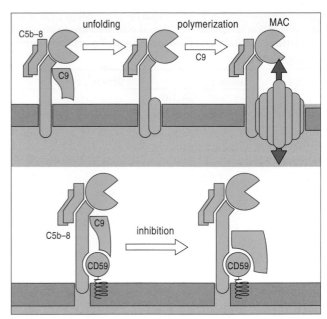

Fig. 4.9 Role of CD59 in protecting host cells from complement damage The *upper diagram* models assembly of the membrane attack complex *(MAC)* in the absence of the regulator CD59; C9 binds C5b–8, unwinds and traverses the membrane and recruits further C9 molecules, which in turn unfold and insert to form the MAC. In the *lower diagram*, CD59 binds the C5b–8 complex and prevents the unfolding and insertion of C9, which is essential for the initiation of MAC pore formation.

CR1, CR2, CR3, and CR4 bind fragments of C3 attached to activating surfaces.

Four different receptors, termed complement receptors 1, 2, 3 and 4 (CR1, CR2, CR3 and CR4), bind fragments of C3 attached to activating surfaces:
* **CR1**, expressed on erythrocytes and leukocytes, binds the largest fragment C3b (and also C4b), an interaction that is crucial to the processing of immune complexes (see later).
* **CR2**, expressed mainly on B cells and follicular dendritic cells (FDCs), binds fragments derived from FI-mediated proteolysis of C3b – iC3b and C3dg.

On B cells, these interactions aid the B-cell immune response to complement-coated particles.

Both CR1 and CR2 are structurally related to the C3 convertase regulators FH, C4bp, MCP and DAF and are encoded in the RCA (Regulators of Complement Activation) cluster on chromosome 1.

  CR3 and **CR4**:
* belong to the integrin family of cell adhesion molecules;
* are expressed on the majority of leukocytes; and
* bind the iC3b fragment, aiding adhesion of leukocytes to complement-coated particles and facilitating phagocytic ingestion of these particles.

Receptors for C3a and C5a mediate inflammation.

C3a, the small fragment released during activation of C3, binds to a receptor (**C3aR**) expressed abundantly on eosinophils and basophils, and at much lower levels on neutrophils and many other cell types.

TABLE 4.3   Cell Receptors for Complement Components and Fragments

Summary of information on the cell surface receptors for complement components and fragments and their biological roles

Ligand	Receptor	Structure	Function	Location
C1q	cC1qR (C1q receptor enhancing phagocytosis)	Acidic 100-kDa trans-membrane glycoprotein	Binds collagenous tail of C1q, enhances phagocytosis	Myeloid cells, endothelia, platelets
	C1qRp (receptor for C1q globular heads)	Acidic 33-kDa glycoprotein	Binds globular heads of C1q, possible role in phagocytosis	All blood cells
C3, C4, and C5 fragments	CR1 (complement receptor 1 – CD35)	SCR-containing trans-membrane glycoprotein, 30 SCRs	Binds C3b and C4b, cofactor and decay accelerating activities, roles in immune complex handling	Erythrocytes, B cells, FDCs, macrophages
	CR2 (complement receptor 2 – CD21)	SCR-containing trans-membrane glycoprotein, 15 SCRs	Binds C3d and iC3b, role in regulating B-cell response to antigen	B cells, FDCs, some T cells, basophils, epithelia
	CR3 (complement receptor 3 – CD11b/CD18)	Integrin family member, heterodimer	Binds iC3b, roles in cell adhesion	Myeloid cells, some B cells and NK cells
	CR4 (complement receptor 4 – CD11c/CD18)	Integrin family member, heterodimer	Binds iC3b, roles in cell adhesion	Myeloid cells, FDCs, activated B cells
	C3aR (receptor for the C3a anaphylatoxin)	G protein-coupled 7-transmembrane spanning receptor	Binds C3a, mediates cell activation	Widely distributed on blood and tissue cells
	C5aR (receptor for the C5a anaphylatoxin – CD88).	G protein-coupled 7-transmembrane spanning receptor	Binds C5a, mediates cell activation and chemotaxis	Myeloid cells, smooth muscle, endothelia, epithelia
	C5L2	G protein-uncoupled 7-transmembrane	Binds C3a, C3a-desArg, C5a, roles uncertain	Leukocytes, adipose tissue

FDC, Follicular dendritic cell.

The C5a fragment released from C5 during activation is closely related to C3a and binds a distinct, but structurally related, receptor, the C5a receptor (**C5aR**), which is present on a wide variety of cell types, including all leukocytes.

The receptors for C3a and C5a are members of the large receptor family of 7-transmembrane segment receptors that signal through association with heterotrimeric G proteins. Receptors for cytokines and chemokines belong to this same family and, in many ways, C3a and C5a behave like chemokines.

Together, C3aR and C5aR are important in orchestrating inflammatory responses and modulating antigen presentation and T-cell activation (see later).

A third receptor, termed C5L2, expressed by leukocytes and in adipose tissue, has binding activity for C3a, its inactivation product C3a-desArg (see later) and C5a. However, this receptor is uncoupled from G proteins and its functional roles are currently the subject of active debate. Recent evidence suggests that this enigmatic receptor mediates anti-inflammatory effects in cells and tissues, perhaps by interfering with C5aR-mediated pro-inflammatory drive.

Receptors for C1q are present on phagocytes, mast cells, and platelets.

Receptors for C1q are less well characterized than C3 receptors but are increasingly recognized as important in homeostasis.

Receptors for the collagen tails (**cC1qR**):
- can recognize C1q attached through its globular head regions to complement-coated particles;

- are present on leukocytes, platelets, and some other cell types; and
- probably play roles in enhancing phagocytosis of C1q-labelled particles.

Receptors for the globular heads (**C1qRp**):
- bind C1q in an orientation that mimics antibody binding;
- are expressed principally on phagocytic cells, mast cells, and platelets; and
- may collaborate with cC1qR to mediate cell activation events.

The bulk of C1q in the circulation is, however, already complexed with C1r and C1s to form intact C1 and it is not clear whether C1q in this C1 complex can interact with its receptors. Specificity for C1q would ensure that the receptors are engaged only in specific circumstances, such as during complement activation when free C1q is available. Some recent evidence suggests that cC1qR on monocytes stably binds intact C1 and utilizes the molecule to capture immune complexes.

The plasma complement regulator FH binds cell surfaces.

The plasma complement regulator FH binds host cell membranes via several heparin (or sugar) binding sites in the molecule. On complement-opsonized surfaces, FH also binds C3b/iC3b through separate sites in the molecule. Surface-bound FH plays important roles in protecting self cells from complement attack. Indeed, a rare but fascinating disease, atypical haemolytic uraemic syndrome (aHUS), which is typified by haemolysis, platelet destruction and renal damage that may progress to renal failure, is caused in many cases by mutations in the C-terminus of FH that ablate a key heparin-binding site, causing reduced surface-binding capacity. Uncontrolled complement activation, as a result of the reduced ability of the mutant FH lacking the membrane-binding site to bind cells and other surfaces, has been demonstrated in patients. Other patients with aHUS have mutations in complement components C3, FB or the membrane regulator MCP, demonstrating that this is a disease of alternative pathway dysregulation.

Some cells also bind FH through cell surface receptors – for example, both CR3 and CR4 on polymorphs binds FH and may contribute to polymorph pathogen recognition.

Many bacteria and other pathogens express specific receptors for FH, enabling them to hijack the protein to protect themselves from complement attack in the plasma.

COMPLEMENT FUNCTIONS

The principal functions of complement are:
- chemotaxis;
- opsonization and cell activation;
- lysis of target cells; and
- priming of the adaptive immune response.

C5a is chemotactic for macrophages and polymorphs. Polymorphs and macrophages express receptors for C3a and C5a. Like other chemokines, these small ($\sim$10 kDa) fragments (i.e. C3a and C5a) diffuse away from the site of injury and complement activation, creating a chemical gradient along which the motile cells migrate to congregate at the site of activation (Fig. 4.10).

Binding of C3a and C5a to their receptors also causes cell activation:
- increasing adhesive properties;
- triggering extravasation; and

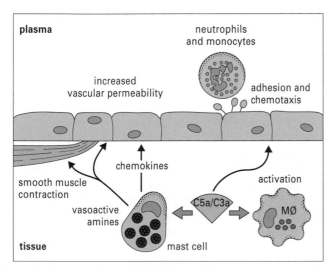

Fig. 4.10 Actions of C5a and C3a C5a and C3a both act on mast cells to cause degranulation and release of vasoactive amines, including histamine and 5-hydroxytryptamine, which enhance vascular permeability and local blood flow. The secondary release of chemokines from mast cells causes cellular accumulation and C5a itself acts directly on receptors on monocytes and neutrophils to induce their migration to sites of acute inflammation and subsequent activation.

- priming phagocytes to release pro-inflammatory molecules, including enzymes, vasoactive amines, reactive oxygen intermediates and inflammatory cytokines.

C3a and C5a enhance adhesion molecule expression on phagocytes, increasing cell stickiness, and may cause increased expression of the C3 fragment receptors CR1 and CR3, thereby enhancing phagocytic capacity for complement-opsonized particles.

C3a and C5a activate mast cells and basophils. Tissue mast cells and basophils also express C3aR and C5aR and binding of ligand triggers massive release of:
- histamine; and
- chemokines (see Fig. 4.10).

Together, these products cause local smooth muscle contraction and increased vascular permeability to generate the swelling, heat and pain that typify the inflammatory response. These effects mirror on a local scale the more generalized and severe reactions that can occur in severe allergic or anaphylactic reactions and for this reason C3a and C5a are sometimes referred to as **anaphylatoxins**.

The actions of C3a and C5a are limited temporally and spatially by the activity of a plasma enzyme, carboxypeptidase-N, which cleaves the carboxy terminal amino acid arginine from both of these fragments. The products, termed C3a-desArg and C5a-desArg (-desArg = without arginine), respectively, have either much reduced (C5a-desArg) or absent (C3a-desArg) chemotactic and anaphylactic activities.

The retention in C5a-desArg of some chemotactic activity enables the recruitment of phagocytes even from distant sites, making C5a and its metabolite the most important complement-derived chemotactic factor.

An important role for C3a-desArg in lipid handling has emerged. A mediator of increased lipid uptake and fat synthesis in adipose tissue, acylation-stimulating protein (ASP) was shown to be identical to C3a-desArg, linking complement activation to lipid turnover. Of note, adipose tissue is the primary site for FD synthesis and also produces C3; a complete alternative pathway can thus be assembled locally to generate C3a-desArg/ASP in adipose tissue.

C3b and iC3b are important opsonins. Complement activation and amplification cause complement fragments to coat efficiently activator surfaces of targets such as bacteria or immune complexes, enhancing their recognition by phagocytes (Fig. 4.11). Phagocytes and other cells carrying receptors for these complement fragments are then able to bind the target, triggering ingestion and cell activation. The key players here are the surface-bound fragments of C3 and the family of C3 fragment receptors described above.

The amplification inherent in the system ensures that bacteria and other activating surfaces rapidly become coated with C3b and its breakdown product **iC3b**, which enhances phagocytosis.

Phagocytes lured by the complement-derived chemotactic factors described above and activated to increase expression

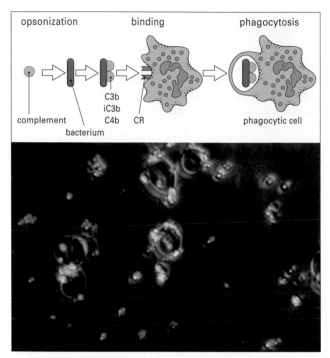

Fig. 4.11 Opsonization, binding and phagocytosis A bacterium is sensitized by the covalent binding of C3b, iC3b, and C4b, which allow it to be recognized by complement receptors *(CR)* on neutrophils and mononuclear phagocytes (upper plate). This promotes phagocytosis and activation of the phagocyte. In humans and primates, erythrocytes also express CR1, which allows them to bind opsonized bacteria and immune complexes. In the *lower panel*, fluorescein-labelled bacteria that have been opsonized with antibody and complement are seen adhering to human erythrocytes. (Courtesy Professor GD Ross.)

of CR1 and CR3 (receptors for C3b and iC3b, respectively) will bind the activating particle and engulf it for destruction in the phagolysosome system.

The importance of complement opsonization for defence against pathogens is illustrated in individuals deficient in complement components. C3 deficiency in particular is always associated with repeated severe bacterial infections that without adequate prophylaxis inevitably lead to early death.

C3b disaggregates immune complexes and promotes their clearance.

Immune complexes containing antigens derived either from pathogens or from the death of host cells form continuously in health and disease. Because they tend to grow by aggregation and acquisition of more components, they can cause disease by precipitating in capillary beds in the skin, kidney and other organs, where they drive inflammation.

Complement activation on the immune complex via the classical pathway efficiently opsonizes the immune complex and helps prevent precipitation in tissues:

- coating with C3b masks the foreign antigens in the core of the immune complex, blocking further growth;
- coating with C3b disaggregates large immune complexes by disrupting interactions between antigen and antibody;

- C3b (and C4b) on immune complexes interact with CR1 on erythrocytes, taking the immune complex out of the plasma – the **immune adherence phenomenon**.

Immune complex adherence to erythrocytes provides an efficient means of handling and transporting the hazardous cargo to sites of disposal (i.e. the resident macrophages in spleen and liver). Importantly, immune complex binding to CR1 is a dynamic process: CR1 binds C3b but this renders the C3b susceptible to cleavage to iC3b by FI; iC3b does not bind CR1 and the complex is released only to be captured again through another C3b. In the spleen and liver, the immune complex is:

- released from the erythrocyte as described; and
- captured by complement and immunoglobulin receptors on the macrophage, internalized and destroyed.

The MAC damages some bacteria and enveloped viruses.

Assembly of the MAC creates a pore that inserts into and through the lipid bilayer, breaching the membrane barrier (see Fig. 4.8). The consequences of MAC attack vary from target to target:

- For most pathogens, opsonization is the most important antibacterial action of complement.
- For Gram-negative bacteria, particularly organisms of the genus *Neisseria*, MAC attack is a major component of host defence and individuals deficient in components of the MAC (e.g. patients with C6 deficiency, which is the second most common deficiency of complement) are susceptible to neisserial infection.

Gram-negative bacteria are protected by a double cell membrane separated by a peptidoglycan wall. Precisely how MAC traverses these protective structures to damage the inner bacterial membrane and causes osmotic lysis of these organisms remains unclear. The MAC:

- may also play roles in the efficient dispatching of other pathogens, including some viruses;
- can also damage or destroy host cells – in some instances, such as autoimmunity, the host cell is itself the target and complement is directly activated on the cell, overwhelming complement regulators and other defence mechanisms leading to MAC-mediated damage;
- can impact neighbouring cells not the target of the initial activation – bystander damage.

Erythrocytes have only a limited capacity to resist and to repair damage and can be lysed, as is seen in autoimmune haemolytic anaemias and some other haemolytic disorders. Although nucleated host cells may escape lysis by MAC, the insertion of pores in the membrane is not without consequence. Ions, particularly Ca^{2+}, flow into the cell and cause activation events with diverse outcomes that may contribute to disease.

Immune complexes with bound C3b are very efficient in priming B cells.

Complement is a key component of the innate immune response. However, it has recently become apparent that complement also plays important roles in adaptive immunity. This realization arose from studies in complement-depleted and complement-deficient mice in which antibody responses to foreign particles were markedly reduced. At least three linked mechanisms contribute to this effect (Fig. 4.12):

- first, immature B cells directly bind foreign particles through the B-cell receptor (BCR) recognizing specific antigen in the particle and through CR2 recognizing attached C3dg – this co-ligation triggers B-cell maturation, with the mature cells migrating to the lymphoid organs;
- second, while in the lymph nodes, mature B cells encounter opsonized antigen and, in the presence of B-cell help, are induced to become activated and to proliferate;
- third, in the lymphoid organs FDCs capture antigen through attached C3 fragments and use this bait to select the correct activated B cells and switch them on to further maturation

and proliferation to form plasma cells and B memory cells (see Chapters 9 and 12).

The overriding principle of this adjuvant effect of C3 opsonization is that simultaneous engagement of CR2 and BCR on the B cell, by recruiting signalling molecules to form an activation complex on the B-cell surface, efficiently triggers the B-cell response. As a consequence, a complement-opsonized particle may be 1000-fold as active as the unopsonized particle in triggering antibody production.

More recently, roles for both C3a and C5a as modifiers of antigen presentation by FDC and other DCs have emerged that help to shape the primary immune response; the physiological relevance of these interactions and the impact of anaphylatoxins on protective immunity in vivo is not yet clear.

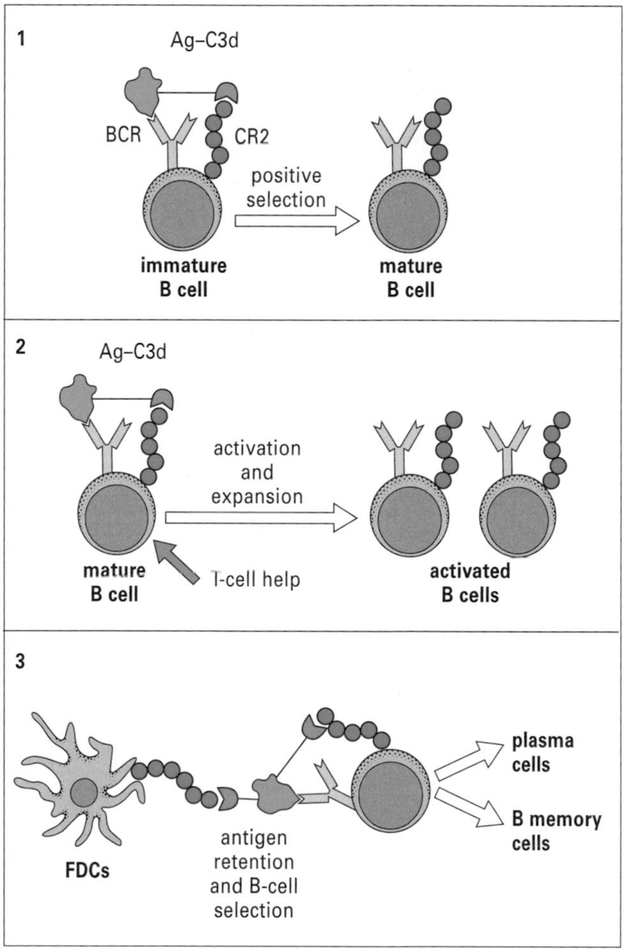

COMPLEMENT DEFICIENCIES

Genetic deficiencies of each of the complement components and many of the regulators have been described and provide valuable experiments of nature, illustrating the homeostatic roles of complement. In general, complement deficiencies are rare, although some deficiencies are much more common in some racial groups.

A variety of assays (Method Box 4.1) are available for detecting:

- the activity of different complement pathways;
- the functional activity of individual components;
- the total amount of individual components (functional or non-functional).

The consequences of a deficiency in part of the complement system depend upon the pathway(s) affected (Fig. 4.13).

Classical pathway deficiencies result in tissue inflammation. Deficiency of any of the components of the classical pathway (C1, C4 and C2) predisposes to a condition that closely resembles the autoimmune disease systemic lupus erythematosus (SLE), in which immune complexes become deposited in capillary networks, particularly in kidney, skin and brain.

Deficiency of any of the C1 subunits (C1q, C1r or C1s) invariably causes severe disease with typical SLE features including skin lesions and kidney damage. The disease usually manifests early in childhood and few patients reach adulthood.

C4 deficiency also causes severe SLE. Total deficiency of C4 is extremely rare because C4 is encoded by two separate genes (*C4A* and *C4B*), but partial deficiencies of C4 are relatively common and are associated with a gene dose-dependent increased incidence of SLE.

C2 deficiency is the commonest complement deficiency in Caucasians. Although it predisposes to SLE, the majority of C2-deficient individuals are healthy.

The large majority of cases of SLE are, however, not associated with complement deficiencies, and autoimmune SLE is discussed in Chapter 20. The historical view of the pathogenesis of immune complex disease in classical pathway deficiency was that it was a result of defective immune complex handling.

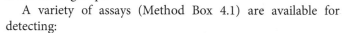

Fig. 4.12 Complement plays important roles in adaptive immunity C3 fragments bound to antigen *(Ag)* bind complement receptors on B cells and follicular dendritic cells *(FDCs)*, enhancing B-cell development at multiple stages in the process. **(1)** B cells bind Ag through the B-cell receptor *(BCR)* and bind Ag-attached C3d through CR2. The combined signals, delivered through these receptors and their co-receptors, markedly enhance positive selection of Ag-reactive B cells and subsequent maturation. **(2)** Binding of C3d-opsonized Ag to mature B cells in the lymphoid follicles (with appropriate T-cell help) triggers B-cell activation and proliferation. **(3)** In the spleen and bone marrow, C3d-opsonized Ag binds complement receptors on FDCs to retain Ag on the FDC, where it is efficiently presented to activated B cells. Ligation of BCR and C3d on the activated B cell triggers differentiation to plasma cells and B memory cells.

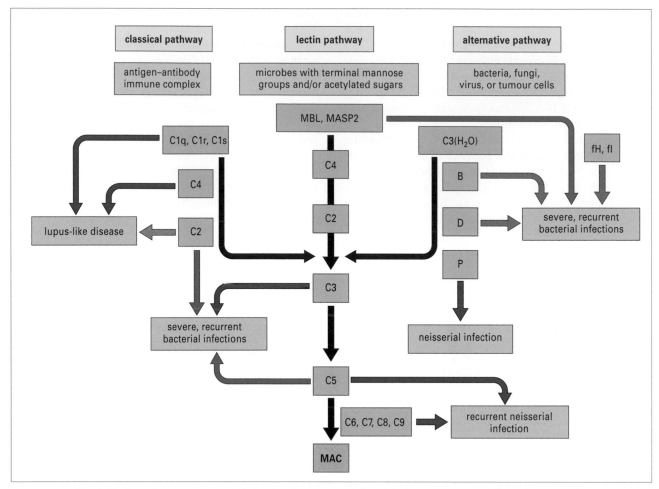

Fig. 4.13 Complement system deficiencies A summary of the clinical consequences of the various complement deficiencies. *Black arrows* denote pathway, *red arrows* show strong effects and *blue arrows* indicate weak effects. *MAC*, Membrane attack complex.

Although these mechanisms of immune complex handling undoubtedly contribute, a new perspective has recently developed that takes a different view of the role of complement in waste management.

Cells continually die by apoptosis in tissues and are removed silently by tissue macrophages. Complement contributes to this essential process because the apoptotic cell binds C1q and activates the classical pathway. In C1 deficiencies, apoptotic cells accumulate in the tissues and eventually undergo necrosis, which releases toxic cell contents and causes inflammation.

This recent observation, emerging from studies in complement deficiencies, has altered the way we think of the handling of waste in the body and moved complement to centre stage in this vital housekeeping role.

Deficiencies of MBL are associated with infection in infants. MBL is a complex multi-chain **collectin**. Each chain comprises a collagenous stalk linked to a globular carbohydrate recognition domain.

The plasma level of MBL is extremely variable in the population and governed by a series of single nucleotide polymorphisms in the *MBL* gene, either in the promoter region or in the first exon, encoding part of the collagenous stalk:

- mutations in the promoter region alter the efficiency of gene transcription;
- mutations in the first exon disrupt the regular structure of the collagenous stalk, destabilizing complexes containing mutated chains and perhaps disrupting association with the MASP enzymes.

At least seven distinct haplotypes arise from mixing of these mutations, four of which yield very low plasma MBL levels. As a consequence, at least 10% of the population have MBL levels below 0.1 µg/mL and are considered to be MBL deficient.

MBL deficiency in infants is associated with increased susceptibility to bacterial infections. This tendency disappears as the individual ages and the other arms of immunity mature.

In adults, MBL deficiency is of little consequence unless there is an accompanying immunosuppression – for example, people with HIV infection who are MBL deficient appear to have more infections than those who have high levels of MBL.

Alternative pathway and C3 deficiencies are associated with bacterial infections.

Deficiencies of either **FB** or **FD** prevent complement amplification through the alternative pathway amplification loop, markedly reducing the efficiency of opsonization of pathogens. As a consequence, deficient individuals are susceptible to bacterial infections and present with a history of severe recurrent infections with a variety of pyogenic (pus-forming) bacteria. Only a few families with each of these deficiencies have been identified, but the severity of the condition makes it imperative to identify affected families so that prophylactic antibiotic therapy can be initiated.

C3 is the cornerstone of complement, essential for all activation pathways and for MAC assembly, and is also the source of the major opsonic fragments C3b and iC3b. Individuals with **C3 deficiency** present early in childhood with a history of severe, recurrent bacterial infections affecting the respiratory system, gut, skin and other organs. Untreated, all die before adulthood. When given broad-spectrum antibiotic prophylaxis, patients do reasonably well and normally survive into adulthood.

Total deficiency of the alternative pathway regulator, FH, results in dysregulation of the alternative pathway and consumption of C3; patients usually present with a kidney disease called dense deposit disease (DDD) where complement deposits in the glomeruli, leading to renal failure.

Terminal pathway deficiencies predispose to Gram-negative bacterial infections.

Deficiencies of any of the terminal complement components (C5, C6, C7, C8 or C9) predispose to infections with Gram-negative bacteria, particularly those of the genus *Neisseria*. This genus includes the meningococci responsible for meningococcal meningitis and the gonococci responsible for gonorrhoea. Gram-negative bacteria are susceptible to MAC lysis because they possess an outer phospholipid membrane that MAC can disrupt. In contrast, Gram-positive bacteria are protected from MAC by their thick cell walls.

Individuals with terminal pathway deficiencies usually present with meningitis, which is often recurrent and sometimes accompanied by septicaemia. Any patients presenting with a second or third episode of meningococcal infection without obvious physical cause should be screened for complement deficiencies because prophylactic antibiotic therapy can be life-saving. Terminal pathway-deficient patients should also be intensively immunized with the best-available meningococcal vaccines.

It is likely that terminal pathway deficiencies are relatively common and under-ascertained in most countries:

- In Caucasians and most other groups investigated, C6 deficiency is the most common.
- In the Japanese population, C9 deficiency is very common, with an incidence of more than 1 in 500 of the population.

C1 inhibitor deficiency causes hereditary angioedema.

Deficiency of the classical pathway regulator C1inh is responsible for the syndrome **hereditary angioedema (HAE)**.

C1inh regulates C1 in the classical pathway and MBL/MASP-2 (or ficolin/MASP-2) in the lectin pathway and also controls activation in the kinin pathway that leads to the generation of bradykinin and other active kinins. The oedema is mediated by two peptides generated by the uninhibited activation of the complement system (C2-kinin) and surface contact systems (bradykinin) (Fig. 4.w1 📶).

C1inh deficiency is a dominant condition.

HAE is relatively common because the disease presents even in those heterozygous for the deficiency (i.e. it is an autosomal dominant disease).

The halved C1inh synthetic capacity in those with HAE cannot maintain plasma levels in the face of continuing consumption of C1inh, which is a **suicide inhibitor** that is consumed as it works. As a consequence, the plasma levels measured are often only 10%–20% of normal, even in periods of apparent good health.

Episodes of angioedema are often triggered in the skin or mucous membranes by minor trauma – occasionally stress may be sufficient to induce an attack. Swelling, which may be remarkable in severity, rapidly ensues as unregulated activation of the kinin and complement systems occurs in the affected area, inducing vascular leakiness. Swelling of mucous membranes in the mouth and throat may block the airways, leading to asphyxia (Fig. 4.14). Involvement of gut mucosa can cause intestinal obstruction, presenting with acute abdominal symptoms.

Episodes of angioedema are transient and usually wane over the course of a few hours without therapy. Emergency treatment for life-threatening attacks involves the infusion of a purified C1inh concentrate. Although available in Europe for over 30 years, C1inh has only recently been approved for therapy of HAE in the United States. Prophylactic treatment usually involves the induction of C1inh synthesis using anabolic steroids or minimizing consumption of C1inh using protease inhibitors; however, C1inh is increasingly being used in prophylaxis.

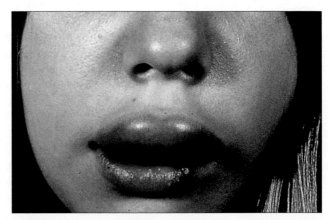

Fig. 4.14 Hereditary angioedema (HAE) This clinical photograph shows the transient localized swelling that occurs in HAE.

Although the majority of cases of HAE involve a mutation that prevents synthesis of C1inh by the defective gene (type I), in about 15% of cases the mutation results in the production of a functionally defective protein (type II). In type II HAE, the plasma levels of C1inh may be normal or even high, but its function is markedly impaired, leading to disease.

A similar syndrome to type II HAE can develop later in life. Acquired angioedema is, in most or all cases, associated with autoantibodies that:

- target C1inh;
- may arise in an otherwise healthy individual or may be associated with other autoimmune diseases, particularly SLE.

Occasionally, acquired angioedema occurs in association with a lymphoproliferative disorder, likely secondary to classical pathway activation and C1inh consumption by the tumour mass.

Deficiencies in alternative pathway regulators cause a secondary loss of C3.

FH or FI deficiency predisposes to bacterial infections. FH and FI collaborate to control activation of the alternative pathway amplification loop. Deficiency of either leads to uncontrolled activation of the loop and near-complete consumption of C3, which is the substrate of the loop. The resultant **acquired C3 deficiency** predisposes to bacterial infections and yields a clinical picture resembling that seen in primary C3 deficiency. As noted earlier, FH-deficient individuals usually present with renal disease.

Properdin deficiency causes severe meningococcal meningitis. Properdin is a stabilizer of the alternative pathway C3 convertase that increases efficiency of the amplification loop. **Properdin deficiency** is inherited in an X-linked manner and is therefore seen exclusively in males. Boys deficient in properdin present with severe meningococcal meningitis, often with septicaemia. The first attack is often fatal and survivors do not usually have recurrent infections because the acquisition of anti-meningococcal antibodies enables a response via the classical pathway in the next encounter. Diagnosis is nevertheless important to identify affected relatives before they get the disease; administration of meningococcal vaccine and antibiotic prophylaxis will prevent infection.

Autoantibodies against complement components, regulators and complexes also cause disease. The association of anti-C1inh autoantibodies with some cases of HAE was mentioned above. Autoantibodies against FH are frequently found in children (and less commonly in adults) with glomerulonephritis, probably causing disease by blocking FH activity. Autoantibodies against the C3 convertase enzyme, termed nephritic factors, are also found in rare patients with renal disease (dense deposit disease, closely resembling that seen in FH deficiency); these antibodies stabilize the convertase, increasing its lifetime and thereby causing complement dysregulation and disease.

COMPLEMENT POLYMORPHISMS AND DISEASE

Common polymorphisms are found in almost all complement proteins and regulators; associations with inflammatory and infectious diseases have been reported, particularly with respect to alternative pathway proteins and regulators. Most strikingly, a common polymorphism in FH (FH$_{Y402H}$) is strongly associated with the common, blinding eye disease, age-related macular degeneration (AMD), homozygosity for the H allele increasing risk of disease up to sevenfold. Polymorphisms in C3 and FB are also linked to AMD, suggesting that dysregulation of the alternative pathway underlies the pathology in this disease. Analysis of the disease-associated coding polymorphisms in the alternative pathway (in components C3, FB and FH) has demonstrated that the single amino acid changes in the variants cause subtle differences in function, variants that lead to more activation associate with inflammatory diseases. Although effects of individual changes are small, in the alternative pathway amplifying loop, these small differences are magnified to deliver large end effects; the combination of complement polymorphisms in an individual, dubbed the complotype, thus predicts plasma complement activity and disease risk.

COMPLEMENT THERAPEUTICS

Although it has been clear for many years that complement dysregulation contributes to many diseases, with the notable exception of C1inh therapy of HAE described earlier, therapeutic targeting of complement was not an option. This changed with the demonstration in 2004 that a C5-blocking antibody, eculizumab, markedly reduced haemolysis and the requirement for transfusions in patients with PNH. This was a game-changing finding that changed outlook not only for this ultra-rare complement dysregulation disease but also for a growing number of other diseases where the membrane attack pathway drives pathology. Eculizumab is currently approved for therapy of PNH and aHUS, both very rare conditions, but recent clinical trials have demonstrated efficacy in myasthenia gravis, neuromyelitis optica, autoimmune haemolytic anaemia and renal transplantation and the list is growing. Alongside the increase in use of eculizumab, there has been an explosion of new anti-complement drugs in preclinical studies and clinical trials, several of which will soon be approved for use in clinics. Although some of these are eculizumab mimics, others target different parts of the complement system (Fig. 4.15) and will undoubtedly mean that more diseases can be treated with an anti-complement approach.

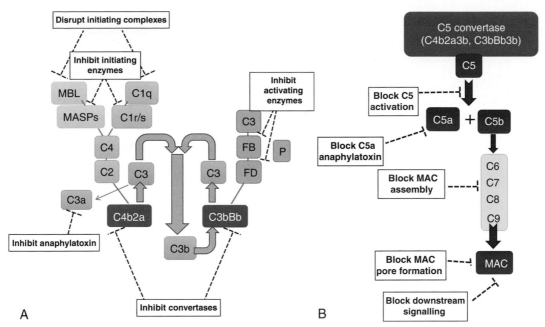

Fig. 4.15 Targets for therapy in the complement system The complement system presents a host of potential targets for therapeutic intervention, inhibiting specific enzymes, blocking cleavage sites or intermolecular interactions or preventing the activities of activation products. These targets are illustrated in the activation pathways (**A**) and terminal pathway (**B**). *MAC*, Membrane attack complex.

CRITICAL THINKING: COMPLEMENT DEFICIENCY

See Critical thinking: Explanations, section 4

A family has been identified in which three of the seven children have had repeated upper respiratory tract infections since early childhood. Of these, one has developed bacterial meningitis and another a fatal septicaemia. In all of the children the levels of antibodies in the serum are within the normal range. When an assay for haemolytic complement (CH50) is carried out, however, the three affected children are all found to be deficient in this functional assay.

1. Why would a deficiency in complement cause the children to be particularly susceptible to bacterial infections? Measurements are made of individual complement components of the classical and alternative pathways to determine which of the components is defective. The results are shown in the table.

Complement component	Normal concentration (µg/mL)	Levels in affected children (µg/mL)
C4	600	480–520
C2	20	15–22
C3	1300	10–80
Factor B (FB)	210	Not detectable
Factor H (FH)	480	200–350
Factor I (FI)	35	Not detectable

2. Using knowledge of the complement reaction pathways, how can you explain the apparent combined deficiencies in C3, FB and FI?

3. What is the fundamental deficiency in this family and how would you treat the affected children?

FURTHER READING

Grumach AS, Kirschfink M. Are complement deficiencies really rare? Overview on prevalence, clinical importance and modern diagnostic approach. Mol Immunol 2014;61:110–117.

Harris CL, Heurich M, Rodriguez de Cordoba S, Morgan BP. The complotype: dictating risk for inflammation and infection. Trends Immunol 2012;33:513–521.

Harrison RA. The properdin pathway: an "alternative activation pathway" or a "critical amplification loop" for C3 and C5 activation? Semin Immunopathol 2018;40:15–35.

Howard M, Farrar CA, Sacks SH. Structural and functional diversity of collectins and ficolins and their relationship to disease. Semin Immunopathol 2018;40:75–85.

Luque A, Serrano I, Aran JM. Complement components as promoters of immunological tolerance in dendritic cells. Semin Cell Dev Biol 2017. pii: S1084–9521(17)30131–3.

Morgan BP. The membrane attack complex as an inflammatory trigger. Immunobiology 2016;221:747–751.

Morgan BP, Boyd C, Bubeck D. Molecular cell biology of complement membrane attack. Semin Cell Dev Biol 2017;72:124–132.

Morgan BP, Harris CL. Complement, a target for therapy in inflammatory and degenerative diseases. Nat Rev Drug Discov 2015;14:857–877.

Sánchez-Corral P, Pouw RB, López-Trascasa M, Józsi M. Self-damage caused by dysregulation of the complement alternative pathway: relevance of the factor H protein family. Front Immunol 2018;9:1607.

Taylor RP, Lindorfer MA. Mechanisms of complement-mediated damage in hematological disorders. Semin Hematol 2018;55:118–123.

Wong EKS, Kavanagh D. Diseases of complement dysregulation – an overview. Semin Immunopathol 2018;40:49–64.

Zanichelli A, Wu MA, Andreoli A, Mansi M, Cicardi M. The safety of treatments for angioedema with hereditary C1 inhibitor deficiency. Expert Opin Drug Saf 2015;14:1725–1736.

5

Mononuclear Phagocytes in Immune Defence

SUMMARY

- **Macrophages: the 'big eaters'.** Macrophages are endowed with a remarkable capacity to internalize material through phagocytosis.
- **Macrophages are widely distributed throughout the body.** Macrophages belong to the family of mononuclear phagocytes, which also include monocytes, osteoclasts and dendritic cells. Phenotypically distinct populations of macrophages are present in each organ.
- **Macrophages are highly effective endocytic and phagocytic cells.** Macrophages have a highly developed endocytic compartment that mediates the uptake of a wide range of stimuli and targets them for degradation in lysosomes.
- **Macrophages sample their environment through opsonic and non-opsonic receptors.** Macrophages express a wide range of receptors that act as sensors of the physiological status of organs, including the presence of infection.
- **Clearance of apoptotic cells by macrophages produces anti-inflammatory signals.** Macrophages produce IL-10 and TGFβ upon internalization of apoptotic cells.
- **Macrophages coordinate the inflammatory response.** Recognition of necrotic cells and microbial compounds by macrophages initiates inflammation, leading to the recruitment of neutrophils. Monocyte recruitment to sites of inflammation is promoted by activated neutrophils and there is a collaborative effort between macrophages and neutrophils to eliminate the triggering insult. Macrophages are actively involved in the resolution of the inflammatory reaction.
- **There are different pathways of macrophage activation.** Cytokines and microbial compounds alter the activation state of macrophages. The TH1 cytokine IFNγ increases anti-microbial activity against intracellular pathogens. TH2 cytokines such as IL-4 and IL-13 induce an alternate activation that promotes tissue repair. TGFβ, corticosteroids and IL-10 can induce an anti-inflammatory phenotype that can contribute to resolution of inflammation. A spectrum of macrophage activation states is likely to occur during the different stages of inflammation.

MACROPHAGES: THE 'BIG EATERS'

Macrophages are cells of haematopoietic origin widely distributed throughout lymphoid and non-lymphoid tissues. They are endowed with a remarkable capacity to internalize material through endocytosis and phagocytosis, which makes them key players in both homeostasis and immune defence. Human macrophages clear approximately 2×10^{11} erythrocytes a day and are also implicated in the removal of cell debris and apoptotic cells, processes critical for normal development and physiology. The machinery mediating this homeostatic uptake also enables macrophages to recognize and to internalize invading microorganisms, a process that facilitates clearance of infectious agents and elicits inflammation. Macrophages are highly heterogeneous and differentiate according to the environmental cues and physiological conditions present in tissues, including the presence of microbes or cellular damage.

Macrophages are heterogeneous. Macrophages belong to the family of mononuclear phagocytes, which also includes monocytes, dendritic cells and osteoclasts. Mononuclear phagocytes are distributed throughout all tissues within the organism where they adapt to their local microenvironment and differentiate into various cell types (Fig. 5.1). Distinctive populations of resident macrophages are found in most tissues of the body; they differ in their life span, morphology and phenotype, for example the microglial cells in the brain appear quite unlike mononuclear phagocytes in other tissues (Fig. 5.2). In the bone marrow, mature macrophages are themselves part of the stromal microenvironment. They associate with developing haematopoietic cells to perform poorly defined non-phagocytic trophic functions, as well as removing effete cells and erythroid nuclei. In bone, osteoclasts, highly specialized multinucleated cells of monocytic origin, mediate bone resorption and their deficiency leads to osteopetrosis.

Secondary lymphoid organs contain several distinct types of macrophages. These macrophages have been better characterized in the mouse (Fig. 5.3) and subsets involved in the clearance of apoptotic lymphocytes (tingible body macrophages) or presentation of naive antigens to B cells (subcapsular sinus macrophages) have been identified. Macrophages involved in clearance of damaged red blood cells contributing to iron recycling are located in the red pulp of the spleen.

Anatomical differences between human and mouse spleen, such as the absence of a well-defined marginal sinus, correlates with phenotypical differences in splenic macrophages (see Fig. 5.3). Macrophages can also be found within interstitial spaces throughout the body. Interestingly, these interstitial macrophages do not differ among different organs to the same extent as bona fide tissue macrophages.

Macrophage Origin

It was considered for a long time that all tissue macrophages derived from circulating blood monocytes originated from haematopoietic stem cells in the bone marrow. This paradigm has

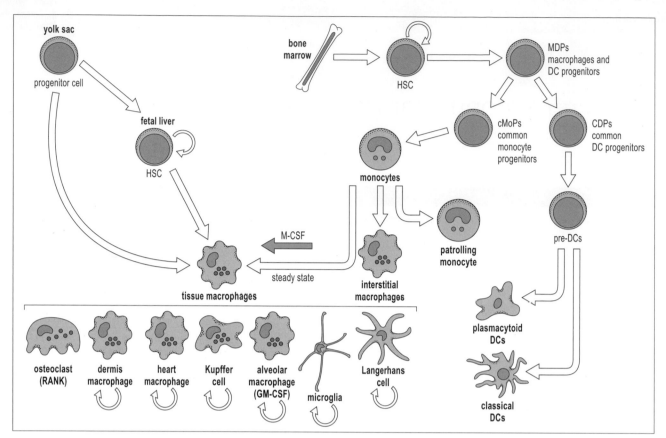

Fig. 5.1 Differentiation of mononuclear phagocytes In mice, precursors in the yolk sac and fetal liver give rise to different populations of tissue macrophages that are maintained through self-replication and monocyte differentiation. The contribution from monocytes is minimal in the case of microglia and alveolar macrophages and higher in the case of macrophages in other organs. Mononuclear phagocytes and some dendritic cells differentiate from a precursor in the bone marrow. Differentiation into monocytes occurs from common monocyte precursors. Monocytes give rise to patrolling monocytes that maintain endothelial integrity and interstitial macrophages in addition to tissue macrophages. *Circular arrows* indicate capacity for self renewal. Granulocyte-macrophage colony stimulating factor *(GM-CSF)* is particularly important for the differentiation of alveolar macrophages and RANK promotes the formation of osteoclasts. *DC*, dendritic cells; *HSC*, hematopoietic stem cells, *M-CSF*, macrophage colony stimulating factor.

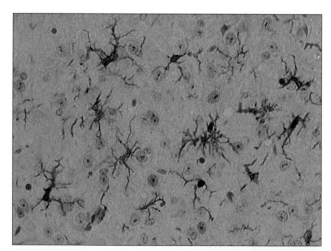

Fig. 5.2 Microglia in mouse brain stained for F4/80 Microglia are widely distributed in non-overlapping fields and show a dendritic morphology – mouse brain stained with antibody to F4/80. (Courtesy Dr Payam Rezaie.)

now been challenged by results showing that most tissue macrophages originate from precursors seeded during fetal development or perinatally and are long lived and replenished through both cell replication and/or monocyte recruitment, depending on the tissue and availability of precursors in different niches of the tissue. Monocytes are immune effector cells in their own right capable of detecting and internalizing pathogens and triggering inflammation. Recently, two subpopulations of monocytes have been described in human and mouse blood. These subpopulations display differential expression of surface receptors; monocytes expressing LY6C in mouse or CD14 in humans are migratory. Migratory monocytes can readily migrate to lymphoid and non-lymphoid tissues without undergoing major phenotypical changes. They can also give rise to interstitial macrophages and, to a lesser extent, to tissue macrophages (Fig. 5.4). Interstitial and tissue macrophages can also be maintained through self-replication. Finally, migratory monocytes also give rise to patrolling monocytes, which in mice lack LY6C expression and express CD43 and in humans express

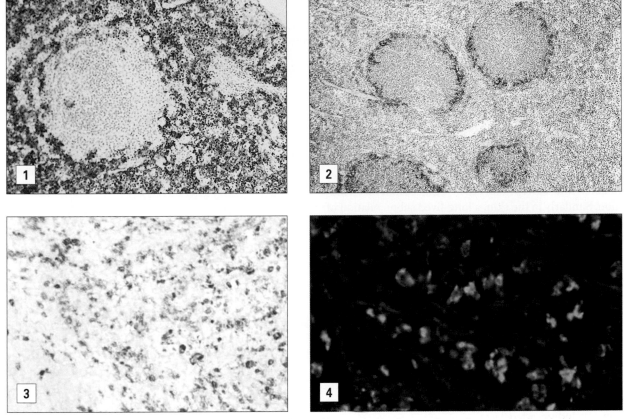

Fig. 5.3 Macrophages in secondary lymphoid tissues Heterogeneity of macrophages in secondary lymphoid organs of mice and humans. (**1**) Red pulp of spleen stained for F4/80. Macrophages stain strongly positive. (**2**) Mouse spleen stained with antibody to sialoadhesin. The marginal metallophils of spleen are strongly sialoadhesin (CD169) positive. (**3**) Human spleen stained for CD68 and (**4**) immunofluorescence staining with anti-CD68 *(green)*, and for the mannose receptor *(red)* indicates staining along sinusoids but most CD68⁺ macrophages lack the mannose receptor. Nuclei are stained *blue*. ((**1**) Courtesy Dr DA Hume. (**2**) Courtesy Dr PR Crocker.)

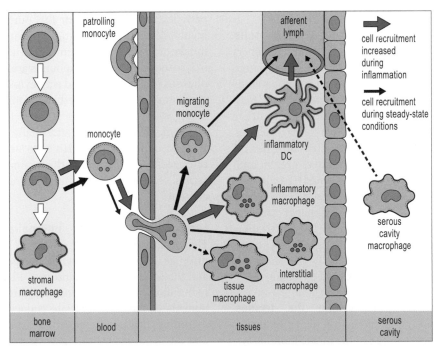

Fig. 5.4 Differentiation and distribution of macrophages Blood monocytes are derived from bone marrow and readily transit tissues with minimal differentiation. Monocytes can give rise to tissue macrophages and interstitial macrophages. At sites of inflammation, monocytes may develop into elicited inflammatory macrophages or dendritic cells, which can migrate through afferent lymph to the local lymph nodes. *Black arrows* indicate recruitment during steady-state conditions. *Red arrows* denote recruitment during inflammation. *White arrow* indicates differentiation of monocytes and resident stromal macrophages from precursors within the bone marrow. *Broken black arrow* denotes the ability of monocytes to differentiate into tissue macrophages and serous cavity macrophages to migrate through lymph.

CD16. Patrolling monocytes interact with the endothelium and are involved in removal of damaged cells and debris from the vasculature, hence contributing to maintenance of endothelial integrity.

Macrophage origin has important consequences during infection. In the lung, alveolar macrophages, located in alveolar spaces, are maintained largely through cell replication, while interstitial macrophages are maintained largely through monocyte recruitment. Phenotypical and metabolic differences between alveolar macrophages and interstitial macrophages underpin differential susceptibility to *Mycobacterium tuberculosis* infection. Similarly in the skin, a long-lived subpopulation of macrophages, not derived from monocytes, that express high levels of mannose receptor are preferentially infected by *Leishmania major*, leading to non-healing chronic lesions.

M-CSF is required for macrophage differentiation.

Macrophage colony stimulating factor (M-CSF) is a major growth, differentiation and survival factor, selective for monocytes and macrophages. It is produced constitutively by fibroblasts, stromal cells, endothelial cells, macrophages and smooth muscle. Most members of the mononuclear phagocyte family express the receptor for M-CSF, CD115, and mice deficient in M-CSF have major defects in different macrophage populations, including osteoclasts.

In contrast, granulocyte-macrophage colony stimulating factor (GM-CSF) primarily regulates myeloid cell production. It is only produced after cell activation and mice deficient in GM-CSF have no major defects in macrophage populations, with only the maturation of alveolar macrophage being altered, leading to pulmonary alveolar proteinosis.

Macrophages can act as antigen-presenting cells.

Macrophages, like dendritic cells, have all the machinery required for antigen processing and presentation of exogenous peptides and endogenous peptides on major histocompatibility complex (MHC) class II and class I, respectively. Cross-presentation, a process by which peptides of exogenous origin are presented on MHC class I, also takes place in macrophages. While dendritic cells are uniquely suited for stimulating naive T cells in secondary lymphoid organs, macrophages present antigen in the periphery to activated (already primed) T cells. This interaction makes macrophages important effector cells during adaptive immunity (Fig. 5.5). Some macrophages can also acquire suppressive characteristics and inhibit T-cell activation. The specialization of dendritic cells for antigen presentation correlates with a reduced degradative capacity that facilitates the generation of MHC-peptide complexes (see Chapter 7).

Macrophages act as sentinels within the tissues.

Macrophages react to a wide range of environmental influences that help to fulfil their role as sentinels of the innate immune system (Fig. 5.6). The presence of cells within tissues with the potential to initiate inflammation through the release of cytokines and chemokines and to cause tissue damage through the production of reactive oxygen species requires control systems capable of down-modulating macrophage activation. One of these systems involves the molecule CD200L, which is an inhibitory receptor

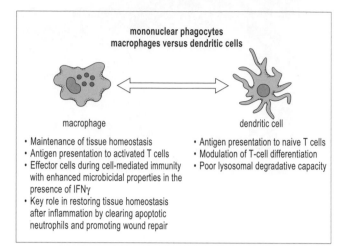

Fig. 5.5 Comparison of the functions of macrophages and dendritic cells

expressed by myeloid cells. CD200L inhibitory signalling is triggered through interaction with CD200 expressed by non-haematopoietic cells and macrophages. The CD200–CD200L interaction is important for the control of macrophage activation by other cells present in tissues.

PHAGOCYTOSIS AND ENDOCYTOSIS

Soluble compounds are internalized by endocytosis.

Macrophages play a key role in the clearance of altered forms of lipoproteins (e.g. acetylated lipoproteins) or glycoproteins (e.g. asialylated mannosylated proteins or proteins bearing advanced glycan products), damaged or apoptotic cells, pollutant particles and microbes. For this purpose, macrophages have a highly developed endocytic compartment that mediates the uptake of a wide range of stimuli and targets them for degradation in lysosomes. Soluble compounds are internalized through fluid phase or receptor-mediated endocytosis (see later), leading to the generation of vesicles called endosomes. Endosomes mature by fusing with different endocytic vesicles from the early and late endocytic compartments and finally the endocytosed material is targeted to lysosomes. This endosomal trafficking is also characterized by a reduction in the luminal pH, which facilitates the action of acid hydrolases and degradation of the endosomal content.

Large particles are internalized by phagocytosis.

Phagocytosis involves the uptake of particulate material (>0.5 μm), its engulfment through the generation of pseudopodia and the formation of phagosomes. Phagosomes follow a similar maturation process to endosomes through the fusion with components of the early and late endocytic compartments so that maturing phagosomes sequentially adopt characteristics of early and late endosomes; this process culminates in the fusion of phagosomes to lysosomes to form phagolysosomes (Fig. 5.7). Phagosomal maturation is accompanied by acidification of the lumen (to between pH 6.1 and 6.5 in early phagosomes and to pH 4.5 in phagolysosomes). Proteins broken down in the acidic endosomes can become associated with MHC class II molecules for presentation to T helper cells as described in Chapter 7.

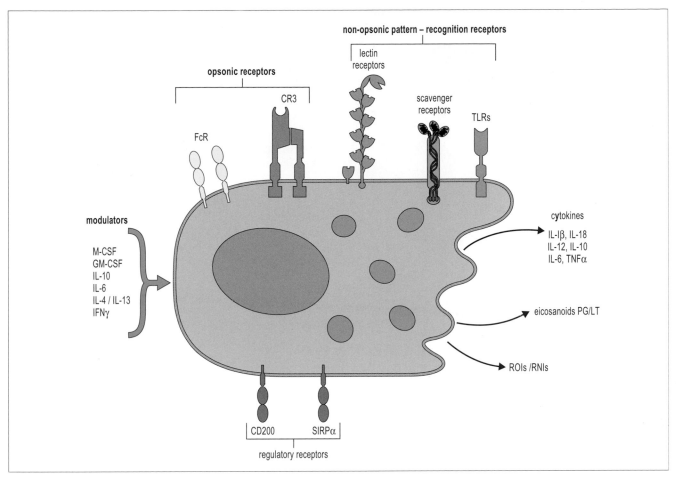

Fig. 5.6 Macrophage phenotype and function Macrophage phenotype and function are modulated by the cytokines shown on the left. They can sense their environment via opsonic receptors for antibody *(FcR)* and complement C3b *(CR3)* and via pattern-recognition receptors. They are also negatively regulated via CD200 and signal regulatory protein-alpha *(SIRPα)*. Macrophages secrete cytokines and eicosanoids (prostaglandins and leukotrienes) and may release reactive oxygen and nitrogen intermediates *(ROIs, RNIs)* at sites of inflammation. *TLRs*, Toll-like receptors.

Acidification also controls membrane traffic and has a direct effect on microbial growth. Other microbicidal mechanisms associated with phagosome maturation are the generation of reactive oxygen and nitrogen species, the presence of antimicrobial proteins and peptides and nutrient sequestration.

Host cells control the phagocytic activity of macrophages by displaying the 'don't eat me' signal CD47. CD47 engages a receptor in macrophages called SIRPα that inhibits the uptake process through its immunoreceptor tyrosine-based inhibitory motif (ITIM) motif. CD47 expression by tumour cells has been proposed as an immunosurveillance escape mechanism.

Macrophages sample their environment through opsonic and non-opsonic receptors. Macrophages have a wide range of receptors that act as sensors of the physiological status of organs, including the presence of infection. These receptors can be categorized as opsonic or non-opsonic, depending on their capacity to interact directly with the stimuli or their need for a bridging molecule such as an antibody or fragments of the complement component C3, which act as opsonins.

Opsonic receptors require antibody or complement to recognize the target. Bacteria opsonized by C3 fragments or antibody engage complement receptors (CR) or Fc receptors (FcR). CR-dependent phagocytosis is not an automatic process but requires additional stimulation such as inflammation. Monocytes and macrophages express a range of receptors (CR1, CR3, CR4) for C3 cleavage products that may become bound to pathogens, immune complexes or other complement activators (see Table 4.3). The role of CR3 in regulated phagocytosis has been well studied and the mechanism of CR3-mediated ingestion differs strikingly from that mediated by Fc receptors.

FcRs belong to the immunoglobulin superfamily (see Fig. 10.15). The best characterized FcR is CD64 (FcγRI), the high-affinity receptor for IgG, which signals through the common γ chain that contains an immunoreceptor tyrosine-based activation motif (ITAM). The common γ chain is also used by some non-opsonic receptors that bind carbohydrates (see later) and it signals through the key kinase Syk. In humans, other activating receptors for IgG are low-affinity FcγRIIa (CD32) and FcγRIII (CD16), which require the recognition of

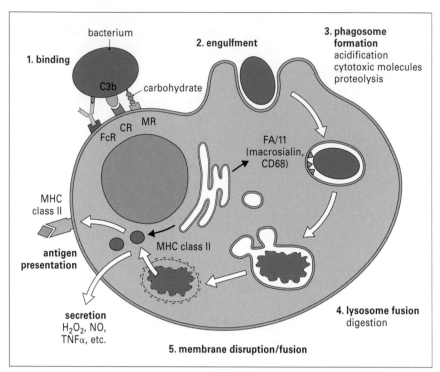

Fig. 5.7 **Phagocytosis mediated by opsonic receptors** *(1)* Pathogens, such as bacteria or fungi, are taken up by binding to opsonic receptors including the Fc receptor *(FcR)*, complement receptors *(CR)* and receptors for carbohydrate, e.g. mannose receptor *(MR)* or dectin-1. *(2)* The particle is engulfed and the phagosome forms *(3)*. Acidification of the phagosome follows as toxic molecules (reactive oxygen and nitrogen intermediates) are pumped into the phagosome. The marker CD68 is located in the phagosome membrane. *(4)* Lysosomes fuse with the phagosome, releasing proteolytic enzymes into the phagolysosome, which digest the pathogen. *(5)* On completion, the membrane of the phagolysosome is disrupted. Antigenic fragments may become diverted to the acidic endosome compartment for interaction with major histocompatibility complex *(MHC)* class II molecules and antigen presentation. The process induces secretion of toxic molecules and cytokines. TNFα, tumour necrosis factor–α.

immune complexes to induce internalization. IgG-opsonized material is readily internalized by macrophages and leads to the production of reactive oxygen species and cellular activation. The activating effect of ITAM-associated FcγRs is regulated by the presence of the inhibitory form of CD32 (FcγRIIb), which bears an ITIM.

The mechanism for ingestion of antibody-coated particles is distinct from that mediated by CR3 (Fig. 5.8). FcR-mediated uptake proceeds by a zipper-like process where sequential attachment between receptors and ligands guides pseudopod flow around the circumference of the particle. In contrast, CR3 contact sites are discontinuous for complement-coated particles, which 'sink' into the macrophage cytoplasm. Small GTPases play distinct roles in actin cytoskeleton engagement by each receptor-mediated process.

The best characterized non-opsonic receptors are the Toll-like receptors. Non-opsonic receptors or pattern recognition receptors (PRRs) recognize unusual features characteristic of damaged, malfunctioning or infected tissues and their general characteristics are described in Chapter 3.

Toll-like receptors (TLRs) are membrane glycoproteins with an extracellular region responsible for ligand binding and a cytoplasmic domain responsible for triggering an intracellular

signalling cascade. They can form hetero- or homodimers with each other or complex with other receptors in order to detect a wide range of microbial components. They are located at the cell surface or within endosomes. In humans, there are 10 of these receptors and together they are able to recognize a wide range of microbes, including Gram-positive bacteria and mycobacteria (see Table 3.2). For example, TLR4 detects Gram-negative bacteria because of its ability to recognize endotoxin (lipopolysaccharide, LPS). It then signals to the cell using similar systems to those mediated by IL-1 (Fig. 5.9). It can also activate the macrophage by a second pathway that is initiated by TRIF which leads to a secondary production of IFNβ and autocrine activation of additional macrophage genes.

CD14 is a glycosylphophatidylinisotol-anchored membrane protein that facilitates the recognition of LPS by TLR4 so that it increases LPS sensitivity (see Fig. 5.9). Recently, CD14 has also been shown to facilitate recognition of ligands by TLR2 and TLR3, which opens the possibility of CD14 acting as a multifunctional adapter protein.

TLR4 also recognizes degraded extracellular matrix and the nuclear protein high mobility group protein B1 (HMGB1), which can be released by necrotic cells. HMGB1 is an example of damage-associated molecules that are released upon tissue damage during trauma or infection.

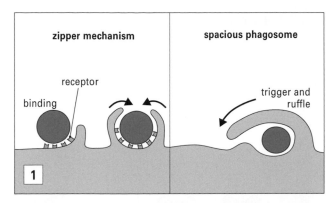

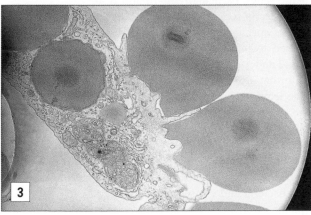

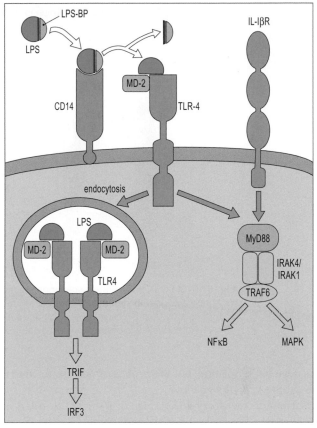

Fig. 5.9 Activation of macrophages by lipopolysaccharide *(LPS)* and IL-1 LPS binds leukocyte CD14 (which is glycosylphophatidylinisotol-anchored to the membrane) through LPS binding protein *(LPS-BP)* and it is transferred to a transmembrane LPS complex composed of Toll-like receptor–4 *(TLR4)* and *(MD-2)*. Binding of LPS to myeloid differentiation factor 2 *(MD-2)* initiates signal transduction both at the plasma membrane and endosomes. Signalling pathways of TLRs at the plasma membrane share elements with the IL-1βR pathway (e.g. IRAK4/IRAK1 – IL-1R-associated kinase). Cell activation proceeds via both the mitogen-activated protein kinase *(MAPK)* pathways and the induction of NFκB. At the endosomes, TLR4 triggers signalling through TIR domain-containing adapter-inducing interferon beta *(TRIF)*, which activates the transcription factor IRF3 (interferon regulatory factor 3).

Fig. 5.8 Zipper model of phagocytosis (1) During phagocytosis, receptor–ligand interactions guide the extension of tightly apposed pseudopods around the particle's total circumference until a fusion of the plasma membrane occurs at the tip. This is known as the zipper mechanism. Alternative trigger mechanisms, in which spacious phagosomes result from flipping over of ruffles back onto the plasma membrane, have also been described. The cytoskeleton of phagocytes plays a key role in engulfment, during which there is extensive remodelling of actin filaments. Some microorganisms and intracellular parasites induce novel mechanisms to recruit cell membranes during entry into phagocytes. (**2** and **3**) Electron micrographs of ingestion of antibody (IgG)-coated sheep erythrocytes by peritoneal macrophage by the zipper mechanism. ((**2**)Scanning electron micrograph courtesy Dr GG MacPherson. (**3**) Transmission electron micrograph courtesy Dr SC Silverstein.)

TLRs activate macrophages through several different pathways. The key adapter molecules that mediate TLR signalling are MyD88 (Fig. 5.w1) and TRIF, both of which interact with the Toll/IL-1R homologous region (TIR) cytoplasmic domain of TLRs either directly or indirectly through an adapter molecule. Most TLRs signal either through MyD88 or TRIF, but

TLR4 is unique in its ability to signal through both. The range of responses elicited by TLRs in macrophages is vast and includes the activation of the NFκB signalling pathway (see Fig. 5.w1) and MAP kinases, responsible for the production of proinflammatory cytokines and induction of microbicidal mechanisms. Signalling through the IL-1 and IL-18 receptors is also mediated by MyD88 (see Fig. 5.9).

The TRIF pathway induces interferon regulatory factor (IRF) transcription factors that will lead to the production of type 1 interferons, which can then stimulate the macrophage to cause a second, delayed wave of gene activation (Fig. 5.w2).

Lectin and scavenger receptors are non-opsonic receptors that recognize carbohydrates and modified proteins directly. In the plasma membrane, members of the scavenger receptor and lectin families mediate the recognition of modified lipoproteins and carbohydrates, respectively. Most of these receptors have signalling and internalization motifs in their cytoplasmic region and are capable of mediating endocytosis and

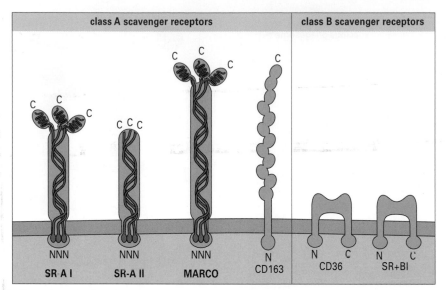

Fig. 5.10 Class A and related scavenger receptors Selected scavenger receptors are shown. Scavenger receptors of macrophages are responsible for the uptake of apoptotic cells, modified lipoproteins, other polyanionic ligands (e.g. LPS and lipoteichoic acids (LTA)) and selected bacteria such as *Neisseria* spp. CD163 is involved in endocytosis of haemoglobin–haptoglobin complexes.

phagocytosis in isolation, but their role is largely confined to the fine-tuning of TLR signalling.

Scavenger receptors (SR) (Fig. 5.10) such as SR-A are involved in LPS clearance, and may serve to downregulate responses induced via the TLR4–CD14 pathway (see Fig. 5.9) and therefore limit the systemic release of TNFα and resultant septic shock. SR-A has also been involved in bacterial uptake. Another member of this family, CD36, collaborates with TLR2 in the recognition of *Staphylococcus aureus* and *M. tuberculosis*.

Dectin-1 (Fig. 5.11), a lectin with a single lectin-like domain and an intracellular ITAM-like motif, is highly specific for the fungi-derived compound β-glucan (Fig. 5.12). Dectin-1-mediated effects are largely mediated by the kinase Syk and the adapter Card 9. Dectin-1 mediates phagocytosis of β-glucan particles and synergizes with TLRs to boost immune responses. It also has a role in TH cell differentiation and β-glucan-treated dendritic cells promote the development of TH17 cells. Humans deficient in dectin-1 are more susceptible to mucosal candidiasis.

The mannose receptor (MR) may play a unique role in tissue homeostasis as well as host defence (see Fig. 5.11). Endogenous ligands include lysosomal hydrolases and myeloperoxidase. The N-terminal cysteine-rich domain of the MR is a distinct lectin for sulfated glycoconjugates, highly expressed in secondary lymphoid organs. The cysteine-rich domain also contributes to the clearance of hormones such as lutropin. MR can internalize collagen, which is recognized through the fibronectin type II domain, and recent evidence suggests that MR promotes TH2 responses, which correlates with its capacity to interact with multiple glycosylated allergens and secreted helminth products.

DC-SIGN, another mannose-binding C-type lectin (see Fig. 5.11), is expressed on some macrophages. It forms tetramers and lacks obvious signalling motifs at its cytoplasmic region. It has been implicated in interactions between APCs and T cells

and in microbial recognition. DC-SIGN has been shown to modulate TLR signalling to promote transcription of various cytokine genes, particularly IL-10 and IL-8.

Other lectin receptors are langerin and dectin-2, which have mannose specificity, and Mincle, which recognizes ligands expressed by necrotic cells in addition to fungal pathogens. Dectin-2 and Mincle (see Fig. 5.11) signal through the common γ-chain that also mediates signalling by the FcγR, CD64.

The lectin receptor DCIR (dendritic cell immunoreceptor) bears an ITIM. Animals deficient in DCIR have altered DC numbers and increased susceptibility to autoimmune diseases.

Cytosolic receptors recognize intracellular pathogens.
Cytosolic receptors include two families of molecules that recognize bacteria and viruses:

- the nucleotide binding and oligomerization domain (NOD)-like receptors (NLR) recognize, among others, bacterial compounds such as peptidoglycan; and
- the retinoic acid-inducible gene I (*RIG-I*)-like helicases (RLHs) recognize nucleic acids such as dsRNA, which are produced during viral replication (Fig. 5.13).

Some of the NLRs form part of a multi-protein complex, the **inflammasome**, which is assembled in the cytoplasm and triggers inflammatory cell death (pyroptosis) of the infected cell. Pyroptosis causes release of cell contents and induces inflammation. Caspase 1 also processes the precursors of IL-1 and IL-18 to produce the active inflammatory cytokines. The composition of the inflammasome varies depending on the initiating stimulus because the NLRs responsible for the formation of the inflammasome complex are activated by different agents (see Fig. 5.13).

The two RLH proteins RIG-1 and MDA5 both recognize viral infection, but they have different specificities. For example RIG-1 is important in the recognition of the influenza virus, whereas MDA5 recognizes the poliovirus. Both RIG-1 and

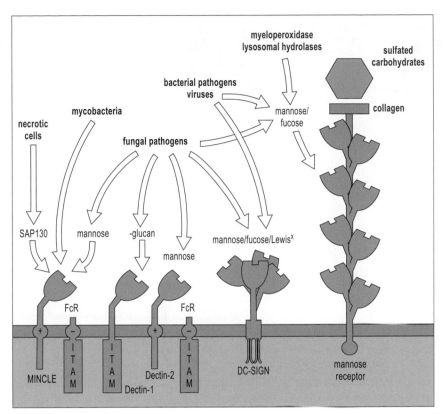

Fig. 5.11 Lectin receptors The mannose receptor contains eight C-type lectin domains involved in binding to mannosylated carbohydrates and related glycoconjugates. A distinct lectin domain located in the distal (C terminal) segment binds sulfated glycoconjugates. The β-glucan receptor (dectin-1) contains a single lectin domain and an intracellular immunoreceptor tyrosine-based activation motif *(ITAM)*. Both dectin-2 and MINCLE recognize mannose and are associated with the common γ chain that is associated with Fc receptors *(FcR)*. DC-SIGN recognizes mannose and fucose through four associated lectin domains. '+' indicates charged amino acid residues.

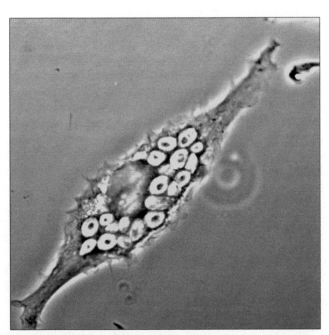

Fig. 5.12 Zymosan particles phagocytosed by a macrophage The micrograph shows zymosan (yeast) particles phagocytosed by a macrophage, a process dependent on dectin-1. Truncation of the cytoplasmic tail prevents phagocytosis.

MDA5 are involved in the recognition of Dengue virus. There are also cytosolic receptors able to recognize DNA.

Mechanism of action of NLRs. All **NLR proteins** have a similar domain structure:

- an N-terminal region that is involved in the recruitment of adapter molecules that link ligand recognition to signal transduction;
- a central nucleotide binding and oligomerization domain (NACHT/NOD) that mediates oligomerization; and
- a C-terminal leucine-rich repeat (LRR) that mediates recognition of pathogen-associated molecular patterns or damage-associated molecular patterns.

Two key members of the NLR family are **NOD-1** and **NOD-2,** which recognize fragments of peptidoglycan generated during the division of Gram-negative and Gram-positive bacteria (Fig. 5.w3). Detection of peptidoglycan through NOD receptors leads to the recruitment of the adapter RICK, activation of NFκB and promotion of inflammation.

NOD-1 polymorphisms are associated with the development of atopic eczema, asthma and increased serum IgE concentrations. Three common mutations of amino acid residues near or within the NOD-2 LRR region are genetic risk factors for the development of Crohn's disease. NOD-2 deficiency leads

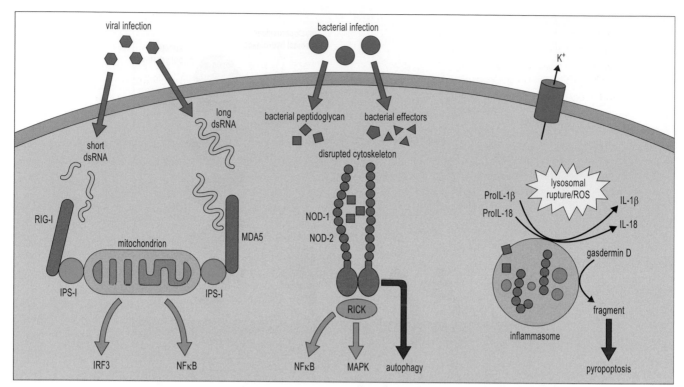

Fig. 5.13 Intracellular pattern recognition receptors (PRRs) Viral nucleic acids are recognized by RIG-1 and MDA-5, which assemble with the adapter protein IPS-1 onto the mitochondrial outer membrane and activate the transcription factors IRF3 and NFκB, which induce genes involved in inflammation. Bacterial peptidoglycans and other effector molecules cause disruption of the actin cytoskeleton, detected by NOD-1 and NOD-2, which signal through RICK to activate NFκB and the MAP-kinase (MAPK) pathway. Molecules of this type form inflammasomes that can lead to the processing of caspase-1. Processed active caspase-1 mediates cleavage of pro-IL-1β and pro-IL-18 into IL-1β and IL-18. Reactive oxygen species (ROS), lysosomal disruption and loss of intracellular K+ ions also signal cell disruption. Caspase-1 also digests gasdermin D and generates a 31 kDa fragment that forms pores in the membrane, leading to pyroptosis.

to increased susceptibility to bacterial infection via the oral route, implying that it may be required for expression of antimicrobial peptides. NOD-1 and NOD-2 can be activated by bacterial effectors in addition to peptidoglycan. It is proposed that the mechanism common to both processes is the disruption of the actin cytoskeleton. In agreement with this hypothesis, cytochalasin D, which blocks actin polymerization, increases NOD1- and NOD2-mediated NFκB activation in the absence of peptidoglycan.

Other NLR proteins, such as NLRP3, NLRP1 and IPAF, are components of multi-protein complexes called inflammasomes that lead to the activation of inflammatory caspases. Inflammatory caspases mediate the processing of pro-IL-1β and pro-IL-18 into their active counterparts and can lead to inflammation (see Fig. 5.13). Inflammatory caspases also cause inflammatory cell death or pyroptosis in which the affected cell dies, alerting the immune system to the presence of DAMPs by releasing its contents. Pyroptosis is caused by the processing of gasdermin D by caspase-1 and generation of a pore-forming 31 kDa fragment that damages the plasma membrane and leads to the release of intracellular components, including processed IL-1β. The assembly of inflammasomes can be induced by pathogens as well as by host-derived molecules, signs of metabolic stress and particles such as uric acid crystals and asbestos.

Mechanisms of action of RLH receptors. The **RLH receptors** include RIG-1 and MDA5. These proteins have an RNA helicase domain with ATPase activity that is activated by ligand binding and is necessary for signalling. After binding, RIG-I and MDA5 interact with the signalling-adapter molecule, IPS-1 (IFNβ promoter stimulator-1), present in the outer membrane of the mitochondria. This unit causes the activation of transcription factors, leading to the expression of IFNβ, IRF3-target genes and NFκB target genes. RNA recognition by RIG-I requires the presence of a free 5′-triphosphate structure, which allows for differential recognition of non-self/viral RNA versus self RNAs, as host RNA is either capped or post-translationally modified to remove the 5′-triphosphate.

The composition of the RNA molecule also has a role:
- MDA5 preferentially binds long dsRNAs (greater than 1 kb in length) and poly I:C;
- RIG-I is responsible for binding shorter dsRNA fragments.

Cytosolic DNA is capable of eliciting pro-inflammatory responses and several pathways can mediate this effect:
- engagement of a DNA receptor;
- detection by RIG-1 of an intermediate RNA molecule produced through the action of RNA polymerase-III;
- activation of the AIM-2 inflammasome. AIM-2 is an IFN-inducible protein and the first example of a non-NLR family member forming an inflammasome scaffold.

Infection can activate autophagy in macrophages.
Autophagy is a cellular process that maintains normal homeostasis by breaking down unrequired proteins (tagged with ubiquitin) and defunct organelles in a double-membrane bound vesicle that fuses with lysosomes. The process is normally linked to the nutritional status of the cell. In macrophages, autophagy can also be induced by ligation of TLRs by PAMPs and activation of MyD88 or TRIF (see Fig. 5.9). Functionally, there is considerable overlap between the breakdown of extracellular material in phagolysosomes and the breakdown of intracellular components in autophagosomes. While macrophages normally deal with bacterial infection by phagocytosis, followed by breakdown in phagolysosomes, intracellular bacteria may become ubiquitinated and directed for breakdown in autophagosomes. However, in the later phases of inflammation, autophagy inhibits inflammation: inflammasomes can become ubiquitinated and broken down in autophagosomes, which limits their activity. There is increasing evidence that impaired autophagy allows continued inflammation and is associated with diseases such as colitis, sepsis and atherosclerosis.

FUNCTIONS OF PHAGOCYTIC CELLS

Clearance of apoptotic cells by macrophages produces anti-inflammatory signals. To maintain appropriate cell numbers during development, normal tissue homeostasis and pathological responses, cells die naturally by apoptosis, which involves activation of non-inflammatory caspases.

Cellular and biochemical pathways resulting in apoptosis are conserved in evolution and apoptotic cells are rapidly and efficiently cleared by macrophages (Fig. 5.14), although they can also be engulfed by non-professional phagocytes. The appearance of phosphatidylserine (PS) in the outer leaflet of the plasma membrane is characteristic of apoptotic cells. PS recognition by PS-binding proteins stimulates the uptake of apoptotic cells and the production of anti-inflammatory mediators, especially

TGFβ, which inhibit production of pro-inflammatory chemokines and cytokines.

There is redundancy in the receptors involved in apoptotic cell recognition. These include a range of scavenger receptors (SR-AI, CD36), T-cell immunoglobulin receptors (Tim) 3 and 4 and stabilin-2, and the complement component C1q, which directly recognize the 'eat-me' signals displayed by the apoptotic cells. PS can also be recognized by the soluble receptors MFG-8, Gas-6 or Protein S that in turn engage TAM receptors, such as MerTK, on macrophages.

Inefficient uptake of apoptotic cells or processing of apoptotic cell contents, such as DNA, may also contribute to autoimmune disorders such as systemic lupus erythematosus and may explain their association with genetic deficiencies of complement components and DNAse II. Lack of DNAse II expression by macrophages causes activation of cytosolic DNA sensors and induction of autoimmunity.

Macrophages coordinate the inflammatory response
Recognition of necrotic cells and microbial compounds by macrophages initiates inflammation. In contrast to the recognition of apoptotic cells, uptake of microbial products and necrotic cells by resident macrophages promotes cellular activation, leading to the production of secreted molecules (Table 5.1). Recognition of PAMPS and molecules from damaged cells through PRRs leads to the activation of the NFκB pathway (see Fig. 5.w1) and the production of cytokines and chemokines. The activation of cytosolic phospholipase A2$_2$ causes the release of arachidonic acid, the precursor of prostaglandins and leukotrienes, through the actions of the cyclooxygenase and lipoxygenase pathways, respectively. Pro-inflammatory prostaglandins control blood flow and vascular dilation and permeability at sites of inflammation. Trafficking of lymphocytes and neutrophils into tissues is induced by leukotriene-B4 (see Table 3.1).

Resident macrophages recruit neutrophils to inflammatory sites. Neutrophils are the first cells recruited to the site of inflammation and play a key role in elimination of the inflammatory insult (Fig. 5.15). Appropriate neutrophil recruitment is essential for successful resolution of the inflammatory response as deficiencies in the clearance of the triggering stimuli will result in chronic inflammation and tissue dysfunction (Fig. 5.16). Although macrophages and neutrophils share the capacity to mediate phagocytosis and intracellular killing, there are key differences between them:
- Neutrophils are short-lived, store a wide range of antimicrobial polypeptides in intracellular granules and readily produce oxygen radicals.
- Resident macrophages are long-lived, less microbicidal and cytotoxic, and display a higher degree of specificity, which makes them better suited as sentinels of the immune system.

Activated tissue macrophages produce chemokines CXCL5 and CXCL8 that promote neutrophil recruitment (see Fig. 5.15) and neutrophil extravasation is also promoted through proteolytic cleavage of chemokines by metalloproteases

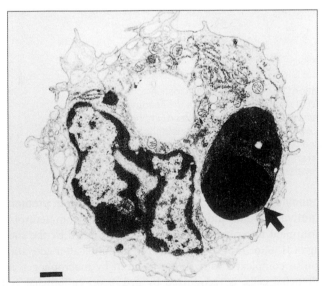

Fig. 5.14 Phagocytosis of apoptotic thymocyte by thymic macrophage Thymic macrophages phagocytose the large numbers of thymocytes that die by apoptosis during T-cell development. The *arrow* indicates the nucleus of a phagocytosed thymocyte. Bar = 1 micrometre.

TABLE 5.1   Secretory Products of Macrophages

Macrophages produce a wide range of secreted molecules

Category	Example	Function
Low-molecular-weight metabolites	Reactive oxygen intermediates, reactive nitrogen intermediates, eicosanoids – prostaglandins, leukotrienes	Killing, inflammation, regulation of inflammation
	Platelet-activating factor (PAF)	Clotting
Cytokines	IL-1β, TNFα, IL-6	Local and systemic inflammation
	IFNα/IFNβ	Antiviral, innate immunity, immunomodulation
	IL-10	Deactivation of MØ, B-cell activation
	IL-12, IL-18	IFNγ production by NK and T cells
	TGFβ	Repair, modulation, inflammation
	CCL2, CCL3, CCL4, CCL5, CXCL8	Chemokines
Adhesion molecules	Fibronectin, thrombospondin	Opsonization, matrix adhesion, phagocytosis of apoptotic cells
Complement	C3, all others	Local opsonization
Procoagulant	Tissue factor	Clotting cascade
Enzymes	Lysozyme	Gram-positive bacterial lysis
	Urokinase (plasminogen activator), collagenase	Fibrinolysis
	Elastase	Matrix catabolism

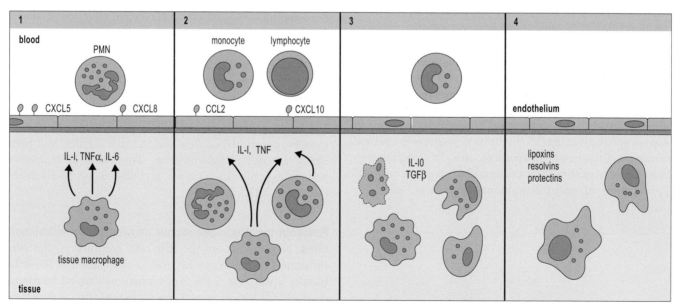

Fig. 5.15 The role of mononuclear phagocytes in inflammation (**1**) Tissue-resident macrophages respond to injury by the release of IL-8, IL-1, tumour necrosis factor–α *(TNFα)* and IL-6, which activate the endothelium and attract neutrophils from the blood. (**2**) As the inflammatory reaction develops, monocytes and lymphocytes are recruited. (**3**) As the inflammation resolves, dead neutrophils are phagocytosed by mononuclear phagocytes and the profile of cytokines switches towards production of IL-10 and TGFβ. (**4**) The production of lipoxins, protectins and resolvins is associated with restoration of normal function and termination of the inflammatory response. *PMN*, polymorphonuclear neutrophils; *TGFβ*, transforming growth factor.

(MMP8 and MMP9), which enhance their chemotactic activity. The primary role of neutrophils in a wound is to eliminate invading pathogens. To aid this goal, recruited neutrophils that fail to encounter bacteria in a short period of time will soon release their microbicidal compounds, leading to the liquefaction of tissue and the formation of pus. Tissue destruction facilitates bacterial clearance by eliminating collagen fibrils that limit cellular movement.

Monocyte recruitment to sites of inflammation is promoted by activated neutrophils. There is a transition from neutrophil recruitment to monocyte influx that is prompted by the shedding of IL-6Rα from the surface of neutrophils after activation. sIL-6Rα complexed with IL-6, produced by macrophages and endothelial cells, is recognized by gp130 on endothelial cells leading to the expression of VCAM-1 (a ligand for the integrin VLA-4 expressed by lymphocytes and monocytes) and CCL2.

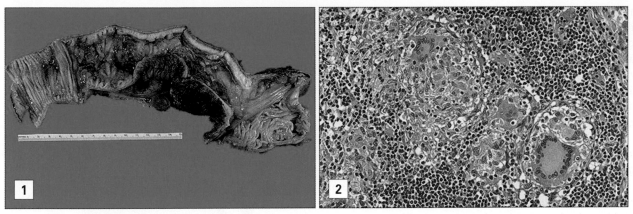

Fig. 5.16 Crohn's disease A section of the gut wall from a patient with Crohn's disease, showing the intense inflammation of the tissue (**1**). The histological section shows a granulomatous reaction with lymphocyte and macrophage infiltration and the formation of giant cells (**2**).

Shedding of IL-6Rα by neutrophils is also induced by apoptosis. Additionally, serine proteases released by neutrophils are capable of modifying chemokines to increase their affinity for CCR1 and to promote the recruitment of inflammatory monocytes.

Macrophages and neutrophils have complementary microbicidal actions. Macrophages and neutrophils complement each other in the clearance of pathogens. After extravasation, neutrophils release preformed proteins stored in granules, in three phases:

- secretory vesicles loaded with membrane-bound receptors are mobilized to the plasma membrane;
- secondary and tertiary granules containing lactoferrin, lipocalin, lysozyme and LL37 are released. These granules also contain matrix metalloproteases MMP-8, MMP-9 and MMP-25, which digest extracellular matrix and facilitate tissue destruction; and

- primary or azurophilic granules containing defensins (see next) and myeloperoxidase are released; myeloperoxidase converts H_2O_2 to hypochlorous acid, which reacts with amines to produce anti-bacterial chloramines (Fig. 5.17).

The defensins are a group of highly cationic polypeptides that contribute to anti-bacterial activities. The defensins:

- are small peptides (30–33 amino acids) found in some macrophages of many species and specifically in human neutrophils, where they comprise up to 50% of the granule proteins;
- form ion-permeable channels in lipid bilayers and probably act before acidification of the phagolysosome;
- are able to kill a range of pathogens, including bacteria (e.g. *S. aureus*, *Pseudomonas aeruginosa*, *Escherichia coli*), fungi (e.g. *Cryptococcus neoformans*) and enveloped viruses (e.g. herpes simplex).

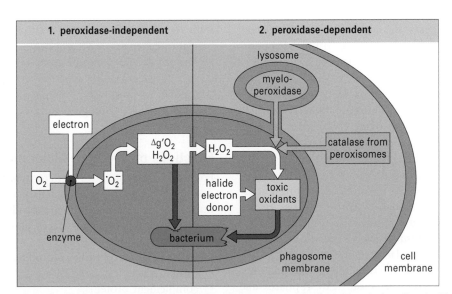

Fig. 5.17 Oxygen-dependent microbicidal activity (**1**) An enzyme (nicotinamide adenine dinucleoide phosphate NADPH oxidase) in the phagosome membrane reduces oxygen to the superoxide anion ($^{\bullet}O_2^-$). This can give rise to hydroxyl radicals ($^{\bullet}OH$), singlet oxygen ($\Delta g'O_2$) and hydrogen peroxide (H_2O_2), all of which are potentially toxic. Lysosome fusion is not required for these parts of the pathway and the reaction takes place spontaneously following formation of the phagosome. (**2**) If lysosome fusion occurs, myeloperoxidase (or, under some circumstances, catalase from peroxisomes) acts on peroxides in the presence of halides (preferably iodide). Then, additional toxic oxidants, such as hypohalites (HIO, HClO), are generated.

The primary granules also contain BPI (LPS-binding bactericidal permeability increasing protein) and serprocidins that include three serine proteases, which in addition to their microbicidal activity, cause tissue destruction.

Cytosolic and nuclear components of neutrophils can also contribute to anti-microbial activity – chromatin from neutrophils forms extracellular nets that associate with proteases from the azurophil granules.

Phagocytes kill pathogens with reactive oxygen and nitrogen intermediates. Phagocytes mediate microbial killing through a wide range of mechanisms, including acidification of the phagosome, through the formation of a H^+ ion gradient by V-ATPase. Acidification has direct microbicidal activity and facilitates the action of enzymes that have acidic pH optima. Additionally the H^+ ion gradient facilitates the extrusion of nutrients needed by the microbes.

Macrophages and neutrophils can also kill pathogens by secreting highly toxic reactive oxygen intermediates (ROIs) and reactive nitrogen intermediates (RNIs) into the phagosome (see Fig. 5.17). The NOX2 NADPH oxidase located at the phagosomal membrane generates ROIs and this property is most prominent in neutrophils. This oxidase transfers electrons from cytosolic NADPH to molecular oxygen, releasing O_2^- into the lumen. ROIs can interact with macromolecules (for instance through sulfur groups) rendering them inactive. Patients with chronic granulomatous disease lacking essential oxidase components suffer from repeated bacterial infections.

One major difference between resting and activated macrophages is the ability to generate hydrogen peroxide (H_2O_2) and other metabolites generated by the respiratory burst. Whereas neutrophils are readily endowed with microbicidal properties, macrophages require activation through the engagement of activating PRRs, reaching maximal microbicidal activity in the presence of IFNγ, which triggers classical activation (see later). Failure of macrophage activation in AIDS contributes to opportunistic pathogen infections and persistence of HIV, as well as reactivation of latent tuberculosis.

Macrophages can also be activated by IFNγ to express high levels of **inducible nitric oxide synthase (i-NOS, NOS2)**, which catalyses the production of nitric oxide (NO) from arginine (Fig. 5.18). ROIs and RNIs can interact to produce peroxynitrites and these reactive species all act within the phagosome to cause toxic effects on intraphagosomal pathogens; they interact with thiols, metal centres and tyrosines, damaging nucleic acids and converting lipids through oxidative damage. In this way, bacterial metabolism and replication are impaired.

Another mechanism that limits bacterial growth involves the sequestration of key nutrients by lactoferrin (Fe^{2+}) or NRAMP1, which extrudes Fe^{2+}, Zn^{2+} and Mn^{2+} from the lumen. Additionally, phagosomes contain endopeptidases, exopeptidases and hydrolases, which break down the pathogens. The proteases are delivered by different granules at different stages during the maturation of the phagosome.

Some pathogens avoid phagocytosis or escape damage. Some pathogens have developed elaborate mechanisms to evade killing within phagosomes. These include the escape of the

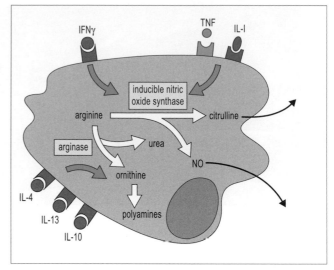

Fig. 5.18 The nitric oxide pathway IFNγ and other inflammatory cytokines cause production of inducible nitric oxide synthase (i-NOS, also known as NOS2). i-NOS combines oxygen with guanidino nitrogen of L-arginine to give nitric oxide (NO•), which is toxic for bacteria and tumour cells. Toxicity may be increased by interactions with products of the oxygen reduction pathway, leading to the formation of peroxynitrites. Cell activation by TH2-type cytokines promotes breakdown of arginine to ornithine and urea. Polyamines are products of ornithine, which promote collagen synthesis and cell proliferation.

bacteria from the phagosome (*Listeria monocytogenes*), promotion of fusion to the endoplasmic reticulum (*Legionella*) and inhibition (*M. tuberculosis*) or delay (*Coxiella burnetii*) of phagosome maturation. This will depend on the mechanism used for internalization; while direct recognition of the pathogen through non-opsonic receptors has limited activating capacity and enables the pathogen to exploit particular escape mechanisms, internalization of antibody-coated pathogens leads to enhanced cellular activation and triggering of microbicidal mechanisms. Macrophages, once activated through PRRs such as TLRs, induce autophagy, which mediates degradation of vacuolar *M. tuberculosis* and *Toxoplasma gondii*. Autophagy is also used by macrophages to sequester and degrade cytosolic pathogens such as *Francisella tularensis* and *Salmonella enterica*.

Functions of Secreted Molecules

Following encounters with microorganisms and antigens, resident macrophages can enhance their transcription and translation of a wide range of gene products, including secreted molecules, which often act locally close to the cell surface.

Secretory products include:
- eicosanoids involved in controlling inflammation;
- cytokines;
- complement proteins;
- antibacterial peptides and enzymes, especially lysozyme.

Lysozyme acts directly on the bacterial cell-wall proteoglycans, present especially in the exposed cell wall of Gram-positive bacteria (Fig. 5.w4). The cell walls of Gram-negative bacteria may also become exposed to lysozyme if they have been damaged by complement membrane attack complexes. Lysozyme is constitutively produced by macrophages.

Cytotoxic products and powerful neutral proteinases such as elastase, collagenase and urokinase (generating plasmin) (Fig. 5.w5) are able to induce tissue injury and contribute to destructive chronic inflammation in joints and lung. Monocyte-derived procoagulant/tissue factor can also induce vascular occlusion and tissue damage.

In addition to their local actions, IL-6 and IL-1 act as circulating mediators of the acute-phase response. Distant targets of these macrophage-derived cytokines include thermoregulatory centres in the central nervous system, muscle and fat stores, liver and the neuroendocrine system.

Resolution of inflammation by macrophages is an active process.

Complete removal of the inflammatory trigger initiates the resolution of inflammation, in which neutrophil infiltration stops and apoptotic neutrophils are phagocytosed. A key event in this process is 'lipid mediator class-switch' in which prostaglandin and leukotriene synthesis is replaced by the synthesis of **lipoxins**, **resolvins** and **protectins** (see Fig. 5.15). Intriguingly, the signalling pathways leading to the pro-inflammatory prostaglandins E_2 and D_2, synthesized early during inflammation, also lead to the transcription of the enzyme responsible for lipoxin synthesis. Lipoxin synthesis by neutrophils occurs through their interaction with platelets and epithelial cells that provide metabolic precursors through a process called **transcellular biosynthesis**. In the case of macrophages, lipoxin synthesis is triggered by uptake of apoptotic cells. Lipoxin A4 reduces neutrophil activity, increases the migration of monocytes, favours uptake of apoptotic neutrophils and inhibits the synthesis of CXCL8. Resolvin E1 and protectin D1 increase the expression of CXCR5 on the surface of apoptotic neutrophils, which facilitates clearance of CXCL3 and CXCL5 (neutrophil chemoattractants) from the inflammatory site. Apoptotic neutrophils produce 'find me' signals (e.g. lysophosphatidylcholine) that attract macrophages. Uptake of these neutrophils by macrophages inhibits production of IL-23, a cytokine involved in promoting granulopoiesis. As described above, recognition of apoptotic cells by macrophages also leads to the production of the anti-inflammatory cytokines IL-10 and TGFβ that, together with factors such as vascular endothelial growth factor, promote tissue repair.

Different pathways of macrophage activation

Previous sections have hinted at the capacity of macrophages to adapt to their surroundings (i.e. macrophages in different anatomical compartments display distinct phenotypes and resident macrophages have lower microbicidal activity compared with recruited macrophages, even after activation). Study of the phenotype of macrophages exposed in culture to different combinations of cytokines further illustrated the plasticity of these cells. Broadly, macrophages can follow classical (M1) or alternative (M2) activation profiles, although it is possible to encounter intermediate phenotypes:

- M1 activation refers to macrophages with enhanced microbicidal activity that can be generated in culture by treating with selected TLR ligands or pathogens in the presence of IFNγ (classical activation) or absence of IFNγ (innate activation).

- M2 activation generally refers to macrophages exposed to IL-4 or IL-13 although, within the spectrum of M2 activation, macrophages with a regulatory phenotype can also be obtained in response to immune complexes and TLR engagement (Fig. 5.19).

Major attempts are being made to correlate the phenotypes observed in vitro with patterns of differentiation in vivo through the analysis of signature markers, some of them having been identified during parasite infection in mice. Classical activation appears to be consistent with the role of macrophages as effector cells during the course of cell-mediated immune responses where IFNγ produced by TH1 T cells will enable the elimination of intracellular pathogens by macrophages (see earlier). Additionally, M1 macrophages promote TH1 responses by producing IL-12 and secreting CXCL9 and CXCL10, which selectively recruit TH1 T cells.

Macrophages treated with IL-4 and IL-13 have a more developed endocytic compartment, produce reduced levels of pro-inflammatory cytokines and IL-12, increased levels of IL-10 and the decoy receptor IL1RA and can recruit regulatory T cells (Tregs) and TH2 cells, eosinophils and basophils through the production of CCL17, CCL22 and CCL24, thereby amplifying TH2-type responses. M2 macrophages are less efficient in producing ROIs and RNIs. In these cells, arginine is processed into ornithine and polyamines through activation of arginase. Arginase activity has been proposed as a way of controlling T-cell activation (see Fig. 5.18). M1- and M2-like macrophages also differ in their metabolic profile (M1 macrophages undergo aerobic glycolysis and M2 oxidative phosphorylation); iron metabolism (M1 macrophages sequester iron and M2 increase iron availability) and phagocytic compartments (M1 produce large quantities of ROS and the luminal pH remains neutral or alkaline and M2 phagosomes generate less ROS because of reduced NOX2 activity and reach lower pH values). In the absence of T cells, other cells at the site of injury collaborate to modulate the phenotype of macrophages. For example, natural killer cells activated by TNFα and IL-12 produced by macrophages will synthesize IFNγ and, under certain conditions, mast cells or early recruited eosinophils will produce IL-4 at sites of inflammation.

There are numerous reports of a role for M2 in parasitic disease models where they exert a regulatory, protective role probably as a result of their capacity to promote tissue repair. Interestingly, some microbes (e.g. *F. tularensis*) exploit the reduced microbicidal activity of M2 macrophages and alter the macrophage activation profile towards this path in order to minimize bacterial killing. Tumour-associated macrophages have also often been shown to display an M2-like phenotype, which promotes tumour survival through their capacity to produce IL-10 and angiogenic mediators.

Macrophages also contribute to TH17-mediated inflammation and macrophages exposed to IL-17 display a pro-inflammatory phenotype with increased transcription of chemokines CCL2, CCL8, CCL20, CXCL1, CXCL2 and CXCL6 and cell surface receptors CD14 and CD163 with substantial overlap with M1 cells.

While the damaging effects of unregulated classical activation are well known and mediate the pathology of chronic

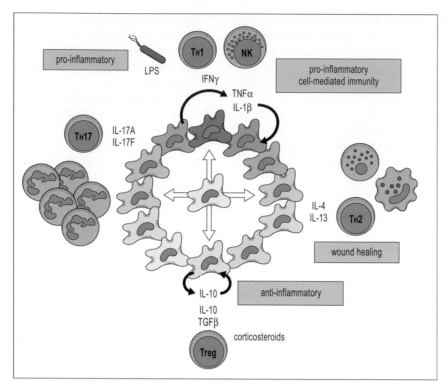

Fig. 5.19 Modulation of macrophage activation Signals from microbial products, phagocytosis and cytokines from T cells and innate cells such as natural killer *(NK)* cells, mast cells and eosinophils result in changes to the surface and secretory properties of macrophages. Broadly, macrophages can be classified as activated, deactivated or, alternatively, activated, but in reality a spectrum of macrophage activation states is likely. *LPS,* Lipopolysaccharide; *MHC,* major histocompatibility complex; *TGFβ,* transforming growth factor–β; *TNFα,* tumour necrosis factor–α.

inflammatory diseases, examples of M2-like activation in some pathological processes, such as fibrosis, have also been described. Because of the strong link between Th17 responses and autoimmune diseases, it is likely that macrophages exposed to Th17 cytokines contribute to the pathology of these disorders.

Macrophages do not readily return to their original naive state after stimuli are discontinued or eliminated. Epigenetic programming in these cells can lead to a state of tolerance. This tolerant phenotype occurs after chronic exposure to LPS, has been associated with immunosuppression during sepsis and is considered a state of M2 activation. In contrast, pre-exposure to agents such as β-glucan induces a state of enhanced responsiveness, termed 'trained', which is also underpinned by epigenetic programming (Fig 5.20) and occurs independently of adaptive immunity. These findings are in line with the developing concept of innate memory, which was originally identified in NK cells.

Macrophages have so many functions in normal physiology and immune defence that it is not surprising that macrophage phenotypes vary both with location in the tissues and in response to cytokines produced in different types of inflammation.

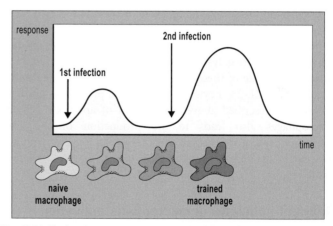

Fig. 5.20 Trained monocytes/macrophages enhance responses to second infections After recovery from first infection, trained monocytes/macrophages respond more strongly to a second infection independently of T-cell involvement. This enhanced ability to respond to infection is temporary and has also been described in natural killer (NK) cells.

CRITICAL THINKING: THE ROLE OF MACROPHAGES IN TOXIC SHOCK SYNDROME

See Critical thinking: Explanations, section 5

In an experimental model of septic shock, mice are infected systemically with bacille Calmette–Guérin (BCG), a non-lethal vaccine strain of mycobacteria. After 12 days, the mice are challenged intraperitoneally with graded doses of LPS. Blood samples are taken at 2 hours and the clinical condition of the mice is monitored for up to 24 hours. Experiments are terminated earlier if mice show severe signs of distress.

1. What cytokines would you measure in the 2-hour serum sample?
2. What clinical signs would be indicative of incipient septic shock?
3. What mechanisms contribute to septic shock?
4. What outcome would you expect if the following knockout mouse strains were used instead of wild-type controls: CD14, scavenger receptor class A (SR-A), IFNγ?
5. Interpret your results.

The role of macrophages in Tн1 and Tн2 responses

Isolated mouse peritoneal macrophages are treated for 2 days with selected cytokines (IFNγ, IL-4, IL-13, IL-10) in culture and a range of assays for cell activation is employed. It is found that IFNγ enhances the respiratory burst (after LPS challenge), MHC class II expression, and pro-inflammatory cytokine production, but downregulates mannose receptor (MR)-mediated endocytosis. IL-10 is an efficient antagonist of the above effects. IL-4 and IL-13 are weak antagonists of respiratory burst and pro-inflammatory cytokine production and markedly induce MHC class II molecules and MR activity.

6. Interpret the significance and possible functional relevance of these results in relation to concepts of Tн1/Tн2 differentiation.
7. What further work could be done to investigate the possibility that macrophage activation could by analogy be classified as M1/M2?
8. How would you investigate the role of macrophages and dendritic cells as possible inducers of CD4+ T-cell subset differentiation?

FURTHER READING

Biswas SK, Lopez-Collazo E. Endotoxin tolerance: new mechanisms, molecules and clinical significance. Trends Immunol 2009;30:475–487.

Biswas SK, Mantovani A. Macrophage plasticity and interaction with lymphocyte subsets: cancer as a paradigm. Nat Immunol 2010;11:889–896.

Blander JM. The many ways tissue phagocytes respond to dying cells. Immunol Rev 2017;277:158–173.

Jakubzick CV, Randolph GJ, Henson PM. Monocyte differentiation and antigen-presenting functions. Nat Rev Immunol 2017;17:349–362.

Dambuza IM, Brown GD. C-type lectins in immunity: recent developments. Curr Opin Immunol 2015;32:21–27.

Flannagan RS, Cosio G, Grinstein S. Antimicrobial mechanisms of phagocytes and bacterial evasion strategies. Nat Rev Microbiol 2009;7:355–366.

Gordon S, Martinez FO. Alternative activation of macrophages: mechanism and functions. Immunity 2010;32:593–604.

Gordon S, Martinez-Pomares L. Physiological roles of macrophages. Pflugers Arch 2017;469:365–374.

Hampton MB, Kettle AJ, Winterbourn CC. Inside the neutrophil phagosome: oxidants, myeloperoxidase, and bacterial killing. Blood 1998;92:3007–3017.

Mosser DM, Edwards JP. Exploring the full spectrum of macrophage activation. Nat Rev Immunol 2008;8:958–969.

Nathan C. Neutrophils and immunity: challenges and opportunities. Nat Rev Immunol 2006;6:173–182.

Netea MG, Joosten LA, Latz E, et al. Trained immunity: a program of innate immune memory in health and disease. Science 2016;352(6284):aaf1098.

Peiser L, Mukhopadhyay S, Gordon S. Scavenger receptors in innate immunity. Curr Opin Immunol 2002;14:123–128.

Soehnlein O, Lindbom L. Phagocyte partnership during the onset and resolution of inflammation. Nat Rev Immunol 2010;10:427–439.

Takahama M, Akira S, Saitoh T. Autophagy limits activation of the inflammasomes. Immunol Rev 2018;281:62–73.

6

T-Cell Receptors and Major Histocompatibility Complex Molecules

SUMMARY

- **The major histocompatibility complex (MHC) is a genetic locus that controls histocompatibility.** In early transplantation experiments, the donor and recipient were found to need the same MHC locus in order to avoid graft rejection. We now know that this occurs because MHC molecules are recognized by T cells, via their T-cell receptors (TCRs).
- **The MHC is polygenic and polymorphic.** The MHC locus consists of three regions. The most important of these are class I, which contains genes encoding six MHC proteins, and class II, which contains a variable number of genes that ultimately encode three heterodimeric MHC proteins. Many of these genes are highly polymorphic, with thousands of different alleles within the human population.
- **MHC molecules allow T cells to recognize antigen.** T cells express TCRs, which recognize peptide antigens being presented by MHC molecules. CD8$^+$ T cells recognize internally derived antigen being presented on MHC class I molecules. CD4$^+$ T cells recognize endocytosed antigen presented on the MHC class II molecules of professional antigen-presenting cells.

- **The TCR is highly variable.** The TCR is a heterodimer consisting of either α and β or γ and δ chains. These chains undergo random rearrangement at the genetic level to generate a wide variety of TCRs.
- **Most T cells express $\alpha\beta$ TCRs, with which they recognize their antigen being presented by MHC.**
- **Some T cells have TCRs of limited diversity, which recognize antigen in other contexts.** $\gamma\delta$ T cells are common at mucosal surfaces and recognize their antigens directly. NKT cells and mucosal associated invariant T cells (MAITs) have $\alpha\beta$ TCRs of limited diversity and recognize non-peptide antigen presented by MHC class I-like molecules.
- **The TCR forms a complex with CD3 molecules in order to signal.** The TCR itself has a short cytoplasmic tail with no signalling capability. It forms a complex with CD3γ, δ, ε and ζ chains. The cytoplasmic tail of CD3ζ contains an immunoreceptor tyrosine-based activation motif (ITAM), which is phosphorylated, allowing it to signal.
- **MHC haplotypes are associated with susceptibility to infectious and autoimmune disease.**

The immune system has evolved to recognize and eliminate invading pathogens. Key to its ability to do this are the interactions between two molecules: the MHC and the TCR.

The MHC is a family of cell surface molecules found in almost all vertebrates. MHC molecules present a selection of peptides made inside the cell (MHC class I) or from endocytosed particles (MHC class II) to TCRs on the surface of T cells. MHC class I is expressed by almost all nucleated cells and allows CD8$^+$ T cells to scan the internal environment of the cells for threats. MHC class II is expressed by professional antigen-presenting cells and allows CD4$^+$ T cells to detect and respond to extracellular pathogens.

MHC GENES

The MHC was originally defined as a genetic locus that controlled histocompatibility, which is the ability to transplant skin grafts between unrelated individuals without graft rejection. Both the donor and recipient had to possess the same MHC in order to avoid graft rejection.

In humans, Jean Dausset identified the MHC locus by injecting leukocytes from an unrelated individual into a volunteer and then tracking the rate at which a panel of skin grafts was rejected. For this reason, MHC genes in humans are also called human leukocyte antigens (HLA). In mice, the MHC locus was identified by Benacerraf and Snell, who performed serial skin grafts and compared the rates of rejection. The mouse MHC is known as H-2 (histocompatibility locus 2).

We now understand that the main purpose of the MHC is not to determine graft rejection. Rather, its involvement in graft rejection occurs as a side effect of its role in presenting antigen to T cells.

The MHC is polygenic and polymorphic. The MHC locus is divided into three regions (Fig. 6.1): class I, class II and class III. The products of the MHC genes are co-dominantly expressed.

The Class I Region

In humans, the class I region contains six genes (Fig. 6.2). Of these, HLA-A, HLA-B and HLA-C are known as classical class I genes. They encode the heavy (or alpha) chains of molecules that present antigen to CD8$^+$ T cells. The classical class I genes are highly polymorphic, with each having thousands of possible variants or alleles. In contrast, there are only a few alleles of each of the non-classical class I (or class Ib) genes, HLA-E, HLA-F

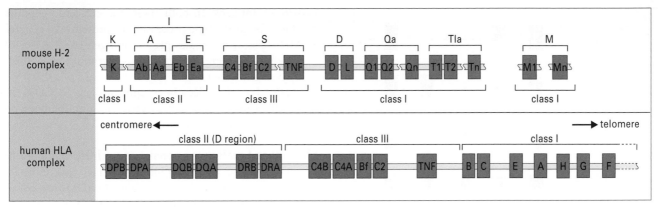

Fig. 6.1 Organization of the murine and human major histocompatibility complexes (MHCs) Diagram showing the locations of subregions of the murine and human MHCs and the positions of the major genes within these subregions. The human organization pattern, in which the class II loci are positioned between the centromere and the class I loci, occurs in every other mammalian species so far examined. The regions span 3–4 Mbp of DNA.

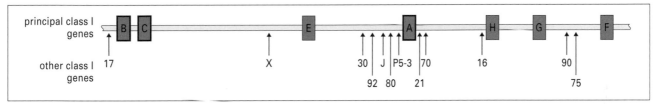

Fig. 6.2 Genes within the human major histocompatibility complex (MHC) class I region The human MHC class I region lies telomeric to the MHC class II region. In addition to the genes encoding the classic transplantation antigens (*HLA-A*, *HLA-B* and *HLA-C*), several other principal class I-like genes have been identified (*HLA-E*, *HLA-F* and *HLA-G*). Mutations in the HLA-H gene are associated with haemochromatosis, a disorder that causes the body to absorb excessive amounts of iron from the diet. A number of other non-classical class I genes and pseudogenes are present, mostly with unknown functions.

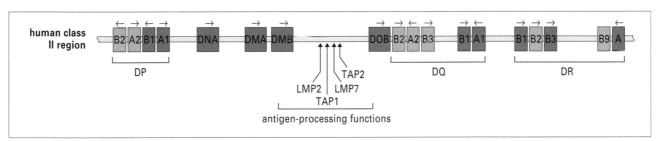

Fig. 6.3 Genes within the human class II region The arrangement of the genes within the human major histocompatibility complex class I region is shown. Expressed genes are coloured *orange* and pseudogenes are shown *yellow*.

and HLA-G. The molecules encoded by these genes do not present antigen to T cells but are instead recognized by natural killer (NK) cells (see Chapter 8).

All class I molecules share a β chain, β$_2$-microglobulin, which is encoded outside the MHC region. β$_2$-Microglobulin is non-polymorphic in humans, but two allelic forms exist in mice.

The Class II Region

The class II region encodes a number of HLA-D genes, as well as some genes involved in antigen presentation that are not expressed at the cell surface (see Chapter 7). The classical class II molecules are HLA-DP, HLA-DQ and HLA-DR (Fig. 6.3). Each of these comprises a less polymorphic α chain, which is expressed together with a highly polymorphic β chain. The heterodimeric complex presents antigen to CD4$^+$ T cells.

The DQ and DP families each have one expressed gene for each of their α and β chains, plus an additional pair of pseudogenes. The DR family comprises a single α gene (DRA) and up to nine β genes (DRB1-9). The organization and length of the DRB region varies in different haplotypes, with different numbers of β chains expressed (Fig. 6.4).

The Class III Region

The genes in the class III region are very diverse. Some encode:

- complement system molecules (C4, C2, factor B);
- enzymes;
- cytokines;
- heat shock proteins;
- molecules involved in antigen processing.

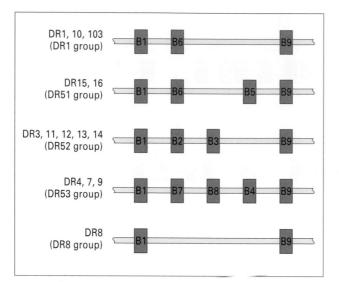

Fig. 6.4 Variations in DRB haplotypes The numbers of DRB loci vary between individuals. For example, a person who has a haplotype producing molecules of the type DR1 has three loci for DRB (top line). Not all of these loci produce mRNA for DR β chains.

Unlike the molecules encoded in the class I and II regions, there are no functional or structural similarities between the gene products encoded in the class III region.

HLA may be defined serologically or by genotyping. HLA molecules were originally defined serologically. For example, HLA-A2 refers to a group of HLA molecules with various amino acid sequences, all of which can be recognized by anti-HLA-A2 antibodies. Modern sequencing technologies mean that it is now faster and easier to define HLA by the sequence of the genes that encode them. When they are defined by genotyping, we call the HLA-A2 group of alleles HLA*A2. Defining alleles by genotyping also yields information about the precise amino acid sequence of the genes. For example, HLA-A*0201 refers to a single molecule within the HLA-A2 serotype, which has a specific sequence of amino acid residues.

Sequencing HLA genes also yields additional information about non-coding substitutions and differences in non-coding regions, which are sometimes conveyed using a longer form of the allele name. Alleles may also be assigned suffixes to show that they are null alleles (N), expressed at a low level (L) or soluble variants (S) (Fig. 6.w1).

MHC molecules

MHC molecules allow T cells to recognize antigens. T cells need to be able to detect:
- endogenous antigens (from viruses or other intracellular pathogens);
- exogenous antigens (antigenic peptides from extracellular pathogens that have been taken up by a professional antigen-presenting cells [APC]).

MHC class I molecules handle endogenous (or intrinsic) antigens and MHC class II molecules handle exogenous

(extrinsic) antigens. In both cases, the antigenic peptides are produced by proteolytic processing of proteins. In general:
- MHC class I molecules present antigen to CD8$^+$ cytotoxic T cells, which are important in controlling viral infections by lysing infected cells.
- MHC class II molecules present antigen to CD4$^+$ helper T cells, which aid B cells in generating antibody responses to extracellular protein antigens.

MHC class I molecules consist of an MHC-encoded heavy chain bound to β$_2$-microglobulin. MHC class I molecules comprise a glycosylated heavy chain (45 kDa) non-covalently associated with β$_2$-microglobulin (12 kDa) (Fig. 6.5).

The class I heavy chain consists of:
- three extracellular domains, designated α$_1$ (N terminal), α$_2$ and α$_3$;
- a transmembrane region; and
- a cytoplasmic tail (Fig. 6.6).

The extracellular portion of the class I heavy chain is glycosylated, the degree of glycosylation depending on the species and haplotype. The three extracellular domains are each about

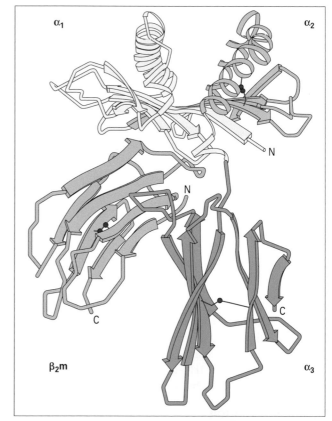

Fig. 6.5 A model of a major histocompatibility complex (MHC) class I molecule The peptide backbone of the extracellular portion of HLA-A2 is shown. The three globular domains (α$_1$, α$_2$ and α$_3$) of the heavy chain are shown in *green* or *turquoise* and are closely associated with the non-MHC-encoded peptide, β$_2$-microglobulin (β$_2$m, *grey*). β$_2$-Microglobulin is stabilized by an intrachain disulfide bond *(red)* and has a similar tertiary structure to an immunoglobulin domain. The groove formed by the α$_1$ and α$_2$ domains is clearly visible.

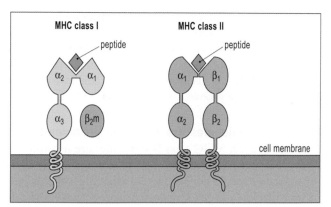

Fig. 6.6 Domain structure of major histocompatibility complex (MHC) class I and II molecules The structures of MHC class I *(left)* and MHC class II *(right)* molecules are shown. The heavy chain of MHC class I consists of three immunoglobulin domains, α_1, α_2 and α_3, a transmembrane domain and a short cytoplasmic domain. The heavy chain associates with an invariant light chain called β_2-microglobulin. The α_1 and α_2 domains form the peptide-binding region and the α_3 and β_2-microglobulin domains are structurally homologous to immunoglobulin constant regions. MHC class II molecules consist of a heavy (α) and light (β) chain. The α_1 and β_1 domains form the peptide-binding region and the α_2 and β_2 domains are structurally homologous to constant regions.

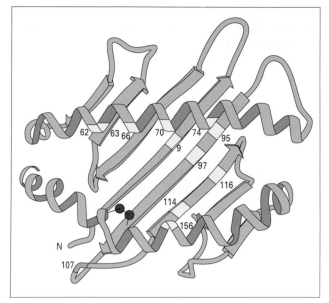

Fig. 6.7 The antigen-binding site of the major histocompatibility complex (MHC) class I molecule HLA-A2 The view of the peptide antigen-binding groove in HLA-A2 as 'seen' by the TCR. The α_1 and α_2 domains each consist of four antiparallel β strands followed by a long helical region. The domains pair to form a single eight-stranded β sheet topped by α helices. The locations of the most polymorphic residues are highlighted. Residues around the binding site are highly polymorphic. For example, HLA-2 and HLA-Aw68 differ from each other by 13 amino acid residues. Ten of these differences occur around the antigen-binding site *(yellow)*. (Modified from Bjorkman et al. Nature 1987;329:512–516, with additional data from Parham P. Nature 1989;342:617–618.)

90 amino acids long. The α_2 and α_3 domains both have intrachain disulfide bonds enclosing loops of 63 and 86 amino acids, respectively. The α_3 domain is structurally homologous to the immunoglobulin constant regions found in TCRs (see Fig. 6.14), B-cell receptors and antibodies (see Chapter 10) and contains a site that interacts with the cytotoxic T-cell co-receptor, CD8.

The transmembrane region comprises 25 amino acid residues and traverses the lipid bilayer, probably in an α-helical conformation. The hydrophilic cytoplasmic domain, 30–40 residues long, may become phosphorylated in vivo.

β_2-Microglobulin is essential for the expression of MHC class I molecules.

Like the α_3 domain, β_2-microglobulin has the structure of an immunoglobulin constant region. It is essential for the expression of all class I molecules at the cell surface: humans and mice lacking β_2-microglobulin do not express MHC class I molecules.

β_2-microglobulin also associates with a number of other molecules that are structurally similar to class I, such as the products of the CD1 genes (see Fig. 6.11) and the neonatal Fc receptor (see Fig. 10.14).

α_1 and α_2 domains form the class I antigen-binding groove.

The α_1 and α_2 domains constitute a platform of eight antiparallel β strands supporting two α helices. The disulfide bond in the α_2 domain connects the N-terminal β strand to the α helix of the α_2 domain. A long groove separates the α helices of the α_1 and α_2 domains (Fig. 6.7).

The original crystal structure of the HLA-A2 molecule revealed diffuse extra electron density in the groove, suggesting the presence of bound peptide.

The groove of an MHC class I molecule typically accommodates a peptide of eight to ten residues.

The ends of the peptide-binding grooves of MHC class I molecules are closed and the peptide is held in the groove as an extended (not α-helical) chain. This limits the length of the peptides that can be bound in the groove to between eight and ten residues.

Variations in amino acid sequence change the shape of the binding groove.

Comparison of the structures of two allelic variants of HLA-A, HLA-A2 and HLA-Aw68 have further refined our understanding of the structural basis for the binding of peptide to class I antigens. The differences between HLA-A2 and HLA-Aw68 result from amino acid side-chain differences at 13 positions. Ten of these differences are at positions lining the floor and side of the peptide-binding groove (see Fig. 6.7). These differences give rise to dramatic differences in the shape of the groove and the antigen peptides that it will bind.

Peptides are held in the binding groove by characteristic anchor residues.

The peptide-binding groove forms a number of ridges and pockets with which the amino acid side chains of the presented peptide can interact. Peptides eluted from a particular MHC class I allele will have different sequences, but the amino acids at certain positions are conserved. The side chains of these conserved amino acids tether the peptide to the pockets in the binding groove and are called anchor residues. Anchor residues need not be identical across all peptides bound by a given MHC molecule but must be related. For example, the anchor residue at position 5 of peptides presented by the mouse class I molecule H-2K^b can be of either the aromatic amino acids phenylalanine (F) or tyrosine (Y) (Fig. 6.8).

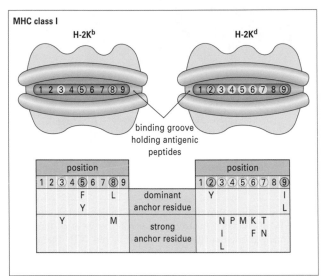

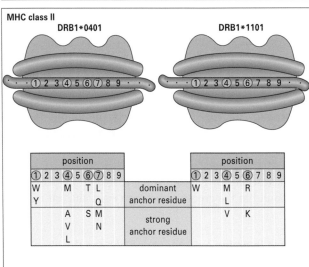

Fig. 6.8 Anchor residues in peptides eluted from major histocompatibility complex (MHC) class I and II molecules Class I MHC molecules from either H-2K^b or H-2K^d haplotypes were isolated *(top)* and peptides bound to these molecules were purified and sequenced. Amino acid residues commonly found at a particular position are classified as dominant anchor residues. Residues that are fairly common at a site are shown as strong. Positions for which no amino acid is shown could be occupied by several different amino acids with equal frequency. The diagram represents the class I MHC molecule-binding groove, viewed from above with anchor positions of each haplotype highlighted. Class II molecules of two haplotypes (DRB1*0401 and DRB1*1101) were purified and incubated with a library of peptides *(bottom)*. After multiple rounds of selection, peptides that bound effectively to the MHC class II molecules were identified and sequenced. Residues having a frequency greater than 20% are shown as dominant anchor residues. Other fairly common residues are shown as strong. Note that the binding site on MHC class II molecules accommodates longer peptides than that on MHC class I molecules. (Data from Hammer J, Valsasnini P, Tolba K, et al. Cell 1993;74:197–203.)

Amino acid variations within the peptide-binding groove vary the shapes and positions of the pockets. This is the structural basis for differences in peptide-binding affinity that in turn govern which peptides can be presented. The majority of polymorphisms in MHC molecules are concentrated in and around the peptide-binding groove.

MHC class II molecules are structurally similar to MHC class I molecules. MHC class II molecules are heterodimers of heavy (α) and light (β) glycoprotein chains. The α chains have molecular weights of 30–34 kDa while the β chains range from 26 to 29 kDa, depending on the locus (Fig. 6.9). The difference in molecular weights is primarily a result of differential glycosylation. The α and β chains have the same overall structures:

- an extracellular portion comprising two domains (α_1 and α_2 or β_1 and β_2);
- a transmembrane region of about 30 residues; and
- a cytoplasmic domain of 10 to 15 residues

The β_1 domain contains a disulfide bond, which generates a 64 amino acid loop. The α_2 and β_2 domains are similar to the class I α_3 domain and β_2-microglobulin and possess the structural characteristics of immunoglobulin constant domains. The β_2 domain also contains the binding site for the T-helper cell co-receptor, CD4.

Despite the differences in length and organization of the polypeptide chains, the overall three-dimensional structure of MHC class II molecules is very similar to that of MHC class I molecules, with a peptide-binding groove formed from a platform of eight antiparallel β strands supporting two α helices (Fig. 6.10).

The MHC class II binding groove accommodates longer peptides than that of MHC class I. The ends of the MHC class II peptide-binding groove are more open than that of MHC class I, allowing the peptide to extend beyond the ends of the groove. This allows MHC class II molecules to bind peptides of 13 to 24 amino acid residues in length.

Similar to MHC class I, the majority of polymorphisms in MHC class II molecules are concentrated in and around the peptide-binding groove. The precise topology of the groove, and thus which peptides can be presented, depends partly on the nature of the amino acid residues that form the groove. Like the grooves of MHC class I molecules, those of MHC class II molecules also contain pockets that bind non-covalently to anchor residues in presented peptides.

CD1 is a class I-like molecule that presents lipid antigens. CD1 molecules are structurally related to MHC class I molecules and are non-covalently bound to β_2-microglobulin. The genes encoding CD1 molecules are located outside the MHC and are not polymorphic. In humans, they consist of five closely linked genes, of which four are expressed (Fig. 6.11), encoding proteins that fall into two separate groups:

HLA-Aw68 (class I)

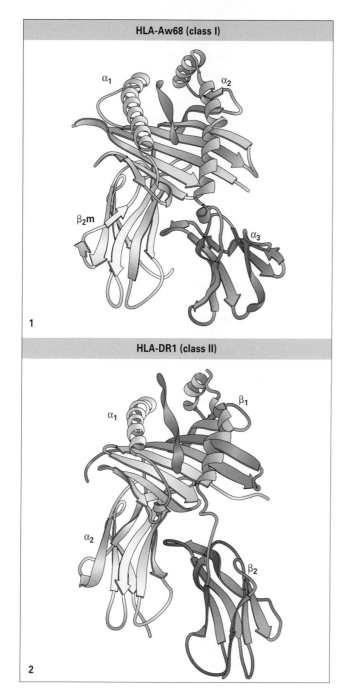

HLA-DR1 (class II)

1

2

Fig. 6.9 Comparison of the extracellular domains of class I and class II molecules Ribbon diagrams of the extracellular domains of class I HLA-Aw68 (**1**) and class II HLA-DR1 (**2**) major histocompatibility complex molecules. The binding cleft is shown with a resident peptide. These diagrams emphasize the similarity in the three-dimensional structures of class I and class II molecules. (Redrawn from Stern LJ. Structure 1994;2:245–251. Copyright 1994 with permission from Elsevier.)

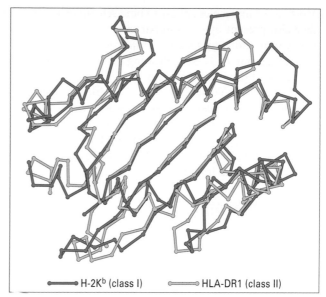

─● H-2K^b (class I)   ○─ HLA-DR1 (class II)

Fig. 6.10 Peptide-binding sites of class I (H-2K^b) and class II (HLA-DR1) major histocompatibility complex (MHC) molecules The peptide-binding sites of class I (H-2K^b) and class II (HLA-DR1) MHC molecules are shown as α carbon atom traces in a top view of the peptide-binding clefts. The similarities between the two sites can clearly be seen, but there are also some differences, some of which account for the difference in peptide length preference between class I (8–10 amino acid residues) and class II (> 12 amino acid residues). (Redrawn from Stern LJ. Structure 1994;2:245–251. Copyright 1994 with permission from Elsevier.)

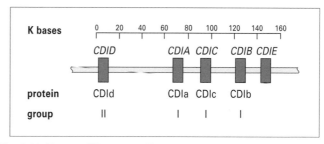

Fig. 6.11 Human CD1 genes The genes of the human CD1 cluster extend over 160 kilobases on chromosome 1. A gene product for CD1E has not yet been identified.

- Group 1 molecules in humans include CD1a, CD1b and CD1c.
- CD1d proteins form the second group.

Analysis of CD1b shows that the molecule has a deep electrostatically neutral antigen-binding groove, which is highly hydrophobic and can accommodate lipid or glycolipid antigens (see Fig. 6.15). One model for the binding places hydrophobic acyl groups of the lipids into the large hydrophobic pockets, leaving the more polar groups of the antigens such as phosphate and carbohydrate on the top, where they can interact with the TCR. The binding requirements of the hydrophobic pockets on CD1 are fairly tolerant because they will accommodate acyl groups of different lengths, but the interactions with the TCR are much more specific – small changes in the structure of the carbohydrate moiety will destroy the ability to stimulate a T cell.

The antigens presented by the group I CD1 molecules and CD1d are different. For example, group I molecules present lipoarabinomannan, a component of the cell wall of mycobacteria whereas CD1d cannot do this.

There is some debate about the physiological functions of the CD1 molecules in host defence:

- Group I CD1 molecules present lipids from mycobacteria and *Haemophilus influenzae* and can stimulate both CD4$^+$ and CD8$^+$ cytotoxic T cells and therefore appear to have a role in antimicrobial defence.

- Most CD1d molecules appear to bind self antigens, although they also present lipids from parasites such as *Plasmodium falciparum* and *Trypanosoma brucei* to T cells that use a restricted group of TCRs, indicating a role in defence against single-celled protozoal parasites.

Another class-1–like molecule is MR1, which presents a limited range of microbial compounds to mucosal-associated invariant T cells (see later). The structure of MR1 is highly conserved, which suggests that it forms part of the pathogen-associated molecular pattern (PAMP) recognition system for anti-microbial innate immunity.

T-CELL RECEPTORS

The MHC was identified as the major barrier to transplantation in the 1950s, but it was a further two decades before its physiological role was understood. In 1974, Zinkernagel and Doherty published their seminal observations that antiviral cytotoxic T cells generated in a mouse are only able to kill virus infected cells in vitro if the mouse and the target cells express the same MHC molecules (Fig. 6.12). From this, they inferred that T cells recognize antigen only in the context of MHC, a concept they called 'MHC restriction'. This is in contrast to B cells, which recognize their antigens in their native conformations (see Chapter 10).

The TCR is a highly variable disulfide-linked heterodimer.

The TCR is a member of the immunoglobulin superfamily and is structurally similar to half an antibody, consisting of a single heavy chain and a single light chain (Fig. 6.13). TCRs are heterodimers (either α and β or γ and δ chains), which

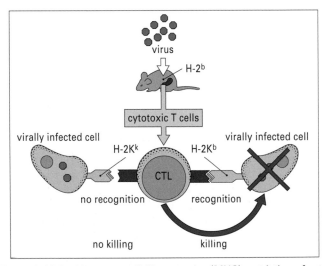

Fig. 6.12 Major histocompatibility complex (MHC) restriction of cytotoxic T cells A mouse of the H-2^b haplotype is primed with virus and the cytotoxic T cells thus generated are isolated and tested for their ability to kill H-2^b and H-2^k cells infected with the same virus. The cytotoxic T cells kill H-2^b, but not H-2^k cells. In this instance, it is the H-2K class I gene product presenting the antigen to the T cells. The T cell is recognizing a specific structure produced by the association of a specific MHC molecule with a specific viral antigen.

are disulfide linked. Each chain contains two immunoglobulin domains: a variable (V) and a constant (C) region. The N-terminal variable region is furthest from the cell membrane; it is the region that contains the greatest amino acid sequence variability and is responsible for binding to antigen presented by MHC molecules. Both chains of the heterodimer contribute to the antigen-binding site. The constant region is closer to the cell membrane, followed by a transmembrane region and a very short cytoplasmic tail. The disulfide bond that links the two chains is found in the peptide sequence located between the constant region and the transmembrane domain.

T cells that express a TCR comprising α and β chains are called αβ T cells and those expressing a TCR with γ and δ chains are called γδ T cells. The majority of T cells throughout the body are αβ T cells. γδ T cells are much less common than αβ T cells in the blood but are more abundant at epithelial surfaces, such as the skin and intestine (see Chapter 2).

αβ TCRs recognize peptides presented by MHC molecules. The αβ TCR consists of α (40–50 kDa) and β (35–47 kDa) subunits. Its structural features have been determined by X-ray crystallography (Fig. 6.14). The variable domains of both the α and β chains have three hypervariable complementarity determining regions (CDRs) that are clustered together to form the antigen-binding site.

- The CDR3 loops (which are the most highly variable regions of the TCR) from both the α and β chains lie at the centre of the antigen-binding site and make extensive contact with antigen presented in the peptide-binding groove of the MHC molecule.
- CDR1 of the α chain interacts with the N-terminal portion of the antigenic peptide.
- CDR1 of the β chain interacts with the C-terminal portion of the antigenic peptide.
- The CDR2 loops of both chains recognize the MHC molecule.

γδ TCRs can recognize antigen without the need for presentation by MHC molecules. γδ T cells are rare in the blood but common in the skin and intestine. Unlike αβ T cells, γδ T cells tend to express a tissue-associated TCR that displays little to no diversity within each tissue.

The γδ TCR is structurally similar to the αβ TCR, consisting of:
- membrane-distal extracellular variable domains in which hypervariable CDRs form the antigen-binding site;
- membrane-proximal constant domains;
- a transmembrane segment; and
- a short cytoplasmic tail.

Unlike the αβ TCRs, most γδ TCRs recognize antigen directly, without the need for presentation by MHC molecules. This is illustrated by the observation that mice deficient in MHC class I and class II lack αβ T cells but have normal numbers of γδ T cells. The ligands of the γδ TCRs have not yet been characterized completely but include:
- MHC class-I–like molecules expressed by stressed cells, such as T10 and T22 in mice and MICA and MICB in humans;

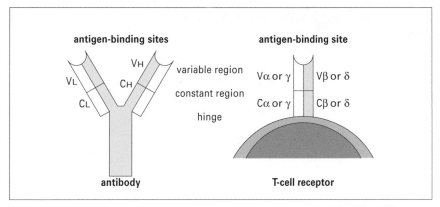

Fig. 6.13 **Similarities and differences between T-cell receptors and immunoglobulins** TCRs are very similar to Fab fragments of B-cell receptors. Both receptor types are composed of two different peptide chains and have variable regions for binding antigen, constant regions and hinge regions. The principal differences are that TCRs remain membrane bound and contain only a single antigen-binding site.

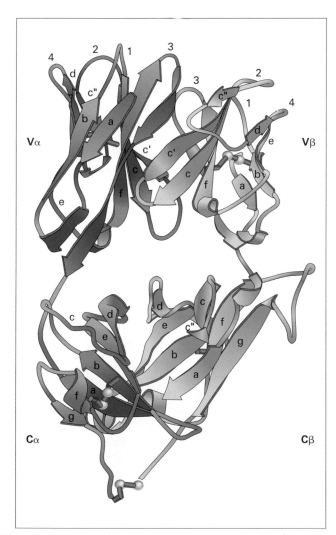

Fig. 6.14 **The T-cell antigen receptor** Three-dimensional structure of an αβ T-cell receptor (only extracellular domains are shown). The α chain is coloured *blue* (residues 1–213) and the β chain is coloured *green* (residues 3–247). The β strands are represented as *arrows* and labelled according to the standard convention used for the immunoglobulin fold. The disulfide bonds (*yellow balls* for sulfur atoms) are shown within each domain and for the C-terminal interchain disulfide. The complementarity determining regions (CDRs) lying at the top of the diagram are numerically labelled (*1–4*) for each chain. These form the binding site for the antigen/MHC molecule. (Adapted from Garcia KC, Degano M, Stanfield RL, et al. Science 1996;274:209–219. Copyright AAAS.)

- the MHC class-I–like molecule CD1d; and
- phosphorylated metabolites including the microbial metabolite 4-hydroxy-3-methyl-but-2-enyl-pyrophosphate (HMBPP) and the eukaryotic metabolite isopentenyl phosphate (IPP).

γδ T cells are early producers of cytokines during infection: they produce IFNγ in response to infection with the bacteria *Listeria monocytogenes* and IL-4 in response to infection with the nematode *Nipostrongylus brasiliensis* days earlier than αβ T cells. They also have a role in maintaining homeostasis at epithelial surfaces. Tcrd-deficient mice, which lack γδ T cells, display delayed wound healing in the skin, reduced proliferation of epithelial cells in the intestine and are more susceptible to chemically induced colitis than wild-type mice.

Some T cells express αβ TCRs with limited diversity, which recognize class-I–like molecules. NKT cells and mucosal-associated invariant T cells (MAITs) express αβ TCRs but, unlike those of conventional T cells, their TCRs display extremely limited diversity. These invariant T cells recognize antigen presented on class-I–like molecules:

- NKT cells are CD1d restricted.
- MAITs are MR1 restricted.

NKT cells are divided into two groups. Of these, the group 1 NKT cells, also known as iNKT cells, are far better understood than the group 2 NKT cells. iNKT cells are found throughout the body but are particularly prominent in the liver, spleen and bone marrow. They express semi-invariant αβ TCRs, which recognize antigen presented by the MHC class-I–like molecule CD1d.

CD1d is structurally very similar to MHC class I and, like MHC class I, associates with β₂-microglobulin. Unlike that of class I, the binding groove of CD1d is lined with hydrophobic residues, which allow it to present lipid, glycolipid and phospholipid, rather than peptide, antigens. The first such lipid antigen to be defined was the synthetic glycolipid α-galactosylceramide (α-GalCer) but the physiological role of CD1d is likely to be in presenting microbial lipid antigens. Several such antigens have been shown to be presented by CD1d and mice lacking CD1d-restricted iNKT cells are more susceptible to infection by *Mycobacterium* and *Pseudomonas* (Fig. 6.15)

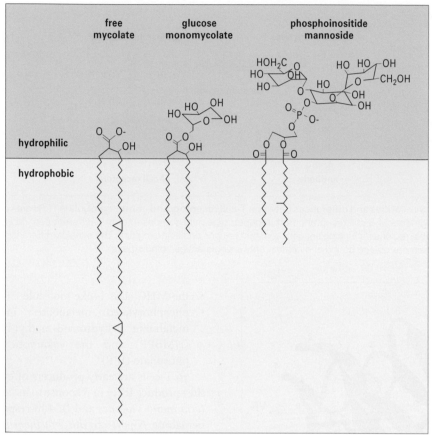

Fig. 6.15 Glycolipid antigens presented by CD1 Some of the antigens presented by CD1b are shown, each of which is a component of mycobacterial cell walls. Each of the antigens has two aliphatic tails, which are thought to be buried in the two hydrophobic binding pockets on CD1b. This leaves the hydrophilic segments exposed in the centre of the binding groove, where they can contact the TCR. (Based on Porcelli SA, Segelke BW, Sugita M, et al. Immunol Today 1998;19:362–368.)

MAITs are most commonly found in the gastrointestinal tract, mesenteric lymph nodes and liver and have a role limiting bacterial infections by rapid production of IFNγ and TNFα. Their invariant TCR recognizes antigen presented by the MHC class-I–like molecule MR1, which also associates with β₂-microglobulin. The complete repertoire of antigens that can be presented by MR1 has not yet been characterized, but it is known to present bacterially derived vitamin D metabolites.

GENERATION OF T-CELL RECEPTOR DIVERSITY

TCR diversity is generated by V(D)J recombination. T and B cells are unique among all the cells of the body, in that they undergo a kind of somatic gene recombination, called V(D)J recombination, that results in the highly diverse repertoire of TCRs found on T cells and BCRs and antibodies expressed by B cells. This process is a defining feature of adaptive immune cells.

V(D)J recombination occurs in developing T and B cells:
- in the thymus, in the case of T cells, and
- in the bone marrow, in the case of B cells.

Variable (V), joining (J) and, sometimes, diversity (D) gene segments are joined in a nearly random manner to form a completed variable region gene (Fig. 6.16). Imprecise joining of V, D and J regions with loss and/or addition of nucleotides is known as junctional diversity and contributes an enormous amount of variability to the T-cell and B-cell repertoires, in addition to the variation that results from the combinatorial assortment of the various gene segments.

Together, VDJ recombination and junctional diversity result in novel amino acid sequences in the antigen-binding regions of TCRs, BCRs and antibodies, with the greatest diversity present within the third CDR of the V region (CDR3). This allows T and B cells to recognize nearly all possible antigens.

Hunkapiller and Hood have calculated that it is possible to construct about:
- 4.4×10^{13} different forms of the V region of the TCR β chain; and
- 8.5×10^{12} forms of the V region of the TCR α chain.

They estimate that if only 1% of the sequences are coded for viable proteins, it would still give 2.9×10^{22} receptors. Even if 99% of these viable receptors were rejected due to autoreactivity or other defects, recombination would still yield 2.9×10^{20} possible murine TCRs. This would seem to be more than enough potential diversity, given that the thymus produces fewer than 10^9 thymocytes over the lifetime of a mouse.

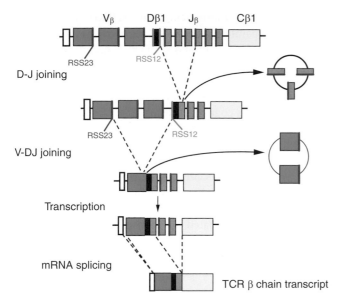

D-J joining

V-DJ joining

Transcription

mRNA splicing

TCR β chain transcript

Fig. 6.16 T-cell receptor diversity is generated by V(D)J recombination V(D)J recombination at the TCRB locus is shown. D-J recombination occurs first. RAG 1 and 2 join a 12 base pair recombination signal sequence (RSS) 3′ of $D_\beta 1$ to a 23 base pair RSS 5′ of a J_β segment, excising the intervening DNA. TdT generates junctional diversity by random addition of nucleotides before the ends are ligated. V-DJ recombination occurs second and is mechanistically similar to D-J recombination. The recombined TCRB gene is transcribed and any remaining J_β segments are removed from the transcript by mRNA splicing before the protein is translated.

V(D)J recombination occurs first in the α and then in the β chain.

The β chain of the TCR, encoded by the TCRB locus, is the first to undergo recombination. D-to-J recombination occurs first, followed by V-to-DJ rearrangements. All gene segments between the V, D and J segments in the newly formed complex are deleted.

The newly synthesized β chain is expressed with an invariant surrogate α chain or preTCRα. If the complex of the β and surrogate α chains is able to signal, the recombination of the second TCRB locus is inhibited in a process called allelic exclusion. If the newly synthesized β chain is unable to complex with the surrogate α chain, the second TCRB locus will undergo rearrangement. If rearrangement at the second TCRB locus does not produce a functional β chain, the developing T cell will be allowed to die.

Once the developing T cell has successfully rearranged the β chain, the α chain undergoes recombination. In the TCRA locus, which encodes the α chain, joining of a V segment to a J segment produces a complete variable region gene, with the large number of potential J segments being the main contributors to the diversity of α chain specificities.

V(D)J recombination relies on recombination activating genes (RAG) 1 and 2.

V(D)J recombination requires a complex of enzymes collectively known as VDJ recombinase. The most important of these are:

- recombination activating genes (RAG) 1 and 2;
- terminal deoxynucleotidyl transferase (TdT); and

- non-homologous end-joining DNA repair factors, especially the Artemis complex.

RAG1 and 2 allow VDJ recombinase to recognize conserved recombination signal sequences (RSS) flanking V, D and J segments (see Fig. 6.16). An RSS consists of:

- a conserved heptamer sequence;
- a spacer sequence of either 12 or 23 base pairs; and
- a conserved nonamer sequence.

RAG1 and 2 pair a 12-base pair spacer RSS with a 23-base pair spacer RSS. This prevents two different segments coding for the same region from recombining so that, for example, each TCR α chain will only have one V region. The RAG enzymes are essential for V(D)J recombination and, by extension, T-cell and B-cell development: RAG-deficient mice lack T and B cells.

The DNA between the two RSSs is excised and the blunt ends of the excised DNA are ligated to form a circular piece of DNA, which is lost during subsequent cell divisions. The cleaved genomic DNA is left with hairpin loops, which are opened by the Artemis complex.

TdT is responsible for the introduction of junctional diversity and mice deficient in this enzyme display limited T-cell and B-cell repertoires. TdT catalyses the random addition of nucleotides to the 3′ ends of the newly opened hairpin loops before the DNA is religated by template-dependent polymerases and DNA ligase.

THE T-CELL RECEPTOR COMPLEX

The CD3 complex associates with antigen-binding αβ or γδ heterodimers to form the complete TCR.

One remarkable feature of the transmembrane portion of the TCR is the presence of positively charged residues in both the α and β chains. Unpaired charges would usually be unfavourable in a transmembrane region, but these positive charges are neutralized by assembly of the complete TCR complex. This complex contains additional polypeptide chains, collectively called the CD3 complex, which bear complementary negative charges.

The CD3 complex allows the antigen-binding domains of the TCR to form a complete, functional receptor that is stably expressed at the cell surface and is capable of transmitting a signal on binding to antigen.

The four chains of the CD3 complex (γ, δ, ε and ζ) are sometimes termed the **invariant chains** of the TCR because they do not show variability in their amino acid sequences. (The γ and δ chains of the CD3 complex should not be confused with the antigen-binding variable chains of the γδ TCR that bear the same names.)

The CD3 γ, δ and ε chains are the products of three closely linked genes and similarities in their amino acid sequences suggest that they are evolutionarily related. All three are members of the immunoglobulin superfamily, containing an external domain followed by a transmembrane region containing negatively charged amino acids and a highly conserved cytoplasmic tail of 40 or more amino acids.

The CD3 ζ gene is on a different chromosome from the CD3 γδε gene complex and the ζ protein is structurally unrelated to the other CD3 components. The ζ chains possess a small extracellular domain (nine amino acids), a transmembrane domain carrying a negative charge and a large cytoplasmic tail.

The CD3 chains are assembled as heterodimers of γε and δε subunits with a homodimer of ζ chains, giving an overall TCR stoichiometry of $(αβ)_2$, γ, δ, $ε_2$ and $ζ_2$, suggesting that the TCR complex exists as a dimer. The negatively charged residues in the transmembrane region of the CD3 chains interact with (and neutralize) the positively charged amino acids in the αβ polypeptides, leading to the formation of a stable TCR complex (Fig. 6.17).

The cytoplasmic domains of ζ chains mediate TCR signalling. The cytoplasmic domains of the CD3 ζ chains contain particular amino acid sequences called immunoreceptor tyrosine-based activation motifs (ITAMs). An ITAM motif contains a tyrosine residue separated from a leucine or isoleucine

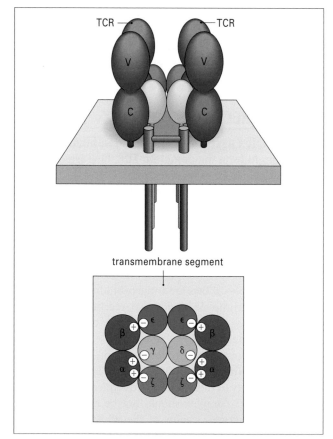

residue by any two amino acid residues. Two of these motifs are typically separated by between six and eight amino acids to constitute the complete ITAM (YxxL/I x_{6-8} YxxL/I). Each ζ subunit contains three ITAMs.

The conserved tyrosine residues in the ITAM motifs are targets for phosphorylation by specific protein kinases. When the TCR is bound to its cognate antigen–MHC complex, the ITAM motifs rapidly become phosphorylated in one of the first steps in T-cell activation. ITAMs are essential for T-cell activation and mutational substitution of the tyrosines in the motif prevents activation from occurring. ITAMs are also present in activating receptors elsewhere in the immune system, including the α and β chains of the B-cell receptor and intracellular adapter molecules associated with activating NK-cell receptors. CD3 ζ itself also functions in another signalling pathway, associating with the low-affinity FcγRIIIa receptor (CD16), which is involved in the activation of macrophages and NK cells (see Fig. 10.15).

Other subunits of the CD3 complex (γ, δ, ε), although lacking in ITAMs, may also become phosphorylated following TCR engagement. Phosphorylation of the CD3 γ chain downregulates TCR expression on the cell surface via a mechanism involving increased receptor internalization. T-cell signalling is discussed in more detail in Chapter 7.

MAJOR HISTOCOMPATIBILITY COMPLEX HAPLOTYPE AND DISEASE SUSCEPTIBILITY

Genetic variations in MHC molecules affect:
- the ability to make an immune response, and therefore
- resistance or susceptibility to infectious diseases and
- resistance or susceptibility to autoimmune diseases and allergies.

This is the key to understanding why the MHC is so polymorphic. The immune system must respond to many different pathogens. By having several different MHC molecules, an individual can present a diverse range of antigens and is more likely to be able to mount an effective immune response. There is therefore a selective advantage in having different MHC molecules.

Certain HLA haplotypes confer protection from infection. Certain MHC class I and class II alleles (HLA-B*5301 and DRB1*1302, respectively) are associated with a reduced risk of severe malaria. DRB1*1302 binds different peptides from the closely related allele DRB1*1301 as a result of a single amino acid difference in the β chain, which is sufficient to influence the response to the malaria parasite. The class I haplotype HLA-B*53 is also associated with protection against childhood malaria and the gene frequency of B*53 is up to 40% in areas affected by malaria, but only 1%–2% in areas where the disease is absent. This demonstrates how infectious agents select for MHC genes that protect against those infections.

HLA-DRB1*1302 has also been associated with an increased clearance of the hepatitis B virus and, consequently, a decreased risk of chronic liver disease.

Fig. 6.17 The T-cell receptor (TCR) complex The TCR α and β (or γ and δ) chains each comprise an external V and C domain, a transmembrane segment containing positively charged amino acids, and a short cytoplasmic tail. The two chains are disulfide-linked on the membrane side of their C domains. The CD3 γ, δ and ε chains comprise an external immunoglobulin-like C domain, a transmembrane segment containing a negatively charged amino acid and a longer cytoplasmic tail. A dimer of ζζ, ηη or ζη is also associated with the complex. Several lines of evidence support the notion that the TCR–CD3 complex exists at the cell surface as a dimer. The transmembrane charges are important for the assembly of the complex. A plausible arrangement that neutralizes opposite charges is shown.

People expressing HLA-A*02 family alleles have a lower risk of developing disease following human T-lymphotropic virus 1 (HTLV1) infection. The viral load is lower in HLA-A*02-positive healthy carriers of HTLV-1, correlating with the presence of large numbers of virus-specific CD8+ T cells.

In HIV-1 infection, a selective advantage has been observed in individuals who have the maximum heterozygosity of MHC class I loci (HLA-A, B and C). This may suggest that the ability to present a broad range of peptides to CD8+ T cells limits the ability of the virus to evade the immune response by mutation. However, some class I alleles are unhelpful in HIV-1 infection: individuals expressing HLA-B*35 or HLA-Cw*04 progress more quickly to AIDS.

Certain HLA haplotypes are associated with autoimmune disease. The association between MHC haplotype and autoimmune disease was among the earliest described genetic associations and MHC haplotype is still one of the strongest risk factors for autoimmune disease. In type I diabetes and celiac disease, for example, HLA-DR and HLA-DQ haplotypes account for 30% of observed variation in phenotype.

Risk of celiac disease is associated with expression of HLA-DQ2.2, HLA-DQ2.5 and HLA-DQ8. MHC mapping identified four amino acids shared by the HLA-DQ alleles associated with the highest risk and these give rise to a pocket in the binding groove that is perfectly tailored to the celiac disease antigen: digested and deamidated gluten. In this case, the molecular structure of the MHC accounts for the link between the antigen, gluten and the autoimmune disease.

Rheumatoid arthritis is associated with a shared epitope at position 70–74 of a number of alleles of HLA-DRB1. MHC mapping locates this variant in the peptide-binding groove of the HLA-DR heterodimer.

CRITICAL THINKING: MHC RESTRICTION

See Critical thinking: Explanations, section 6

SM/J mice were immunized with the λ repressor protein, which is 102 amino acids long. One week later, T cells were isolated from the animals and set up in culture with APCs and antigen. The ability of the APCs to activate the T cells was determined in a lymphocyte proliferation assay.

When APCs from SM/J mice were used in culture, the T cells were activated, but when APCs from Balb/c mice were used, they were not.

1. Why were the APCs from the Balb/c mice unable to activate the T cells?
2. What do you predict would happen if you used APCs from an F1 SM/J × Balb/c mouse?

In order to identify the immunogenic peptide, the investigators repeated the experiment using the primed T cells, APCs from an SM/J mouse and a variety of peptides made from the λ repressor protein, rather than intact antigen. The table shows the sequences of some of these peptides and their ability to activate T cells when included in culture at a concentration of 10 μM.

Peptide	Amino acid sequence	T-cell activation
12–36	QLEDARRLKAIYEKKKNELGLSQESV	−
80–102	SPSIAREIYEMYEAVSMQPSLRS	+++
73–88	ILKVSVEEFSPSIAREIY	−
80–94	**S**PSIAREIYEMYEAVS	++
84–98	AREIYEMYEAVSMQP	−

3. Why do peptides 80–102 and 80–94 activate the T cells, while the others do not?

The investigators make a mutated version of peptide 80–94 by substituting aspartate for serine at position 80 *(bold)*. The mutated peptide is unable to stimulate T cells.

4. Why might this be the case?

The investigators make another version of peptide 80–94 in which aspartate is substituted for isoleucine at position 87 *(underlined)*. The mutated peptide is able to stimulate the T cells as well as the original peptide, even at lower concentrations (1 μM).

5. What would you predict about the binding affinity of this peptide within the TCR-MHC-peptide complex?

FURTHER READING

Alcover A, Alarcón B, Di Bartolo V. Cell biology of T cell receptor expression and regulation. Annu Rev Immunol 2018;36:103–125.

Castro CD, Luoma AM, Adams EJ. Coevolution of T-cell receptors with MHC and non-MHC ligands. Immunol Rev 2015;267:30–55.

Chien YH, Meyer C, Bonneville M. γδ T cells: first line of defense and beyond. Annu Rev Immunol 2014;32:121–155.

Kaufman J. Unfinished business: evolution of the MHC and the adaptive immune system of jawed vertebrates. Annu Rev Immunol 2018;26:383–409.

La Gruta NL, Gras S, Daley SR, Thomas PG, Rossjohn J. Understanding the drivers of MHC restriction of T cell receptors. Nat Rev Immunol 2018;18:467–478.

Matzaraki V, Kumar V, Wijmenga C, Zhernakova A. The MHC locus and genetic susceptibility to autoimmune and infectious disease. Genome Biol 2017;18:76.

Salio M, Silk JD, Jones EY, Cerundola V. Biology of CD1- and MR1-restricted T cells. Annu Rev Immunol 2014;32:323–366.

Schatz DG, Ji Y. Recombination centres and the orchestration of V(D)J recombination. Nat Rev Immunol 2011;11:251–263.

Thorsby E. A short history of HLA. Tissue Antigens 2009;74:101–116.

Zinkernagel RM, Doherty PC. The discovery of MHC restriction. Immunol Today 1997;18:14–17.

7

Antigen Presentation

SUMMARY

- **T cells recognize peptide fragments that have been processed and bound to major histocompatibility complex (MHC) class I or II molecules.** These MHC-antigen complexes are presented at the cell surface.
- **The professional antigen-presenting cells (APCs) include dendritic cells (DCs), macrophages, B cells and some innate lymphoid cells.** Of these, DCs are most important for initiating the immune response. The others can enhance a response that is already underway.
- **MHC class I molecules most often associate with endogenously synthesized peptides, produced by degradation of proteins in the cytoplasm.** This type of antigen processing is carried out by proteasomes, which cleave the proteins, and transporters, which allow the fragments to access the endoplasmic reticulum (ER).
- **MHC class II molecules bind to peptides produced after the breakdown of proteins that the cell has endocytosed.** The peptides produced by degradation of these external antigens are loaded onto MHC class II molecules in a specialized endosomal compartment called the MIIC.
- **Some DCs can present internalized antigen on MHC class I.** This process is known as cross-presentation.
- **Co-stimulation is essential for T-cell activation.** CD80 and CD86 on the APC bind to CD28 on the T cell to cause activation. Co-stimulatory molecules are upregulated when APCs are activated, to ensure T cells only respond to antigens when there is infection or tissue damage. Antigens presented without co-stimulation usually induce T-cell anergy.
- **Ligation of CTLA-4 or PD-1 on the T cell limits activation.** Both of these ligands inhibit the co-stimulatory signal the T cell receives from CD28.
- **CD4 binds MHC class II and CD8 binds MHC class I.** These interactions increase the affinity of T-cell binding to its MHC-antigen complex and stabilize the immune synapse.
- **The immune synapse is a highly ordered signalling structure.** The TCR, co-receptor, CD2 and CD28 are found in the centre of the synapse, surrounded by a ring of adhesion molecules. CD45 is excluded from the synapse, which allows signalling.
- **The T-cell signalling cascade leads to the production of IL-2, which drives T-cell division.**

T cells can only recognize their antigens as peptides held, or presented, in the binding grooves of major histocompatibility complex (MHC) molecules (see Chapter 6). Antigen presentation refers to the processes by which peptides are generated from the original protein antigen and loaded onto MHC molecules. T-cell receptors (TCRs) on the T cell can then recognize their cognate antigen and, where appropriate, make a response (Fig. 7.1). The nature of the T-cell response is affected by a number of factors, including:

- the kind of antigen-presenting cell (APC). Dendritic cells (DCs) are important for activating T cells at the beginning of the immune response, but antigen presentation is also involved in the processes by which B cells receive help from CD4$^+$ T cells and by which CD8$^+$ T cells recognize and kill virally infected and cancerous cells (see Chapter 8).
- whether the APC is expressing co-stimulatory molecules. Co-stimulatory signals delivered by APCs result in T-cell activation only when appropriate, such as during infection.
- whether the antigen-presenting cell is producing cytokines. In the final stages of the initiation of the immune response, the actions of cytokines on the T cells drive cell division. The precise cytokines produced may also alter the nature of the immune response (see Chapter 12).
- The activation status of the T cell. For example, a CD8$^+$ T cell that has already been activated by a DC is likely to kill a

somatic cell presenting its cognate antigen on MHC class I, whereas a T cell that has not been activated will not.

ANTIGEN-PRESENTING CELLS

It is important to distinguish between professional and non-professional APCs. Almost all nucleated cells present antigen to CD8$^+$ T cells on MHC class I, allowing the T cells to survey their internal environment. These are non-professional APCs and are not able to initiate an immune response.

Professional APCs, which are often simply called APCs, specialize in presenting antigen to T cells. They are efficient at internalizing antigens, processing them into peptide fragments and presenting the peptides to T cells, bound to either MHC class I or class II. Professional APCs are able to initiate an immune response by expressing co-stimulatory molecules alongside the MHC. The expression of MHC class II and co-stimulatory molecules are defining features of professional APCs.

The professional APCs include dendritic cells, macrophages, B cells and some innate lymphoid cells.

Dendritic cells are crucial for priming T cells. Activation of naive T cells on first encounter with antigen on the surface of an APC is called priming to distinguish it from the responses of

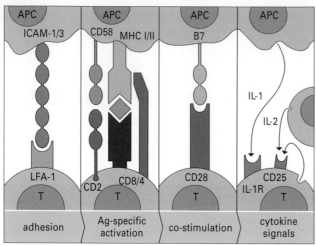

Fig. 7.1 Summary of the key intercellular signals in T-cell activation Association of antigen-presenting cells (APCs) and T cells first involves non-specific, reversible binding through adhesion molecules, such as Leukocyte function-associated antigen 1 (LFA-1) with intercellular adhesion molecule (ICAM)-1 or ICAM-3. Antigen-specific recognition of the peptide antigen in the MHC molecule by the T-cell receptor, provides the specificity of the interaction and results in prolonged cell–cell contact. A second signal (co-stimulation) is necessary for the T cell to respond efficiently, otherwise tolerance may result. Cytokine signals result in upregulation of cytokines and their receptors, including IL-2 and the IL-2 receptor (CD25), which drive T-cell division. Expression of IL-2 receptor is enhanced by IL-1 from the APC.

effector T cells to antigen on the surface of their target cells and the responses of memory T cells.

DCs are found in abundance in the T-cell areas of lymph nodes and spleen and are the most effective cells for the initial activation of naive T cells. They pick up antigens in peripheral tissues. If, at the same time, the DC is activated via its pattern

recognition receptors (see Chapter 3), it will migrate to the lymph nodes, increasing its expression of MHC class I and II molecules, adhesion and co-stimulatory molecules in transit, which allows it to interact with T cells. Once they have migrated, DCs stop synthesizing new MHC molecules but maintain high levels of the MHC molecules containing peptides from the antigens derived from the tissue where they originated.

The majority of DCs enter lymph nodes via afferent lymphatics. DCs arriving from the periphery in this way transport antigen and process it for presentation to T cells. As they mature, DCs express CCR7, which allows them to localize to lymphoid tissues. There is also some evidence that DCs from skin and the gut have distinctive chemokine receptors, which allow them to recirculate selectively to their own lymphoid organs.

A minority of the DCs in lymph nodes arrive from the blood across the HEV, using the same route as T and B cells (Fig. 7.2). However, these cells have not acquired antigen in the periphery and they can only acquire it from lymph or transfer from other cells.

Macrophages, B cells and some innate lymphoid cells present antigen to primed T cells. Macrophages and B cells are less effective than DCs at presenting antigen to naive T cells, partly because they express lower levels of co-stimulatory molecules, even when they have been activated. Although they migrate to lymph nodes, the numbers of macrophages in afferent lymph is relatively few by comparison with DCs and this too limits their effectiveness in activating T cells.

Macrophages:
* ingest microbes and particulate antigens;
* digest them in phagolysosomes; and
* present fragments at the cell surface on MHC molecules.

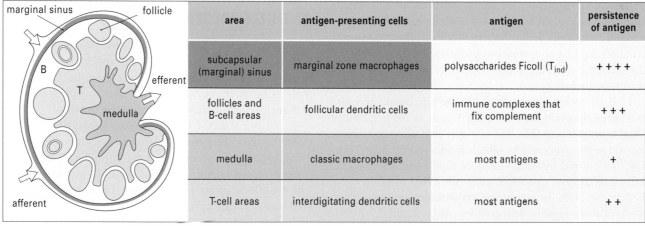

area	antigen-presenting cells	antigen	persistence of antigen
subcapsular (marginal) sinus	marginal zone macrophages	polysaccharides Ficoll (T_{ind})	+ + + +
follicles and B-cell areas	follicular dendritic cells	immune complexes that fix complement	+ + +
medulla	classic macrophages	most antigens	+
T-cell areas	interdigitating dendritic cells	most antigens	+ +

Fig. 7.2 Localization of antigen-presenting cells (APCs) in lymph nodes A lymph node represented schematically showing afferent and efferent lymphatics, follicles, the outer cortical B-cell area and the paracortical T-cell area. Different APCs predominate in these areas and selectively take up different types of antigen, which then persist on the surface of the cells for variable periods. Polysaccharides are preferentially taken up by marginal zone macrophages and may persist for months or years, whereas antigens on recirculating macrophages in the medulla may last for only a few days or weeks. The recirculating veiled cells (Langerhans cells and dermal dendritic cells), which originally come from the skin, change their morphology to become interdigitating dendritic cells within the lymph node. Both these cells and the follicular dendritic cells have long processes, which are in intimate contact with lymphocytes.

In mice that lack DCs, there is some evidence that macrophages can initiate CD8$^+$ T-cell responses to viruses that infect macrophages. However, in most circumstances, macrophages present antigen to T cells in order to amplify a response that has already been initiated by DCs.

B cells:

- bind to their specific antigen through surface IgM or IgD;
- internalize it;
- degrade it into peptides, which associate with MHC class II molecules.

If antigen concentrations are very low, B cells with high affinity antigen receptors (IgM or IgD) are the most effective APC because other APCs simply cannot capture enough antigen. Therefore, for secondary responses, when the number of antigen-specific B cells is high, B cells may be the major APC.

B-cell antigen presentation to CD4$^+$ T cells is also a critical part of the mechanism by which B cells receive T-cell help (see Chapter 9).

Among the innate lymphoid cells (ILC), subsets of both ILC2 and ILC3 express MHC class II molecules and are able to present model antigens to CD4$^+$ T cells in vitro, although they do so less efficiently than DCs. Their expression of co-stimulatory molecules suggests that, similar to macrophages and B cells, they are most able to present antigen to T cells that have already been activated. In mice whose ILC2 or ILC3 lack MHC class II, CD4$^+$ T-cell responses were impaired, suggesting that ILC2 and 3 can present antigens to T cells, but it is not yet clear how these ILCs internalize their antigen.

The properties and functions of some APCs are summarized in Fig. 7.3 and Table 7.1.

ANTIGEN PROCESSING

Antigen processing involves degrading the antigen into peptide fragments. The vast majority of epitopes recognized by T cells are fragments from a peptide chain. Only a minority of peptide fragments from a protein antigen are able to bind to a particular MHC molecule. Furthermore, different MHC molecules bind different sets of peptides, depending on the amino acid sequence of the peptide and the peptide-binding groove of the MHC molecule (see Fig. 6.8). For example, the vast majority of the human immune response against the HIV protein gag is directed against a single immunodominant region, which is recognized by a large number of T cells. However, exactly which part of this region is recognized depends on the MHC haplotypes of the individual (Table 7.2).

CD8$^+$ T cells recognize antigen presented by MHC class I, which is usually, but not always, derived from endogenous antigens synthesized within the APC or target cell. The peptide fragments from endogenous proteins are produced in a cytoplasmic organelle, the proteasome.

CD4$^+$ T cells recognize exogenous antigen, which has been internalized and broken down in endosomal compartments.

Manipulation of the location of a protein can determine whether it elicits an MHC class I- or class II-dependent response. For example, influenza virus hemagglutinin (HA), a glycoprotein associated with the membrane of an infected host cell, normally elicits only a weak CD8$^+$ T cell response, but if the

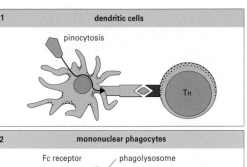
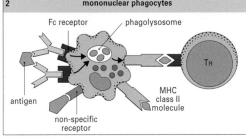
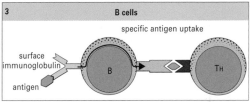
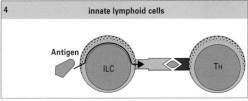

Fig. 7.3 Antigen presentation Dendritic cells (DCs) (**1**), mononuclear phagocytes (**2**), B cells (**3**) and some innate lymphoid cells (**4**) can all present antigen to major histocompatibility complex *(MHC)* class II restricted T helper *(TH)* cells. DCs constitutively express MHC class II molecules and take up antigen by pinocytosis. Macrophages take up bacteria or particulate antigen via non-specific receptors or as immune complexes, process it and return fragments to the cell surface in association with MHC class II molecules. Activated B cells can take up antigen via their surface immunoglobulin and present it to T cells associated with their MHC class II molecules. Some innate lymphoid cells are able to take up antigen via pathways that have not yet been defined and present it to T cells on MHC class II.

part of the protein's sequence that encodes the N-terminal signal peptide (required for translation across the membrane of the endoplasmic reticulum (ER)) is deleted, HA accumulates in the cytoplasm. This produces a strong CD8$^+$ T cell response to HA. Similarly, the introduction of ovalbumin into the cytoplasm of a target cell by osmotic shock generates CD8$^+$ T cells recognizing ovalbumin, whereas the addition of extracellular ovalbumin generates an exclusively CD4$^+$ T-cell response.

MAJOR HISTOCOMPATIBILITY COMPLEX CLASS I PATHWAY

Proteasomes partially degrade cytoplasmic proteins for presentation by MHC class I molecules. Although the assembly and peptide loading of MHC class I molecules occurs in the ER, peptides destined to be presented by MHC class I molecules

TABLE 7.1 Antigen-Presenting Cells

	Phagocytosis	Type	Location	Class II Expression
Phagocytes (monocyte/ macrophage lineage)	+	Monocytes, macrophages, marginal zone macrophages, Kupffer cells, microglia	Blood, tissue, spleen and lymph node, liver brain	(+)→ + + + inducible
Non-phagocytic constitutive APCs	–	Langerhans cells, interdigitating DCs (IDCs)	Skin, lymphoid tissue	+ + constitutive
		Follicular DCs	Lymphoid tissue	–
Lymphocytes	–	B cells and T cells	Lymphoid tissues and at sites of immune reactions	– → + + inducible
	?	Innate lymphoid cells	Mucosal tissues	– → + + inducible
Facultative APCs	+	Astrocytes	Brain	Inducible
	–	Follicular cells	Thyroid	Inducible
		Endothelium	Vascular and lymphoid tissue	– → + + inducible
		Fibroblasts	Connective tissue	
		Other types in appropriate tissue		

APCs, Antigen-presenting cells; *DC*, dendritic cell; *IFNγ*, interferon-γ; *MHC*, major histocompatibility complex.
Many APCs are unable to phagocytose antigen but can take it up in other ways, such as by pinocytosis. Endothelial cells (not normally considered to be APCs) that have been induced to express MHC class II molecules by IFNγ are also capable of acting as APCs, as are some epithelial cells. Another example is the thyroid follicular cell, which acts as an APC in the pathogenesis of Graves' autoimmune thyroiditis.

TABLE 7.2 Recognition of HIV Protein Gag

Recognition of HIV Protein Gag	HLA-Restriction
LQTGSEELRSLYNTVATLYCVHQRI	**A*29 B*44**
LQTGSEELRSLYNTVATLYCVHQRI	**A*02**
LQTGSEELRSLYNTVATLYCVHQRI	**A*01**
LQTGSEELRSLYNTVATLYCVHQRI	**A*11**
LQTGSEELRSLYNTVATLYCVHQRI	**B*08**

Overlapping polypeptide fragments from an immunodominant region of the matrix protein (p17) of the HIV protein gag are presented by different variant major histocompatibility complex (MHC) molecules. The amino acid sequence is given in single letter code and the peptide presented by each MHC molecule is shaded in blue.

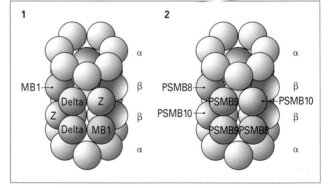

Fig. 7.4 Generation of immunoproteasomes by replacement of active subunits The 20S proteasome, shown in cartoon form, is composed of four stacked disks, two identical outer disks of α subunits, and two similar inner disks comprised of β subunits. Each disk has seven different subunits. Peptides enter the body of the proteasome for cleavage into peptides. Only three of the β subunits are active. In normal proteasomes, these are called MB1, delta and Z (**1**). Interferon-γ treatment of cells results in replacement of these three subunits by the two major histocompatibility complex–encoded proteins, PSMB8 and PSMB9, as well as a third inducible protein, PSMB10 (**2**). These subunits are shown adjacent to each other here, whereas they are actually in separate parts of the β ring and some would be hidden at the back of the structure shown.

are generated from cytosolic proteins. The initial step in this process involves the proteasome – a multi-protein complex that forms a barrel-like structure (Fig. 7.4).

Proteasomes provide the major proteolytic activity within the cytosol. They have a range of different endopeptidase activities that allow them to degrade denatured or ubiquitinated protein to peptides of about 5–15 amino acids long (ubiquitin is a protein that tags other proteins for degradation).

Two genes, PSMB8 and PSMB9, located in the class II region of the MHC (Fig. 7.5) encode proteasome components that subtly modify the range of peptides produced by proteasomes. The expression of these genes is induced by IFNγ. The proteins displace constitutive subunits of the proteasome and along with a third inducible proteasome component (PSMB10 encoded on a different chromosome) influence processing of peptides by creating a wider range of peptide fragments suitable for binding

MHC class I molecules. Additional subunits associated with the ends of core (20S) proteasomes may also influence antigen processing. These include interferon-inducible PA28 (proteasome-activator-28) molecules as well as a complex of proteins that result in a larger (26S) particle.

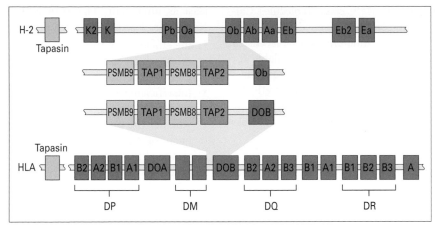

Fig. 7.5 Major histocompatibility complex (MHC) genes involved in antigen processing and presentation Genes encoding the two subunits of the peptide transporter *(TAP)* and two components (PSMB8 and 9) of the multi-subunit proteasome (see Fig. 7.6) are located in the murine and human class II regions. The Tapasin gene is located just centromeric of the MHC.

Proteasomes may not be the only proteases involved in producing peptides for presentation by MHC class I molecules. There is also evidence for the involvement of enzymes, such as the giant tripeptidyl aminopeptidase II (TPPII) complex.

Transporters move peptides into the ER. The products of two genes, TAP1 and TAP2, located in the MHC region (see Fig. 7.5) function as a heterodimeric transporter called TAP that translocates peptides into the lumen of the ER. TAP is a member of the large ATP-binding cassette (ABC) family of transporters localized in the ER membrane. Microsomes from cells lacking TAP1 or TAP2 could not take up peptides in experiments in cell culture. Using a similar system, it was

shown that the most efficient transport occurred with peptide substrates of 8–15 amino acids. Although this size is close to the length preferred by MHC class I molecule-binding grooves, it is slightly longer, suggesting that some additional trimming occurs in the lumen of the ER. One enzyme that is important for this trimming is ER-associated aminopeptidase (ERAAP).

A multimeric complex loads peptides onto MHC class I molecules. Once the peptides have been transported to the lumen of the ER, they are loaded onto MHC class I molecules by a large multimeric complex that consists of TAP, tapasin, calnexin, calreticulin and Erp57 (Fig. 7.6). Calnexin is a chaperone that stabilizes MHC class I heavy chains before they bind to

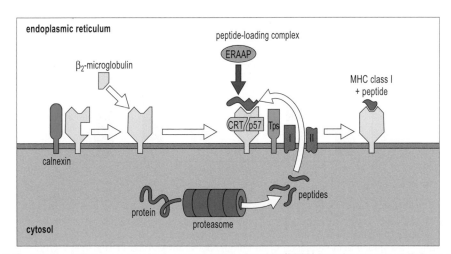

Fig. 7.6 Peptide loading onto major histocompatibility complex *(MHC)* class I molecules MHC class I alpha chains (α) are initially held in the endoplasmic reticulum associated with the chaperone protein calnexin. After combining with β_2-microglobulin to form a complete MHC class I molecule, they are released from calnexin and join a peptide-loading complex, consisting of tapasin *(Tps)*, ER-protein-p57 and calreticulin *(CRT)*. Tapasin also associates with the TAP transporters (I and II). Proteins are degraded in the cytosol by proteasomes to produce polypeptide, which are transported into the endoplasmic reticulum (ER) and loaded onto the MHC class I molecule. The peptides may be trimmed by ER-associated aminopeptidases (ERAAP). The MHC class I molecule with a bound peptide is finally released from the peptide-loading complex to be transported to the plasma membrane.

β₂-microglobulin to form complete MHC class I molecules. Calnexin then dissociates from the complex.

Empty MHC class I molecules are inherently unstable, ensuring that only functionally useful complexes are available for interaction with TCRs. During peptide loading, the empty class I molecule is stabilized by binding to the chaperones calreticulin and Erp57. Tapasin forms a bridge between the MHC and the TAP proteins, which allows peptides to be loaded onto the class I molecule.

Antigen processing affects which peptides are presented.

It was originally thought that the MHC haplotype of an individual largely controlled which sets of antigenic peptides would be presented to T cells. We now know that antigen processing is at least as important. The availability of peptides to load onto MHC class I molecules in the ER depends upon:

- the efficiency of the proteasome in generating different peptides, which varies if the proteasome contains interferon-inducible components;
- the efficiency of the transporters in taking peptides from the cytosol to the ER;
- whether the peptides can be trimmed by ERAAP.

Each of these factors also depends on the amino acid sequence of the original protein and to some extent on genetic variations in molecules involved in antigen processing (Fig. 7.7). All of these considerations are important in developing vaccines where the aim is to identify an immunodominant region of a pathogen to stimulate T cells.

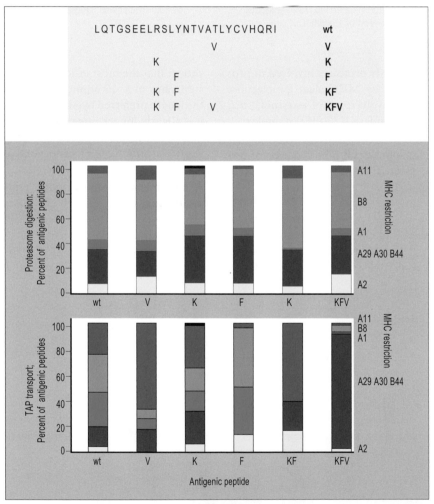

Fig. 7.7 Production of antigenic peptides Production of antigenic peptides by the proteasome and their transport to the endoplasmic reticulum (ER) varies, depending on the amino acid sequence of the epitope. The *upper diagram* shows the amino acid sequence of an immunodominant epitope of HIV matrix protein p17 and 5 mutants that often emerge during HIV infection. The sequence is shown in single amino acid code and the variants indicate single, double or triple mutations in the wild-type sequence *(wt)*. The *lower diagram* shows how efficiently these different mutants are digested by proteasomes and transported to the ER by binding to transporter associated with antigen processing *(TAP)* transporters. The bars show the proportion of peptides generated that are presented by different MHC molecules (A11, B8, etc.). For example, the KFV mutant produces peptides (red, recognized by HLA-A29, -A30 and -B44) that have a high affinity for the transporters and are transported well to the ER. Conversely, the KFV mutant generates some HLA-A11-binding peptides *(dark blue)* but they are not well transported compared with peptides of the wild-type sequence. (Data from Tenzer et al. Nature Immunology 2009;10:636–646.)

In some animals, antigen-processing genes are genetically linked to the MHC. The vaccination of chickens is important for global food production and because of this the chicken MHC region has been extensively studied. In chickens, both MHC genes and the genes involved in peptide loading are polymorphic and closely genetically linked. It is thought that this arrangement represents the ancestral organization of the MHC region and that, in mammals, a gene rearrangement resulted in the class III region being inserted between the class I and class II regions. This separated the MHC class I molecules from their antigen-processing genes, TAP, tapasin and the inducible proteasome components, which ended up in the class II region. As a result of the broken genetic linkage, the mammalian class I antigen-processing genes became less polymorphic, such that they could work with any MHC class I molecule. However, in some mammals, notably rats, there is some evidence that alleles of TAP are linked to alleles of class I that are most suited to receiving the peptides that they transport (Fig. 7.8).

The non-classical class I molecule HLA-E presents leader peptides from other class I molecules. HLA-E molecules bind a restricted set of peptides consisting of hydrophobic leader sequence peptides from classical class I molecules. Although these leader sequences are generated by signal peptidases within the ER, HLA-E nevertheless requires TAP transporters.

By binding and presenting sequences from classical class I molecules, HLA-E acts as a single signal summarizing the overall level of classical class I expression by the cell. HLA-E is recognized by the inhibitory receptor NKG2A, which is expressed by NK cells (see Chapter 8). HLA-E expression therefore indicates to NK cells that the target cell is expressing normal global class I levels. A number of viruses can evade recognition by cytotoxic T cells by downregulating MHC class I expression in infected cells. However, lack of presentation of the leader peptides by HLA-E can still alert the immune system that normal cell function has been altered.

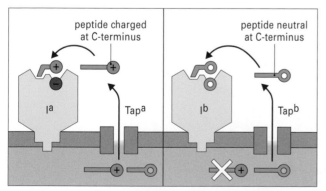

Fig. 7.8 Linkage of TAP and class I alleles Different major histocompatibility complex class I molecules in rats can accommodate peptides *(blue bars)* with either a positive charge at the C-terminus (+) or a neutral amino acid (o). Similarly, TAP molecules *(orange)* come in two forms, which differ in the types of peptide they preferentially transport into the ER. Most rat strains have the appropriate TAP allele on the same haplotype as the class I gene that it serves best.

Cross-presentation allows exogenous antigen to be presented on class I molecules. In general, MHC class I molecules present endogenously derived antigens. However, if this were exclusively the case, it would not be possible for professional APCs to initiate CD8+ T-cell responses by presenting viral or cancer antigen on MHC class I molecules, unless the APCs were themselves diseased. The process by which professional APCs can take up antigen from extracellular sources but present it on MHC class I molecules is known as cross-presentation.

In vitro, a number of cell types have the ability to cross-present, at least to some extent, but the main cross-presenting cells in vivo are XCR1+ DCs, sometimes called cDC1. Mice lacking these DCs produce weakened CD8+ T-cell responses and as a result are more susceptible to viral infection than wild-type mice.

The mechanism by which cross-presentation occurs is not yet entirely clear and indeed may differ depending on the cross-presenting cell and the source of antigen. For example, ERAAP is required for cross-presentation of antigen given as immune complexes, but not for soluble antigen. Most studies agree that cross-presentation always requires the proteasome, implying that antigen must at some point travel through the cytosol. It is not yet clear whether exogenous antigen escapes the phagosome via an unknown transporter and then undergoes processing and presentation on class I molecules via the conventional class I loading pathway, if some loading within the phagolysosome occurs, or if both can occur, depending on the circumstances.

MAJOR HISTOCOMPATIBILITY COMPLEX CLASS II PATHWAY

Professional APCs endocytose and partially degrade antigen. APCs phagocytose antigens and the phagosomes containing endocytosed antigen fuse with lysosomes to form phagolysosomes. In the phagolysosome, a number of proteases break down the proteins into smaller fragments. These proteases include:

- cathepsins B and D; and
- an acidic thiol reductase, γ-interferon-inducible lysosomal thiol reductase (GILT), which acts on disulfide bonds.

The efficiency by which the APC degrades internalized antigen has an effect on antigen presentation. Macrophages degrade antigen more efficiently than DCs. This leads to a smaller pool of partially degraded antigen and therefore less efficient antigen presentation.

Peptide loading onto class II molecules occurs in the MIIC. The phagolysosome fuses with an intracellular compartment called the MHC class II compartment (MIIC), which appears as a multivesicular body and is specialized for the transport and loading of MHC class II molecules. The compartment has characteristics of both endosomes and lysosomes with an

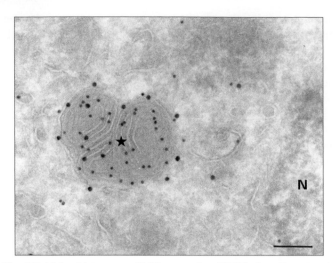

Fig. 7.9 Major histocompatibility complex (MHC) class II molecule processing compartment Electron micrograph of ultrathin cryosections from B cells showing a multilaminar MHC class II compartment vesicle (star). The bar represents 100 nm. MHC class II molecules are revealed by antibodies coupled to 10 nm gold particles and human leukocyte antigen DM. by large gold particles (15 nm). *N*, Nucleus.

onion-skin appearance under the electron microscope, comprising multiple membrane structures (Fig. 7.9).

MHC class II molecules are produced in the ER, complexed with a polypeptide called the invariant chain (Ii) (encoded

outside the MHC), which stabilizes the complex and prevents the inappropriate binding of endogenous antigen within the ER. The αβ-Ii complex is transported from the ER, through the Golgi network to the MIIC, where peptide loading occurs. The αβ complex spends 1–3 hours in this compartment before travelling to the cell surface (Fig. 7.10).

Non-classical class II molecules mediate peptide loading onto classical class II. The MIIC is acidic, allowing the proteases cathepsin S and cathepsin L to be activated and digest Ii, leaving a small fragment called CLIP (class II-associated invariant peptide) in the binding groove of the class II molecule. CLIP is then exchanged for antigenic peptides and this exchange is orchestrated by the non-classical class II molecule HLA-DM, which acts as a chaperone (see Fig. 7.10). HLA-DM binds to the αβ-CLIP complex to stabilize it until it has bound a suitable antigenic peptide. In cell lines lacking HLA-DM, the class II molecules are unstable and the cells no longer process and present proteins. Their class II molecules end up at the cell surface occupied by CLIP.

Another non-classical class II molecule, HLA-DO, is associated with HLA-DM and appears to fine-tune peptide loading by inhibiting the selection of immunodominant epitopes by HLA-DM.

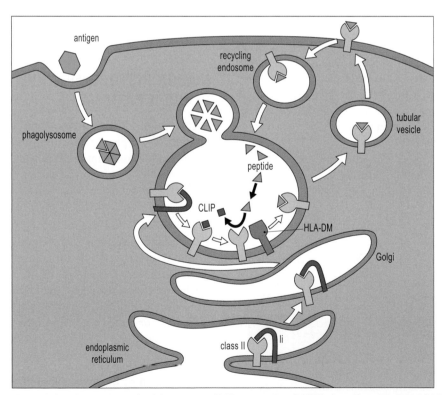

Fig. 7.10 Peptide loading onto major histocompatibility complex (MHC) class II molecules MHC class II molecules are produced in the endoplasmic reticulum, where their peptide-binding groove is occupied by the invariant chain, Ii. The complex is transported through the Golgi network to the MHC class II compartment *(MIIC)*. Here, cathepsins digest Ii, leaving a small fragment called CLIP in the peptide-binding groove of the class II molecule. Antigens are taken up and partially degraded in the phagolysosome to generate peptides. The phagolysome fuses with the MIIC to deliver its cargo of peptides for loading onto MHC class II. HLA-DM acts as a chaperone, stabilizing the class II molecule as CLIP is exchanged for the antigenic peptide. The peptide-loaded class II molecule then traffics to the cell surface.

Class II-peptide complexes recycle from the plasma membrane. Class II-peptide complexes are released from the multivesicular bodies as tubular/vesicular structures that fuse with the plasma membrane. The complexes tend to cluster on the cell surface in lipid rafts, which probably favours the formation of the immunological synapse (see later). There is a continuous recycling of complexes from the plasma membrane to endosomes and the proportion of complex that is present on the plasma membrane is regulated by ubiquitination, which varies between cells. For example, mature DCs tend to maintain more of the class II-peptide complexes on the cell surface than immature DCs.

CD1 PATHWAY

CD1 molecules present lipids and glycolipids. CD1 molecules, encoded outside the MHC on chromosome 1 (see Fig. 6.11), are a family of non-polymorphic MHC class-I–like molcules that present lipids and glycolipids to subsets of T cells. Humans have five CD1 genes whereas mice have two.

CD1 heavy chains are synthesized in the ER. Like class I molecules, they assemble with $\beta_2$microglobulin and are stabilized by the chaperones calnexin, calreticulin and ERp75 during loading. ER-derived lipids are loaded onto CD1 molecules by a lipid transfer protein called MTP. The loaded CD1 molecules are then transported to the cell surface, except for CD1e, which is transported to endosomes.

CD1 molecules on the cell surface are internalized via motifs in their cytoplasmic tails, which allow them to enter various intracellular compartments, where the ER-derived lipid in their binding grooves is replaced with internalized lipid antigen. This process is mediated by a variety of lipid transfer proteins, including CD1e, saposins and GM2 activator. Following loading, the CD1 molecules are recycled back to the cell surface (see Fig. 7.11). Thus, like those of MHC class II, the intracellular trafficking pathways of CD1 molecules involve recycling between the plasma membrane and endosomes. However, unlike the class II pathway, antigen presentation on CD1 molecules does not improve as the cell matures.

CO-STIMULATION

Danger signals enhance T-cell activation. For appropriate immune responses to be generated, T cells must respond to infection, but not to high levels of harmless antigen that may fluctuate in the environment. Mucosal tissues in the gut are in contact with high concentrations of harmless food antigens, while respiratory mucosa contacts many airborne antigens such as pollen, but strong immune responses against these antigens are undesirable.

APC activation is generally a response to infection or at least the presence of substances, such as constituents of bacterial cell walls, that are characteristic of infection. This explains the mechanism of action of adjuvants derived from bacterial

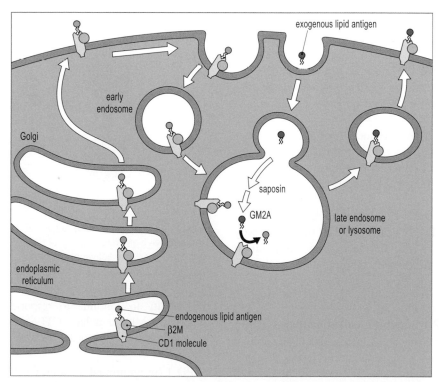

Fig. 7.11 Lipid-antigen loading onto CD1 molecules CD1 heavy chains assemble with β_2-microglobulin *(β2M)* in the endoplasmic reticulum (ER) and their binding grooves are loaded with ER-derived lipids. The loaded CD1 molecules are transported through the Golgi network to the cell surface, where they are internalized and directed to either the recycling endosome (CD1a), late endosome (CD1c and d) or lysosome (CD1b). In the late endosome and lysosome, CD1e, saposins and GM2 activator mediate the exchange of ER-derived lipid for lipid antigen. CD1 molecules loaded with exogenous lipid antigen then return to the cell surface.

components, which can be used to enhance the immune response experimentally.

The concept of immune activation only in response to infection (or adjuvant as a surrogate for infection), and not to other antigens, has been promoted as the danger hypothesis. This proposes that the immune system does not merely distinguish between self and non-self (see Chapter 12) but responds to clues that an infection has taken place before responding strongly to antigens. In other words, foreign substances may be invisible to the immune system unless accompanied by danger signals provided by pattern recognition receptors on APCs, such as the Toll-like receptors (TLRs), which recognize microbial products. These cause increased antigen presentation by upregulating MHC and adhesion molecules, but also boost T-cell activation by increasing the expression of co-stimulatory molecules.

Co-stimulation by CD80/86 binding to CD28 is essential for T-cell activation.

T-cell recognition of antigen presented on MHC molecules, although necessary, is not sufficient to activate the T cell fully. A second signal, referred to as co-stimulation, is of crucial importance for T-cell activation.

The most potent co-stimulatory molecules are B7s, which are homodimeric members of the immunoglobulin superfamily. They include CD80 (B7.1) and CD86 (B7.2). These are constitutively expressed by DCs and are upregulated when the DC is activated by inflammatory cytokines or by the interaction of microbial products with pattern recognition receptors. Monocytes, B cells and other APCs do not constitutively express co-stimulatory molecules, but can upregulate them following activation.

CD80 and CD86 bind to CD28 and its homologue CTLA-4 (CD152), which is expressed after T-cell activation. CD28 is the main co-stimulatory ligand expressed on naive T cells. CD28 ligation:

- prolongs and augments the production of IL-2 and other cytokines; and
- prevents the induction of anergy, a condition in which the T cell is not activated and is subsequently unable to respond to antigen.

Many cells can be induced to express MHC class II molecules and present antigen to CD4$^+$ T cells. However, they are mostly ineffective at inducing T-cell activation and proliferation because they lack the necessary co-stimulatory molecules (Fig. 7.12).

Ligation of CTLA-4 and PD-1 inhibit T-cell activation.

CTLA-4 is an alternative ligand for CD80 and CD86, with a higher affinity than CD28. CTLA-4 is not a conventional inhibitory receptor, since it lacks a bona fide immunotyrosine-based inhibition motif (ITIM), which recruits phosphatases that inhibit signalling. It has been proposed that it can recruit phosphatases indirectly or it may prevent T-cell activation by preferentially binding CD80 and CD86, so that they are unavailable to bind CD28. Following activation, T cells express higher levels of CTLA-4, which dampens

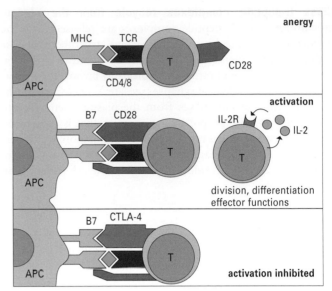

Fig. 7.12 Dual signalling is necessary for full T-cell activation A T cell requires signals from both the T-cell receptor *(TCR)* and CD28 for activation. In the absence of co-stimulatory molecules, inactivation or anergy results. If CD28 is bound by B7 on the surface of a professional antigen-presenting cell *(APC)*, the T cell is activated and produces IL-2 and its receptor (IL-2R). The cell divides and differentiates into an effector T cell, which no longer requires signal 2 for its effector function. However, if CTLA-4 on the T cell binds to B7, activation is inhibited.

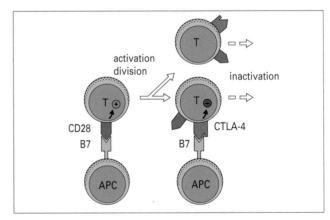

Fig. 7.13 Role of CTLA-4 in controlling T-cell activation Before activation, T cells express CD28, which ligates B7-1 and B7-2 on antigen-presenting cells *(APCs)*. After activation, CTLA-4 is expressed, which is an alternative high-affinity ligand for B7. CTLA-4 binds to B7 so the T cells no longer receive an activation signal.

their ability to continue to respond to antigen presentation (Fig. 7.13). Mice that lack CTLA-4 suffer from an aggressive lymphoproliferative disorder because their T cells cannot be inactivated.

PD-1 (programmed death-1, CD279) is an inhibitory receptor expressed by T cells, which belongs to the same family as CD28 and CTLA-4. Its expression is associated with an exhausted T-cell phenotype, i.e. cells that are incapable of producing cytokines and undergoing further division. PD-1 is ligated by PD-L1 and PD-L2 (CD273 and CD274) on APCs and signals negatively through its ITIM to inhibit the co-stimulatory signal from CD28.

There is therefore a balance in the co-stimulatory and inhibitory signals that a T cell receives, which determines whether it remains in an active state.

T-CELL SIGNALLING

The interaction between a T cell and an APC develops over time, in three phases.

The initial encounter between T cells and APCs is by non-specific binding through adhesion molecules, particularly Intercellular adhesion molecule 1 (ICAM-1; CD54) on the APC and the integrin Leukocyte function-associated antigen 1 (LFA-1; CD11a/18), which is present on all immune cells. Transient binding permits the T cell to interact with many APCs; T cells in vivo are highly active and a single T cell may contact up to 5000 DCs in 1 hour. Adhesion between the cells is enhanced by the interaction of CD2 (LFA-2) on the T cell with CD58 (LFA-3) on the APC. In rodents, CD48 performs a similar function to CD58. CD2 contributes to the initial activation signal for the T cell but more importantly, it stabilizes the interaction between the T cell and the APC, allowing the TCR time to recognize specific peptide antigen being presented by the APC. The initial phase of antigen presentation may last for several hours, but in the absence of a specific interaction, the APC and the T cell dissociate.

When the T cell encounters the appropriate antigen, a conformational change in LFA-1 on the T cell, signalled via the TCR, results in tighter binding to ICAM-1 and prolonged cell–cell contact. The joined cells can exist as a pair for up to 12 hours and this marks the second phase of interaction. At this stage, an immunological synapse forms and the T cell may be activated.

In the third phase, the APC and the T cell dissociate and the activated T cell undergoes division and differentiation.

CD4 binds to MHC class II and CD8 binds to MHC class I. Productive T-cell proliferation depends on the formation of a stable cluster of TCRs interacting with MHC molecules. The affinity of the binding of a single TCR to its MHC-peptide is not high and so the formation of this cluster requires the concerted action of a number of additional molecules, including the co-receptors CD4 and CD8. CD4 enhances the binding of helper T cells to class II, whereas CD8 enhances the binding of cytotoxic T cells to MHC class I. Both of these increase the sensitivity of a T cell for its target antigen by ~100-fold. Although signalling efficiency of CD8$^+$ T cells and thymocytes relates closely to the affinity of their TCR for the MHC-peptide, this is only partly true for CD4$^+$ T cells.

The immunological synapse is a highly ordered signalling structure. The interactions between APCs and T cells have been studied extensively in vitro, where the cells form a bulls-eye structure at the point of contact (Fig. 7.14). This immune synapse is thought to reflect, in idealized conditions, the events that

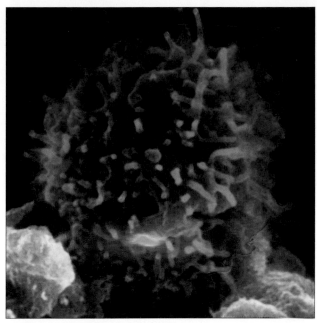

Fig. 7.14 Colour-enhanced reconstruction of an immunological synapse A live-cell fluorescence image, showing the peripheral zone of adhesion molecules *(red)* surrounding the core containing T-cell receptors *(green)*, is superimposed on a scanning electron micrograph of a T cell *(purple)* interacting with a DC *(dark green)*. Courtesy Dr Mike Dustin and (the journal) *Science*.

occur within a lymph node when T cells and DCs interact. In vitro, high doses of antigen can be used, which makes the synapse larger and more stable than it is likely to be under normal conditions.

TCRs, CD4, CD28 and CD2, which have relatively small extracellular domains, cluster in the centre of the synapse (or central supramolecular activation cluster; cSMAC) and the adhesion molecule LFA-1 forms a ring around the outside in the pSMAC (peripheral SMAC). CD45, the common leukocyte antigen, is a phosphatase with a large extracellular domain and is excluded from the synapse (Fig. 7.15). It is thought that the size-based exclusion of this phosphatase allows the balance of enzymatic activity within the synapse to be tipped in favour of phosphorylation, which triggers T-cell signalling. T cells in which the molecules that usually segregate in the cSMAC are artificially made to be the same size as CD45 cannot exclude CD45 from the synapse and are unable to signal.

T-cell signalling requires phosphorylation of ITAMs. The ζ chains of the TCR, CD4 and CD28 all contain immunoreceptor tyrosine-based activation motifs (ITAMs) in their cytoplasmic tails (see Chapter 6, the TCR complex). When they are clustered together in the absence of the phosphatase CD45, the ITAMs initiate signalling by recruiting tyrosine kinases. The most important of these are:

- Lck, which is recruited by CD4 and phosphorylates ITAMs on the ζ chains of the TCR.
- Fyn, which is recruited to the ζ chains and phosphorylates phospholipase C (PLCγ). Phosphorylated PLCγ cleaves a

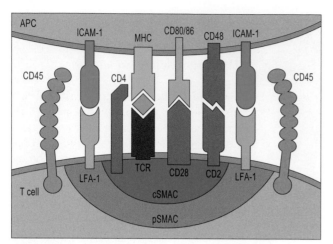

Fig. 7.15 Molecular interactions in the immunological synapse T-cell receptor *(TCR)*, the co-receptor (which may be CD4 or CD8), CD28 and CD2 are molecules with relatively small extracellular domains, and contact their ligands on the antigen-presenting cell *(APC)* in the centre of the immune synapse, or cSMAC. The adhesion molecule leukocyte function-associated antigen 1 (LFA-1) moves to the periphery, or pSMAC, where it contacts interceullar adhesion molecule 1 (ICAM-1) on the APC. CD45 is a phosphatase with a large, stiff extracellular domain and is excluded from the synapse. It is thought that the exclusion of CD45 allows phosphorylation, and thus signalling, to occur within the synapse.

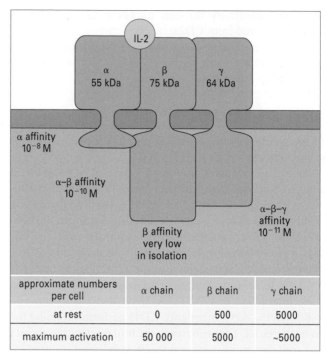

approximate numbers per cell	α chain	β chain	γ chain
at rest	0	500	5000
maximum activation	50 000	5000	~5000

Fig. 7.16 Expression of the high-affinity IL-2 receptor on T cell The high-affinity IL-2R consists of three polypeptide chains, shown schematically. Resting T cells do not express the α chain, but after activation they may express up to 50 000 α chains per cell. Some of these associate with the β chain to form the high-affinity IL-2R. (The γc chain is a common signalling chain of several cytokine receptors.)

phospholipid component of the cell membrane into two products, one of which promotes Ca^{2+} release from the ER and influx from outside the cell. This is required for the activation of the transcription factors NF-κB and NF-AT (see later).

- ZAP-70, which is recruited to the ζ chain and phosphorylates a transmembrane protein called LAT, which localizes to lipid rafts. Once phosphorylated, LAT acts as a docking site for molecules that integrate signals from the TCR and CD28.

Intracellular signalling pathways activate transcription factors. Immune synapse formation and the subsequent recruitment of signalling tyrosine kinases initiates a cascade of intracellular signals, which ultimately terminates in the activation of the transcription factors NF-κB, NF-AT and AP1 (Fig. 7.w1).

The IL-2 enhancer contains binding sites for NF-AT, hence NF-AT induces IL-2 production. Two widely used immunosuppressive drugs, ciclosporin and tacrolimus, work by preventing NF-AT from translocating to the nucleus.

Interleukin-2 drives T-cell division. T-cell activation leads to the production of IL-2 and IL-2 receptors and a T cell can act on itself and on its surrounding cells. In most CD4⁺ and some CD8⁺ T cells, there is transient production of IL-2 for 1–2 days. During this time, the interaction of IL-2 with the high-affinity IL-2R results in T-cell division.

On resting T cells, the IL-2R is predominantly present as a low-affinity form consisting of two polypeptide chains, a β chain (CD122) that binds to IL-2 and a common γc chain (CD132) that signals to the cell. When the T cell is activated, it produces

an α chain (CD25), which contributes to IL-2 binding and, together with the β and γc chains, forms the high-affinity receptor (Fig. 7.16). IL-2 is internalized within 10–20 minutes and the β and γc chains aree degraded in lysosomes while the α chain is recycled to the cell surface. Sustained IL-2 signalling over several hours is needed to drive T-cell division.

The transient expression of the high-affinity IL-2R for about 1 week after stimulation of the T cell, together with the induction of CTLA-4, helps limit T-cell division. In the absence of positive signals, most of the T cells will die by apoptosis. However, a few remain alive to become memory cells. The life span of memory cells can be more than 40 years in humans.

In view of the importance of IL-2 in T-cell division, it was surprising that the rare patients who lack CD25 (and CD25 knockout mice) develop an immunoproliferative condition. These observations led to an awareness that IL-2 also has a regulatory function in T-cell development. Regulatory T cells (Tregs) are characterized by high CD25 expression and IL-2 is required for their generation in the thymus and maintenance in the periphery (see Chapters 2 and 12).

Other cytokines contribute to activation and division. As T-cell division and immune responses are not ablated in mice lacking the IL-2 or IL-2Rα genes, it suggests that other cytokines may support T-cell division. The cytokine IL-15 is structurally similar to IL-2, acts on a receptor that shares the β and γc chains of the IL-2 receptor and causes the expansion of T- and NK-cell populations. IL-15 is produced by APCs and may therefore be important in initial T-cell activation before IL-2 is produced.

Although it was originally defined as a B-cell growth and differentiation factor, IL-4 can also induce division of naive T cells. The relative importance of these other cytokines will vary depending on the state of the T cell and these cytokines may partly overlap in their functions with IL-2.

Other cytokines contribute indirectly to T-cell proliferation. For example, IL-1 and IL-6 induce the expression of IL-2R on resting T cells and may thus enhance their responsiveness to IL-2. IL-1 and IL-6 are produced by mononuclear phagocytes and may therefore enhance their antigen-presenting function.

Activated T cells signal back to APCs. Antigen presentation is not a unidirectional process. Activated T cells:

- release cytokines such as IFNγ and granulocyte-macrophage colony stimulating factor (GM-CSF), which activate APCs;
- express CD40 ligand (CD40L; CD154), which binds to the co-stimulatory molecule CD40 on the APC. In macrophages, this increases their production of microbicidal substances, including reactive oxygen species and nitric oxide. In B cells, CD40 ligation is important for class switching and differentiation to plasma cells (see Chapter 9).

CRITICAL THINKING: ANTIGEN PROCESSING AND PRESENTATION

See Critical thinking: Explanations, section 7

Two T-cell clones have been produced from a mouse infected with influenza virus. One of the clones reacts to a virus peptide when it is presented on APCs that have the same MHC class I (H-2K) locus as the original mouse (i.e. the clone is MHC class I restricted). The other clone is MHC class II restricted. The two clones are stimulated in tissue culture using syngeneic macrophages as APCs. The macrophages have been either infected with live influenza virus or treated with inactivated virus. The patterns of reactivity of the two clones are shown in the table. In the last two lines of the table the macrophages are pretreated with either emetine or chloroquine before they are infected with virus. Emetine is a protein synthesis inhibitor. Chloroquine inhibits the fusion of lysosomes with phagosomes.

1. Why does the live influenza virus stimulate both clones, whereas the inactivated virus stimulates only the MHC class II-restricted clone?
2. What result would you expect if you used infected fibroblasts as the antigen-presenting cell?
3. What result would you expect if you used XCR1+ DCs?
4. Why does emetine prevent the macrophages from presenting antigen to the MHC class I-restricted T cells, whereas chloroquine prevents them from presenting to MHC class II-restricted cells?
5. One of these clones expresses CD4 and the other CD8. Which way round is it?

REACTIVITY OF CLONE

Antigen	APCs Treated With	Clone 1	Clone 2
None	—	—	—
Live virus	—	+	+
Inactivated virus	—	—	+
Live virus	Emetine	—	+
Live virus	Chloroquine	+	—

FURTHER READING

Blander JM. Regulation of the cell biology of antigen cross-presentation. Annu Rev Immunol 2018;26:717–753.

Davis SJ, van der Merwe PA. The kinetic-segregation model: TCR triggering and beyond. Nat Immunol 2006;7:803–809.

Gaud G, Lesourne R, Love PE. Regulatory mechanisms in T cell receptor signaling. Nat Rev Immunol 2018;19:1–13.

Grotzke JE, Sengupta D, Lu Q, Cresswell P. The ongoing saga of the mechanism(s) of MHC class I-restricted cross-presentation. Curr Opin Immunol 2017;46:89–96.

Malissen B, Bongard P. Early T cell activation: integrated biochemical, structural, and biophysical cues. Annu Rev Immunol 2015;33:539–561.

Sharpe AH, Pauken KE. The diverse function of the PD1 inhibitory pathway. Nat Rev Immunol 2018;18:153–167.

Van Kaer L, Wu L, Joyce S. Mechanisms and consequences of antigen presentation by CD1. Trends Immunol 2016;37:738–754.

van Kasteren SI, Overkleeft H, Ovaa H, Neefjes J. Chemical biology of antigen presentation by MHC molecules. Curr Opin Immunol 2014;26:21–31.

Walker LS, Sansom DM. Confusing signals: recent progress in CTLA-4 biology. Trends Immunol 2015;36:63–70.

Withers DR. Innate lymphoid cell regulation of adaptive immunity. Immunology 2016;149:123–130.

8

Cell-Mediated Cytotoxicity

SUMMARY

- **Cell-mediated cytotoxicity is an essential defence against intracellular pathogens, including viruses, some bacteria and some parasites.**
- **Cytotoxic T lymphocytes (CTLs) and natural killer (NK) cells are the lymphoid effectors of cytotoxicity.** Most CTLs are CD8$^+$ and respond to non self antigens presented on major histocompatibility complex (MHC) class I molecules. Some virally infected and cancerous cells try to evade the CTL response by downregulating MHC class I. NK cells recognize these MHC class I negative targets.
- **NK cells recognize cells that fail to express MHC class I.** NK cells express a variety of inhibitory receptors that recognize MHC class I molecules. When these receptors are not engaged, the NK cell is activated. Killer immunoglobulin-like receptors (KIRs) recognize classical MHC class I molecules. CD94 interacts with HLA-E. LILRB1 recognizes a wide range of class I molecules.
- **Cancerous and virally infected cells express ligands for the activating receptor NKG2D.** Stressed cells, including cancerous and virally infected cells, upregulate ULBP1–3, MICA and MICB, which are ligands for NKG2D. This results in NK-cell activation.

- **NK cells can also mediate ADCC.** They recognize antibody-coated targets using the Fc receptor CD16 (FcγRIII).
- **The balance of inhibitory and activating signals determines NK-cell activation.**
- **Cytotoxicity is effected by direct cellular interactions, granule exocytosis and cytokine production.** Fas ligand and tumour necrosis factor (TNF) can induce apoptosis in the target cell. Granules containing perforin and granzymes are also released. Perforin forms a pore in the cell membrane, allowing granzymes access to the cytosol. Granzymes trigger the cell's intrinsic apoptosis pathways.
- **Macrophages, neutrophils and eosinophils are non-lymphoid cytotoxic effectors.** Macrophages and neutrophils usually destroy pathogens by phagocytosis but can sometimes also release the contents of their granules into the extracellular environment. Eosinophils release cytotoxic granules in response to antibody-coated cells.

Cytotoxicity describes the ways in which leukocytes can recognize and destroy other cells. It is an essential defence against intracellular pathogens, including viruses, some bacteria and some parasites. Tumour cells and even normal host cells may also become the targets of cytotoxic cells. Cytotoxicity is important in the destruction of allogeneic tissue grafts.

Several types of cells have cytotoxic potential, including:
- cytotoxic T lymphocytes (CTLs);
- natural killer (NK) cells; and
- some myeloid cells.

The two cytotoxic lymphoid effector cells recognize their targets in different ways but use similar mechanisms to kill them. The myeloid cells use different recognition and killing mechanisms from the lymphoid cells and indeed these also differ between different types of myeloid cell.

CYTOTOXIC LYMPHOCYTES

CTLs and NK cells mediate cytotoxicity. T cells and NK cells belong to the lymphoid lineage and are more closely related to each other than they are to B cells. CTLs and NK cells all induce apoptosis in their targets by production of TNF family molecules, cytokines and cytotoxic granules, but they recognize their targets in different ways. CTLs recognize foreign antigens being presented on major histocompatibility complex (MHC) class I, whereas NK cells respond to cells that

fail to express class I. NK cells are also able to recognize stressed or antibody-coated target cells directly (Fig. 8.1).

Effector CTLs home to peripheral organs and sites of inflammation. Naive CTLs circulate in the blood and lymphatic system but, in order to kill specific target cells, they must be activated and become effector cells. This process is mediated by antigen-presenting cells (APCs) in the lymph nodes. Naive T cells in the lymph nodes use their T-cell receptor (TCR) to recognize specific antigens being presented by MHC molecules on APCs. Most CTLs are CD8$^+$ and therefore recognize antigen presented on MHC class I molecules. Like nearly all nucleated cells, APCs may present endogenous peptide on MHC class I, but some APCs also have the ability to present exogenous peptide from phagocytosed particles on MHC class I. This process is called cross-presentation and is extremely important for an effective CD8$^+$ CTL response (see Chapter 7).

A minority of CD4$^+$ cells are cytotoxic and these recognize antigen presented on MHC class II molecules.

If, in addition to signalling through the TCR, the APC also delivers a co-stimulatory signal through CD28, the CTL becomes activated and proliferates. Activated CTLs downregulate the sphingosine phosphate receptor, allowing them to exit the lymph node. They also downregulate molecules associated with homing to the lymph node, such as L-selectin and CCR7, and upregulate molecules that allow them to home to sites of inflammation, such

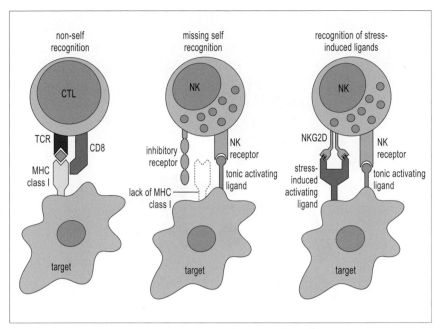

Fig. 8.1 Cytotoxic T lymphocytes *(CTLs)* and natural killer *(NK)* cells mediate cytotoxicity CTLs recognize processed antigen presented on the target cell by major histocompatibility complex *(MHC)* molecules, using their T-cell receptor *(TCR)*. Most CTLs are CD8+ and recognize antigen presented by MHC class I molecules, but a minority are CD4+ and recognize antigen presented on MHC class II molecules. In contrast, NK cells have receptors that recognize MHC class I on the target and inhibit cytotoxicity. NK cells also express a number of activating receptors to identify their targets positively, including NKG2D and their Fc receptor (CD16).

as CD44 and LFA-1. Effector T cells may also express adhesion molecules that allow them to home to specific tissues. Circulating CD8+ memory T cells appear to migrate preferentially to the tissue in which they first encountered their antigen and some CD8+ memory T cells become resident in the tissue and are called resident memory T cells, or T_{RM}.

CTLs recognize antigen presented on MHC class I molecules. The most important role of CTLs is the elimination of virally infected cells. CTLs recognize specific antigens (e.g. viral peptides on infected cells) presented by MHC class I molecules, which are expressed by nearly all nucleated cells. Cellular molecules that have been partly degraded by the proteasome are transported to the endoplasmic reticulum, where they become associated with MHC class I molecules and are transported to the cell surface. Normal cells therefore present a sample of all the antigens they produce to CD8+ T cells.

Like CD4+ T cells, CD8+ CTLs form an immunological synapse with their target. Signalling molecules, including the TCR and CD3, are found in the central zone of the supra-molecular activation cluster (cSMAC) and adhesion molecules segregate in the peripheral zone (pSMAC). In contrast to CD4+ T cells, the cSMAC of CTLs and NK cells is divided into signalling and secretory domains (Fig. 8.2). After signalling has occurred, the microtubule-organizing centre polarizes towards the synapse, directing cytotoxic granules to the secretory domain of the cSMAC. Early CTL signalling occurs within 10 seconds of cell–cell contact and granule release follows some 2 minutes later.

CTLs and NK cells are complementary in the defence against virally infected and cancerous cells. NK cells were first identified as a subset of immune cells that were able to kill tumour cells in vitro without prior immunization of the host, even in T-cell-deficient mice. In 1981, Klas Kärre made the seminal observation that targets killed by NK cells tend to be spared by T cells and vice versa. From this, he reasoned that NK cells must recognize targets that are not expressing a full complement of self molecules. Kärre's 'missing self' hypothesis postulates that unlike T cells, which recognize non-self (foreign peptide or foreign MHC), NK cells respond to the absence of MHC class I.

Several viruses (particularly herpes viruses) have evolved mechanisms to avoid recognition by CTLs. They reduce the expression of MHC class I molecules on the cell surface to reduce the likelihood that processed viral peptides can be presented to CTLs. Cancerous cells may evade the CTL response in a similar way. NK cells specifically recognize cells that have lost their MHC class I molecules. Therefore, NK cells and CTLs act in a complementary way. In effect:
- NK cells check that cells of the body are carrying their identity card (MHC class I);
- CTLs check the specific identity (antigen specificity) on the card.

Human peripheral blood contains two kinds of NK cells. NK cells in human blood are defined as CD3− CD56+. Within this group, there are CD56Lo cells (usually called CD56dim NK cells) and CD56Hi cells (usually called CD56bright NK cells).

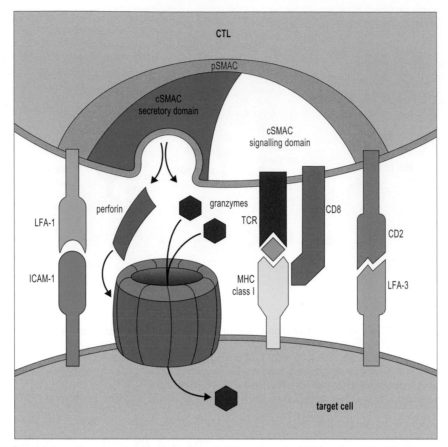

Fig. 8.2 Some interactions involved in the cytotoxic T-lymphocyte *(CTL)* **synapse** The T-cell receptor *(TCR)* and CD8 localize to the signalling domain in the centre of the synapse *(cSMAC)*; degranulation occurs in the secretory domain. Adhesion molecules that stabilize the cell–cell interactions are located at the periphery of the supramolecular activation complex *(pSMAC)*.

- CD56^{Lo} cells account for 90% of circulating NK cells. They are highly cytotoxic and recognize their targets using the Fc receptor CD16, killer immunoglobulin-like receptors (KIRs) and to a lesser extent NKG2A.
- CD56^{Hi} cells account for 10% of circulating NK cells. They are less cytotoxic than CD56^{Lo} cells but more able to produce IFNγ. They do not express CD16 or KIRs but express high levels of NKG2A. There is some evidence that CD56^{Hi} cells are immature NK cells that can differentiate into CD56^{Lo} NK cells.

NK-CELL RECEPTORS

NK cells recognize cells that fail to express MHC class I. NK cells express inhibitory receptors that bind to MHC class I molecules. When they encounter a target cell that is not expressing MHC class I, this inhibitory signal is lost and tonic activating signals cause the NK cell to degranulate or to produce cytokines in response to the target cell.

Many of the inhibitory receptors expressed by NK cells have activating counterparts, many of which recognize the same ligands but with lower affinity (Table. 8.1). In some cases where NK-cell receptors recognize MHC class I molecules, the peptide being presented affects binding affinity and it may be that these activating receptors can only recognize their ligands when a specific peptide is being presented. For example, the inhibitory receptor CD94-NKG2A recognizes HLA-E with high affinity; its activating counterpart CD94-NKG2C recognizes HLA-E with high affinity only when it is presenting human cytomegalovirus (HCMV)-derived peptides.

KIRs recognize MHC class I. The KIRs are members of the immunoglobulin superfamily. They are present on the majority of CD56^{Lo} NK cells, with each individual NK cell expressing a random selection of KIRs. Almost none of the CD56^{Hi} NK cells express KIRs.

KIRs fall into two main subsets:
- KIR2D (CD158) have two immunoglobulin domains;
- KIR3D have three immunoglobulin domains.

The KIRs are then further classified by whether they have a long (L) or short (S) cytoplasmic tail. KIRs with long tails are inhibitory and those with short tails are activating (Fig. 8.3). For example, the inhibitory receptor KIR2DL1 has two immunoglobulin domains and a long cytoplasmic tail. It binds alleles of HLA-C that have a lysine residue at position 80 (HLA-C2 alleles). Its activating counterpart, KIR2DS1 also binds HLA-C2 alleles, but with lower affinity.

TABLE 8.1 NK-Cell Receptors With Well-Defined Ligands

Family	Receptor	Ligands	
KIR	KIR2DL1	HLA-C2	Inhibitory
	KIR2DS1	HLA-C2,	Activating
	KIR2DL2/L3	HLA-C1 (high affinity), HLA-C2 (low affinity)	Inhibitory
	KIR2DS2	HLA-C1	Activating
	KIR3DS1	HLA-F	Activating
	KIR3DL1	HLA-Bw4	Inhibitory
	KIR3DL2	HLA-A3 and A11	Inhibitory
C-type lectin-like	CD94-NKG2A	HLA-E	Inhibitory
	CD94-NKG2C	HLA-E	Activating
	CD94-NKG2E	HLA-E	Activating
	NKG2D	MICA, MICB, ULBPs	Activating
NCRs	NKp30	BAT3, B7-H6, PfEMP1, heparan sulfates	Activating
	NKp44	Viral haemagglutinins, viral envelope glycoproteins, heparan sulfates	Activating
	NKp46	Viral haemagglutinins, PfEMP1, complement factor P, heparan sulphates	Activating
LILR	LILRB1	Broad MHC-I	Inhibitory
Others	LAIR1	Collagens	Inhibitory
	Siglec-7	Sialic acid	Inhibitory
	KLRG1	Cadherins	Inhibitory
	CEACAM1	CEACAM1	Inhibitory
	CD16	IgG	Activating
	CD58 (LFA-3)	CD2 (LFA-2)	Activating
	2B4	CD48	Activating

KIR, Killer immunoglobulin-like receptors; *MHC*, major histocompatibility complex; *NCR*, natural cytotoxicity receptor; *NK*, natural killer.

Fig. 8.3 Killer immunoglobulin-like receptors *(KIRs)* KIRs consist of either two or three extracellular immunoglobulin superfamily domains. The inhibitory forms have long cytoplasmic tails that contain immunoreceptor tyrosine-based inhibitory motifs *(ITIMs)*. The activating forms have short cytoplasmic tails and a charged lysine residue *(K)* in their transmembrane domains, which allows them to associate with an immunoreceptor tyrosine-based activation motif (ITAM)-containing adapter molecule.

Inhibitory KIRs therefore allow NK cells to recognize and respond to cells that have downregulated specific HLA molecules. This is likely to explain genetic associations whereby those individuals who have both a particular KIR and its cognate HLA molecule experience better outcomes in some viral diseases, such as hepatitis B and C.

Because activating KIRs bind to MHC class I molecules with such low affinity, it has been difficult to define their ligands and the normal functions of most activating KIRs are still unknown. However, some clues about their function have come from genetic studies. For example, patients who have both KIR3DS1 and its putative ligand HLA-Bw4 experience slower progression to AIDS in HIV infection and women who have the activating KIR2DS1 experience better outcomes in pregnancy when the fetus expresses its ligand, HLA-C2. Similarly, the presence of activating KIR in the donor is associated with better outcomes following haematopoietic stem-cell transplantation for myeloid malignancies.

NK cells in mice do not express KIRs. Instead, they use Ly49 receptors, which are members of the lectin-like receptor family. Like KIRs, Ly49 receptors come in inhibitory and activating forms, bind to specific MHC class I molecules and are expressed stochastically. Unlike KIRs, which recognize the top of the peptide-binding groove of MHC class I, Ly49 receptors recognize the underside of the molecule. Ly49 and KIRs are unrelated molecules that perform the same function in different species, demonstrating convergent evolution in NK-cell function between species.

The lectin-like receptor CD94 recognizes HLA-E. The lectin-like receptor CD94 is present on the majority of CD56^Hi NK cells, a large subset of CD56^Lo NK cells, and is also found on a small subset of CTLs. It covalently associates with different members of another group of lectin-like receptors called NKG2 and the heterodimers are expressed at the cell membrane.

There are at least six members of the NKG2 family (NKG2A–F), of which all except NKG2D associate with CD94. NKG2A-CD94 is an inhibitory receptor that blocks NK-cell activation. By contrast, CD94-NKG2C is an activating receptor (Fig. 8.4). The ligand for both CD94-NKG2A and CD94-NKG2C is HLA-E, although under most circumstances the inhibitory CD94-NKG2A has greater affinity for HLA-E than its activating counterpart. CD94-NKG2A allows NK cells to recognize and to respond to cells, such as those that are virally infected or cancerous, and are expressing low levels of MHC class I molecules.

The *HLA-E* gene locus encodes an MHC class I-like molecule. These are sometimes called non-classical class I molecules, or class Ib molecules, to distinguish them from the classical MHC molecules that present antigen to CTLs. HLA-E presents peptides from other MHC class I molecules. The leader peptides from other MHC molecules are transported to the endoplasmic reticulum and are loaded into the peptide-binding groove of HLA-E molecules, stabilizing them and allowing them to be transported to the plasma membrane (Fig. 8.5). Cells lacking classical MHC class I molecules do not express HLA-E at the cell surface. Thus, surface HLA-E levels provide a sensitive mechanism for monitoring global MHC class I expression by the cell.

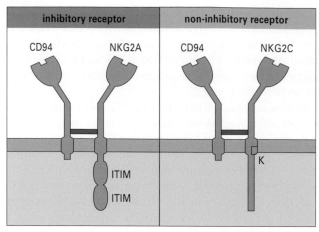

Fig. 8.4 Lectin-like receptors of natural killer (NK) cells CD94 associates with members of the NKG2 family via a disulfide bond. NKG2A contains intracellular immunoreceptor tyrosine-based inhibitory motifs *(ITIMs)* and so forms an inhibitory receptor. NKG2C lacks ITIMs but has a charged lysine residue *(K)* in its transmembrane segment, which allows it to interact with immunoreceptor tyrosine-based activating motif (ITAM)-containing adapter molecules.

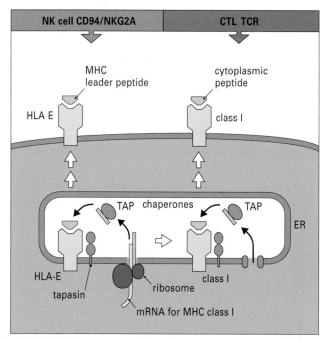

Fig. 8.5 HLA-E presents peptides of other major histocompatibility complex *(MHC)* **class I molecules** Leader peptides from MHC class I molecules are loaded onto HLA-E molecules in the endoplasmic reticulum *(ER)*, a process that requires transporters associated with antigen-processing *(TAP)* and tapasin to assemble functional HLA-E molecules. These are presented at the cell surface for review by CD94 receptors on natural killer *(NK)* cells. The MHC class I molecules meanwhile present antigenic peptides from cytoplasmic proteins that have been transported into the ER. These complexes are presented to the T-cell receptor *(TCR)* on CD8+ cytotoxic T lymphocytes *(CTLs)*.

LILRB1 recognizes all MHC class I molecules including HLA-G.
LILRB1 belongs to the LILR family of type I transmembrane proteins with multiple extracellular immuno-globulin domains (previously called the ILT family or CD85).

Of this family, only two inhibitory receptors, LILRB1 and LILRB2, have well-defined ligands and these interact with a broad spectrum of MHC class I molecules. LILRB1 is expressed by a proportion of NK cells and some T cells, B cells and all monocytes, whereas LILRB2 is only expressed by monocytes and dendritic cells. Thus LILRB1, like CD94-NKG2A, allows NK cells to detect target cells that are expressing low levels of any MHC class I molecule.

LILRB1 recognizes both classical and non-classical MHC class I molecules, but it has a particularly high affinity for the non-classical molecule HLA-G, whose expression is restricted to extravillous trophoblast cells in the placenta. Interaction of LILRB1 with HLA-G inhibits NK-cell cytotoxicity more strongly than that with other class I molecules, although the significance of this observation is not yet clear.

NK cells are self-tolerant.
The MHC and NK receptor loci are polygenic, polymorphic and unlinked. Furthermore, NK cells are highly heterogeneous with respect to their receptor repertoire, with some NK cells failing to express any inhibitory receptors that recognize self MHC class I molecules. Since they cannot be inhibited by self MHC class I molecules, these NK cells are potentially autoreactive. Therefore, similar to the cells of the adaptive immune system, there must be some mechanism by which NK-cell tolerance to self is established and maintained.

The mechanisms that maintain NK tolerance to self have not yet been defined, but some simple rules are clear:
- An NK cell lacking an inhibitory receptor that recognizes a self MHC class I molecule cannot carry out cytotoxicity or cytokine production in response to target cells.
- An NK receptor that has an activating receptor that recognizes a self MHC class I molecule is also unable to carry out effector functions. Such NK cells are referred to as hyporesponsive.
- Hyporesponsive NK cells may still be able to carry out effector functions in some situations, such as when activated by IL-2 or when they recognize an antibody-coated cell using their Fc receptors.
- NK cells can tune their responsiveness when they move between environments. A classic experimental demonstration of this is that NK cells adoptively transferred from a wild-type mouse to one that lacks MHC class I rapidly reduce their responsiveness. Physiologically, this may occur as NK cells move between tissues with different levels of MHC class I expression. For example expression of MHC class I is very low or absent from neurons and some glial cells in the CNS, but these cells are not targeted by NK cells.

Cancerous and virally-infected cells are recognized by NKG2D.
Like other NKG2 receptors, NKG2D is a member of the C-type lectin receptor family, but unlike other NKG2 molecules, NKG2D does not associate with CD94, instead forming a disulfide-linked homodimer (Fig. 8.6). It is an activating receptor expressed by all circulating NK cells.

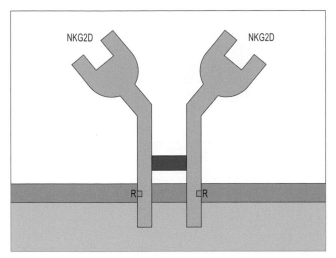

Fig. 8.6 NKG2D forms disulfide-linked homodimers NKG2D forms disulfide-linked homodimers. Its transmembrane domain contains an arginine residue *(R)*, which allows it to recruit the adapter protein DAP10.

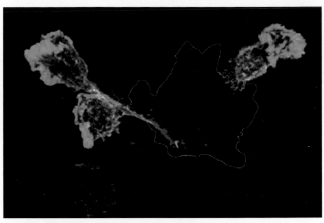

Fig. 8.7 Fluorescence micrograph of two natural killer cells attacking a tumour cell F-actin is stained *red* and perforin *green*. (Courtesy Dr Pedro Roda Navarro and Dr Hugh Reyburn.)

In humans, the ligands for NKG2D are the MHC class-I–like molecules ULBP1–3, MICA and MICB. Expression of these molecules is upregulated by a variety of cellular stresses, including heat shock, oxidative stress, proliferation and viral infection. Thus, NKG2D allows NK cells to recognize cells that are stressed, including virally infected and cancerous cells. For this reason, some viruses encode immune evasion proteins that interfere with NKG2D ligand expression and some cancers produce soluble NKG2D ligands that block NKG2D recognition of its ligands at the cell surface.

The natural cytotoxicity receptors (NCRs) recognize a variety of ligands.
The natural cytotoxicity receptors, NKp30, NKp44 and NKp46, recognize a variety of ligands that are associated with virally infected and cancerous cells.

Heparan sulfate proteoglycans are differentially expressed in cancerous versus healthy tissues, and all three NCRs are able to recognize these ligands. NKp30 recognizes two additional tumour-associated ligands, B7-H6 and BAT3.

NKp44 and NKp46 recognize viral haemagglutinins and some viral envelope glycoproteins, providing a mechanism through which NK cells can detect virally infected cells directly.

NK cells can also recognize antibody on target cells using Fc receptors.
The Fc receptor CD16 (FcγRIII) is expressed by all CD56^{Lo} NK cells, but not by CD56^{Hi} cells. CD16 binds antibody bound to target cells, activating the NK cell so that it degranulates, mediating antibody–dependent cell-mediated cytotoxicity (ADCC) (Fig. 8.7). NK-cell–mediated ADCC requires both an adaptive immune stimulus (cells coated with antibody) and an innate immune effector mechanism (NK cells) and is thus an example of cross-talk between the innate and adaptive immune systems.

The balance of inhibitory and activating signals controls NK cell activation.
During an interaction with a target cell, an NK cell must decide between cytotoxic action and inaction. This decision depends on the co-ordination of intracellular signalling pathways and may involve the balance between activating and inhibitory signals.

- Inhibitory receptors contain an immunoreceptor tyrosine-based inhibitory motif (ITIM) in their cytoplasmic tails. These recruit inhibitory phosphatases, which disrupt phosphorylation of activating receptors and intracellular signalling molecules and prevent NK-cell activation. All NK-cell inhibitory receptors contain an ITIM.
- CD94-NKG2C and activating KIR associate with intracellular proteins that have an immunoreceptor tyrosine-based activation motif (ITAM). This allows them to phosphorylate and to recruit tyrosine kinases, including ZAP-70, which lead to cellular activation. CD16, NKp46, NKp44 and NKp30 also associate with ITAM-bearing intracellular molecules.
- Some other activating receptors recruit an intracellular adapter that has an ITAM-like motif. For example, NKG2D recruits the adapter molecule DAP10, which bears the ITAM-like motif, YXXM.

In addition to inhibitory receptors that recognize MHC class I, NK cells express inhibitory receptors for collagens (LAIR1, CD305) and sialic acid (Siglecs). These may affect the balance of activation and inhibition at locations where they are present in large amounts, such as in tissues.

To degranulate, NK cells require a longer contact period with their targets than CTLs do and this reflects the more complex processing that must occur to integrate activating and inhibitory signals at the NK-cell immunological synapse (Fig. 8.8).

NK cells display some features of adaptive immune cells.
NK cells have traditionally been thought of as members of the innate immune system, but it has recently emerged that they do display some features of adaptive immune cells.

Rag-deficient mice, which lack T and B cells, can be protected against death when infected with a large dose of mouse cytomegalovirus (MCMV) if they are first exposed to a small dose. The protective effect can be transferred between animals by transferring NK cells, suggesting that NK cells mediate the effect. NK cells expressing the activating receptor Ly49H, which

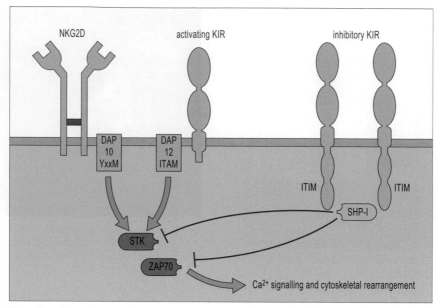

Fig. 8.8 Signalling through activating and inhibitory receptors Signalling through activating receptors leads to the recruitment of adapter molecules *(DAP10, DAP12)* that contain either an ITAM- or ITAM-like motif. These recruit and phosphorylate intracellular signalling molecules, leading to NK-cell activation. Signalling through inhibitory receptors recruits inhibitory phosphatases *(SHP-1)*, which inhibit the phosphorylation of activating signalling molecules. *ITAM*, Immunoreceptor tyrosine-based activation motif; *ITIM*, immunoreceptor tyrosine-based inhibitory motif; *STK*, signalling tyrosine kinase.

recognizes the MCMV protein m157, expand on MCMV infection. After infection, the Ly49H NK cells contract, but a small number are retained, becoming long-lived, and this population is able to re-expand rapidly in response to a second infection. This is reminiscent of a T-cell or B-cell memory response, although unlike a T-cell or B-cell response, the critical receptor in this case is germline encoded and can only respond to MCMV.

Similarly, an NK-cell population expressing the activating receptor NKG2C expands during human cytomegalovirus (HCMV) infection and population studies point to these cells being long-lived. These cells recognize peptides from the viral protein UL40, presented by HLA-E.

CYTOTOXICITY

Cytotoxicity is effected by direct cellular interactions, granule exocytosis and cytokines. CTLs and NK cells use a variety of different mechanisms to kill their targets. These include:

- direct cell–cell signalling via TNF family molecules;
- pore formation, which allows apoptosis-inducing proteins to access the target cell cytoplasm;
- indirect signalling via cytokines.

All of these mechanisms culminate in target-cell death by apoptosis. Apoptosis is a form of programmed cell death in which the nucleus fragments and the cytoplasm, plasma membranes and organelles condense into apoptotic bodies and are digested. Any remnants are phagocytosed by tissue macrophages.

Apoptosis can be triggered in one of three ways (Fig 8.9):

- the extrinsic pathway begins outside the cell. Recognition of pro-apoptotic proteins by cell surface receptors initiates the caspase cascade;
- the intrinsic pathway is initiated from within the cell. Pro-apoptotic proteins are released from the mitochondria and initiate the caspase cascade;
- DNA damage in the nucleus can cause apoptosis via a caspase-independent pathway.

The target cell remains in control of its internal processes throughout apoptosis. Thus, CTLs and NK cells effectively instruct their targets to commit suicide.

Cytotoxicity may be signalled via TNF receptor family molecules on the target cell. CTLs and NK cells can initiate apoptosis in their targets via the extrinsic pathway using members of the tumour necrosis factor (TNF) family of molecules. These include:

- TNFα, which binds to TNFR1;
- Fas ligand, which binds to Fas (CD95);
- TRAIL, which binds to TRAIL receptors.

Although TNFα is predominantly produced by macrophages, activated CD4+ T cells, CD8+ T cells and NK cells are also able to produce this cytokine, which can induce apoptosis in target cells by binding to and cross-linking its receptor. The cross-linked receptor forms a trimer, which recruits caspases 8 and 10 via an intracellular adapter protein called TRADD (TNF receptor associated death domain), leading to apoptosis.

Fas ligand and TRAIL are membrane-bound TNF family molecules. Fas ligand is expressed by CD4+ T cells, CD8+ T cells and NK cells and binds to the widely expressed cell surface

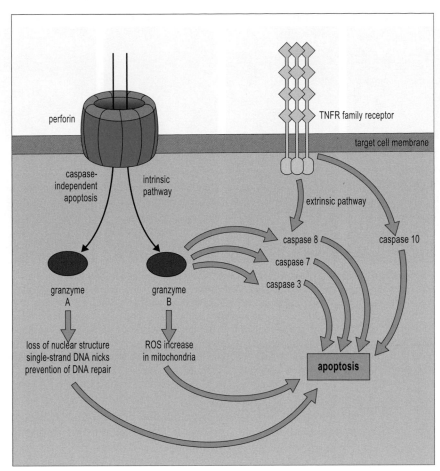

Fig. 8.9 Cytotoxic T lymphocytes (CTLs) and natural killer (NK) cells can trigger apoptosis CTLs and NK cells can trigger apoptosis in their targets by signalling through molecules of the tumour necrosis factor (TNF) receptor *(TFNR)* family, which activate caspases 8 and 10, to initiate apoptosis via the extrinsic pathway. CTLs and NK cells also trigger apoptosis in their targets by releasing cytotoxic granules. Perforin forms a pore in the target cell membrane, allowing granzymes access to the cytoplasm. Granzyme B activates caspases 3, 7 and 8, triggering apoptosis via the intrinsic pathway. Granzyme A initiates a caspase-independent pathway of apoptosis. *ROS,* Reactive oxygen species.

protein Fas. TRAIL (TNF-related apoptosis-inducing ligand) is expressed by CD8$^+$ T cells and NK cells, but not usually by CD4$^+$ T cells, and binds to a family of cell surface molecules called TRAIL receptors. Cross-linking and trimerization of Fas and TRAIL receptors leads to the recruitment of the intracellular adapter protein, FADD (Fas-associated protein with death domain), which recruits caspases 8 and 10, leading to apoptosis.

Apoptotic signals delivered by members of the TNF family are Ca^{2+} independent.

CTL and NK cell granules contain perforin and granzymes.

Activated CTLs and resting CD56^{Lo} NK cells contain numerous cytoplasmic granules called lytic granules. Upon recognition of a target cell, these granules polarize to the site of contact, the immunological synapse, releasing their contents into a small cleft between the two cells (Fig. 8.10). The lytic granules contain the pore-forming protein perforin and a series of granule-associated enzymes, called granzymes.

Perforin is a monomeric pore-forming protein that is inactive when located within granules, but undergoes a conformational activation, which is Ca^{2+} dependent. It is

related both structurally and functionally to the complement component C9, which forms the membrane attack complex. Like C9, perforin is able to form homopolymers, inserting into the membrane to form a circular pore of approximately 16 nm diameter. Unlike C9, perforin is able to bind membrane phospholipids directly in the presence of Ca^{2+} (Fig. 8.11).

Perforin-deficient mice show greatly reduced cytotoxicity. The fact that some cytotoxicity remains demonstrates that other mechanisms contribute to CTL- and NK-cell–mediated death. Some of the residual killing is likely to come from TNF family molecules.

Granzymes are serine proteases that are released from the lytic granules alongside perforin. Once perforin has formed a pore in the cell membrane, granzymes may enter the target cell cytoplasm and cleave a number of substrates, leading to apoptosis via the intrinsic pathway:

- Granzyme B cleaves pro-caspases 3, 7 and 8, triggering apoptosis in the target cell. Granzyme B-deficient mice show delayed but not ablated cytotoxicity, illustrating the importance of other pathways.

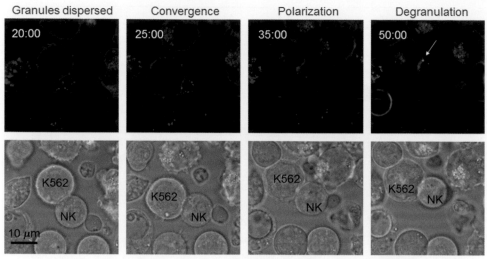

Fig. 8.10 Polarization of granules during natural killer *(NK)* cell–target cell interaction A human NK-cell line (NK92) expressing the degranulation indicator LAMP1-pHluorin *(green)* and with lytic granules shown in *red* (LysoTracker Red) were incubated with NK targets (K562) labelled with yellow membrane dye, then imaged by confocal microscopy. A representative image is shown without *(top)* and with *(bottom)* bright-field micros copy. At 20 minutes, the NK cell has made contact with the target cell but the granules are dispersed. Shortly after contact, at 25 minutes, the lytic granules have converged around the microtubule-organizing centre (not shown) and at 35 minutes they have tightly polarized towards the target cell. At 50 minutes, a single lytic event is shown *(arrow, top right)* (Courtesy Emily Mace, PhD, and Jordan Orange, MD, PhD).

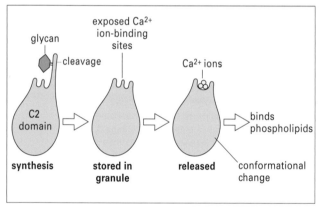

Fig. 8.11 Perforin undergoes a conformational activation Perforin is synthesized with a tailpiece of 20 amino acid residues with a large glycan residue attached. In this form, it is inactive. Cleavage of the tailpiece within the granules allows Ca^{2+} ions to access a site associated with the C2 domain of the molecule, but the molecule is thought to be maintained in an inactive state by the low Ca^{2+} concentration in the granules. Following secretion, the increased Ca^{2+} concentration permits a conformational change, which exposes a phospholipid-binding site, allowing the perforin to bind to the target membrane as a precursor to polymerization.

- Granzyme A triggers apoptosis via a caspase-independent pathway. It targets the endoplasmic reticulum (ER)-associated protein complex SET, activating DNAse, which nicks the target cell DNA. It also cleaves nuclear laminins, leading to loss of nuclear structure, and acts on the mitochondria to increase reactive oxygen intermediates (ROI) production.

Granzymes other than A and B have been identified, although mice with these genes knocked out are less severely affected than granzyme A and B knockout mice, suggesting that A and B are the most important death-inducing granzymes. The large number of granzymes is likely to provide multiple pathways to trigger apoptosis, ensuring that cell death ensues.

Some cell types are resistant to cell-mediated cytotoxicity.

A number of cell types display some resistance to cell-mediated cytotoxicity, including the CTLs and NK cells themselves. CTLs and NK cells can be killed by other cytotoxic effector cells but do not destroy themselves when they kill a target cell. A number of mechanisms contribute to this protection:

- Both perforin and granzymes are synthesized as inactive precursors that must be activated by cleavage.
- Activation takes place only after perforin and granzymes have been released from the granules. Inside granules, low pH, low Ca^{2+} levels and the presence of proteoglycans that bind perforin and granzymes keep them inactive.
- During degranulation, a membrane-bound form of cathepsin B lines the granule membrane and cleaves perforin on the CTL or NK side of the synapse.
- CTL and NK express cFLIP, a protein that inhibits the cleavage of caspase 8 and prevents apoptosis via the caspase 8 pathway.
- They also express a protease inhibitor 8 (PI-8), a serpin that can inhibit granzyme B activity.

Neurons, hepatocytes and some placental cell populations are resistant to CTL and NK-cell attack under normal circumstances. These cells express little or no MHC class I and for this reason, they are largely resistant to CTL-mediated cytotoxicity. They would, however, be expected to be susceptible to killing by NK cells. They evade NK cell killing in a number of ways:

- Neurons, as well as cells in other immune privileged sites, such as the cornea and testes, express FasL. NK and T cells themselves express Fas and this induces apoptosis in the immune cells as they enter the tissue.

- Tissue-resident NK cells are generally not efficient killers. In non-pathological situations, neurons, hepatocytes and most placental extravillous trophoblast cells are only exposed to tissue-resident and not blood NK cells. Placental extravillous trophoblasts also express HLA-C, HLA-E and HLA-G, all of which inhibit NK-cell activation.
- Placental villous trophoblast cells express no MHC class I molecules and are in direct contact with peripheral blood NK cells. They form a syncytium and this may confer some resistance to killing, but other mechanisms, as yet undefined, are also likely to be important.

Cytokine-stimulated CTL and NK cells are able to kill these cell types in vitro, and under inflammatory conditions, CTL and NK cells can kill neurons and hepatocytes in vivo. Therefore, these cell types are only resistant to cell-mediated cytotoxicity in the absence of inflammation or infection.

NON-LYMPHOID CYTOTOXIC CELLS

A number of non-lymphoid cells may be cytotoxic to other cells or to invading microorganisms, such as bacteria or parasites. Macrophages and neutrophils may phagocytose cells and debris in a non-specific way but also express FcγRI and FcγRII, which allow them to recognize antibody-coated target cells. Eosinophils also recognize antibody-coated targets via Fc receptors, triggering degranulation.

Macrophages and neutrophils primarily kill target cells by phagocytosis.

In general, macrophages and neutrophils destroy pathogens by internalizing them and barraging them with toxic molecules and enzymes within the phagolysosome. These include:

- the production of reactive oxygen species, toxic oxidants and nitric oxide;
- the secretion of molecules such as neutrophil defensins, lysosomal enzymes and cytostatic proteins (Fig. 8.12).

If the target is engaged by surface receptors but is too large to phagocytose, the phagosome may fail to internalize its target. In this case, molecules from the phagolysosome may be released into the extracellular environment and contribute to localized cell damage. This is called 'frustrated phagocytosis'. Frustrated phagocytosis can be considered a type of ADCC, but unlike ADCC mediated by NK cells, the mediators produced by the phagocyte damage the target cell, inducing necrosis rather than apoptosis. Activated macrophages also secrete TNFα, which induces apoptosis (see Fig. 3.4). Macrophages can therefore induce necrosis, apoptosis or a combination of both, depending on the state of activation of the macrophages and the target cell involved.

Eosinophils kill target cells by ADCC.
Mature eosinophils contain two types of granules: specific granules are unique to eosinophils and have a crystalloid core that binds the dye eosin, whereas primary granules are similar to those found in other cells of the granulocyte lineage. Eosinophils are only weakly phagocytic. They are capable of ingesting some bacteria following activation but are less efficient than neutrophils at intracellular killing.

The major function of eosinophils is the secretion of various toxic granule constituents following activation. They are effective at extracellular killing of microorganisms, particularly of large parasites such as schistosomes (see Fig. 16.11).

Eosinophil degranulation can be triggered in a number of ways:

- FcγRII binding to IgG-coated targets;
- FcεRII binding to IgE-coated targets;
- activation by cytokines, including IL-3, IL-5, granulocyte-macrophage colony stimulating factor (GM-CSF), TNFα, IFNβ and platelet-activating factor (PAF). These cytokines also enhance ADCC-mediated degranulation.

The components of the eosinophil specific granule include:

- major basic protein (MBP);
- eosinophil peroxidase (EPO);
- eosinophil cationic protein (ECP).

MBP is the major component of the granules, forming the crystalloid core. It increases membrane permeability, causing damage to, and sometimes killing, parasites. It can also damage host cells.

EPO is a cationic heterodimeric haemoprotein distinct from the myeloperoxidase of neutrophils and macrophages. In the presence of H_2O_2, which is also produced by eosinophils, EPO oxidizes a variety of substrates, including halide ions and nitric oxide, to produce highly toxic oxidant species. These products may represent the eosinophil's most potent killing mechanism for some parasites, but they are also toxic to host cells.

ECP is an eosinophil-specific protein that is toxic to many parasites, particularly *Schistosoma mansoni* schistosomula. It is a ribonuclease that binds avidly to negatively charged surfaces. ECP binds and aggregates on the cell surface, altering cell membrane permeability and intracellular ion equilibrium, which ultimately leads to apoptosis via both caspase-dependent and caspase-independent pathways.

Eosinophils also produce eosinophil-derived neurotoxin (EDN), another ribonuclease but with strong neurotoxic activity. The ribonuclease activity of ECP and EDN is not required for their toxicity.

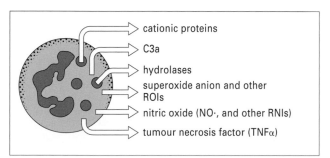

cationic proteins

C3a

hydrolases

superoxide anion and other ROIs

nitric oxide (NO·, and other RNIs)

tumour necrosis factor (TNFα)

Fig. 8.12 Mechanisms that may contribute to the cytotoxicity of myeloid cells Reactive oxygen intermediates *(ROIs)* and reactive nitrogen intermediates *(RNIs)*, cationic proteins, hydrolytic enzymes and complement proteins released from myeloid cells may damage the target cell, in addition to cytokine-mediated attack.

Eosinophils are prominent in the inflammatory lesions of a number of diseases, particularly atopic disorders of the gut, skin and respiratory tract: for example, atopic eczema, asthma and inflammatory bowel disease. Although eosinophils may play some regulatory role in these conditions, such as inactivating histamine, their toxic products and cytotoxic mechanisms are a major cause of the tissue damage. In asthma, MBP can kill some pneumocytes and tracheal epithelial cells and EPO kills type II pneumocytes. MBP can also induce mast cells to secrete histamine, exacerbating allergic inflammation.

CRITICAL THINKING: MECHANISMS OF CYTOTOXICITY

See Critical thinking: Explanations, section 8

Lymphocytes from a normal individual were stimulated in vitro by co-culture with irradiated T lymphoma cells. (Irradiation of these stimulator cells prevents them from dividing in culture.) After 7 days, the lymphocytes were harvested and sorted to obtain a population of CTLs (CD3$^+$CD8$^+$) and a population of NK cells (CD56^{Lo}CD16$^+$). These effector cells were set up in a cytotoxicity assay with two tumour cell lines as targets: Tumour line 1 and Tumour line 1 S, which is derived from Tumour line 1. The percentage of cells displaying DNA fragmentation in each condition is shown in the table.

Treatment	Tumour line 1	Tumour line 1 S
No effector cells	1%	2%
CTLs	84%	2%
NK cells	15%	88%
Anti-class I antibody	2%	1%
CTLs + anti-class I antibody	6%	1%
NK cells + anti-class I antibody	46%	85%

1. Why is target cell DNA fragmentation a good indication of CTL and NK-cell activity?
2. From the cultures with CTLs or NK cells alone, what can you deduce about Tumour lines 1 and 1 S?
3. How can you account for the observation that NK cells cause some DNA fragmentation in Tumour line 1? How would you test your hypothesis?
4. The cultures were repeated including an antibody that recognizes MHC class I molecules, and blocks their interactions. How can you account for the effects on DNA fragmentation observed in Tumour line 1?

FURTHER READING

Boudreau JE, Hsu KC. Natural killer cell education and the response to infection and cancer therapy: stay tuned. Trends Immunol 2018;39:222–239.

Cullen SP, Martin SJ. Mechanisms of granule-dependent killing. Cell Death Differ 2008;15:251–262.

Dustin ML, Long EO. Cytotoxic immunological synapses. Immunol Rev 2010;235:24–34.

Finlay D, Cantrell DA. Metabolism, migration and memory in cytotoxic T cells. Nat Rev Immunol 2011;11:109–117.

Kärre K. Natural killer cell recognition of missing self. Nat Immunol 2008;9:477–480.

Kruse PH, Matta J, Ugolini S, Vivier E. Natural cytotoxicity receptors and their ligands. Immune Cell Biol 2014;92:221–229.

Long EO, Kim HS, Liu D, Peterson ME, Rajagopalan S. Controlling natural killer cell responses: integration of signals for activation and inhibition. Annu Rev Immunol 2013;31:227–258.

Parham P, Guethlein LA. Genetics of natural killer cells in human health, disease and survival. Annu Rev Immunol 2018;26:519–548.

Rothenberg ME, Hogan SP. The eosinophil. Annu Rev Immunol 2006;24:147–174.

Tscarke DC, Croft NP, Doherty PC, La Gruta NL. Sizing up the key determinants of the CD8(+) T cell response. Nat Rev Immunol 2015;15:705–716.

B-Cell Development and the Antibody Response

SUMMARY

- **The primary development of B cells is antigen independent.** Pre-B cells recombine genes for immunoglobulin heavy and light chains to generate their surface receptor for antigen. Initially, a B cell produces IgM; later it may switch to production of another immunoglobulin isotype, but with the same antigen specificity.
- **B-cell activation, proliferation and differentiation follow contact with antigen.** Activated B cells proliferate and differentiate into plasma cells (antibody-forming cells).
- **T-dependent antigens taken up by B cells are processed and presented to TH2 cells,** which provide direct cell–cell signals and secrete cytokines that control B-cell development.
- **B-cell activation requires signals from the B-cell receptor and co-stimulation.** CD40 is the most important co-stimulatory molecule on B cells. Ligation of the B-cell–co-receptor complex can lower the threshold of antigen needed to trigger the B cell. Intracellular signalling pathways are analogous in B cells and T cells.
- **T-independent (TI) antigens activate B cells without requiring T-cell help.** They can be divided into two groups. TI-1 antigens can act as polyclonal stimulators, while TI-2 antigens are polymers that activate by cross-linking the B-cell receptor.
- **Antibody responses to T-dependent antigens show class switching and an increase in antibody affinity over time.** These processes are a consequence of mutation and recombination events affecting the immunoglobulin gene loci in individual B cells, followed by selection of B-cell clones producing high-affinity antibornmdies.
- **Class switching is effected by somatic recombination occurring within the heavy chain genes.** Somatic hypermutation and class switching by recombination are linked processes, which require selective targeting of DNA-modification and DNA-repair enzymes to the heavy chain gene locus. The cytokines produced by different T-cell populations determine which class switch will occur.

The production of antibodies is the final stage in the development and differentiation of B cells.

In mammals, all serum antibodies (immunoglobulins) belong to one of five different classes (IgM, IgD, IgG, IgA and IgE), each of which has a distinct set of activities. Some classes have subclasses although these vary between different species. For example, in humans the IgG class has four subclasses (IgG1, IgG2, IgG3 and IgG4) and these too have slightly different functions, which are described in Chapter 10. Each antibody subclass is an isotype, meaning that it is encoded by its own gene. Initially, an individual B cell produces an antigen receptor (BCR) consisting of cell surface IgM, associated with signalling molecules, which is analogous to the T-cell antigen receptor (TCR).

As it develops, an individual B cell may switch the class of antibody that it produces by a process of somatic cell gene recombination, called class-switch recombination (CSR) (Fig 9.1). At the same time the immunoglobulin genes may undergo somatic hypermutation (SHM), sometimes resulting in an immunoglobulin with higher affinity for its target antigen. These events are driven by contact with antigen and interactions with T cells in the germinal centres of secondary lymphoid tissues (lymph nodes, Peyer's patches, etc.) where memory B cells also develop. The class switching that takes place in individual B cells is reflected in an overall switch in the class of secreted antibodies in serum, as the immune response develops (Fig 9.2). At the same time, the overall affinity of the serum antibodies increases, a process called affinity maturation.

B-CELL DEVELOPMENT

In adults, B-cell development occurs in the bone marrow and does not require contact with antigen. During this time, the B cells rearrange the genes for their immunoglobulin heavy and light chains, in a similar way to the recombination that occurs in the TCR β chain genes (see Fig 6.16). Each B cell undergoes its own unique set of gene rearrangements to produce a combination of one heavy chain and one light chain, which determine the structure and antigen-binding specificity of the antibodies that will be produced by that clone of B cells. It is the genes encoding the variable (V) domains of the heavy chain and the light chain that undergo recombination during early B-cell development. First, the heavy chain genes are rearranged to form a functional gene for a μ heavy chain. This heavy chain is expressed at the cell surface of the developing B cell in association with a surrogate light chain (Fig. 9.w1). If a functional heavy chain has been generated, the cell will proceed to rearrange genes for the κ chain. If this is unsuccessful, the cell will attempt to rearrange its other set of light chain genes, encoding λ chains. Since these recombination events occur within a single chromosome, an individual B cell uses either the maternal or the paternal chromosome to generate its recombined heavy and light chain genes – an example of allelic exclusion within each B cell.

B-Cell receptor diversity is generated by V(D)J recombination. The germline human heavy chain locus

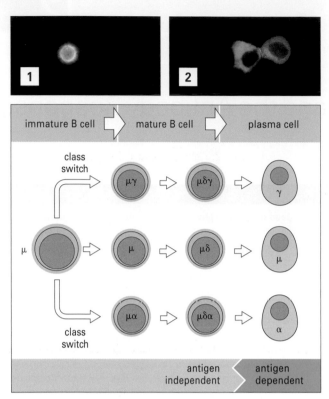

Fig. 9.1 B-cell differentiation – class diversity Immature B cells produce IgM only, but mature B cells can express more than one cell surface antibody because mRNA and cell surface immunoglobulin remain after a class switch. IgD is also expressed during clonal maturation. Maturation can occur in the absence of antigen, but the development into plasma cells (which have little surface immunoglobulin but much cytoplasmic immunoglobulin) requires antigen and (usually) T-cell help. The photographs show B cells stained for surface IgM (*green*, **1**) and plasma cells stained for cytoplasmic IgM and IgG (*green and red*, **2**).

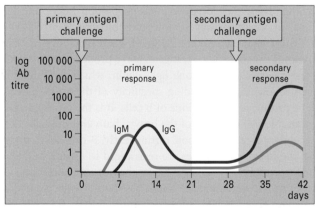

Fig. 9.2 Primary and secondary antibody responses In comparison with the primary antibody response, the antibody level after secondary antigenic challenge in a typical immune response appears more quickly, persists for a longer period of time, attains a higher titre and consists predominantly of IgG.

(IGH) on chromosome 14 contains a library of ~50 functional VH gene segments that encode the N-terminal 95 residues of the heavy chain variable domain. The remaining residues of the VH domain are encoded by 23 DH and 6 JH gene segments (Fig 9.3). The first event in the rearrangement is recombination between a

JH gene segment and a DH segment, which is then followed by recombination with a VH segment. The exact position of the recombination is variable and this can add additional nucleotide sequence diversity at the junctions. Moreover, the DH segments:

- are highly variable, both in the number of codons and nucleotide sequence;
- may be read in all three possible reading frames without generating stop codons;
- may be used singly or in combination.

Productive recombination between VH, DH and JH segments forms a contiguous VDJ segment, which encodes the whole of the heavy chain V domain. The recombined region itself forms a hypervariable loop (HV3) in the antigen-binding site. Since each B cell will use a different combination of V, D and J genes, there is the potential to produce millions of different VH domains from the initial germline gene set.

The germline human κ light chain locus on chromosome 2 contains about 35 functional Vκ gene segments that encode the N-terminal 95 residues of the κ chain V domain. The remaining residues are encoded by one of five Jκ gene segments (Fig. 9.4). Recombination in this locus brings together one Vκ and one Jκ gene segment, possibly with variation in the splice point, which can create additional diversity (Fig. 9.w2). If recombination in the κ light chain locus fails, the cell may attempt a rearrangement in the λ chain locus by a similar mechanism (Fig. 9.w3).

The enormous diversity of antibodies in naive B cells is therefore generated by several mechanisms:

- There are multiple genes encoding V, D and J segments.
- VDJ or VJ recombinations occur at random.
- Recombinational inaccuracies and nucleotide insertions in the recombined segments add additional diversity.
- The combination of heavy and light chains multiplies the number of heavy + light variants.
- Either the maternal or paternal chromosome can be used in any one B cell.

The mechanism by which immunoglobulin V, D and J gene segments undergo somatic recombination is essentially similar to the mechanisms underlying the recombination in the TCR variable region gene loci (see Chapter 6).

The initial BCR complex includes:

- membrane-bound IgM immunoglobulin – two IgM heavy chains, at first associated with surrogate light chains and later with one of the regular light chains, either kappa or lambda;
- the signalling chains Igα and Igβ (CD79a and CD79b).

Immature transitional B cells exit the bone marrow and enter the periphery where they further mature in secondary lymphoid organs. If these cells do not encounter antigen, they die within a few weeks by apoptosis. If, however, these mature B cells encounter specific antigen, they undergo activation, proliferation and differentiation, leading to the generation of plasma cells and memory B cells.

Pro-B cells develop into immature and then mature B cells.

The earliest stage of antigen-independent B-cell development is the progenitor B (pro-B) cell stage. Pro-B cells can be divided into three groups based on the expression of:

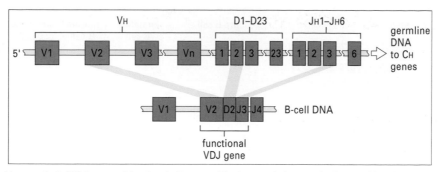

Fig. 9.3 Heavy chain VDJ recombination in humans The heavy chain gene loci recombine three segments to produce a VDJ gene, which encodes the VH domain. There are about 50 functional VH genes, which may recombine with one or more DH genes and one of the six JH gene segments to produce a single functional VDJ gene in the B cell. The recombination illustrated is only one of the many possible gene rearrangements. IGH genes show allelic exclusion within one B cell, i.e. if the maternal chromosome is expressed, the paternal chromosome is not expressed and vice versa.

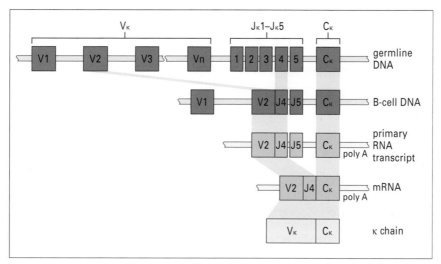

Fig. 9.4 κ-Chain production in humans During differentiation of pre-B cells one of several Vκ genes is recombined with one of the five Jκ gene segments. The recombination illustrated is only one of the many possible gene rearrangements. The B cell transcribes this VJ gene segment together with the exon for the constant domain of the light chain (Cκ). The primary RNA transcript is processed into mRNA by removal of the intervening intron and this is exported for the nucleus to be translated into a κ light chain.

- terminal deoxynucleotidyl transferase (TdT), an intranuclear enzyme uniquely expressed during VH gene rearrangement; and
- B220, a splice variant of leukocyte common antigen (CD45R in humans), a tyrosine phosphatase that appears to be important in regulating B-cell receptor signalling.

Early pro-B cells express TdT alone, intermediate pro-B cells express both TdT and B220 and late pro-B cells express B220 and lose TdT. B220 remains expressed on the surface throughout the remainder of B-cell ontogeny.

As the cells progress through the pro-B cell stage and rearrange their Ig heavy chain genes they begin to express CD43 (leukosialin), CD19, RAG (recombination-activating gene)-1 and RAG-2. The markers expressed during B-cell development are shown in Figure 9.5.

As immature B cells develop further into mature B cells, they begin to express both IgM and IgD on their surface. These mature B cells are then free to exit the bone marrow and migrate into the periphery.

IL-3, IL-4, IL-7 and BAFF are important for B-cell development. Several cytokines affect B-cell development. Common lymphoid progenitors are responsive to IL-7, which promotes B-cell lineage development. Mice deficient in IL-7 or IL-7R exhibit an early arrest in B-cell development at the pro-B cell stage.

B-cell activating factor (BAFF), which is also called Blys (B-lymphocyte stimulator), signalling through its receptor BR3 is important for the survival of pre-immune B cells from the transitional stage onwards. This is supported by the observation of a developmental block at the transitional B-cell stage in BAFF-deficient animals. BAFF is also required for the later survival of mature B cells (see Fig. 9.13).

In addition, a number of growth and differentiation factors are required to drive the B cells through early stages of development. Receptors for these factors are expressed at various stages of B-cell differentiation. IL-4, IL-3 and low-molecular-weight B-cell growth factor (L-BCGF) are important in initiating the process of B-cell differentiation, whereas other factors are active in the later stages (see Fig. 9.12).

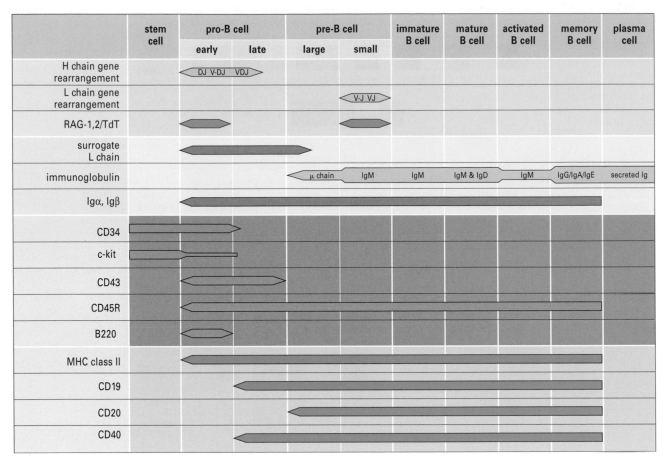

Fig. 9.5 Markers expressed during B-cell development and differentiation B cells differentiate from lymphoid stem cells into naive B cells and may then be driven by antigen to become memory cells or plasma cells. Upon antigen stimulation, the B cell proliferates and develops into a plasma cell or a memory cell. The cellular location of immunoglobulin during differentiation is shown in *yellow*. Pre-B cells express cytoplasmic μ chains only. The immature B cell has surface IgM and the mature B cell has other immunoglobulin isotypes. During early B-cell development, the heavy chain gene (IgH) undergoes a DJ recombination, followed by a VDJ recombination. The recombined heavy chain is initially expressed with a surrogate light chain and the Igα and Igβ chains (CD79) to produce the pre-B-cell receptor. Later, light chain genes undergo a VJ recombination and surface IgM is produced as the B-cell receptor. Recombination events are associated with expression of the recombination activating genes (Rag-1 and Rag-2), but TdT expression only occurs during heavy chain recombination. The diagram also shows the time of expression of a number of other B-cell markers.

B-CELL ACTIVATION

Follicular dendritic cells act as antigen depots for B cells.

Follicular dendritic cells (FDCs) are key components of the lymphoid follicle. These cells are of mesenchymal (not haematopoietic) origin and are called dendritic cells because of their morphology. They are not related to the dendritic cells that are involved in antigen processing and presentation. They express the complement receptors CR1 and CR2 and the Fc receptor FcγRIIb, which allows them to retain unprocessed antigen on their surface for prolonged periods of time as immune complexes (see Fig. 2.14).

BCR binding to the antigen in such complexes leads to BCR signalling. The B cell may also internalize antigen bound to the BCR and present it to CD4 T cells, in order to receive help.

B-cell activation and T-cell activation follow similar patterns. In B cells, the signalling function that in T cells is achieved by CD3 is instead carried out by a heterodimer of Igα and Igβ. The cytoplasmic tails of Igα and Igβ carry **immunoreceptor tyrosine-based activation motifs (ITAMs)**.

Cross-linking of surface Ig leads to activation of the Src family kinases, which in B cells are Fyn, Lyn and Blk. Syk is analogous to ZAP-70 in T cells and binds to the phosphorylated ITAMs of Igα and Igβ (Fig. 9.6). This leads to activation of a kinase cascade and translocation of nuclear transcription factors analogous to the process that occurs in T cells.

B-cell activation is also markedly augmented by the co-receptor complex comprising three proteins:
• CD21 (complement receptor-2, CR2);
• CD19; and
• CD81 (target of anti-proliferative antibody, TAPA-1) (Fig. 9.7).

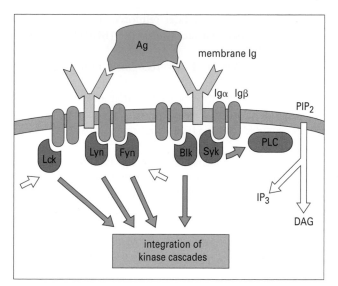

Fig. 9.6 Intracellular signalling in B-cell activation B-cell activation is similar to T-cell activation. If membrane Ig becomes cross-linked (e.g. by a T-independent antigen), tyrosine kinases, including Lck, Lyn, Fyn and Blk, become activated. They phosphorylate the ITAM domains in the Igα and Igβ chains of the receptor complex. These can then bind another kinase, Syk, which activates phospholipase C *(PLC)*. This acts on membrane PIP₂ to generate IP₃ and diacylglycerol *(DAG)*, which activates protein kinase C. Signals from the other kinases are transduced to activate nuclear transcription factors.

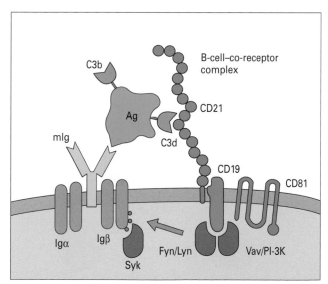

Fig. 9.7 B-cell–co-receptor complex The B-cell–co-receptor complex consists of CD21 (the complement receptor type-2), CD19 and CD81 (a molecule with four transmembrane segments). Antigen *(Ag)* with covalently bound C3b or C3d can cross-link the membrane Ig to CD21 of the co-receptor complex. This greatly reduces the cell's requirement for antigen to activate it. CD19 can associate with tyrosine kinases including Lyn, Fyn, Vav and PI-3 kinase *(PI-3 K)*. Compare this with CD28 on the T cell. Receptor cross-linking causes phosphorylation of the Igα and Igβ chains of the antigen–receptor complex and recruitment and activation of Syk.

CD21 allows the B cell to bind antigens in immune complexes via the complement molecule C3d. Notably, animals depleted of complement C3 have a greatly reduced secondary immune response.

Phosphorylation of the cytoplasmic tail of CD19 leads to binding and activation of Fyn/Lyn. These kinases enhance the activation signal of the BCR through the phospholipase C and PI-3 kinase pathways, particularly when antigen concentration is low.

T-Independent antigens do not require T-cell help to stimulate B cells. The immune response to most antigens depends on both T cells and B cells recognizing the antigen in a linked fashion. This type of antigen is called a **T-dependent (TD) antigen**.

A small number of antigens, however, can activate B cells without major histocompatibility complex (MHC) class II-restricted T-cell help and are referred to as **T-independent (TI) antigens** (Table 9.1).

Importantly, many TI antigens are particularly resistant to degradation. TI antigens can be divided into two groups (TI-1 and TI-2) based on the manner in which they activate B cells:

- TI-1 antigens are predominantly bacterial cell wall components, e.g. lipopolysaccharide (LPS), a component of the cell wall of Gram-negative bacteria;
- TI-2 antigens are predominantly large polysaccharide molecules with repeating antigenic determinants, e.g. Ficoll, dextran, polymeric bacterial flagellin and poliomyelitis virus.

Many TI-1 antigens possess the ability in high concentrations to activate B-cell clones that are specific for other antigens – a phenomenon known as polyclonal B-cell activation. However, in lower concentrations they only activate B-cells specific for themselves. TI-1 antigens do not require a second signal.

TI-2 antigens, on the other hand, are thought to activate B cells by clustering and cross-linking immunoglobulin molecules on the B-cell surface, leading to prolonged and persistent signalling. TI-2 antigens require residual non-cognate T-cell help, such as cytokines.

T-independent antigens induce faster responses but poor memory. Primary antibody responses to TI antigens in vitro are generally slightly weaker than those to TD antigens. They

TABLE 9.1 T-Independent Antigens

Antigen	Polymeric	Polyclonal Activation	Resistance to Degradation
Lipopolysaccharide (LPS)	+	+++	+
Ficoll	+++	–	+++
Dextran	++	+	++
Levan	++	+	++
Poly-D amino acids	+++	–	+++
Polymeric bacterial flagellin	++	++	+

The major common properties of some of the T-independent antigens are listed. T-independent antigens induce the production of cytokines IL-1, TNFα and IL-6 by macrophages. (Note: both poly-L amino acids and monomeric bacterial flagellin are T-dependent antigens, demonstrating the role of antigen structure in determining T-independent properties.)

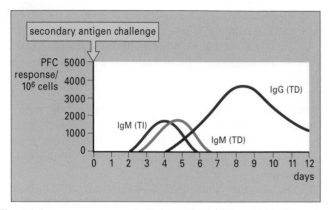

Fig. 9.8 Immune response to T-dependent *(TD)* and T-independent *(TI)* antigens in vitro The secondary response to T-dependent antigens is stronger and induces a greater number of IgG-producing cells.

peak fractionally earlier and both generate mainly IgM. However, the secondary responses to TD and TI antigens differ greatly (Fig. 9.8). The secondary response to TI antigens resembles the primary response, whereas the secondary response to TD antigens is far stronger and has a large IgG component. It seems, therefore, that TI antigens do not usually induce the maturation of a response leading to class switching or to an increase in antibody affinity, as seen with TD antigens. This is most likely a result of the lack of co-stimulation via CD40L and lack of IL-2, IL-4 and IL-5, which T cells produce in response to TD antigens. Memory induction to TI antigens is also relatively poor.

There are advantages if the immune response to bacteria does not depend on complex cell interactions, because it could be more rapid. Moreover, many bacterial antigens bypass T-cell help because they are very effective inducers of cytokine production by macrophages: IL-1, IL-6 and tumour necrosis factor-α (TNFα).

TI antigens predominantly activate the B-1 subset of B cells found mainly in the peritoneum. These B-1 cells can be identified by their expression of CD5, which is induced upon binding of TI antigens. In contrast to conventional B cells, B-1 cells have the ability to replenish themselves.

T-dependent B cells require T-cell help for activation. In the late 1960s and early 1970s, studies by Mitchison and others, using chemically modified proteins, led to significant advances in understanding of the different functions of T cells and B cells. To induce an optimal secondary antibody response to a small chemical group or hapten (which is immunogenic only if bound to a protein carrier), it was found that the experimental animal must be immunized and then challenged using the same hapten–carrier conjugate – not just the same hapten. This was referred to as the carrier effect.

By manipulating the cell populations in these experiments, it was shown that:
• TH cells are responsible for recognizing the carrier; whereas
• the B cells recognize hapten.

These experiments were later reinforced by details of how:
• B cells use their surface antibody (BCR) to recognize epitopes; while
• T cells use their TCR to recognize processed antigen fragments.

One consequence of this system is that an individual B cell can receive help from T cells specific for different antigenic peptides provided that the B cell can present those determinants to each T cell.

In an immune response in vivo, the interactions between T and B cells that drive B-cell division and differentiation involve T cells that have already been stimulated by contact with the antigen on other antigen-presenting cells (APCs), for example dendritic cells.

This has led to the basic scheme for cell interactions in the antibody response set out in Figure 9.9. Antigen is processed by APCs and presented in a highly immunogenic form to the TH and B cells. The T cells recognize determinants on the antigen that are distinct from those recognized by the B cells, which

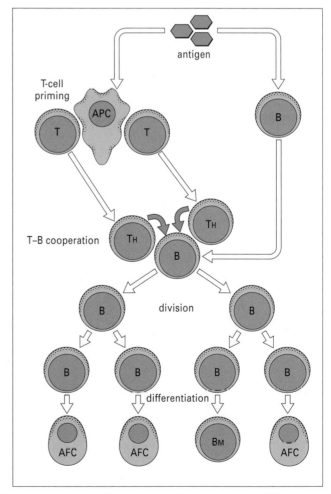

Fig. 9.9 Cell cooperation in the antibody response Antigen is presented to virgin T cells by antigen-presenting cells *(APCs)* such as dendritic cells. B cells also take up antigen and present it to the T cells, receiving signals from the T cells to divide and to differentiate into antibody-forming cells *(AFCs)* and memory B *(BM)* cells.

differentiate and divide into plasma cells. Therefore, two processes are required to activate a B cell:

- antigen interacting with the B-cell receptor (BCR) – this involves native antigen;
- stimulating signal(s) from Tн cells that respond to processed antigen bound to MHC class II molecules.

T-follicular helper cells provide help to B cells in germinal centres. T cells in the lymph node are primarily found within the T-cell zone. However, one group of T cells, called T-follicular helper (Tғн) cells is found in the B-cell zone, where they provide help for B cells.

Tғн develop from naive CD4 T cells in the T-cell zone, which receive ICOS and IL-21 signalling alongside TCR stimulation. This causes them to express the Tғн lineage defining transcription factor Bcl6, the chemokine receptor CXCR5, which allows them to enter the B-cell follicle, and more IL-21. IL-21 and its receptor are critical for germinal centre formation and class switching.

Tғн cells provide help for developing B cells by expressing co-stimulatory molecules and producing cytokines, most often IL-4 or IFNγ. Regulatory Tғн cells have also been described. Tғн cells express inhibitory molecules, such as PD-1, which prevent them from expanding in response to TCR signalling. This limits the amount of help that can be provided. B cells must compete for help, so that only those that are able to take up antigen using high-affinity BCRs will receive help.

Direct interaction of B cells and T cells involves Co-stimulatory molecules. Antigen-specific T-cell populations can be obtained by growing and cloning T cells with antigens, APCs and IL-2. It is thus possible to visualize directly B-cell and T-cell clusters interacting in vitro:

- the T cells become polarized, with the T-cell receptors concentrated on the B-cell side;
- the B cells also become polarized and express most of their MHC class II molecules and ICAM-1 in proximity to the T cells.

The interactions in these clusters strongly suggest an intense exchange of information, which leads to two important events in the B-cell life cycle:

- induction of proliferation; and
- differentiation into plasma cells.

The initial interaction between a naive B cell and a cognate antigen via the BCR in the presence of cytokines or other growth stimuli induces activation and proliferation of the B cell. This then leads to processing of the T-dependent antigen and presentation to T cells. The interaction between B cells and T cells is a two-way process in which B cells present antigen to T cells and receive signals from the T cells for division and differentiation (Fig. 9.10).

The central, antigen-specific interaction is between the MHC class II–antigen complex and the TCR. This interaction is augmented by interactions between LFA-3 and CD2 and between ICAM-1 or ICAM-3 and LFA-1.

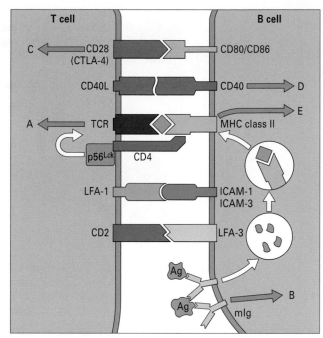

Fig. 9.10 Cell surface molecules involved in the interaction between B and Tн cells Membrane immunoglobulin *(mIg)* takes up antigen *(Ag)* into an intracellular compartment where it is degraded and peptides can combine with major histocompatibility complex *(MHC)* class II molecules. Other arrows show the discrete signal transduction events that have been established. *A* and *B* are the antigen–receptor signal transduction events involving tyrosine phosphorylation and phosphoinositide breakdown. The antigen receptors also regulate LFA-1 affinity for ICAM-1 and ICAM-3. CD28 also sends a unique signal to the T cell *(C)*. In the later phases of the response CTLA-4 can supplant CD28 to cause downregulation. In the B cell, stimulation via CD40 is the most potent activating signal *(D)*. In addition, class II MHC molecules appear to induce distinct signalling events *(E)*.

The interaction between B and T cells activates both cells:

- CD40, a member of the TNF receptor family, delivers a strong activating signal to B cells, more potent even than signals transmitted via the BCR;
- upon activation, T cells transiently express a ligand, termed CD40L (a member of the TNF family), which interacts with CD40;
- CD40–CD40L interaction helps to drive B cells into cell cycle;
- transduction of signals through CD40 induces upregulation of CD80/CD86 and therefore helps to provide further co-stimulatory signals to the responding T cells via CD28.

Signalling through CD40 is also essential for germinal centre development and antibody responses to TD antigens.

Type 2 cytokines guide B-cell proliferation and differentiation. During B-cell–T-cell interaction, T cells can secrete a number of cytokines that have a powerful effect on B cells (Fig. 9.11). IL-2, for example, is an inducer of proliferation for B cells as well as T cells.

In particular, type 2 cytokines produced strongly promote B-cell activation and the production of IgG1 and IgE. These cytokines include IL-4, IL-5, IL-6, IL-10, IL-13 and BAFF:

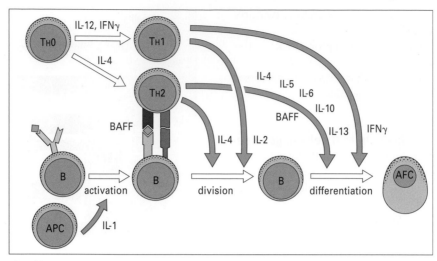

Fig. 9.11 Cytokines and B-cell development B-cell development is influenced by cytokines from T cells and antigen-presenting cells *(APCs)* and by direct interactions with TH2 cells. IL-4 is most important in promoting cell division and a variety of other cytokines including IL-4, IL-5, IL-6, IL-10 and IFNγ influence development into antibody-forming cells *(AFCs)* and affect the isotype of antibody that will be produced.

- IL-4 acts on B cells to induce activation and differentiation. It also acts on T cells as a growth factor and promotes differentiation of TH2 cells, thus reinforcing the antibody response; excess IL-4 plays a part in allergic disease, causing production of IgE.
- IL-5 in humans is chiefly a growth and activation factor for eosinophils and is responsible for the eosinophilia of parasitic disease. In the mouse it also acts on B cells to induce growth and differentiation.
- IL-6 is produced by many cells including T cells, macrophages, B cells, fibroblasts and endothelial cells and acts on many cell types, but it is particularly important in inducing B cells to differentiate into plasma cells. IL-6 is an important growth factor for multiple myeloma, a malignancy of plasma cells.
- IL-10 acts as a growth and differentiation factor for B cells in addition to modulating cytokine production by TH1 cells.
- IL-13, which shares a receptor component and signalling pathways with IL-4, acts on B cells to produce IgE.
- BAFF is important in controlling early differentiation of B cells, as well as their later development in germinal centres.

Cytokines can also influence antibody affinity. Antibody affinity to most TD antigens increases during an immune response and a similar effect can be produced by certain immunization protocols. For example, high-affinity antibody subpopulations are potentiated after immunization with antigen and IFNγ.

In addition to the effects of cytokines on B-cell proliferation and differentiation, cytokines are capable of influencing the class switch from IgM to other immunoglobulin classes (see Table 9.2).

BAFF is important for B-cell development in germinal centres. Receptors for the many growth and differentiation factors required to drive the B cells through early stages of

development are expressed at various stages of B-cell differentiation. Receptors for IL-7, IL-3 and low-molecular-weight B-cell growth factor are important in the initial stages of B-cell differentiation, whereas other receptors are more important in the later stages (Fig. 9.12).

BAFF is particularly important in B-cell development and survival in germinal centres. The protein is present as a membrane-bound form (CD257) on dendritic cells and monocytes and may be released as a secreted cytokine. BAFF belongs to the superfamily of TNF-like cytokines and it acts through a family of three receptors that can activate NF-κB and MAP kinase to promote B-cell differentiation and survival. The principal receptor for BAFF, BR3, belongs to the TNF receptor superfamily (it is also known as TNFRSF-13C) and is expressed in mature B cells. Animals deficient in BAFF or its receptor produce low levels of antibody; conversely, high production is associated with high levels of antibody synthesis in some autoimmune conditions.

Memory B cells lose their BR3 but retain one of the other receptors for BAFF (TNFRSF-13B or TACI) when they differentiate into memory B cells. Mutations in TACI are associated with common variable immunodeficiency (CVID).

Long-lived plasma cells also lose BR3 but retain another BAFF receptor: B-cell maturation antigen (TNFRSF-17 or BCMA). Another ligand for TACI and BCMA is a proliferation-inducing ligand (APRIL, TNFSF-13, CD256), which supports long-lived plasma cells. Like BAFF, this is a cell surface molecule that may be cleaved to become a soluble cytokine. Hence mature cells of the B-cell lineage can all respond to BAFF and/or APRIL but do so through different receptors (Fig. 9.13)

Anergy limits the activation of self-reactive B cells. APC–T-cell interaction may yield two diametrically opposing results: namely, activation or inactivation (clonal anergy). In the same

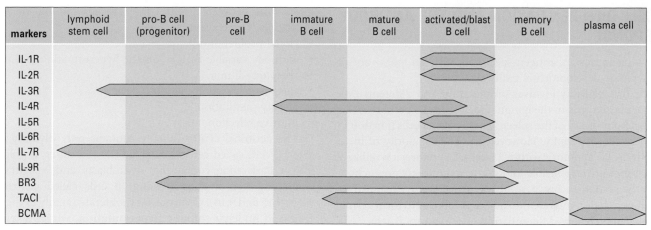

Fig. 9.12 Cytokine receptor expression during B-cell development The whole life history of B cells from stem cell to mature plasma cell is regulated by cytokines. Receptors for these cytokines are selectively expressed by B cells at different stages of development. Some of these receptors now have CD designation.

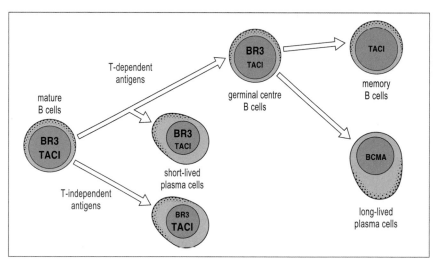

Fig. 9.13 Receptors for BAFF and APRIL B-cell activating factor (BAFF) and a proliferation-inducing gland *(APRIL)* support development of mature B cells and survival of plasma cells in bone marrow. They act on a set of three related receptors (BR3, TACI and BCMA) expressed at different levels as the B cells differentiate.

way, B cells frequently become anergic. This is an important process because up to 50% of naive B cells may have generated a self-reactive BCR and even in mature populations up to 20% are self-reactive. Additionally, affinity maturation of B cells during the immune response, as a result of rapid mutation in the genes encoding the antibody variable regions, could easily result in new auto-antibodies or higher-affinity auto-antibodies.

Clonal anergy and other forms of tolerance in the periphery are therefore important for silencing these potentially damaging clones.

A number of mechanisms have been identified that can lead to anergic B cells. They include:
- lack of co-stimulation via CD40;
- chronic low-level stimulation/cross-linking of the BCR, possibly leading to clonal exhaustion;
- reduction of CD21 (B-cell co-receptor) so that B-cell activation requires higher levels of antigen.

These mechanisms imply ineffective signalling via the BCR complex or lack of co-stimulation can result in clonal anergy.

In addition, experiments suggest that the life span of self-reactive B cells in germinal centres is much shorter than other B cells – a few days, compared with more than 30 days. This implies self-reactive B cells undergo apoptosis, either by inability to compete for limiting amounts of BAFF or by direct interaction with cytotoxic T cells. Thus, self-reactive B cells are unable to respond (anergy) and they die relatively quickly (apoptosis).

Another question has arisen about the role of IgD in maintaining anergy. During development, IgM is produced first as part of the BCR, as described earlier, but IgM may later be co-expressed with IgD on the B-cell surface (see Fig. 9.1). It was noted that IgM is reduced on anergic B cells, while IgD levels are maintained and it was therefore proposed that IgD is less effective as a component of the BCR, for inducing B-cell activation. However, the relative importance of these two cell surface receptors for antigen on B cells is still not fully understood in terms of activation or inactivation.

B-CELL DIFFERENTIATION AND THE ANTIBODY RESPONSE

Following activation, antigen-specific B cells can follow one of two separate developmental pathways:

- The first pathway involves proliferation and differentiation into plasma cells in the lymph nodes or in the peri-arteriolar lymphoid sheath of the spleen. These plasma cells function to clear antigen rapidly. However, the great majority of these cells die via apoptosis within 2 weeks. Therefore, it is unlikely that they are responsible for long-term antibody production.
- In the second pathway, some members of the expanded B-cell population migrate into adjacent follicles to form germinal centres before differentiating into memory B cells.

The development of memory B cells and their rate of exit from the germinal centre are controlled by IL-9, produced by TFH. While most studies on memory cell formation have focused on events in the germinal centre, there is some evidence for memory B-cell development in other sites that is independent of TFH cells.

Affinity maturation and class switching occurs in germinal centres. The germinal centre is important because it provides a micro-environment where B cells can undergo developmental events that ultimately result in long-lived memory B cells (Fig. 9.14). These developmental events are a result of complex interactions between B cells, CD4$^+$ TH cells and follicular dendritic cells. These events include:

- clonal proliferation;
- antibody variable region somatic hypermutation (SHM);
- receptor editing;
- class-switch recombination (CSR);
- affinity maturation;
- positive selection.

The germinal centre initially contains only dividing, activated B cells called centroblasts. Shortly thereafter, it polarizes into a dark zone containing centroblasts and a light zone containing non-dividing (resting) B cells called centrocytes (Figs. 9.15 and 9.16). Centroblasts proliferate rapidly in the dark zone and undergo **somatic hypermutation**, which diversifies the rearranged variable region genes. Somatic hypermutation allows a single B cell to give rise to variants with different affinities for the antigen.

Class-switch recombination occurs following somatic hypermutation and requires cell cycling. Receptor editing of immunoglobulin light chain genes also occurs in centroblasts.

Following these developmental changes, the centroblasts remove their old cell surface immunoglobulin. Those that have made a crippling mutation in one of their immunoglobulin genes undergo apoptosis and are removed by macrophages. Those cells that still have a fully functional set of antibody genes

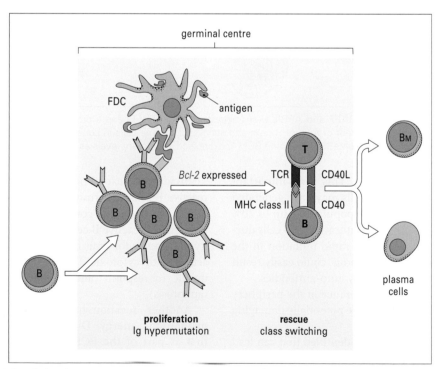

Fig. 9.14 B-cell development in germinal centres A B cell enters a germinal centre and undergoes rapid proliferation and hypermutation of its immunoglobulin genes. Antigen is presented by the follicular dendritic cell *(FDC)*, but only B cells with high-affinity receptors will compete effectively for this antigen. High-affinity B cells express Bcl-2 and are rescued from apoptosis by interaction with T cells (i.e. the B cell presents antigen to the T cell). Interaction with T cells promotes class switching. The class switch that takes place depends on the T cells present, which partly relates to the particular secondary lymphoid tissue and the type of immune response current (TH1 versus TH2). B cells leave the germinal centre to become either plasma cells or B memory cells *(BM)*. *MHC*, Major histocompatibility complex; *TCR*, T-cell receptor.

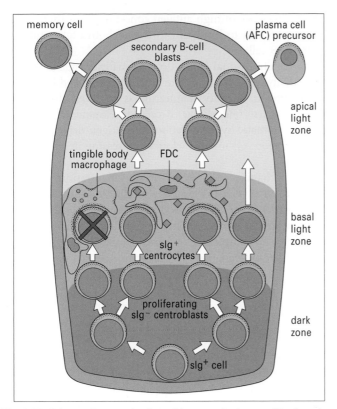

Fig. 9.15 Schematic organization of the germinal centre The functions of the germinal centre are clonal proliferation, somatic hypermutation of Ig receptors, receptor editing, isotype class switching, affinity maturation and selection by antigen. The germinal centre is composed of three major histologically identified zones: a dark zone, a basal light zone and an apical light zone. These zones are predominantly occupied by centroblasts, centrocytes and secondary blasts, respectively. Primary B-cell blasts carrying surface immunoglobulin receptors *(sIg⁺)* enter the follicle and leave as memory B cells or antibody-forming cells *(AFCs)*. Antigen-presenting follicular dendritic cells *(FDCs)* are mainly found in the two deeper zones, and cell death by apoptosis occurs primarily in the basal light zone where tingible body macrophages are also located. Blue squares are antigen-containing iccosomes on FDC.

reduce expression of chemokine receptor CXCR4, which allows them to migrate into the lymphoid follicle.

The B cells express their new BCR and contact FDC in the light zone of the germinal centre, where they give rise to centrocytes. In the light zone, centrocytes encounter antigen bound to the FDCs and antigen-specific T_H2 cells. FDCs and T cells interact with centrocytes through:

- surface molecules such as the BCR, CD40, CD80 (B7-1), CD86 (B7-2), LFA-1, VLA-4 and CD54 (ICAM-1); and
- cytokines such as IL-2, IL-4, IL-5, IL-6, IL-9, IL-10, IL-13, BAFF and lymphotoxin-α.

After the centrocytes have stopped dividing, they are selected according to their ability to bind antigen. Those with high-affinity receptors for foreign antigen are positively selected, while those without adequate affinity are induced to undergo apoptosis by ligation of the surface molecule Fas.

Self-reactive B cells generated by somatic mutation are deleted. Centrocytes that respond to soluble antigen or do not receive T-cell help are negatively selected and undergo Fas-independent apoptosis. In this way, selection provides a mechanism for elimination of self-reactive antibodies that may be generated during somatic hypermutation.

Positively selected centrocytes can re-enter the dark zone for successive rounds of expansion, diversification and selection. Somatic hypermutation and selection improve the average affinity of the germinal centre B-cell population for presented antigen.

Following these B-cell developmental stages, the centrocytes exit the germinal centre and lose their susceptibility to apoptosis by downregulating Fas and increasing the expression of Bcl-2. Three possible outcomes are associated with exit from the germinal centre:

- antibody-secreting bone marrow homing effector B cells;
- marginal zone memory B cells;
- recirculating memory B cells.

SOMATIC HYPERMUTATION AND CLASS-SWITCH RECOMBINATION

Somatic hypermutation and class switching require activation-induced cytidine deaminase. Somatic hypermutation is a common event in antibody-forming cells during T-dependent responses and is important in the generation of high-affinity antibodies. Somatic hypermutation introduces mutations at a very high rate into the V regions of the rearranged heavy and light chain genes (Fig. 9.17). Mutants that bind antigen with higher affinity than the original surface immunoglobulin provide the raw material for the antigen-dependent selection processes outlined above.

Somatic hypermutation occurs at the same time as class switching and both processes involve an enzyme, **activation-induced cytidine deaminase (AID)**, which is highly expressed in germinal centres and is induced by IL-4 and ligation of CD40. AID introduces point mutations into the DNA of the

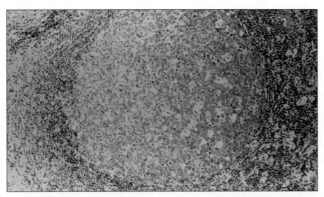

Fig. 9.16 Zoning of the germinal centre of a lymph node The Giemsa-stained section shows the light zone *(left)* and the more actively proliferating dark zone *(right)*. There is a well-developed mantle of small resting lymphocytes that have less cytoplasm and therefore appear more densely packed. (Courtesy Dr K McLennan.)

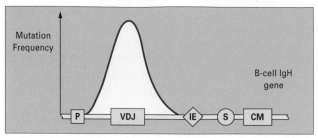

Fig. 9.17 Somatic hypermutation Somatic hypermutation is confined to the area immediately around the recombined VDJ or VJ genes. In this region, the mutation rate may be as high as 10^{-3} per base pair in comparison with the normal rate of 10^{-6} per base pair per round of replication. Note that the promotor *(P)*, intronic enhancer *(IE)*, the switch region *(S)* and the C region genes *(CM)* are outside the zone of hypermutation.

V regions. Animals lacking this enzyme have deficient somatic hypermutation and class-switch recombination.

Affinity maturation depends on somatic hypermutation and cell selection.

The antibodies produced in a primary response to a TD antigen generally have a low average affinity. However, during the course of the response, the average affinity of the antibodies increases or matures. As antigen becomes limiting, the clones with the higher affinity will have a selective advantage. This process is called **affinity maturation**.

The degree of affinity maturation is inversely related to the dose of antigen administered. High antigen doses produce poor maturation compared with low antigen doses (Fig. 9.18). It is thought that:

- in the presence of low antigen concentrations, only B cells with high-affinity receptors bind sufficient antigen and are triggered to divide and to differentiate;

- in the presence of high antigen concentrations, there is sufficient antigen to bind and to trigger both high- and low-affinity B cells.

Although individual B cells do not usually change their overall specificity, the affinity of the antibody produced by a clone may be altered. Affinity maturation is achieved through the cellular events underlying B-cell development, described earlier: i.e. somatic hypermutation and antigen-driven selection and expansion of mutant clones expressing higher-affinity antibodies.

The mechanism by which affinity maturation occurs is thought to involve B-cell progeny binding to antigen held on FDCs in order to proliferate and to differentiate further. Unprocessed antigen in immune complexes is captured by the FDCs via their Fc and complement receptors and held there. As B cells encounter the antigen, there is competition for space on the surface of the FDC, leading to selection. When a B cell with higher affinity arises, it will stay there longer and be given a stronger signal. In addition, B cells with higher-affinity receptors will internalize more antigen and therefore they have a greater potential of presenting it to T cells and receiving T-cell help. Hence, B cells with higher-affinity antibodies have a selective survival advantage.

B cells recombine their heavy chain genes to switch immunoglobulin isotype.

Humans have nine different subclasses (isotypes) of antibody – IgM, IgD, IgG1, IgG2, IgG3, IgG4, IgA1, IgA2 and IgE. Each terminally differentiated plasma cell is derived from a specific B cell and produces antibodies of just one isotype. The first B cells to appear during development carry surface IgM as their antigen receptor. Upon activation, other classes of immunoglobulin are seen, each associated with different effector functions. When a mature B cell switches antibody class, all that changes is the constant region of the heavy chain. The expressed V(D)J region and light chain do not change. Antigen specificity is therefore retained. The arrangement of the constant genes in humans is shown in Figure 9.19.

Upstream of the μ genes is a switch sequence (S), which is repeated upstream to each of the other constant region genes except δ. These sequences are important in the recombination events that occur during class switching, as explained later.

Class switching occurs during maturation and proliferation.

Most class switching occurs in mature B cells during proliferation. However, it can also take place before encounter with exogenous antigen during early clonal expansion and maturation of the B cells. This is known because some of the progeny of immature B cells synthesize antibodies of other immunoglobulin classes, including IgG and IgA.

Further evidence that some class switching occurs independently of antigen comes from experiments with vertebrates raised in germ-free environments where exposure to exogenous antigens is severely restricted.

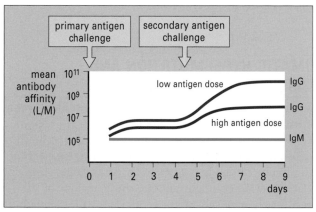

Fig. 9.18 Affinity maturation This figure shows the average affinity of the IgM and IgG antibody responses after primary and secondary challenge with a T-dependent antigen. The affinity of the IgM response is constant throughout. The affinity maturation of the IgG response depends on the dose of the secondary antigen. Low antigen doses produce higher-affinity immunoglobulin than do high antigen doses, because the high-affinity clones compete effectively for the limiting amount of antigen.

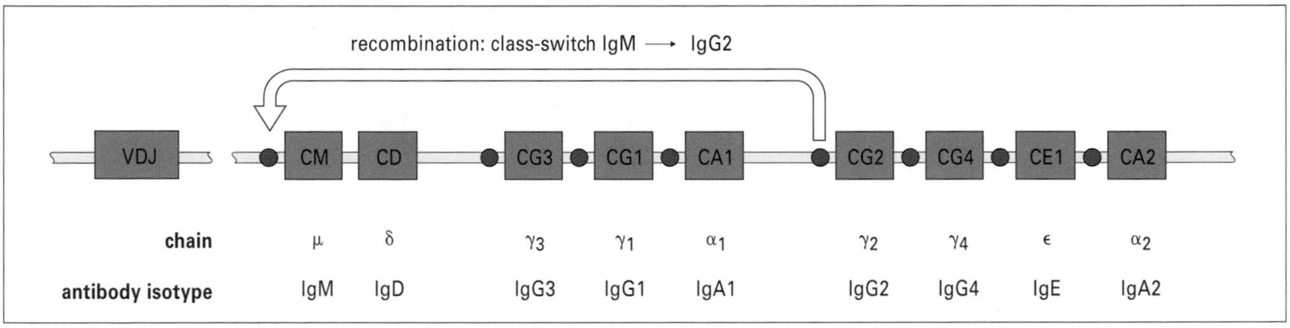

recombination: class-switch IgM ⟶ IgG2

VDJ		CM	CD		CG3	CG1	CA1		CG2	CG4	CE1	CA2

chain	μ	δ		γ₃	γ₁	α₁	γ₂	γ₄	ε	α₂
antibody isotype	IgM	IgD		IgG3	IgG1	IgA1	IgG2	IgG4	IgE	IgA2

Fig. 9.19 Constant-region genes and class switching in humans The human immunoglobulin heavy chain gene locus (IGH) is shown. Initially, B cells transcribe a VDJ gene and a μ heavy chain that is spliced to produce mRNA for IgM. Under the influence of T cells and cytokines, class switching may occur, illustrated here as a switch from IgM to IgG2. Each heavy chain gene except CD (which encodes IgD) is preceded by a switch region. When class switching occurs, recombination between these regions takes place, with the loss of the intervening C genes – in this case CM, CD, CG3, CG1 and CA1.

Class switching may be achieved by differential splicing of mRNA.
Initially, a complete section of DNA that includes the recombined VDJ region and the δ and μ constant regions is transcribed. Two mRNA molecules may then be produced by differential splicing, each with the same VDJ segment, but having either μ or δ constant regions (Fig. 9.20).

Class switching is mostly achieved by gene recombination.
The principal mechanism of class switching is by recombination, which occurs immediately before the B cells enter the germinal centres. B cells switch from IgM to the other immunoglobulin classes or subclasses by an intra-chromosomal deletion process that involves the excision of intervening genetic material between highly repetitive switch regions 5′ to each chain (Fig. 9.21). Switching requires cytokine-dependent transcription of DNA in the region of the new constant region, which occurs before recombination of the 5′ switch regions that precede the C genes for each of the heavy chain isotypes.

Immunoglobulin class expression is influenced by cytokines.
During a TD immune response, there is a progressive change in the predominant immunoglobulin class of the specific antibody produced, usually to IgG. This class switch is not seen in TI responses, in which the predominant immunoglobulin usually remains IgM (see Fig. 9.8). There is now considerable evidence for the involvement of T-cell cytokines in determining exactly which isotype switch will be made (Table 9.2). This can be related to the underlying CSR events occurring in the B cells. In order to make a switch, it is necessary for the new C region genes to be transcribed before the recombination actually takes place. These transcripts are not translated into protein and are referred to as germline transcripts. Critically, transcription allows AID to access the transcribing switch region, to initiate the switch for that immunoglobulin isotype. Each of the switch regions has a 5′ promoter with target sites that bind to transcription factors induced by specific cytokines. Consequently, a cytokine can induce transcription factors that initiate germline transcription from a specific switch region, which results in class switching to that isotype.

Immunoglobulin class expression is influenced by the site of synthesis.
Isotype switching is greatly affected by the tissue environment. This can partly be accounted for by the cytokines released by the T cells at different sites. For example, T cells at mucosal sites tend to promote a switch to IgA production and this can be correlated with the production of IL-5 from TH2 cells, which predominate in mucosal tissues.

Equally important are the subsets of APCs and tissue cells, which are present in each of the lymphoid tissues or mucosal sites. Tissue cells attract particular lymphocyte subsets into the tissue by release of appropriate chemokines and this selective migration is further reinforced by the chemokines released by the lymphocytes. The interaction of appropriate lymphocyte subsets then promotes selective class switching and antibody synthesis in different tissues.

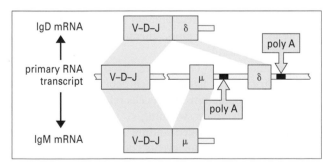

IgD mRNA

primary RNA transcript

IgM mRNA

Fig. 9.20 Isotype switching by differential RNA splicing Single B cells produce more than one antibody isotype from a single long primary RNA transcript. A transcript containing μ and δ is shown here. Polyadenylation *(poly A)* can occur at different sites, leading to different forms of splicing, producing mRNA for IgD *(top)* or IgM *(bottom)*. Even within this region, there are additional polyadenylation sites that determine whether the translated immunoglobulin is the secreted or membrane-bound form.

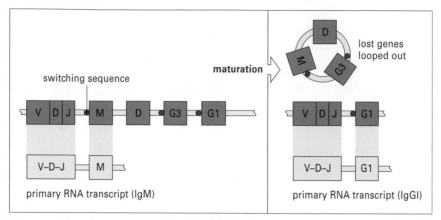

Fig. 9.21 Class switching by gene recombination Initially the VDJ region is transcribed together with the M gene for the IgM heavy chain *(left)*. After removal of introns during processing, mRNA for secreted IgM is produced. During B-cell maturation, class-switch recombination occurs between the Sμ recombination region and a downstream switch region (G1 in this example). The intervening region (containing genes for IgM, IgD and IgG3 in this instance) is looped out and then cut, with deletion of the intervening regions and joining of the two switch regions.

TABLE 9.2 Isotype Regulation by Human T-Cell Cytokines

T Cells	Cytokines	IMMUNOGLOBULIN CLASSES					
		IgG1	IgG2	IgG3	IgG4	IgA	IgE
TH2	IL-4	↑		↓	↑		↑
	IL-5					↑	
TH1	IFNγ	↓		↑			↓
Treg	TGFβ			↓		↑	
	IL-10	↑		↑			

Cytokines can cause an increase (↑) or decrease (↓) in the frequency of isotype-specific B cells.

Events in B-cell development shape the antibody response.

It is now possible to understand the features of the antibody response in vivo in terms of the underlying cellular events, although the events can best be understood by viewing the B-cell population as a whole, rather than as a collection of individual cells. Features of the antibody response in vivo include:

- the enhanced secondary response, which follows from the expansion of antigen-specific B-cell populations during the primary immune response;
- class switching, which is a consequence of the gene recombination (CSR) occurring in the secondary lymphoid tissues;
- affinity maturation, which results from somatic hypermutation (SHM) of immunoglobulin V region genes, followed by selective survival of B-cell clones producing high-affinity antibodies;
- the development of long-lived memory B cells, which depends on their survival during maturation in the lymphoid follicles and results in development of B cells with a distinct profile of cytokine receptors, chemokine receptors and co-stimulatory molecules; and
- differentiation of B-cell clones producing different Ig isotypes in different tissues, which depends on interactions with distinct populations of TH cells releasing cytokines that promote selective class switching.

In each case an understanding of the antibody response can be related to events occurring during B-cell development.

CRITICAL THINKING: DEVELOPMENT OF THE ANTIBODY RESPONSE

See Critical thinking: Explanations, section 9

A project is underway to develop a vaccine against mouse hepatitis virus, a pathogen of mice, which may become a serious problem in colonies of mice. The vaccine consists of capsid protein of the virus, which is injected subcutaneously as a depot in alum on day 0. At days 5 and 14, blood is taken from the six mice and their serum is tested for the presence of antibodies against the viral capsid protein. Separate assays are performed for each of the immunoglobulin classes IgM, IgG and IgA. The amounts, expressed in μg/mL of antibody, are shown in Figure 9.22.

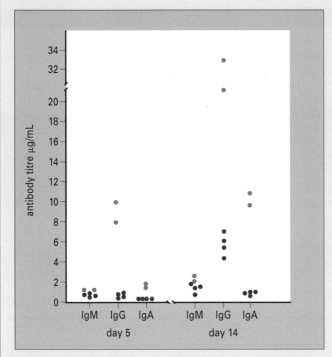

Fig. 9.22 Antibody titres at days 5 and 14 in immunised mice.

When the data are analysed, it appears that two of the animals *(green spots)* have high titres of antibody, particularly of IgG and IgA, at days 5 and 14.

1. Why do the titres of IgG antibodies increase more rapidly between days 5 and 14 than IgM antibodies, in all animals?
2. Propose an explanation for the high titres of IgG antibodies in the two animals indicated at day 5. Can this explanation also account for the relatively high levels of IgA antibodies also seen in these mice?

   The spleens from mice taken at day 14 are used to produce B cells making monoclonal antibodies against the viral protein. Of the clones produced, 15 produce IgG, three produce IgM and none produces IgA.
3. Why do you suppose there are no IgA-producing clones, despite the good IgA response?
4. You want a high-affinity antibody for use in an assay. Which of the clones you have produced are likely to be of higher affinity?

FURTHER READING

Hardy RR, Hayakawa K. B cell development pathways. Annu Rev Immunol 2001;19:595–621.

Khan WF. B cell receptor and BAFF receptor signaling regulation of B cell homeostasis. J Immunol 2009;183:3561–3567.

Peled JU, Kuang FL, Iglesias-Ussel MD, et al: The biochemistry of somatic hypermutation. Ann Rev Immunol 2008;26:481–511.

Quách TD, Manjarrez-Orduño N, Adlowitz DG, et al. Anergic responses characterize a large fraction of human autoreactive naive B cells expressing low levels of surface IgM. J Immunol 2011;186:4640–4648.

Smith KG, Fearon DT. Receptor modulators of B cell receptor signaling – CD19/CD22. Curr Top Microbiol Immunol 2000;245:195–212.

Stavenezer J, Guikema JEJ, Schrader CE. Mechanisms and regulation of class switch recombination. Ann Rev Immunol 2008;26:261–292.

Stewart I, Radtke D, Phillips B, McGowan SJ, Bannard O. Germinal center B cells replace their antigen receptors in dark zones and fail light zone entry when immunoglobulin gene mutations are damaging. Immunity 2018;49:477–489.

Suan D, Sundling C, Brink R. Plasma cell and memory B cell differentiation from the germinal center. Curr Opin Immunol 2017;45:97–102.

Wang Y, Shi J, Yan J, et al. Germinal-center development of memory B cells driven by IL-9 from follicular helper T cells. Nat Immunol 2017;18:921–930.

Yarkoni Y, Getahun A, Cambier JC. Molecular underpinning of B-cell anergy. Immunol Revs 2010;237:249–263.

10

Antibodies

SUMMARY

- **Antibodies (immunoglobulins) are glycoproteins that specifically recognize and bind foreign bodies (antigens) that have gained access to the body, e.g. microorganisms.** They are present in blood and tissue fluids as soluble molecules and as membrane-bound receptors on B lymphocytes. They establish an immune response that neutralizes and eliminates foreign antigens.
- **There are five classes of antibody in most mammals:** IgM, IgD, IgG, IgA, and IgE. In humans, four subclasses of IgG and two of IgA are also defined. Thus, collectively, there are nine **isotypes**, in order of their genes: IgM, IgD, IgG3, IgG1, IgA1, IgG2, IgG4, IgA2, IgE.
- **Antibodies are composed of four polypeptide chains:** two light chains of identical sequence and two heavy chains of identical sequence. Complex oligosaccharide moieties are covalently linked to the heavy chains. The N-terminal $\sim$110 amino acid residues of the light and heavy chains of each specific antibody are unique, i.e. they vary between antibody specificities and are referred to as light (VL) and heavy (VH) variable regions, respectively. The unique sequences of paired VL/VH regions form the specific antigen-binding site **(paratope)**. The C-terminal sequences of each light (CL) and heavy (CH) isotype are relatively constant and contribute to the activation of effector functions that eliminate antigen/antibody complexes.
- **Antigen-binding sites of antibodies are specific for the three-dimensional shape (conformation) of their target**: the antigenic determinant or **epitope**.
- **Antibody affinity** is a measure of the strength of the interaction between an antibody paratope and its epitope. The avidity, functional affinity, of an antibody depends on the number of paratopes (2 for IgG, 5–10 for IgM) and their ability to engage multiple epitopes on the antigen to form antigen/antibody complexes: the more epitopes bound, the greater the avidity.
- **Receptors for antibody heavy chain constant regions (Fc receptors)** may be expressed by mononuclear cells, neutrophils, natural killer cells, eosinophils, basophils or mast cells. The receptors are specific for the constant (Fc) region of an antibody isotype and promote activation of effector functions, e.g. phagocytosis, tumour cell killing, mast cell degranulation, etc.
- **Therapeutic antibodies are used as treatments for many conditions.** Antibody engineering has resulted in reduced immunogenicity in humans and improvements in antibody functions and activity in different subcellular compartments.

Antibodies and B-cell receptors. Specific recognition of antigen is the hallmark of the adaptive immune response. Two principal molecules are involved in this process:
- B-cell antigen receptors (BCRs); and
- T-cell antigen receptors (TCRs).

Recognition specificity and structural diversity are defining characteristics of these antigen receptor molecules. The primary immune repertoire composed of IgM or IgM + IgD is produced by gene recombination in the gene loci encoding the antibody heavy and light chains as described in Chapter 9.

Antibodies are a family of glycoproteins. Five classes and nine isotypes of antibody molecule are present in most mammals. Whilst sharing the basic four-chain structure (Fig. 10.1), they differ in size, e.g. the number of polypeptide chains, charge, amino acid sequence, carbohydrate content, etc.

In humans, four subclasses of IgG and two of IgA are defined. Each isotype is defined by the amino acid sequence of the heavy chain constant region that is encoded by a unique gene. Antibodies present in blood (serum) are polyclonal, i.e. structurally heterogeneous, reflecting their ability to recognize and bind different epitopes expressed by multiple antigens; each antibody is the product of a unique plasma cell clone.

All antibody isotypes are bifunctional. Antibodies are bifunctional molecules that:
- recognize and bind antigen;
- promote activation of the effector mechanisms, resulting in the removal and degradation of antibody/antigen (pathogen) immune complexes (Fig. 10.2).

Whilst the variable region of an antibody determines its antigen specificity, the constant region of the heavy chain (Fc) determines the effector functions activated.

Effector functions include binding of the Fc regions to:
- Fc receptors (FcR) expressed on host tissues (e.g. FcγRI on phagocytic cells);
- activation of the classical or alternate pathways of complement (see Chapter 4).

Antibody class and subclass is determined by the sequence of the genetically encoded heavy chain. The basic structure of each antibody molecule is a unit consisting of:
- two light polypeptide chains ($\sim$25 kDa); and
- two heavy polypeptide chains (IgG, IgA, IgD: $\sim$55 kDa; IgM, IgE: $\sim$70 kDa).

In an individual antibody molecule, the amino acid sequences of the two light chains are identical, as are the

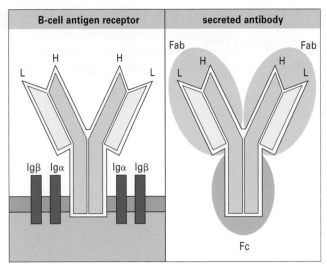

Fig. 10.1 Surface and secreted antibodies The B-cell antigen receptor *(left)* consists of two identical heavy *(H)* chains and two identical light *(L)* chains. In addition, secondary components (Igα and Igβ) are closely associated with the primary receptor and couple it to intracellular signalling pathways. Circulating antibodies *(right)* are structurally identical to the primary B-cell antigen receptors except they lack the transmembrane and intracytoplasmic sections. Many proteolytic enzymes cleave antibody molecules into three fragments: two identical Fab (antigen-binding) fragments and one Fc (crystallizable) fragment.

sequences of the two heavy chains. Both light and both heavy chains are folded into a series of discrete domains composed of ~110 amino acid residues. The sequence of the constant region of the heavy chain determines the isotype (class, subclass) of the antibody. The heavy chains are designated:

- mu: μ, (IgM);
- gamma: γ1, γ2, γ3 and γ4 (IgG1, IgG2, IgG3, IgG4);
- alpha: α1 and α2 (IgA1, IgA2);
- delta: δ (IgD);
- epsilon: ε (IgE).

There are no subclasses of IgM, IgD or IgE (Table 10.1).

Different antibody isotypes activate different effector systems. The human IgG subclasses (IgG1–IgG4) are present in serum in the approximate proportions of 66%, 23%, 7% and 4%, respectively. They arose after the evolutionary divergence that led to humans, during which each subclass gained or lost interaction with various Fc receptors and complement. Consequently, the subclasses differ in their functional capacity. Antibody subclasses in other species have no direct functional correlation to the four human subclasses even when they have the same nomenclature For example, human IgG1 and mouse IgG1 are not direct analogues.

IgG is the predominant antibody isotype present in normal human serum. IgG accounts for 70%–75% of the total serum antibody pool with a normal concentration range of 6–16 g/L.

IgM accounts for about 10% of the serum antibody pool. Serum IgM consists of five monomer four-chain structures covalently bound, through a J (joining) polypeptide chain of mass ~15 kDa, to form a pentameric structure of mass ~970 kDa. Normal concentration range: 0.5–2.0 g/L. A transmembrane monomeric form (mIgM) is present as an antigen-specific receptor on mature B cells (BCR).

IgA is present in serum and seromucous secretions. The IgA1 subclass antibody predominates in serum and accounts for approximately 15%–20% of the serum antibody pool. In

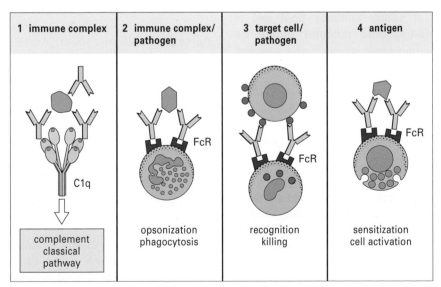

Fig. 10.2 Antibodies act as adapter molecules for immune effector systems Antibodies act as adapter molecules for different immune effector systems, linking antigens to receptor molecules (C1q and FcR) of the immune system. **(1)** Immune complexes can activate the complement classical pathway. **(2)** Antibodies bound to the surface of pathogens opsonize them for phagocytosis. **(3)** Antibodies bound to cells can promote their recognition and killing by natural killer cells. (Similarly, recognition of some parasitic worms by eosinophils, mediated by antibodies, targets them for killing.) **(4)** Antibody bound to Fc receptors sensitizes cells so that they can recognize antigen and the cell becomes activated if antigen binds to the surface antibody.

TABLE 10.1   Physicochemical Properties of Human Immunoglobulin Classes

Property	IMMUNOGLOBULIN TYPE									
	IgG1	IgG2	IgG3	IgG4	IgM	IgA1	IgA2	sIgA	IgD	IgE
Heavy chain	γ_1	γ_2	γ_3	γ_4	μ	α_1	α_2	α_1/α_2	δ	ε
Mean serum conc. (mg/mL)	9	3	1	0.5	1.5	3.0	0.5	0.05	0.03	0.00005
Sedimentation constant	7s	7s	7s	7s	19s	7s	7s	11s	7s	8s
Mol. wt (kDa)	146	146	170	146	970	160	160	385	184	188
Half-life (days)	21	20	7	21	10	6	6	?	3	2
% Intravascular distribution	45	45	45	45	80	42	42	trace	75	50
Carbohydrate (%)	2–3	2–3	2–3	2–3	12	7–11	7–11	7–11	9–14	12

Each immunoglobulin class has a characteristic heavy chain. Thus IgG possesses γ chains; IgM, μ chains; IgA, α chains; IgD, δ chains; and IgE, ε chains. Variation in heavy chain structure within a class gives rise to immunoglobulin subclasses. For example, the human IgG pool consists of four subclasses reflecting four distinct types of heavy chain. The properties of the immunoglobulins vary between the different classes. In secretions, IgA occurs in a dimeric form (sIgA) in association with a protein chain termed the secretory component. The serum concentration of sIgA is very low, whereas the level in mucosal secretions can be very high.

humans, over 80% of serum IgA has a four-chain monomer structure with a normal concentration in the range 0.8–4.0 g/L. However, it is present in the sera of most other species as a dimer.

IgA2 is the predominant antibody isotype present in seromucous secretions (secretory IgA, sIgA), e.g. saliva, colostrum, milk and tracheobronchial and genitourinary secretions. sIgA is produced by plasma cells at mucosal sites and secreted as a J-chain-mediated dimer. It is transported across the epithelial cell boundary by transcytosis following binding to the polymeric immunoglobulin receptor (pIgR). During this process, the pIgR is cleaved to produce a major fragment termed secretory component (SC), which becomes covalently attached to the IgA dimer.

IgD accounts for 1 % of serum antibody pool and is expressed as an antigen-specific receptor (mIgD) on mature B cells. IgD has a four-chain structure and a normal serum concentration range: 2–100 mg/L.

IgE has a low serum concentration. IgE has a four-chain structure with very low (0–90 IU/mL) serum concentrations relative to the other antibody isotypes. However, basophils and mast cells express the high-affinity IgE-specific receptor (FcεRI), resulting in saturation binding. The low-affinity IgE receptor (FcεRII) is expressed on B cells.

The basic four-chain structure consists of a series of folded domains. The basic four-chain structure and folding of antibody molecules is illustrated for IgG1 (Fig. 10.3). The **light chains** (~25 kDa) are bound to the heavy chains (~55 kDa) by inter-chain disulfide bonds and multiple non-covalent interactions. The **heavy chains** are similarly bound to each other by inter-chain disulfide bridges and multiple non-covalent interactions.

Each segment of ~110 amino acids folds to form a compact domain, which is stabilized through multiple non-covalent interactions and a covalent intra-chain disulfide bond. Thus: the light chain has two domains and an intra-chain disulfide

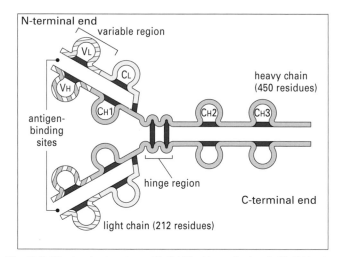

Fig. 10.3 The basic structure of IgG1 The N-terminal end of IgG1 is characterized by sequence variability (V) in both the heavy and light chains, referred to as the VH and VL regions, respectively. The rest of the molecule has a relatively constant (C) structure. The constant portion of the light chain is termed the CL region. The constant portion of the heavy chain is further divided into three structurally discrete regions: CH1, CH2 and CH3. These globular regions, which are stabilized by intrachain disulfide bonds, are referred to as domains. The sites at which the antibody binds antigen are located in the variable domains. The hinge region is a segment of heavy chain between the CH1 and CH2 domains. Flexibility in this area permits the two antigen-binding sites to operate independently. There is close pairing of the domains except in the CH2 region (see Fig. 10.4). Carbohydrate moieties are attached to the CH2 domains.

bond in each of the VL and CL domains; the IgG heavy chain (γ) has four domains VH, CH1, CH2 and CH3 ($C_\gamma1$, $C_\gamma2$, $C_\gamma3$) each having an intra-chain disulfide bridge enclosing a peptide loop of 60–70 amino acid residues.

There is significant amino acid sequence homology between antibody domains, which is reflected in a common conformational motif, referred to as the **immunoglobulin fold**. This characteristic fold defines members of the immunoglobulin gene superfamily (Fig. 10.w1).

Antibodies are prototypes of the immunoglobulin superfamily. The three-dimensional (tertiary) structure of each ~110 amino acid homology region (domain) provides a scaffold for the generation of a multiplicity of structural and functional variants, which may or may not have an overt immune function. Examples include:

- the adhesion molecules ICAM-1 and VCAM-1 (see Chapter 3);
- the TCR and MHC molecules (see Chapter 6);
- cellular receptors for antibodies.

Such molecules are said to belong to the **immunoglobulin supergene family (IgSF)**.

The principal elements of the domain are two opposed β-pleated sheets, stabilized by one or more disulfide bonds between the β-pleated sheets. This structure is sometimes referred to as a **β barrel**.

The three-dimensional structure of an antibody molecule varies with class and subclass. X-ray crystallography has provided structural data on full-length IgG molecules (Fig. 10.4). Mobility around the hinge region of IgG allows for the generation of the Y- and T-shaped structures visualized by electron microscopy. All antibody isotypes exhibit pairing between V$_H$/V$_L$ and C$_H$1/C$_L$ domains, through extensive non-covalent interactions, to form the antigen binding (Fab) region and the antigen-binding paratope.

Whilst the sequence homology between the IgG-Fc subclass regions exhibits >95% sequence homology, each IgG subclass exhibits a unique profile of effector activities.

The hinge regions are structurally distinct and determine the independent mobilities of the IgG-Fab and IgG-Fc moieties that facilitate FcγR and C1 binding. A structural equivalent of the IgG hinge region is present in IgA and IgD but not in IgM or IgE.

In addition to the pairing of the V$_H$/V$_L$ and C$_H$1/C$_L$ domains, the C$_H$3 domains of the IgG-Fc are also paired through non-covalent interactions.

The C$_H$2 domains in IgG do not physically interact through protein–protein interactions but are kept apart by an amphipathic N-linked oligosaccharide moiety. Although accounting for only 2%–3% of the mass of the IgG molecule, the N-linked oligosaccharide influences the conformation of the IgG-Fc and interactions with effector ligands. The oligosaccharide exhibits structural heterogeneity within and between IgG antibody molecules and may modulate effector functions, depending on the oligosaccharide structure of individual IgG molecules (glycoform).

Assembled IgM molecules have a 'Star' conformation. IgM is present in human serum as a pentamer of the basic four-chain structure (Fig. 10.w2). Each heavy chain consists of a V$_H$ and four C$_H$ (Cμ) domains. One advantage of this pentameric structure is that it provides 10 identical binding sites, which can dramatically increase the avidity with which IgM binds its cognate antigen. Given that serum IgM commonly functions to eliminate bacteria containing low-affinity polysaccharide antigens, the increased avidity provided by the pentameric structure provides an important functional advantage.

Covalent disulfide bonds between adjacent C$_H$2 and C$_H$3 domains and the C-terminal 18-residue peptide sequence, referred to as the tailpiece, and J chain link the subunits to form a pentamer.

The J chain is synthesized within plasma cells, has a mass of ~15 kDa and folds to form an immunoglobulin domain. Each heavy chain bears four N-linked oligosaccharide moieties. However, the oligosaccharides are not integral to the protein structure in the same way as in IgG-Fc. IgM activates the classical complement pathway and the presence of high mannose oligosaccharides may activate complement via the mannose binding lectin pathway (see Chapter 4).

Electron micrographs of the IgM molecule reveal a star conformation with a densely packed central region and radiating arms (Fig. 10.5). However, electron micrographs of IgM antibodies bound to poliovirus show molecules adopting a staple or crab-like configuration (see Fig. 10.5), which suggests that flexion readily occurs between the C$_H$2 and C$_H$3 domains, although this region is not structurally homologous to the IgG hinge. Distortion of this region, referred to as **dislocation**, results in the staple configuration of IgM required to activate the classical complement pathway.

Secretory IgA is a complex of IgA, J chain and secretory component. IgA present in serum is produced by plasma cells and secreted as a monomer with the basic four-chain structure. Each heavy chain consists of a V$_H$ and three C$_H$ domains.

The IgA1 and IgA2 subclasses differ substantially in the structure of their hinge regions: the hinge of IgA1 is extended and bears O-linked oligosaccharides; the hinge of IgA2 is truncated, relative to IgA1.

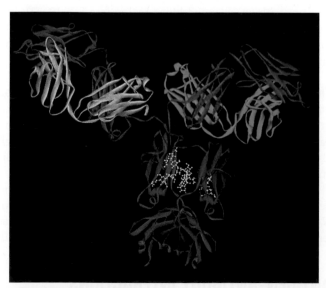

Fig. 10.4 Model of an IgG molecule A model of an IgG molecule showing the polypeptide backbones of the four chains as a ribbon. Heavy chains are shown in *dark blue* and *dark green*. The antigen-binding sites are at the tips of the arms of the Y-shaped molecule and are formed by domains from both the heavy and light chains. The extended, unfolded hinge region lies at the centre of the molecule. Carbohydrate units are shown as ball and stick structures covalently linked to the Fc region.

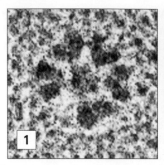
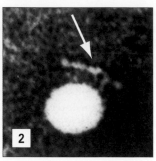

Fig. 10.5 Electron micrographs of IgM molecules (**1**) In free solution, deer IgM adopts the characteristic star-shaped configuration. ×195 000. (**2**) Rabbit IgM antibody *(arrow)* in crab-like configuration with partly visible central ring structure bound to a poliovirus virion. × 190 000. ((**1**) Courtesy Dr E Holm Nielson, Dr P Storgaard and Professor S-E Svehag. (**2**) Courtesy Dr B Chesebro and Professor S-E Svehag.)

A deficit in the addition of O-linked sugars within the hinge region of IgA1 protein has been linked with the disease IgA nephropathy.

IgA is the predominant antibody isotype in external secretions and is present as a complex secretory form. IgA is secreted by gut-localized plasma cells as a dimer in which the heavy chain tailpiece is covalently bound to a J chain, through a disulfide bond (Fig. 10.w2).

Electron micrographs of IgA dimers show double Y-shaped structures, suggesting that the monomeric subunits are linked end-to-end through the C-terminal Cα3 regions (Fig. 10.6).

The dimeric form of IgA binds a **poly-Ig receptor** (pIgR) (Fig. 10.7) expressed on the basolateral surface of epithelial cells. The complex formed is internalized, transported to the apical surface where the poly-Ig receptor is cleaved to yield the secretory component (SC) that is released bound to the IgA dimer. The released secretory form of IgA is relatively resistant to cleavage by enzymes in the gut and consists of two units of IgA, J chain and a secretory component (mass 70 kDa) (see Figs. 10.w2 and 10.7).

Serum IgD exhibits antigen specificity and an IgG-like four-chain structure. Serum IgD accounts for less than 1% of the total serum immunoglobulin. Recent studies have demonstrated that IgD antibody may enhance mucosal homeostasis and

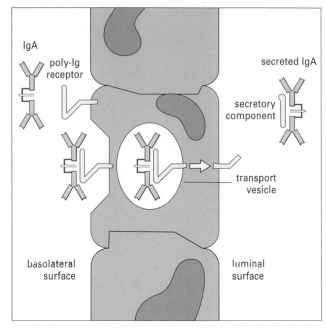

Fig. 10.7 Transport of IgA across the mucosal epithelium IgA dimers secreted into the intestinal lamina propria by plasma cells bind to poly-Ig receptors on the internal (basolateral) surface of the epithelial cells. The sIgA–receptor complex is then endocytosed and transported across the cell while still bound to the membrane of transport vesicles. These vesicles fuse with the plasma membrane at the luminal surface, releasing IgA dimers with bound secretory component derived from cleavage of the receptor. The dimeric IgA is protected from proteolytic enzymes in the lumen by the presence of this secretory component.

immune surveillance by arming myeloid effector cells such as basophils and mast cells with IgD antibodies specific for mucosal antigens, including commensal and pathogenic microbes. Each heavy chain consists of a VH domain and three CH (Cδ) domains with an extended hinge region (see Fig. 10.w2). IgD also functions as an antigen-specific receptor on mature B cells, together with IgM and, as such, exhibits the same diversity and antigen specificity.

The heavy chain of IgE consists of four constant region domains. It is estimated that ~50% of total body IgE is present in the blood, with the remainder being bound to mast cells and basophils through their high-affinity IgE receptor (FcεRI). IgE also binds the low affinity receptor (FcεRII) expressed on B cells and cells of the myeloid lineage.

Each heavy chain consists of a VH and four CH domains and bears six N-linked oligosaccharides (see Fig. 10.w2). An N-linked oligosaccharide, present in the CH3 domain, equivalent to CH2 in IgG, influences binding to FcεRI but not FcεRII.

ANTIGEN–ANTIBODY INTERACTIONS

The conformations of the epitope and the paratope are complementary. Protein molecules are not rigid structures but exist in a dynamic equilibrium between structures that may differ in their ability to form a **primary interaction** with specific **ligands.**

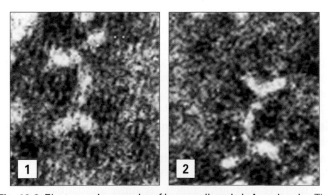

Fig. 10.6 Electron micrographs of human dimeric IgA molecules The double Y-shaped appearance suggests that the monomeric subunits are linked end-to-end through the C-terminal Cα3 domain. × 250 000. (Courtesy Professor S-E Svehag.)

Following a primary interaction, each partner may influence the final **conformation** within the complex. This concept approximates to the induced fit model of protein–protein interactions.

An examination of the interaction between the Fab fragment of the mouse D1.3 monoclonal antibody and hen egg white lysozyme (HEL) reveals the complementary surfaces of the epitope and the antibody's combining site (paratope), comprising 17 amino acid residues of the antibody and 16 residues of the lysozyme molecule (Fig. 10.8). All hypervariable regions of the heavy

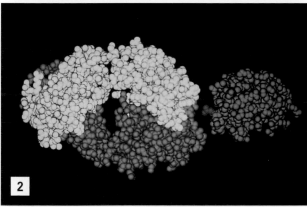

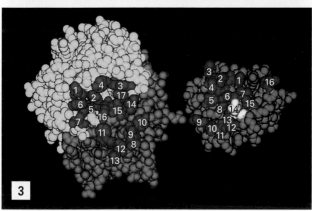

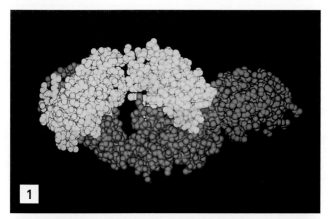

Fig. 10.8 The Fab–lysozyme complex **(1)** Lysozyme *(green)* binds to the hypervariable regions of the heavy *(blue)* and light *(yellow)* chains of the Fab fragment of antibody D1.3. **(2)** The separated complex with Glu121 visible *(red)*. This residue fits into the centre of the cleft between the heavy and light chains. **(3)** The same molecules rotated 90 degrees to show the contact residues that contribute to the antigen– antibody bond. (Reprinted with permission from Poljak RJ, Science. 1986;233:747–753. Copyright 1986 AAAS and reprinted with permission from Garcia KC et al., Science. 1996; 274:209–219.)

and light chains contribute, although the third hypervariable region in the heavy chain appears to be dominant. The paratope of the D1.3 monoclonal antibody may be regarded as classical. The structures of other lysozyme–antibody complexes show differing involvement of hypervariable and framework residues.

Classic studies of antibody variability showed three hypervariable regions in the antibody V domains (Fig 10.w4). The first two of these regions (HV1 and HV2) are germline encoded (V genes) while the third region (HV3) is generated by gene recombination and shows the highest level of variability.

Such structural studies are essential when engineering antibody molecules (e.g. when humanizing a mouse antibody to generate an antibody therapeutic; see Method Box 10.2).

Antibody affinity is a measure of the strength of interaction between a paratope and its epitope.

The affinity of a protein–protein interaction is a thermodynamically defined measure of the strength of interaction between reciprocal binding sites, i.e. as between the paratope of a Fab fragment and the epitope of an antigen. Since an antibody has two Fab moieties and an antigen may express multiple epitopes, three-dimensional complexes can be formed; thus, the apparent affinity is enhanced and is referred to as the avidity.

Antibodies form multiple Non-covalent bonds with antigen.

The antigen–antibody interaction results from the formation of multiple non-covalent bonds. These attractive forces consist of: hydrogen bonds; electrostatic bonds; van der Waals forces; and hydrophobic forces. Each bond is relatively weak in comparison with a covalent bond, but cumulatively they generate high-affinity interactions.

The strength of a non-covalent bond is critically dependent on the distance (d) between the interacting groups, being proportional to $1/d^2$ for electrostatic forces and to $1/d^7$ for van der Waals forces.

Thus, interacting groups must be in intimate contact before these attractive forces come into play.

For a paratope to combine with its epitope, the interacting sites must be complementary in shape, charge distribution and hydrophobicity and, in terms of donor and acceptor groups, capable of forming hydrogen bonds.

Close proximity of two protein surfaces can also generate repulsive forces (proportional to $1/d^{12}$) if electron clouds overlap.

In combination, the attractive and repulsive forces have a vital role in determining the specificity of the antibody molecule and its ability to discriminate between structurally similar molecules.

The great specificity of the antigen–antibody interaction is exploited in a number of widely used assays (see Method Box 10.1).

Antigen–antibody interactions are reversible.

The affinity of an antibody is the sum of the attractive and repulsive forces resulting from binding between the paratope of a monovalent Fab fragment and its epitope. This interaction will be reversible and at equilibrium the Law of Mass Action can be applied and an equilibrium constant, K (the association constant), can be

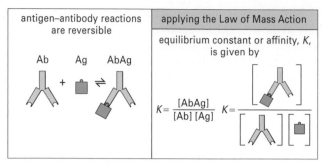

Fig. 10.9 Calculation of antibody affinity All antigen–antibody reactions are reversible. The Law of Mass Action can therefore be applied and the antibody affinity (given by the equilibrium constant, K) can be calculated. (Square brackets refer to the concentrations of the reactants.)

determined (Fig. 10.9). In practice, because of the divalency of antibody and multiple epitopes expressed on some antigens, large three-dimensional complexes may be formed that do not readily dissociate; when a paratope–epitope interaction is broken, both the antibody and antigen remain in proximity due to other paratope–epitope interactions, thus re-association is favoured.

Avidity is likely to be more relevant than affinity. Because each antibody unit of four polypeptide chains has two antigen-binding sites, antibodies are potentially divalent or multivalent (IgM, IgA) in their reaction with antigen.

In addition, antigen can be monovalent (e.g. a small chemical group) or multivalent (e.g. microorganisms).

The strength with which a multivalent antibody binds a multivalent antigen is termed **avidity** to differentiate it from the **affinity**, which is determined for a univalent antibody fragment (Fab) binding to a single antigenic determinant.

The avidity of an antibody for its antigen is dependent on the affinities of the individual antigen-combining sites for the epitopes on the antigen. Avidity will be greater than the sum of these affinities if both antibody-binding sites bind to the antigen because all antigen–antibody bonds would have to be broken simultaneously for the complex to dissociate (Fig. 10.10).

In physiological situations, avidity is likely to be more relevant than affinity because all antibodies, except human IgG4, are functionally divalent and most naturally occurring antigens are multivalent.

In practice, we determine the association constant at equilibrium when the rate of formation of complex (k_a) is equal to the spontaneous rate of dissociation (k_d). The association or equilibrium constant is defined as $K = k_a/k_d$.

It has been suggested that B-cell selection and stimulation during a maturing antibody response depend upon selection for the ability of antibodies to bind to antigens both rapidly (kinetic selection) and tightly (thermodynamic selection).

Cross-reactive antibodies recognize more than one antigen. The specificity of an antibody is defined by the antigen (epitope) provoking its generation; however, an antibody can exhibit **cross-reactivity**, i.e. binding to a structurally related but different antigen (Fig. 10.11). Thus, monoclonal antibodies raised to the antigen hen egg lysozyme (HEL) may also bind structurally homologous duck egg lysozyme (DEL). A polyclonal antiserum

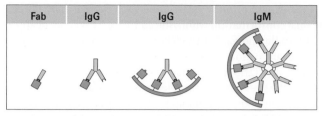

antibody	Fab	IgG	IgG	IgM
effective antibody valence	1	1	2	up to 10
antigen valence	1	1	n	n
equilibrium constant (L/mol)	10^4	10^4	10^7	10^{11}
advantage of multivalence	–	–	10^3-fold	10^7-fold
definition of binding	affinity	affinity	avidity	avidity
	intrinsic affinity		functional affinity	

Fig. 10.10 Affinity and avidity Multivalent binding between antibody and antigen (avidity or functional affinity) results in a considerable increase in stability as measured by the equilibrium constant, compared with simple monovalent binding (affinity or intrinsic affinity, here arbitrarily assigned a value of 10^4 L/mol). This is sometimes referred to as the 'bonus effect' of multivalency. Thus there may be a 10^3-fold increase in the binding energy of IgG when both valencies (combining sites) are used and a 10^7-fold increase when IgM binds antigen in a multivalent manner.

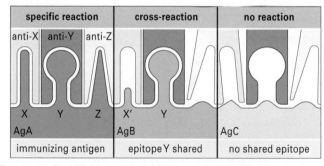

Fig. 10.11 Specificity, cross-reactivity and non-reactivity Antiserum specificity results from the action of a population of individual antibody molecules (anti-X, anti-Y, anti-Z) directed against different epitopes (X, Y, Z) on the same or different antigen molecules. Antigen A *(AgA)* and antigen B *(AgB)* have epitope Y in common. Antiserum raised against AgA (anti-XYZ) not only reacts specifically with AgA, but cross-reacts with AgB (through recognition of epitopes Y and X'). The antiserum gives no reaction with AgC because there are no shared epitopes.

to HEL will contain populations of antibodies specific for HEL and others that cross-react with DEL.

Antibodies recognize the conformation of antigenic determinants. Analysis of antibodies to protein antigens reveals that the epitope may be formed by a contiguous stretch of amino acids (**a continuous epitope**) or of two or more stretches of sequence separated in the primary structure but adjacent in the folded conformation (**discontinuous** or **conformational epitopes**).

Continuous epitopes are unique three-dimensional structures and discontinuous epitopes may be formed of a flexible peptide that assumes a unique conformation when bound to

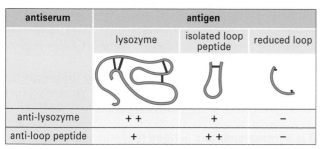

antiserum	antigen		
	lysozyme	isolated loop peptide	reduced loop
anti-lysozyme	+ +	+	–
anti-loop peptide	+	+ +	–

Fig. 10.12 Configurational specificity The lysozyme molecule possesses an intrachain bond *(red)*, which produces a loop in the peptide chain. Antisera raised against whole lysozyme (anti-lysozyme) and the isolated loop (anti-loop peptide) are able to distinguish between the two. Neither antiserum reacts with the isolated loop in its linear reduced form. This demonstrates the importance of tertiary structure in determining antibody specificity.

a paratope, i.e. the paratope may influence the conformation of the epitope by an induced-fit mechanism.

Antibodies are capable of expressing remarkable specificity and are able to distinguish small differences in the shape and chemical properties (e.g. charge, hydrophobicity) of epitopes. Small changes in the epitope, even a single side chain, can therefore abolish binding (Fig. 10.12).

ANTIBODY EFFECTOR FUNCTIONS

Antibodies are bifunctional molecules that specifically bind antigen to form large complexes, thus limiting the spread of pathogens in vivo, and elicit host responses to facilitate their removal and destruction.

The isotype/allotype of the constant region determines the possible effector functions activated, e.g. complement activation, phagocytosis.

In antibody–antigen complexes, the antibody molecules are essentially aggregated such that the multiple Fc regions are able to engage, cross-link and activate ligands or receptors (e.g. FcγR and C1q) (Table 10.2). Thus, an antibody may be an opsonin (from the Greek *opsōneîn*, meaning to prepare for eating): immune complexes formed with antigen are tasty and ingested (eaten) by phagocytes.

IgM predominates in the primary immune response. IgM is the first antibody produced in the primary immune response and is largely confined to the intravascular pool. It is frequently associated with the immune response to antigenically complex, blood-borne infectious organisms.

When bound to its target, IgM is a potent activator of the classical pathway of complement.

Although the pentameric IgM antibody molecule consists of five Fcμ regions, it does not activate the classical pathway of complement in its soluble form. However, when bound to an antigen with repeating identical epitopes, it forms a staple structure (see Fig. 10.5), undergoing a conformational change referred to as **dislocation**, and the multiple Fcμ presented in this form are able to initiate the classical complement cascade.

IgG is the predominant isotype of secondary immune responses. The four IgG subclasses are highly homologous in structure, but each exhibits a unique profile of effector

TABLE 10.2 Biological Properties of Human Immunoglobulins

Isotype	IgG1	IgG2	IgG3	IgG4	IgA1	IgA2	IgM	IgD	IgE
Complement Activation									
Classical pathway	++	+	+++	-	-	-	+++	-	-
Alternative pathway	Varies with epitope density and antibody/antigen ratio								
Lectin pathway	Varies with glycosylation status								
Fc-Receptor Binding									
FcγRI (monocytes)	+++	-	+++	++	-	-	-	-	-
FcγRIIa (monocytes, neutrophils, eosinophils, platelets)	+	±[a]	+	-	-	-	-	-	-
FcγRIIb (lymphocytes)	+	±	+	-					
FcγRIII (neutrophils, eosinophils, macrophages, LGLs, NK cells,T cells)	+	-	+	±	-	-	-	-	-
FcεRI (mast cells, basophils)	-	-	-	-	-	-	-	-	+++
FcεRII (monocytes, platelets, neutrophils, B and T cells, eosinophils)	-	-	-	-	-	-	-	-	++
FcαR (monocytes, neutrophils, eosinophils, T and B lymphocytes)	-	-	-	-	+	+	-	-	-
FcμB (T cells, macrophages)	-	-	-	-	-	-	+	-	-
FcδR(T and B cells)	-	-	-	-	+	-	-	+	-
pIgR, poly-Ig receptor; mucosal transport	-	-	-	-	+	+	+	-	-
FcRn, placental transport and catabolism	+	+	+	+	-	-	-	-	-
Products of Microorganisms									
SpA, staphylococcal protein A	+	+	-	+	-	-	-	-	-
SpG, streptococcal protein G	+	+	+	+	-	-	-	-	-

[a]Dependent on the allotype of FcγRIIa.
LGLs, Large granular lymphocytes; *NK cells,* natural killer cells.
The biological functions of different antibody classes and subclasses depend on which receptors they bind to and the cellular distribution of those receptors mediated by acting as adapters that bind via their Fc region to Fc receptors on different cell types.

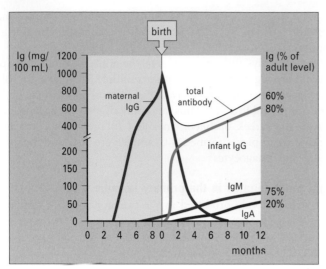

Fig. 10.13 Immunoglobulins in the serum of the fetus and newborn IgG in the fetus and newborn is derived solely from the mother. This maternal IgG has disappeared by the age of 9 months, by which time the infant is synthesizing its own IgG. The neonate produces its own IgM and IgA; these classes cannot cross the placenta. By the age of 12 months, the infant produces 80% of its adult level of IgG, 75% of its adult IgM level and 20% of its adult IgA level.

functions. Thus, in activating the classical pathway of complement, complexes formed with IgG1 and IgG3 antibodies are efficient; those formed with IgG2 antibodies are less effective; and those formed with IgG4 antibodies are largely inactive.

The IgG subclasses also interact with a complex array of cellular Fc receptors (FcγR) expressed on various cell types (see Table 10.2 and later). IgG equilibrates between the intravascular and extravascular pools, providing comprehensive systemic protection.

In humans, the newborn infant is not immunologically competent and the fetus is protected by maternal IgG selectively transported across the placenta (Fig. 10.13). Transport is mediated by the neonatal Fc receptor (FcRn): all IgG subclasses are transported but the cord/maternal blood ratios differ, being approximately 1.2 for IgG1 and approximately 0.8 for IgG2.

In some species (e.g. the rat), maternal IgG is present at high concentrations in colostrum or milk and is transferred to the offspring in the postnatal period through selective transport of IgG across the gastrointestinal tract via the FcRn receptor.

Serum IgA is produced during a secondary immune response. Serum monomeric IgA is a product of a secondary immune response. Immune complexes of serum IgA opsonize antigens and activate phagocytosis through cellular Fc receptors (FcαRI).

A predominant role for IgA antibody is in its secretory dimeric form, affording protection of the respiratory, gastrointestinal and reproductive tracts.

The IgA1 subclass predominates in human serum (approximately 90% of total IgA) and secretions such as nasal mucus, tears, saliva and milk (70%–95% of total IgA).

In the colon, IgA2 predominates (approximately 60% of the total IgA). Many microorganisms that can infect the upper respiratory and gastrointestinal tracts have adapted to their environment by releasing proteases that cleave IgA1 within the extended hinge region, whereas the short hinge region of IgA2 is not vulnerable to these enzymes.

Dimeric IgA is also actively transported by the polymeric Ig receptor to the colostrum or milk and may passively provide immune protection in the postnatal period.

IgD is a transmembrane antigen receptor on B cells. The co-expression of membrane IgM and IgD is a marker for mature circulating B cells. Cellular receptors binding IgD have only recently been described. Serum IgD expresses predominantly lambda light chains. A presence of high serum IgD levels is associated with an inflammatory condition, designated as hyper IgD syndrome.

IgE may Have evolved to protect against helminth parasites infecting the gut. Despite its low serum concentration, the IgE class is characterized by its ability to bind avidly to the high-affinity FcεRI receptor expressed on circulating basophils, tissue mast cells and cells on mucosal surfaces such as the conjunctival, nasal and bronchial mucosae.

IgE may have evolved to provide immunity against helminth parasites, but in developed countries it is now more commonly associated with allergic diseases such as asthma and allergies: e.g. sensitivity to peanuts, eggs, fish, etc.

Fc RECEPTORS

Antibodies may protect simply by binding a pathogen to prevent it from attaching to cells and infecting them. More often, antibodies act as adapters that bind antigen, via the paratope, to form immune complexes that bind, via their Fc regions, to Fc receptors (FcRs) are expressed on multiple cell types, to activate downstream inflammatory killing and clearance mechanisms. Fc receptors specific for the Fc region of each antibody isotype have been identified, FcμR, FcδR, FcγR, FcαR and FcεR; within each class of FcR there are several different types and subtypes, e.g. FcγRI, FcγRIIa, FcγRIIb, FcγRIIIa, FcγRIIIb, etc. A structurally and functionally distinct receptor referred to as the neonatal Fc receptor (FcRn) was first identified as facilitating transport of IgG from rat milk to the newborn.

FcRn: The structure of FcRn is similar to that of major histocompatibility complex (MHC) class I molecules and consists of two α domains in complex with β2-microglobulin (Fig. 10.14). FcRn is expressed by multiple cell types and functions to effect the pharmacokinetics of IgG and transport of maternal IgG across the human placenta to provide immune protection for the early life of the newborn. The IgG/FcRn interaction is pH sensitive, binding at pH 6.5 (the pH within vacuoles) and dissociating at pH 7.4 (the pH of blood).

pIgR: The poly-Ig receptor containing 5 IgSF domains is found on mucosal epithelia, where it actively binds IgM and dimeric IgA and transports them from the basolateral to the apical side (see Fig. 10.7). In this way, it actively transports these isotypes to mucosal surfaces and mothers' milk. After transport, the extracellular domain is proteolytically cleaved, forming the secretory component (SC), which remains covalently bound to

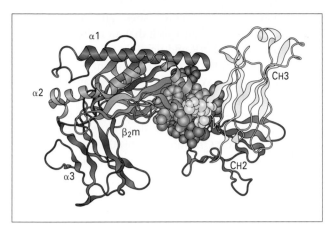

Fig. 10.14 Neonatal rat intestinal Fc receptor FcRn Principal interactions between neonatal rat intestinal FcRn and the Fc of maternal IgG (derived from milk) are illustrated by ribbon diagrams of FcRn (domains α1, α2, α3 and β₂m are shown in *red, light green, purple* and *grey*, respectively) and of Fc (CH2 and CH3 domains are shown in *blue* and *yellow*). The main contact residues of the FcRn (α1 domain, 90; α2, 113–119 and 131–135; β₂m, 1–4 and 86) are depicted as space-filling structures. (Reproduced from Ravetch JV, Margulies DH. New tricks for old molecules. Nature. 1994;372:323–324.)

IgA, but not IgM, whereby it enhances the proteolytic resistance of IgA in secretions.

The three types of Fc receptor for IgG are FcγRI, FcγRII and FcγRIII.

Three types of cell surface receptor for IgG (FcγR) are defined in humans:

- FcγRI (CD64);
- FcγRII (CD32); and
- FcγRIII (CD16).

Each FcγR receptor is characterized by a transmembrane glycoprotein **α** chain and extracellular Ig superfamily domains (Fig. 10.15); FcαR and FcεR are structurally similar receptors to FcγR. Many FcγRs are expressed constitutively but differentially on a variety of cell types. Some FcγR may be upregulated or induced by environmental factors (e.g. cytokines).

Biological activation results from aggregation (cross-linking) of the FcγR on the cell surface with consequent signal transduction and activation of **immunoreceptor tyrosine-based activation (ITAM)** or **immunoreceptor tyrosine-based inhibitory (ITIM)** motifs in the cytoplasmic sequences.

Phosphorylation of ITAM triggers activities such as phagocytosis, antibody-dependent cell-mediated cytotoxicity (ADCC), apoptosis, mediator release and enhancement of antigen presentation. In contrast, phosphorylation of ITIM blocks cellular activation.

FcγRI is involved in phagocytosis of immune complexes and mediator release.

It is common practice to refer to FcγR as being of high, medium or low affinity. However, these descriptions are imprecise, relative and vary considerably depending on the methods of determination.

FcγRI (CD64) binds monomeric IgG1 and IgG3 with high affinity, IgG4 with low affinity; IgG2 does not have detectable binding affinity. FcγRI has a restricted cellular distribution

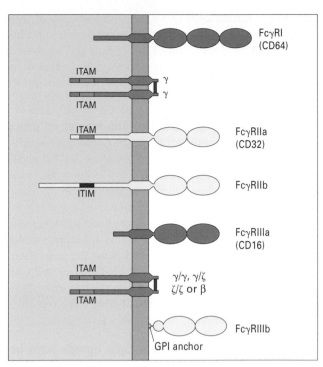

Fig. 10.15 Fcγ receptors Receptors for Fcγ in humans belong to the immunoglobulin superfamily and have either two or three extracellular immunoglobulin domains. Motifs (ITAM, ITIM) on the intracellular segments or on associated polypeptides are targets for tyrosine kinases involved in initiating intracellular signalling pathways.

but is expressed on all cells of the mononuclear phagocyte lineage and is involved in the phagocytosis of immune complexes, mediator release, etc. The extracellular region of the α chain consists of three immunoglobulin domains; the cytoplasmic domain is associated with a γ chain that bears an ITAM motif.

FcγRIIa and FcγRIIb: FcγRIIa is an activating receptor and FcγRIIb is an inhibitory receptor.

FcγRIIa (CD32a) has a wide cellular distribution. The α chain of FcγRIIa has moderate affinity for monomeric IgG1 and IgG3 and binds complexed (multivalent, aggregated) IgG with high avidity. An ITAM motif is expressed within the cytoplasmic tail. Polymorphisms in the FCGR2A gene determine the presence of histidine or arginine at position 131 in the extracellular domains: the His[131] allotype binds IgG1 and IgG3 with slightly higher affinity than Arg[131] and is also activated by immune complexes of IgG2.

FcγRIIb (CD32b) expresses an ITIM motif within its cytoplasmic tail and when cross-linked inhibits cellular activation, particularly on B cells (see Fig. 12.17).

FcγRIII is expressed as FcγRIIIa and FcγRIIIb.

FcγRIIIa **(CD16a)** is structurally and functionally distinct from FcγRIIIb (CD16b). They have different cellular distributions and both are extensively glycosylated.

FcγRIIIa is a transmembrane protein and FcγRIIIb is GPI (glycosyl phosphatidylinositol) anchored (see Fig. 10.15).

The α chains of FcγRIIIa have a moderate affinity for monomeric IgG and may be associated with γ/ξ and/or β chains bearing ITAM motifs. FcγRIIIa is expressed on monocytes, macrophages, natural killer (NK) cells and a fraction of T cells; FcγRIIIb is expressed on neutrophils and basophils and has a low affinity for monomeric IgG. Engagement and cross-linking of FcγRIIIb can result in cellular activation as a result of lipid raft formation and association with other membrane proteins bearing signalling motifs.

Polymorphism in FcγRIIIa and FcγRIIIb may affect disease susceptibility.
Polymorphism in the FCGR3A gene results in the presence of phenylalanine (Phe) or valine (Val) at position 158 in the extracellular domains; the Val[158] allotype is associated with higher binding affinity for IgG1/IgG3 and consequently more efficient NK-cell activation.

Polymorphism in the FcγRIIIB gene results in expression of FcγRIIIb-NA1 and FcγRIIIb-NA2 forms exhibiting multiple amino acid sequence differences, including the generation of an N-linked glycosylation motif in FcγRIIIb-NA2 and consequently the extent of glycosylation. The relative expression of the FcγRIIIb-NA1 and FcγRIIIb-NA2 forms are reported to be associated with differing susceptibility to infection.

Interaction sites of IgG-Fc for multiple ligands have been identified.
Application of state-of-the-art genetic engineering and physicochemical techniques has allowed elucidation of the molecular topography of two distinct IgG-Fc regions interacting with multiple ligands. Thus, FcRn, staphylococcal protein A (SpA) and streptococcal protein G (SpG) bind at overlapping non-identical sites at the CH2/CH3 interface whilst the FcγR and the C1 component of complement bind at overlapping non-identical sites at the hinge proximal region of the CH2 domain (Fig. 10.16) The crystal structure of IgG-Fc/FcγR complexes

reveals asymmetric interaction sites embracing the CH2 domains of both heavy chains such that an individual IgG molecule is univalent for FcγR and possibly C1.

IgM–antigen complexes are very efficient activators of the classical complement system, but the mechanism by which IgM binds C1q appears to be different from that of IgG. The conformational change from a 'star' to a 'staple' conformation observed upon binding to multivalent antigen is thought to unveil a ring of occult C1q-binding sites that are not accessible in the star-shaped configuration (see Fig. 10.5).

Glycosylation of both the IgG-Fc and FcγR is essential for receptor binding to IgG.
N-linked glycosylation of the IgG Cγ2 domain is essential for the binding and activation of FcγRI, FcγRII, FcγRIII and C1q, but not FcRn, SpA, SpG, etc. The oligosaccharide is of the complex diantennary type both between and within IgG antibody populations. It is sequestered between the two heavy chain CH2 domains. The precise oligosaccharide structure of an IgG molecule (glycoform) influences affinity and downstream responses elicited by IgG immune complexes. The glycoform of an IgG antibody-based therapeutic drug is identified as a critical quality attribute (CQA) and glycoform fidelity must be maintained throughout the lifetime of the drug. Glycosylation is a species- and tissue-specific post-translational modification that challenges biopharmaceutical companies producing IgG antibody therapeutics in non-human cell lines, e.g. Chinese hamster cells (CHO) (see Method Box 10.2).

The FcR for IgA is FcαRI.
The transmembrane IgA receptor FcαRI (CD89) consists of two Ig superfamily ecto-domains and is associated with a γ chain bearing an ITAM sequence. It binds both IgA1 and IgA2, is expressed on myeloid cells and can trigger phagocytosis, cell lysis and the release of inflammatory mediators.

The two types of Fc receptor for IgE are FcεRI and FcεRII.
FcεR is the classical high-affinity receptor that is expressed on mast cells and basophils. The α chain is a glycoprotein composed of two immunoglobulin-like extracellular domains and is a member of the immunoglobulin superfamily. The low-affinity FcεRII is not a member of the immunoglobulin superfamily but has substantial structural homology with several animal C-type lectins (e.g. mannose-binding lectin, MBL).

Cross-linking of IgE bound to FcεRI results in histamine release.
The FcεRI is expressed on the surface of mast cells and basophils as a complex with a β (33 kDa) and two γ (99 kDa) chains to form the αβγ2 receptor unit (Fig. 10.17). FcεRI binds IgE with an affinity of approximately 10^{10} L/mol such that, although the serum concentration of IgE is very low, the receptors are permanently saturated. Cross-linking of the IgE bound to these receptors results in the activation and release of histamine and other vasoactive mediators.

FcεRII is a type 2 transmembrane molecule.
FcεRII is the low-affinity (CD23) receptor and is a type 2 transmembrane molecule (i.e. one in which the C-termini of the polypeptides

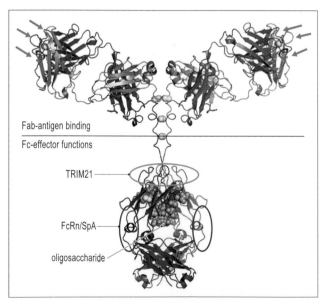

Fig. 10.16 Ligand binding sites on IgG1 and IgG3 antibody molecules Antigen binds to the hypervariable loops in the V domains of the Fab region. Fc receptors and C1q bind to a region close to the hinge of IgG1 and IgG3. The placental receptor FcRn and SpA (protein-A from *Staphylococcus aureus*) bind to a region between the two domains of the Fc region. (Based on Jefferis R. Arch Biochem Biophys 2012;526:159-166.)

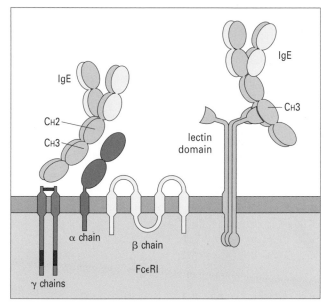

Fig. 10.17 Models for FcεRI and FcεRII Models for the high-affinity IgE receptor (FcεRI), which binds to IgE via its α chain, and the low-affinity receptor (FcεRII), which binds using its lectin domains. Both receptors are shown with IgE bound.

are extracellular; see Fig. 10.17). The two forms of human CD23 are **CD23a**, which is expressed in antigen-activated B cells and influences IgE production, and **CD23b**, whose expression is induced in a wide range of cells exposed to IL-4.

CD23a and CD23b differ in their cytoplasmic N termini, by a stretch of seven or six amino acids, respectively, and contain different signalling motifs that modify their functions.

IgE receptors bind to IgE by different mechanisms. Decades of research and controversy surround the identification of the interaction site on IgE for the high-affinity FcεRI receptor. Recent crystal structures of a Cε2Cε3Cε4 fragment and a Cε3Cε4–FcεRI complex seem to have resolved the issue revealing a striking structural homology between this site and the site on IgG Fc that binds FcγR. Possible models for the interaction of IgE with the FcεRI and FcεRII receptors are illustrated in Figure 10.17.

ANTIBODY ENGINEERING

The vast functional range of antibodies is poised to recognize a plethora of foreign antigens and provide protection from infectious diseases. The capacity of antibodies for highly specific targeting is increasingly being explored for treatment of various human ailments. Examples range from neutralization of immune mediators such as cytokines, to killing of tumour cells. The origin of these antibodies is often immortalized B-cell hybridomas derived from immunized animals, but also from humans. After cloning, the resulting recombinant antibody may be further improved and equipped with new functions. The challenges associated with production of therapeutic antibodies in quantity are outlined in Method Box 10.2.

Human therapeutic antibodies have low immunogenicity. Antibody-based therapeutics have been used since the late 1890s in the form of anti-serum (obtained from immunized horses) that neutralizes bacterial toxins. Pooled human serum antibodies have been used since the 1960s as replacement therapy for humoral immune deficiencies.

The first versions of monoclonal antibody therapeutics were mouse derived, but these have become fully human to reduce the immunogenicity through several means (Fig. 10.18):
- generation of chimeric antibodies by fusing the antibody variable regions to human constant regions;
- generation of humanized antibodies by engrafting antibody CDRs onto human framework regions;
- generation of human antibodies through recombinatory libraries in vitro (phage display);
- generation of fully human antibodies by cloning from immunized humans or mice expressing human antibodies.

Generally, humanized and fully human antibodies are less immunogenic than chimeric antibodies, whereas the difference between the former two is less pronounced.

Several strains of mice have been generated that do not express mouse antibodies but instead have been equipped (knocked-in) for part or even the full range of both heavy chain and light chain V-gene loci.

Engineering for tailored antibody-effector function. Antibody treatments for humans are mostly formulated on the backbone of human IgG1, IgG4 or IgG2, thereby exploring the natural functionality of human immune responses. However, attempts have been made to improve upon nature by engineering useful qualities of antibodies (Fig. 10.19). For example, these are:
- increase affinity to C1q to ensure enhanced complement activity;
- increase affinity to FcγR for augmented myeloid and NK-cell activity towards targets;
- eliminate binding to effector molecules to avoid side-effects;
- optimize FcRn-binding to either reduce or increase half-life and bioavailability;
- incorporate new biological functions.

Some of these engineering feats can be combined to generate even more potent drugs or research tools. The most successful are likely to be changes that do not also introduce immunologically foreign epitopes, although in some cases these cannot be avoided.

Alterations that affect effector functions. Early adaptations to reduce effector functions include the choice of an IgG2 or IgG4 backbone or even a combination of these two (eculizumab). More advanced engineering includes changes to the protein backbone. Several different variations to the amino acid sequence of the hinge-proximal region of the CH2 domain (see Fig. 10.19) have been devised that eliminate binding to both C1q and FcγR receptors.

On the other hand, antibodies have also been engineered which enhance effector functions, including mutations to increase binding to one or even all FcγR and/or enhance

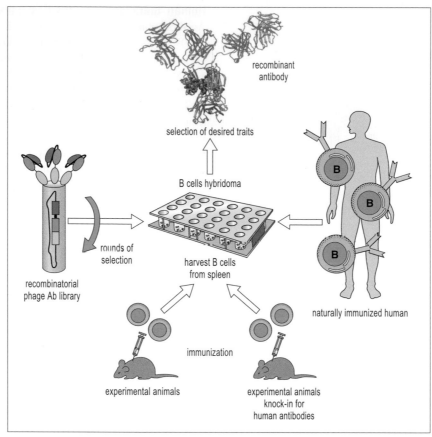

Fig. 10.18 Production of therapeutic antibodies Monoclonal and recombinant antibodies can be generated by two different means: through immunization in animals (including humans) or by artificial combinatory libraries of a pair of variable regions, often expressed on bacterial phages. Human antibodies can be generated from human B-cell clones in vitro or they may be produced from mice transfected with the genes needed to produce the human antibodies.

complement activity. The mutations are primarily focused on amino acid changes; however, engineering of the IgG-glycan can also be used, e.g. through deglycosylation or afucosylation (e.g. obinutuzumab anti-CD20), which eliminates effector functions or increases ADCC, respectively. Mutations that alter the potential of IgG1 to form multimeric structures through lateral-C$_H$2/C$_H$3 interactions between several IgG, forming for example hexamers that enable efficient docking with the hexameric structure of C1q, are also being explored.

Alterations that affect half-life and biodistribution. One important aspect of using antibodies for human therapy is the exceptionally long half-life of IgG of 3 weeks compared with approximately 1 week for IgA. This is because of the unique ability of IgG to interact with FcRn within acidic recycling compartments in cells, which then transports IgG back to the surface. Several attempts have been made to engineer this by:
- eliminating FcRn binding (which may be favourable if short exposure is required because of toxicity or for enhanced contrast for imaging);
- enhancing binding at slightly acidic pH, while eliminating binding at neutral pH. This ensures binding in recycling compartments and efficient release at the cell surface.

Engineering of this type is also likely to affect biodistribution of IgG because FcRn also seems to provide transport of IgG to mucosal surfaces and affect transport of such drugs across the placenta. In addition, the effector function of such drugs, and even immunogenicity towards their targets, may also be altered as a result of high expression of these receptors in myeloid cells, including dendritic cells, where FcRn also facilitates antigen presentation of IgG-containing immune complexes.

Engineering of variable regions. Variable domains mediate target binding and confer specificity. As such, variable domains of each monoclonal antibody are unique, making engineering challenging. Several aspects may be addressed:
- humanization, i.e. grafting CDRs onto human (germline) framework regions to minimize immunogenicity;
- elimination of possible (strong) T-cell epitopes to minimize immunogenicity;
- introducing mutations to enhance affinity;
- removing regions that may affect aggregation behaviour;
- modifying net charge of the variable domains, which impacts on the in vivo half-life by affecting FcRn-mediated recycling.

It can be challenging to humanize variable regions without compromising affinity or stability of a given antibody. Certain

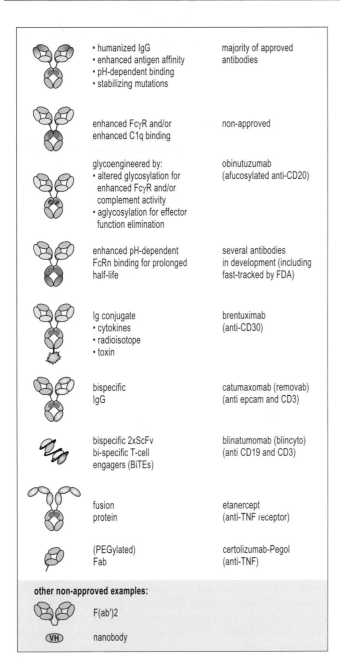

• humanized IgG • enhanced antigen affinity • pH-dependent binding • stabilizing mutations	majority of approved antibodies
enhanced FcγR and/or enhanced C1q binding	non-approved
glycoengineered by: • altered glycosylation for enhanced FcγR and/or complement activity • aglycosylation for effector function elimination	obinutuzumab (afucosylated anti-CD20)
enhanced pH-dependent FcRn binding for prolonged half-life	several antibodies in development (including fast-tracked by FDA)
Ig conjugate • cytokines • radioisotope • toxin	brentuximab (anti-CD30)
bispecific IgG	catumaxomab (removab) (anti epcam and CD3)
bispecific 2xScFv bi-specific T-cell engagers (BiTEs)	blinatumomab (blincyto) (anti CD19 and CD3)
fusion protein	etanercept (anti-TNF receptor)
(PEGylated) Fab	certolizumab-Pegol (anti-TNF)

other non-approved examples:

	F(ab')2
	nanobody

Fig. 10.19 Production of therapeutic antibodies Antibody biology can be improved from nature by engineering one or more of the seven main areas of an IgG. These are the variable regions affecting antigen binding, the upper part of the C_H2 domain, the glycans affecting binding to FcγR and C1q, the glycans also affecting binding to the same effector molecules, the C_H2/C_H3 interface affecting half-life and possibly complement activation, the C_H3 domains affecting dimerization of the two halves of the IgG, and the C-terminus and the hinge for fusion to other proteins or drugs. The two heavy chains are coloured *orange*, light chains *cyan* and the CDR *red*. The glycan is colour-coded by glycan adduct (fucose *red*, GlcNAc *blue*, mannose *green*, galactose *yellow*). *FDA*, US Food and Drug Administration.

non-human framework residues may be needed for functionality but are still immunogenic.

An interesting novel concept are so-called sweeping antibodies, which have high affinity at neutral pH but low affinity at lower pH found in endosomes. This results in dissociation of soluble targets (such as a cytokine) during FcRn-mediated recycling of antibody and facilitates target clearance.

Alternative forms. The long half-life and good yield of IgG antibodies in engineered cell factories has inspired the generation of so-called fusion proteins, which generally consist of a protein fused to the Fc portion of IgG, often replacing the antibody Fab region by fusion to the hinge, or by fusion to the C-terminus leaving the Fab region intact. The Fc portion provides a bivalent mode of action through the symmetry of the antibody and provides a prolonged binding to FcRn and long-half life. A good example of such a drug is the fusion of tumour necrosis factor (TNF) receptor 2, which blocks the inflammatory effect in various autoimmune patients. Various platforms have been developed to make bispecific antibodies by introducing mutations that favour asymmetrical assembly of two different heavy chains.

If the mode of action of an antibody is simply to block a target (e.g. TNF-blocking agents), it may be sufficient to retain only one Fab portion. It may also even be desirable to prevent FcRn binding as this also results in transcytosis through the placenta. This enables autoimmune patients requiring anti-TNF therapy to continue therapy during pregnancy without exposing the unborn fetus to high doses of the drug. An example is certolizumab pegol, a TNF inhibitor, which is further PEGylated to prevent renal removal because of its small size, thereby giving a longer half-life, which the Fc tail would have otherwise provided.

Conjugates. So-called antibody-drug conjugates (ADCs) consist of a cytotoxic substance coupled to an antibody for the targeted killing of cancer cells. The combination of an antibody and a cytotoxic drug allows more specific killing of cancer cells and spares healthy tissue. The linker can either be chemically stable, non-cleavable or cleavable with, for example, local enzyme activity being responsible for release of the cytotoxic payload.

Production of antibodies as drugs. The success of antibodies such as infliximab (anti-TNFα) and rituximab (anti-CD20) has resulted in demands for their production in metric tonnes. The biopharmaceutical industry has met the challenge with the construction of mammalian cell culture facilities (10 000–20 000-litre capacities) to produce recombinant monoclonal antibodies (rMAbs). Productivity has been greatly enhanced in recent years such that downstream processing is now the bottleneck. The cost of treatment with these drugs remains very high. All full-length antibody therapeutics currently licensed have been produced by mammalian cell culture using CHO cells or the mouse NSO or Sp2/0 plasma cell lines; a Fab therapeutic is produced in *Escherichia coli*. Other systems under development and evaluation include transgenic animals, yeast and plants.

The efficacy of an antibody therapeutic is critically dependent on appropriate post-translational modifications (PTMs) and each production system offers a different challenge because PTMs show species, tissue and site specificity. Essential human PTMs are relevant to potency; non-human PTMs may increase the potential immunogenicity of the products, some of which, like glycosylation, may alter the effector functions of antibodies. The most frequent cell lines used today are the CHO cells, which produce human IgG heavy chains largely bearing human type glycoforms, but with minor fractions containing foreign sialic acids and galactose-alpha-1,3-galactose. These may be immunogenic; therefore specific glycosyltransferases have been 'knocked-out'. This technique is also used to generate more effective antibodies, because non-fucosylated antibodies have enhanced ADCC, compared with the fucosylated form. Thus, the cell lines used to produce antibodies are also being engineered to produce pre-selected glycoforms, depending on the effector activities considered to be optimal for a given application.

CRITICAL THINKING: THE SPECIFICITY OF ANTIBODIES

See Critical thinking: Explanations, section 10

The human rhinovirus HRV14 is formed from four different polypeptides: one of them (VP4) is associated with viral RNA in the core of the virus, while the other three polypeptides (VP1–VP3) make up the shell of the virus – the capsid.

1. When virus is propagated in the presence of neutralizing antiviral antiserum it is found that mutated forms of the virus develop. Mutations are detected in VP1, VP2 or VP3, but never in VP4. Why should this be so? The most effective neutralizing antibodies are directed against the protein VP1 – this is termed an immunodominant antigen. Two different monoclonal antibodies against VP1 were developed and used to induce mutated forms of the virus. When the sequences of the mutated variants were compared with the original virus, it was found that only certain amino acid residues became mutated (see table below).

2. What can you tell about the epitopes that are recognized by the two different monoclonal antibodies?

3. When the binding of the antibody VP1-a is measured against the different mutant viruses, it is found that it binds with high affinity to the variant with glycine (Gly) at position 138, with low affinity to the variant with Gly at position 95, and does not bind to the variant with lysine (Lys) at position 95. How can you explain these observations?

Antibody	Amino acid number	Residue in wild type	Observed mutations
VP1-a	91	Glu	Ala, Asp, Gly, His, Asn, Val, Tyr
VP1-a	95	Asp	Gly, Lys
VP1-b	83	Gln	His
VP1-b	85	Lys	Asn
VP1-b	138	Glu	Asp, Gly
VP1-b	139	Ser	Pro

FURTHER READING

Gutzeit C, Chen K, Cerutti A. The enigmatic function of IgD: some answers at last. Eur J Immunol 2018;48:1101–1113.

Hayes JM, Cosgrave FJ, Struwe WB, Wormald M, Davey GP, Jefferis R, Rudd PM. Glycosylation of immunoglobulins and their Fc receptors. Curr Top Microbiol Immunol 2014;382:165–199.

Jefferis R. Glycosylation as a strategy to improve antibody-based therapeutics. Nat Rev Drug Discov 2009;8:226–234.

Kaplon H, Reichert JM. Antibody-based therapeutics to watch in 2018. MAbs 2018;10:183–203.

Kiyoshi M, Tsumoto K, Ishii-Watabe A, Caaveiro JMM. Glycosylation of IgG-Fc: a molecular perspective. Int Immunol 2017; 29(7):311–317.

Lefranc MP, Lefranc G. Human Gm, Km, and Am allotypes and their molecular characterization: a remarkable demonstration of polymorphism. Methods Mol Biol 2012;882:635–680.

Litman GW, Rast JP, Fugmann SD. The origins of vertebrate adaptive immunity. Nat Rev Immunol 2010;10:543–553.

Monteiro RC. Role of IgA and IgA Fc receptors in inflammation. J Clin Immunol 2010;30:1–9.

Ramsland PA, Hutchinson AT, Carter PJ. Therapeutic antibodies: discovery, design and deployment. Mol Immunol 2015;67(2 Pt A): 1–3.

Schroeder HW Jr., Cavacini L. Structure and function of immunoglobulins. J Allergy Clin Immunol 2010;125:S41–S52.

Shukla AA, Thömmes J. Recent advances in large-scale production of monoclonal antibodies and related proteins. Trends Biotechnol 2010;28:253–261.

Sutton BJ, Davies AM. Structure and dynamics of IgE-receptor interactions: FcεRI and CD23/FcεRII. Immunol Rev 2015;268:222–235.

Vidarsson G, Dekkers G, Rispens T. IgG subclasses and allotypes: from structure to effector functions. Front Immunol 2014;5:520.

11

Immunological Tolerance

SUMMARY

- **Immunological tolerance is the state of unresponsiveness to a particular antigen**. The clonal receptors of lymphocytes are generated by random recombination of the many genes that code for the antigen-binding regions. This creates the need to control cells that could recognize and destroy self tissues. The breakdown of immunological tolerance to self antigens is the cause of autoimmune diseases.
- **Immunological tolerance is achieved by many different mechanisms** operating on different cell types.
- **Central tolerance refers to the selection processes that T-cell precursors undergo in the thymus**. Thymic epithelial cells and dendritic cells present self antigens to the immature T-cell precursors. T-cell precursors that respond strongly to the self antigens presented in the thymus undergo apoptosis. This is called negative selection. A specialized population of thymic epithelial cells can express genes that are normally only expressed in a strictly organ-specific or time-restricted manner.
- **Peripheral tolerance refers to the diverse mechanisms that enforce and maintain T-cell tolerance outside the thymus.** These include the prevention of contact between autoreactive T cells and their target antigens **(immunological ignorance)**, the **peripheral deletion** of autoreactive T cells by activation-induced cell death or cytokine withdrawal, the incapacity of T cells to mount effector responses upon recognizing their target antigen **(anergy)** and the suppression of immune responses by **regulatory T cells**.
- **B-cell tolerance** is established by several mechanisms, including clonal deletion of autoreactive B cells, mostly in the bone marrow; the rearrangement of autoreactive B-cell receptors **(receptor editing)** or by **B-cell anergy**. In addition, B-cell tolerance is maintained by tolerant T cells. The production of high-affinity class-switched antibodies depends on T-cell help. Therefore, if tolerance to a particular antigen is firmly established in the T-cell compartment, B cells that recognize this antigen will usually remain tolerant.
- **To establish or to re-establish tolerance** is a major goal for innovative treatments for autoimmunity, allergy and transplantation. In contrast, to overcome immunological tolerance is one major goal for innovative treatments against cancer.

GENERATION OF AUTOREACTIVE ANTIGEN RECEPTORS DURING LYMPHOCYTE DEVELOPMENT

The specificity of the antigen receptors of T cells and B cells is the result of random shuffling of the many gene segments that encode the antigen-binding site of these receptors. Theoretically, this process could generate more than 10^{15} different T-cell receptors (TCRs), including some that can bind to autoantigens (Fig. 11.1). Similar considerations apply to B-cell receptors. Cells expressing such receptors are called self-reactive lymphocytes. The immune system has to fulfil two contradictory requirements: on the one hand, the repertoire of different antigen receptors needs to be as large as possible to avoid 'holes in the repertoire' that could be exploited by pathogens to evade immune detection; on the other hand, the receptor repertoire must be shaped to prevent the immune system from attacking the organism that harbours it. Any disturbance in this delicately balanced system can have pathogenic or even lethal consequences, either from infections or from the unwanted reaction with autoantigens or harmless external antigens as in allergy. This paradox was recognized by Paul Ehrlich, who coined the term 'horror autotoxicus' for the possibility of reactions against self components. Tolerance is the process that eliminates or neutralizes such autoreactive lymphocytes and a breakdown of this system can cause autoimmunity. To avoid autoreactivity, the randomly generated repertoire of T-cell and B-cell receptors is censored by several different mechanisms.

T-CELL TOLERANCE

T-cell tolerance is established at two levels. Immature thymocytes undergo harsh selection processes in the thymus. This is often called **central tolerance** and results in the deletion of most T cells with high affinity for self antigens. Mature T cells are also regulated to avoid self reactivity. The mechanisms that reinforce T-cell tolerance outside the thymus are collectively called **peripheral tolerance**.

Central T-cell tolerance develops in the thymus. The chief mechanism of T-cell tolerance is the deletion of self-reactive T cells in the thymus. Immature T-cell precursors migrate from the bone marrow to the thymus. There, they proliferate, differentiate and undergo selection processes before a selected few re-enter the blood stream as mature naive T cells. These differentiation and selection processes depend on interactions with thymic epithelial cells and dendritic cells in specialized microenvironments within the thymus (Fig. 11.2, see also Figs. 2.26 and 2.28).

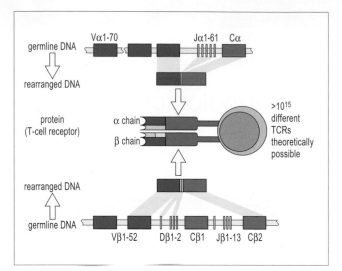

Fig. 11.1 The need for immunological tolerance Lymphocyte receptors are produced by random recombination of the many genes encoding for their heterodimeric receptors. Humans possess more than 70 different T-cell receptor *(TCR)* Vα gene elements, 61 Jα gene elements and one Cα gene element in germline configuration. One Vα, Jα and Cα gene element is used to code for an individual TCRα chain. For the TCR β chain, there are 52 Vβ, 2 Dβ, 13 Jβ and 2 Cβ gene elements. Additional combinatorial possibilities are created by random insertion of N regions (V–J for the TCRα and V–D, D–J for the TCRβ). The random combinations of these different elements allow for the generation of more than 10^{15} different TCRs. Similar numbers apply to B-cell receptor heavy and light chains.

Generation of their clonal TCR is the first step in T-Cell development. In the thymus, the T-cell precursors, also called thymocytes, start to express the recombinase-activating gene (RAG) products and begin to rearrange their αβ TCR genes. The randomly rearranged TCRs expressed by the double-positive (DP) CD4⁺8⁺ thymocytes collectively constitute the organism's unselected TCR repertoire, which is also called the germline repertoire. These thymocytes undergo processes of **positive and negative selection.** Less than 5% of them survive these selection events and are allowed to exit the thymus as naive mature T cells.

In addition to αβ T cells, other lineages including γδ T cells also develop in the thymus. These cells rearrange their TCR genes and therefore could potentially become autoreactive, but they do not normally interact with major histocompatibility complex (MHC) class I and class II molecules for antigen presentation. Consequently, it is uncertain whether selection of the receptor repertoire of these cells occurs in the thymus.

Natural killer (NK) T cells also rearrange their antigen receptor and may be autoreactive. There is some evidence that they have undergone both positive and negative selection in the thymus, although the ligand(s) that drive this process have not been identified.

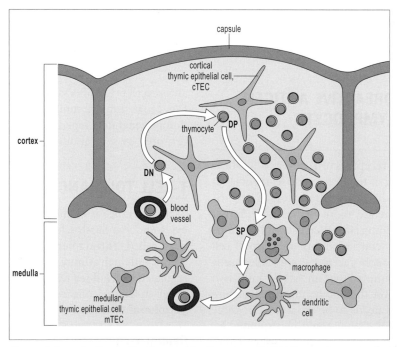

Fig. 11.2 T-cell repertoire selection in the thymus T-cell precursors, the thymocytes, enter the thymic cortex through blood vessels. At this stage, the thymocyte cells are called double-negative *(DN)* because they express neither CD4 nor CD8. They proliferate and express recombinase activating gene products to assemble their TCRs. Thymocytes that have successfully rearranged a T-cell receptor (TCR) β chain express both CD4 and CD8 (double-positive, *DP*) and these reassemble α chains to form the TCR. They interact with cortical thymic epithelial cells *(cTECS)*. Recognition of a selecting ligand is necessary for thymocytes' survival, so-called positive selection. Positive selection also induces commitment to either the CD4⁺ or the CD8⁺ lineage, the cells become single-positive *(SP)* and move to the thymic medulla. Here they interact with antigen-presenting cells, including medullary thymic epithelial cells *(mTECs)*, capable of expressing tissue-restricted antigens. Thymocytes that react strongly with ligands presented by antigen-presenting cells in the thymic medulla undergo apoptosis. This is called negative selection. (Adapted from Kyewsky B, Klein L. Ann Rev Immunol 2006;24:571–606.)

Thymocytes are positively selected for their ability to interact with self MHC molecules. The DP T cells interact with thymic cortical epithelial cells that present peptides derived from endogenous proteins bound to MHC molecules. Recognition of self-peptide/MHC complexes is vital for the DP T cells for two reasons:

- in the DP T cells, RAG is active and TCR α chains are continuously rearranged to maximize the chance of producing a TCR capable of interacting with self MHC;
- only upon recognition of a peptide/MHC complex via the TCR is RAG expression halted and the cell is committed to express a particular αβ TCR.

Moreover, recognition of a peptide/MHC complex via the TCR is necessary for the DP T cell to receive a survival signal. This is called **positive selection** (see Fig. 11.2). Experiments have shown that T cells are positively selected by interaction with self-MHC to prepare them for subsequent activation by non-self-peptide/self-MHC complexes, indicating the biological benefit of positive selection. Accordingly, mice that do not express MHC class II molecules lack CD4$^+$ T cells and mice that do not express MHC class I molecules lack CD8$^+$ T cells.

Positive selection occurs predominantly in the thymic cortex. Specialized antigen-presenting cells (APCs), the cortical thymic epithelial cells (cTECs), are pivotal for positive selection. Given that the number of different peptides that can be presented by any particular MHC molecule is much smaller than the number of different TCRs that undergo positive selection, each peptide must be involved in positively selecting many different T cells. Accordingly, experiments have demonstrated that the peptide on which a TCR is positively selected does not need to share sequence similarity with the peptides recognized by that same TCR in the periphery.

Note that positive selection depends on the recognition of self-peptides bound to self-MHC. The TCRs that are positively selected based on low-affinity interactions with self-peptide/MHC form the selected repertoire that ultimately recognizes microbial antigens to protect the organism from infectious diseases. This is one illustration of the flexibility of antigen recognition by T cells. The peptides that mediate positive selection in the thymus are also presented outside the thymus, where they support survival of mature T cells and may also act as co-agonists that enhance T-cell activation by agonist peptides.

An immediate question is why T cells that were selected based upon self-recognition do not usually cause damage to the organism? One answer is that the threshold for TCR signalling is lower in immature DP T cells in the thymus than in mature T cells in the periphery. Thus, DP T cells can respond to low-affinity interaction with peptide/MHC complexes that would not trigger mature T cells. One important regulator of this TCR signalling threshold is the microRNA miR-181a that regulates the expression of several phosphatases involved in TCR signalling. DP T cells express much higher levels of miR-181a than mature single-positive (SP) T cells.

Lack of survival signals leads to death by neglect. DP T cells whose receptors have a very low affinity for the peptide/MHC

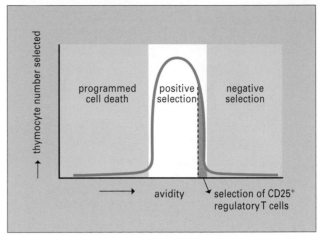

Fig. 11.3 The correlation between avidity and thymocyte selection The avidity of a T cell's interaction with antigenic peptide presented by an antigen-presenting cell (APC) will depend on the level of expression of the major histocompatibility complex (MHC)–peptide complex [MHC + peptide] on the APC and both the affinity and surface expression of TCR on the T cell. MHC + peptide depends on the affinity of peptide for MHC and the stability of the complex once formed. T cells with an intermediate affinity for MHC undergo positive selection and those with high affinity for MHC + self peptides undergo negative selection. Current evidence suggests that CD25$^+$ regulatory T cells are selected in the thymus and have a relatively high affinity for MHC + peptide.

complexes they encounter during their approximately 3–4-day life span in the thymic cortex do not receive survival signals and undergo apoptosis in the thymus (Fig. 11.3). This is called **death by neglect**. Accordingly, T cells do not progress beyond the DP stage in mice that have been manipulated to lack expression of MHC molecules. Analyses of the germline repertoire of TCRs have revealed that this unselected repertoire contains more self-MHC reactive TCRs than expected by chance. In other words, co-evolution of TCR and MHC molecules has shaped the germline αβ TCR repertoire to favour the generation of receptors that can interact with self-MHC.

Thymocytes are negatively selected if they bind strongly to self peptides on MHC molecules. After positive selection and commitment to the CD4 or CD8 lineage in the thymic epithelium, thymocytes express the chemokine receptor CCR7 and migrate towards the medulla, where the CCR7 ligands CCL19 and CCL20 are produced. In the thymic medulla, the thymocytes are probed for another 4–5 days. T cells whose receptors have a high affinity for the peptide/MHC complexes encountered in the medulla are potentially autoreactive and undergo apoptosis. This is called **negative selection** (see Figs. 11.2 and 11.3). Experimental evidence suggests that the majority of the DP T cells that were positively selected are later eliminated by negative selection.

The relevance of negative thymic selection can be demonstrated by neonatal thymectomy. Mice that are thymectomized within the first 3 days after birth develop an autoimmune syndrome that includes sialadenitis, diabetes, autoimmune gastritis and hepatitis.

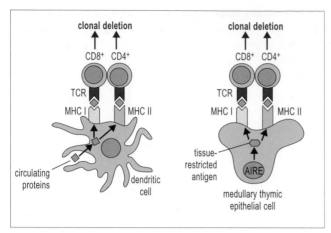

Fig. 11.4 Medullary thymic epithelial cells express and present tissue-restricted antigens Different antigen-presenting cell populations induce thymic tolerance. Dendritic cells and other conventional antigen-presenting cells (APCs) present phagocytosed or endogenously synthesized proteins to T lymphocytes. T cells that express high-affinity receptors for these ubiquitous proteins will undergo apoptosis. Medullary thymic epithelial cells (mTECs) express the transcriptional autoimmune regulator *AIRE* and, therefore, possess the unique capacity of expressing tissue-restricted antigens (TRAs) ectopically in the thymus. This allows for intrathymic clonal deletion of T cells expressing high-affinity T-cell receptors *(TCRs)* for tissue-restricted antigens. *MHC,* Major histocompatibility complex. (Adapted from Sprent J, Surh CD. Nature Immunol 2003;4:303–304.)

A library of self antigens is presented to developing T cells in the thymus.

The induction of central tolerance requires the presence of autoantigens in the thymus. This poses an obvious problem for thymic selection: some autoantigens (e.g. insulin) are expressed in a tissue-specific manner and are called tissue-restricted antigens (TRAs). The question, then, is how do TRAs get into the thymus for presentation to developing T cells? Some might be brought into the thymus by immigrating antigen-presenting cells, but it is highly unlikely that this would yield a reliable representation of the organism's TRAs. Moreover, developmentally regulated TRAs, e.g. antigens that are only expressed after puberty, would not gain access to the fetal thymus. The answer is that specialized cells in the thymus, the medullary thymic epithelial cells (mTECs), express proteins that are otherwise strictly tissue restricted. This has been called ectopic or **promiscuous gene expression** (Fig. 11.4).

mTECS express several hundreds or even thousands of structurally diverse antigens that represent almost all tissues in the body. Importantly, mTECs express not only tissue restricted antigens but also developmentally regulated antigens. Thus, gene expression in mTECs is uncoupled from spatial and developmental regulation, but not all mTECs express all TRAs: any particular TRA is expressed by less than 5% of mTECs.

AIRE controls promiscuous expression of genes in the thymus.

mTECs express the transcriptional regulator **AIRE (autoimmune regulator)**, which controls the expression of a large number of TRAs. Mice with a targeted disruption of the AIRE gene have reduced promiscuous gene expression in mTECs and suffer from various autoimmune conditions. Similarly, in humans, point mutations in the gene coding for AIRE are the cause of the rare monogenic autosomal recessive autoimmune polyendocrinopathy–candidiasis–ectodermal dystrophy (APECED) syndrome. APECED is characterized by high titres of several different autoantibodies that cause disease, mainly in endocrine organs. Together, these findings strongly suggest that the autoimmune manifestations are caused by diminished expression of TRAs in thymic mTECs due to the AIRE deficiency.

AIRE appears to act by removing stops on transcriptional machinery. Small clusters of genes are activated in concert in different mTECs, suggesting that AIRE acts by epigenomic action to allow transcription of sets of linked genes that would normally be silent. The activated gene clusters vary between different cells, which explains why each mTEC only expresses a small set of the available TRAs.

Subtle quantitative alterations in the thymic expression of TRAs can be consequential. Murine intrathymic expression levels of autoantigens, including insulin and myelin antigens, correlate inversely with susceptibility to autoimmune diseases, type 1 diabetes and experimental autoimmune encephalitis (EAE), respectively. Similarly, in humans, genetic variants resulting in low levels of intrathymic insulin expression are strongly associated with susceptibility to type 1 diabetes.

Qualitative variations in TRAs expressed in mTECs have also been associated with autoimmune disease models. Differential splicing or the expression of embryonic, rather than mature, variants of myelin autoantigens have been associated with strain-specific susceptibility to EAE and may well play a role in the pathogenesis of multiple sclerosis in humans.

Thymic dendritic cells can also cause negative selection.

Whereas mTECs are the only cells known to be capable of promiscuous gene expression, they are not the only cells important for negative selection. Thymic dendritic cells can take up TRAs expressed by mTECs and cross-present these TRAs to T cells. Recent intravital imaging studies have yielded the estimate that a thymocyte makes contact with approximately 500 dendritic cells during its sojourn in the thymic medulla. Although we do not have experimentally based quantitative estimates for thymocyte:mTEC contacts, the purging of self-reactive T cells in the thymic medulla is a remarkable achievement.

Peripheral T-cell tolerance.

Despite the intricate mechanisms of central tolerance induction in the thymus, approximately one-third of the autoreactive clones are not deleted. Thus, a large number of low-avidity self-reactive T cells escape into the periphery. For example, T cells that recognize insulin or myelin basic protein can be isolated from people without diabetes or multiple sclerosis. Despite their low avidity for self antigens, these cells are potentially dangerous and could cause autoimmune tissue destruction.

Immunological ignorance is maintained as long as autoreactive T lymphocytes do not enter the tissue in which the autoantigen that they recognize is expressed. The autoreactive naive T cells are not tolerized and can be activated upon recognizing their cognate antigen.

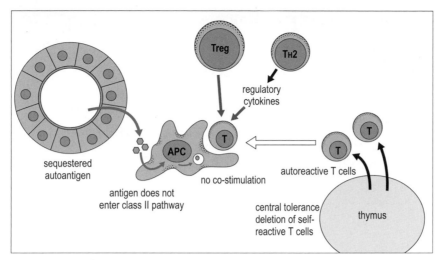

Fig. 11.5 Mechanisms of peripheral T-cell tolerance Many autoreactive T cells escape central tolerance induction in the thymus, but their activity is controlled by other mechanisms. Some antigens are normally sequestered in particular organs and are not released to enter the lymphatic system unless damage to the tissue occurs. Only antigens that are processed and presented by antigen-presenting cells can activate autoreactive T cells, and this also requires co-stimulatory signals. Even if an autoantigen is presented to an autoreactive cell, its activation can still be controlled by Tregs and cytokines released by other T-cell populations. *APC*, Antigen-presenting cell.

Even if these autoreactive T cells encounter their antigen, auto-immune diseases are the exception and it follows that other peripheral tolerance mechanisms must exist to prevent these T cells from causing harm (Fig 11.5).

Some self antigens are sequestered in immunologically privileged tissues.
One explanation for lack of activation of auto-reactive cells is the **sequestration** of potentially harmful T cells from the tissues in which their target self antigens are expressed. Sequestration can be achieved when antigens are physically separated from T cells (e.g. by the blood–brain barrier, see Chapter 13). The blood–brain barrier can be surmounted by activated lymphocytes, however, and many organs do not possess a physical barrier to prevent lymphocytes entering from the blood stream. Instead, lymphocyte migration is controlled by chemokines, selectins and their receptors.

Lymphocyte activation enhances their migration into non-lymphoid tissues.
Upon activation in secondary lymphatic organs, naive T cells acquire effector functions and express a different set of chemokine receptors and adhesion molecules which then enables them to enter other organs, particularly in the context of inflammation. Naive T cells lacking those surface molecules, however, are excluded from non-lymphoid tissues so that, under normal conditions, potentially autoreactive T cells will ignore their antigens, thereby maintaining self tolerance. Should such cells be activated accidentally they would pose a permanent threat to the organism. Dendritic cells (DCs) that are activated during infection are likely to present not only microbial but also self antigens. The T cells activated in this process would gain the capacity to enter tissues and thus would have lost their ignorance. Consequently, additional mechanisms must ensure the maintenance of immunological self tolerance.

The amount of released self antigen critically affects sensitization.
How does the immune system decide which autoreactive T cells may survive and which need to be deleted? Antigen dose and TCR avidity play a major role (Fig. 11.6). One key experiment used two different strains of mice that expressed ovalbumin (OVA) specifically in the pancreas. One strain expressed OVA at low levels and the other expressed it at high levels. Only in the high-expressing strain was OVA presented to T cells in the draining lymph nodes, resulting in the deletion of adoptively transferred OVA-specific Tc cells. In the low-expressing cells, the OVA-specific T cells remained ignorant. Further in vitro assays revealed that the low-level OVA expression was still sufficient to allow recognition and killing of the OVA-expressing pancreatic β cells by the OVA-specific CTL. Therefore, tissue restricted self antigens need to be expressed at sufficiently high levels to be presented in the draining lymph nodes. These experiments also clearly showed that self-reactive T cells are potentially dangerous even if they are temporarily ignorant. In fact, destruction of pancreatic islet cells can induce the release of sufficient amounts of self antigen to activate OVA-specific CTL in the OVA-low expressing mice.

Antigen-presenting cells reinforce self tolerance.

Dendritic cells can present antigen in a tolerogenic manner.
Experiments designed to analyse CD4 and CD8 T-cell responses to antigens that were expressed in a tissue-restricted manner (e.g. exclusively in the pancreas or the skin) revealed that self antigen-specific T cells accumulated in the draining lymph nodes as a result of reaction with self antigen transported by DCs. Depending on the information received from the DC in addition to peptide presentation, the TH cells may become:
- activated;
- anergic;

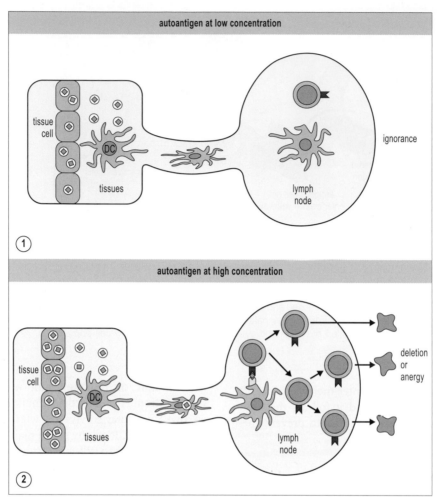

Fig. 11.6 Abundant self antigens induce peripheral deletion (**1**) Immunological ignorance predominantly works if the self antigen is present at relatively low concentrations. The antigen remains in the tissue in which it is expressed and is not transported into the draining lymph node under steady-state conditions. (**2**) If tissue antigens are present at high concentrations, they will be brought to draining lymph nodes by dendritic cells *(DCs)* even under non-inflammatory conditions. Under these conditions, the DCs are not immunogenic but tolerogenic and induce apoptosis or anergy in T cells that recognize the self antigen.

- converted into a regulatory T cell; or
- undergo apoptosis.

The critical importance of DCs for the maintenance of tolerance has also been shown in experiments in which conditional DC depletion in mature mice resulted in spontaneous autoimmunity.

Functional maturation of DCs, characterized by strong expression of MHC and co-stimulatory molecules, is induced by microbial or self-derived stimuli, which are sometimes called danger signals (Fig. 11.7). In the absence of such stimuli, immature DCs express MHC and co-stimulatory molecules (CD80/86) at low levels and antigen presentation induces T-cell anergy or deletion depending upon the expression of high or low levels of self antigen, respectively. Several molecules have already been identified that are necessary for tolerogenic DC:T cell interactions. These include surface molecules such as E-cadherin, PDL-1L, CD103, CD152 (CTLA-4) and ICOS-L (CD275) and cytokines, including IL-10 and TGFβ.

Tolerogenic DCs mature under steady-state conditions. DC maturation under steady-state conditions can be triggered by disrupting DC–DC adhesion, which is mediated by E-cadherin. Similar to DC maturation induced by microbial products, the disruption of DC–DC contacts induces upregulation of MHC class II, co-stimulatory molecules and chemokine receptors and this process requires the activation of β-catenin. In contrast to DCs that have matured upon sensing microbial products, the DCs that have matured under steady-state conditions do not produce pro-inflammatory cytokines. Consequently, when they present antigen to naive TH cells these DCs induce regulatory T cells rather than effector T cells.

REGULATORY T CELLS

Regulatory T cells (Treg) specialize in preventing and suppressing immune responses and are central for the prevention of autoimmune diseases. Usually, Tregs comprise approximately 10% of all CD4+ T cells. An inborn lack of Treg cells is the cause of severe autoimmune inflammation in patients suffering from the IPEX (immunodysregulation, polyendocrinopathy, enteropathy, X-linked) syndrome. Treg cells do not only limit

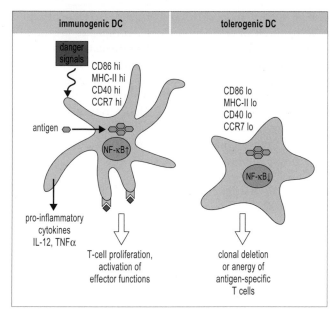

Fig. 11.7 Critical role of antigen-presenting cells (APCs) for T-cell tolerance APCs are critical for the decision between T-cell activation or tolerance. Upon antigen uptake, the APCs become activated if they sense exogenous or endogenous danger signals. Such classically activated APCs present antigen in an immunogenic manner to T lymphocytes and induce T-cell proliferation and effector functions. Such immunogenic dendritic cells (DCs), which have matured under inflammatory conditions (i.e. they have received signals via their TLRs or other pattern recognition receptors), upregulate co-stimulatory molecules (e.g. CD86, CD40), major histocompatibility cells class II (MHC-II) molecules and CCR7. These changes increase their capacity to present antigen to T cells in an immunogenic manner. They also activate NF-κB and express pro-inflammatory cytokines (e.g. IL-12), which instruct T-cell effector functions. If, in contrast, the APCs do not receive danger signals, they can still undergo homeostatic maturation. Such APCs present antigen in a non-immunogenic manner to T cells and induce clonal deletion or anergy. Tolerogenic DCs, which are either immature or have matured under steady-state conditions, express only low amounts of co-stimulatory and MHC-II molecules and do not secrete pro-inflammatory cytokines.

autoimmune responses, they also dampen responses against microbial and viral antigens, allergens, tumours and allografts and protect fetuses (semi-allografts) during pregnancy.

Regulatory T cells suppress immune responses. Neonatal thymectomy in mice results in an autoimmune syndrome that affects a number of different organs, including the thyroid, stomach, ovaries and testes. Adoptive transfer of $CD4^+$ T cells or $CD4^+CD8^+$ thymocytes from non-thymectomized syngeneic mice prevents autoimmune disease manifestations. These findings have three important implications:

- normal mice harbour self-reactive cells, which can cause autoimmune damage;
- normal mice produce $CD4^+$ T cells in the thymus, which can suppress the autoreactive cells;
- depletion of these suppressive cells can cause autoimmune disease.

It was, therefore, important to identify the $CD4^+$ subset capable of suppressing autoimmune disease. Subsequent experiments revealed that adoptive transfer of $CD4^+$ cells induced a range of autoimmune diseases in immunodeficient hosts

provided that the transferred $CD4^+$ cells had been purged of cells that co-express CD25 (the IL-2 receptor alpha chain). Cotransfer of $CD4^+CD25^+$ cells prevented autoimmunity. Accordingly, these $CD4^+CD25^+$ cells were named **regulatory T cells** (Treg). Further experiments demonstrated that the majority of these cells constitute a distinct, thymus-derived lineage of $CD4^+$ T cells.

Since the seminal report of these findings, numerous reports have confirmed that Tregs suppress immune responses against both self and non-self antigens in vivo and in vitro. When cultured in vitro Tregs do not proliferate and do not produce effector cytokines such as IL-2, TNFα, IFNγ or IL-4 upon stimulation via their TCR. This anergic state is not overcome by co-stimulatory signals.

When co-cultured with $CD25^-$ effector cells in vitro, Tregs can suppress the proliferation of the effector cells. To be able to suppress, Tregs need to be stimulated via their TCR.

In addition to Treg cells, various other cell types can help to suppress immune responses by distinct effector mechanisms. Moreover, not all $CD4^+CD25^+$ T cells are Tregs. Therefore, Tregs cannot be discriminated from activated TH effector cells based on the expression of CD25 alone.

The transcription factor FoxP3 controls Treg development. Regulatory T cells express the transcription factor forkhead box P3 (FoxP3), a member of the forkhead/winged-helix family of transcription factors. A lethal X-linked mutation occurs in the FoxP3 gene in scurfy mice, which results in hyperactivation of $CD4^+$ T cells, overproduction of numerous cytokines and extensive lymphocyte infiltration of multiple organs. The same manifestations occur in FoxP3-null mice. Both scurfy mice and FoxP3-null mice are deficient in $CD4^+CD25^+$ regulatory T cells. In normal mice, only $CD4^+CD25^+$ peripheral T cells and $CD4^+CD25^+$ thymocytes express FoxP3. Forced expression of FoxP3 can convert $CD4^+CD25^-$ T cells into $CD4^+CD25^+$ T cells that can suppress the activation of other T cells. Thus, FoxP3 is essential for Treg differentiation and maintenance and is important for Treg effector functions. Consequently, the co-expression of CD4, CD25 and FoxP3 is widely used to identify murine Treg cells.

Defects in FoxP3 result in multi-system autoimmune diseases. Since the discovery of FoxP3, a multitude of studies in animal models of autoimmunity have proved that a deficiency in $CD4^+CD25^+FoxP3^+$ Tregs can accelerate the development or increase the severity of autoimmune disease. Conversely, in some models, disease could be prevented or even reversed through adoptive transfer of Tregs.

Similarly, Tregs isolated from human peripheral blood can suppress T-cell proliferation and cytokine production in vitro. The human counterpart of the scurfy mutation, the IPEX (immune dysregulation, polyendocrinopathy, enteropathy, X-linked) syndrome, has similar clinical manifestations to those observed in scurfy mice. IPEX patients suffer from autoimmune diseases, most prominently autoimmune diabetes (type 1 diabetes, T1D), thyroiditis, haemolytic anaemia, inflammatory bowel disease and allergic manifestations such as eczema. More than

90% of IPEX patients die from autoimmune diabetes at an early age. This demonstrates that (almost) all individuals harbour potentially diabetogenic autoreactive T cells in their peripheral repertoire. Usually, in healthy people, these autoreactive T cells are controlled by Tregs.

In contrast to murine T cells, human T cells express FoxP3 readily and transiently upon TCR signalling. Most of these cells do not possess immunosuppressive capacities. Thus, FoxP3 expression alone is not a reliable marker for human Treg cells.

Natural Treg cells differentiate in the thymus. During thymic development, FoxP3 expression starts in CD4$^+$CD8$^+$ double-positive thymocytes. Approximately 5% of the more mature CD4$^+$CD8$^-$ single-positive thymocytes express FoxP3. These Treg cells, which acquire their phenotype and functional capacities in the thymus and are released into the periphery as CD4$^+$CD25$^+$FoxP3$^+$ T cells, are called thymic Tregs (**tTreg**) or natural Treg cells (**nTregs**) (Fig. 11.8).

The number of FoxP3$^+$ thymocytes is drastically reduced in mice that lack MHC class I or II expression. Thus, the nTregs

must be subject to positive and negative selection based on the recognition of self-peptide/MHC complexes presented by thymic APCs. The same cell types that mediate negative selection are also relevant for Treg generation. How, then, are nTregs selected during thymic development? TCR repertoire analyses do not support the notion that the Treg repertoire was skewed towards self-reactivity. Current evidence rather suggests that high-affinity interactions of the TCR with self-peptide/MHC complexes in the thymus favour the recruitment of thymocytes into the Treg lineage.

Selection of nTregs is partly related to the affinity for antigen/MHC. Double transgenic mice that express both a transgene-encoded antigen and a transgene-encoded TCR that recognizes that antigen are instructive. In such mice, a large percentage of transgenic T cells will develop into nTregs if either:
- the antigen is expressed at high levels in the thymus; or
- the TCR possesses a high affinity for the transgenic antigen.

In contrast, if the TCR's affinity for the transgenic peptide is low or if the transgenic peptide is present in low concentration

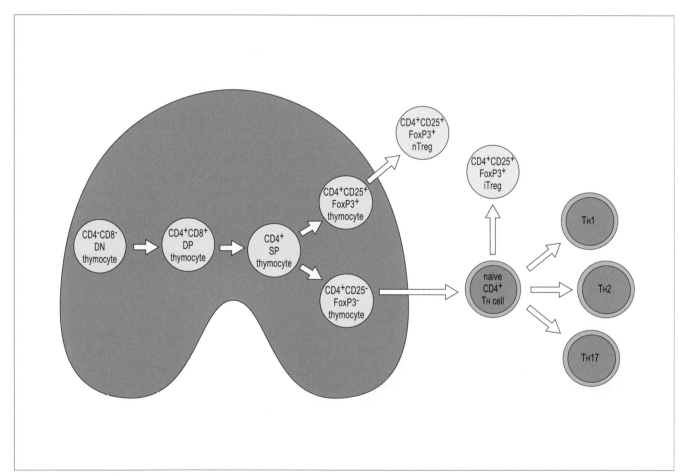

Fig. 11.8 Natural and induced Tregs In mice, CD4$^-$CD8$^-$ double-negative *(DN)* T-cell precursors enter the thymus and undergo several selection processes. At the CD4 single-positive stage, a population of thymocytes starts expressing FoxP3 and CD25. These cells leave the thymus as natural regulatory T cells (Tregs), which comprise approximately 5%–10% of all peripheral CD4$^+$ T cells. The CD4$^+$FoxP3$^-$CD25$^-$ thymocytes emigrate from the thymus as naive effector T$_H$ cells. Upon activation by APCs, they can assume different effector functions, broadly characterized as T$_H$1, T$_H$2 or T$_H$17 cells. Some of the naive CD4$^+$FoxP3$^-$CD25$^-$ T$_H$ cells can also develop into CD4$^+$FoxP3$^+$CD25$^+$ induced Treg cells. These iTregs exert similar functions to the nTregs; however, their FoxP3 expression is less stable. *DP*, Double-positive

in the thymus, few T cells bearing the transgene-encoded TCR will develop into nTregs (see Fig. 11.3). It is currently a matter of debate whether these findings reflect positive selection of T cells with strongly self-reactive TCRs to the Treg lineage or the resistance of FoxP3$^+$ thymocytes to negative selection.

Repertoire analyses have revealed considerable overlap between the TCR repertoires of FoxP3$^+$ Treg cells and conventional FoxP3$^-$ T cells. Therefore, the TCR's affinity for self-peptide/MHC is not the only determinant for Treg selection in the thymus. Co-stimulatory signals from the antigen-presenting cells are critically important as demonstrated by the fact that mice deficient in co-stimulatory ligands or receptors such as CD28, CD80, CD86, CD40 or LFA-1 (CD11a/CD18) have massively reduced numbers of Tregs.

IL-2 is required for the development of Tregs. The Treg marker CD25 is the IL-2R α chain and is critically important for the development and maintenance of Treg; FoxP3 expression is supported by IL-2. Mice that lack IL-2, CD25, CD122 (the IL-2R β chain) or CD132 (the γc chain which is shared by the IL-2R, IL-4R, IL-7R, IL-9R, IL-21R and IL-15R) suffer from lymphocytic infiltration of internal organs and autoimmune disease manifestations such as haemolytic anaemia. These mice also display a profound reduction of FoxP3$^+$ Tregs. Similarly, CD25 deficiency in humans is clinically indistinguishable from the IPEX syndrome. Moreover, administration of a neutralizing antibody against IL-2 to neonatal mice results in a profound reduction of FoxP3$^+$ Tregs and autoimmune disease manifestations. Therefore, IL-2 is essential for the development and maintenance of Treg cells.

iTreg cells differentiate in the periphery. In addition to the natural Tregs, which differentiate in the thymus, mature T cells outside the thymus can also acquire Treg phenotype and function. These are called induced Treg cells (**iTregs**) (see Fig. 11.8). FoxP3 expression can be induced in naive CD4$^+$ cells in vitro by antigen recognition in the presence of TGFβ. There is a close developmental relationship between iTregs and TH17 cells. Antigen recognition in the presence of TGFβ induces FoxP3 expression if IL-6 is not present. In contrast, antigen recognition in the presence of TGFβ and IL-6 prevents FoxP3 expression, induces expression of the retinoic acid receptor (RAR)-related orphan nuclear receptor RORγt expression and, therefore, TH17 differentiation. The transcription factor IRF4 is necessary for the downregulation of TGFβ-induced FoxP3 expression in response to IL-6 (Fig. 11.9).

Chronic antigen stimulation, particularly with suboptimal doses, in vivo, also induces FoxP3 expression and iTreg differentiation.

The phenotype of Treg cells. Based on studies in mice, distinct populations of Tregs are found in different tissues, having phenotypes and functions related to their location. Tissue Tregs may include both thymic-derived (nTreg) and peripherally induced (iTreg) populations. There is some debate as to the extent that phenotype is established before the Tregs enter

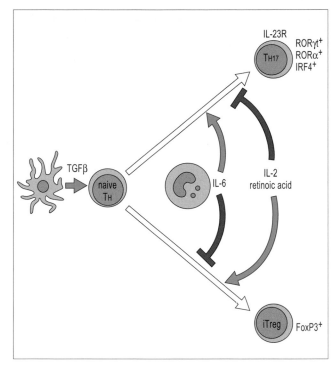

Fig. 11.9 Close lineage relationship between TH17 and induced Tregs T-cell differentiation depends largely on instructing cytokines provided by the antigen-presenting cell upon T-cell activation. TGFβ is an important instructive signal for the development of both TH17 and iTregs. If, in response to IL-6, the transcription factor IRF4 suppresses FoxP3 expression while increasing RORγt expression, development of TH17 rather than iTreg cells ensues. In contrast, IL-2 or retinoic acid favours the development of iTreg and inhibits TH17 differentiation. The major transcription factors for the functional differentiation of TH17 and iTreg are shown.

the tissue, versus induction by local signals. In this sense local differentiation of Tregs may be analogous to the tissue-specific development of mononuclear phagocyte populations. It is not therefore possible to identify a single phenotype for Tregs. The fact that human Tregs differ from those in mice and are less well characterized complicates the issue.

Treg effector functions. Treg effector functions can be analysed in vivo either by depletion or transfer of Treg cells or in vitro. When cultured in vitro, Tregs proliferate poorly upon stimulation via their TCR unless IL-2 is also added to the culture. Nevertheless, Treg proliferation can be demonstrated in vivo. Tregs need stimulation via their TCR to exert their immunosuppressive functions. Once activated, Treg cells suppress immune responses independent of their own antigen specificity. This antigen non-specific immunosuppression has been called **bystander suppression**. Another characteristic of Treg action has long been known as **infectious tolerance**. The concept of infectious tolerance is based on in vivo transfer studies in which the adoptive transfer of Tregs induced the differentiation or selective outgrowth of Tregs in the host. These endogenous Tregs would maintain tolerance even after the transferred Tregs were no longer detectable in the host.

Tregs can act on a number of different target cells, including effector T cells and DCs, but also on numerous other cell types, including B cells, macrophages, NK cells, NKT cells, mast cells,

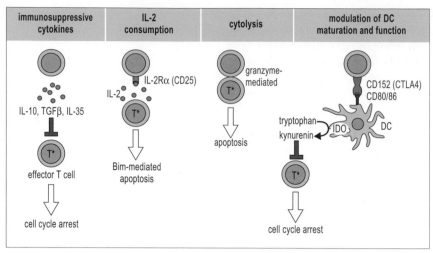

Fig. 11.10 Treg effector mechanisms Treg cells use different mechanisms to control effector T cells (T*). These include the secretion of immunosuppressive cytokines, the consumption of IL-2, leading to a lack of IL-2 to sustain proliferation and survival of effector T cells leading to Bim-mediated apoptosis, cytolysis of effector T cells and the modulation of dendritic cell (DC) maturation and function. Treg cells can induce DCs to express indoleamine 2,3-dioxygenase (IDO), which depletes tryptophan resulting in the suppression of effector T-cell responses. This interaction also depends on the interaction between CD152 and CD80/86. (Adapted from Shevach EM. Immunity 2009;30:636 and Vignali DAA et al. Nat Rev Immunol 2008;8:523.)

osteoblasts and osteoclasts. They produce or consume cytokines to modulate their target cells and Tregs are also capable of lysing target cells (Fig. 11.10).

Tregs secrete immunosuppressive cytokines. One possible mechanism of immunosuppression by Tregs is the secretion of immunosuppressive cytokines (see Fig. 11.10). Indeed, three inhibitory cytokines, IL-10, TGFβ and IL-35, are produced by Tregs and are important for Treg development or effector function. However, most in vitro studies found IL-10 or TGFβ produced by Tregs to be non-essential for Treg-mediated suppression.

IL-10 is a potent suppressor of macrophage and T-cell effector functions and critically important to dampen immune responses. Many cell types, including TH2, TH17 and some tissue cells, normally produce IL-10. Therefore, the production of IL-10 by Tregs is not critically required in many experimental settings. Mice that lack IL-10 expression specifically in Tregs do not develop autoimmune disease manifestations spontaneously. Nevertheless, experimentally induced airway hypersensitivity is more severe in these mice than in their wild-type littermates and Treg-produced IL-10 seems to be most critical for the control of mucosal immune responses to environmental stimuli. The importance of Treg-produced IL-10 seems to depend on the triggers and localization of the immune response.

TGFβ has immunosuppressive functions and is critically required for the differentiation of precursors into Treg cells in vivo and in vitro. TGFβ is also necessary to maintain FoxP3 expression of nTreg cells and thus for Treg-cell homeostasis. In contrast, the relevance of Treg-cell-produced TGFβ as a mediator of Treg effector function in vivo remains unproven.

IL-35 is a heterodimeric member of the IL-12 family, which is selectively expressed by a subpopulation of Tregs and required for their optimal effector function. Interestingly, this subpopulation does not overlap with the IL-10-producing Tregs.

Tregs can deplete IL-2. One important effect of Tregs on responder T cells is to inhibit the induction of mRNA for cytokines, including IL-2: FoxP3 binds to the promoter of the IL-2 gene. Importantly, the addition of exogenous IL-2 does not rescue IL-2 mRNA production in the responder cells.

The consumption of IL-2 by Tregs can induce IL-2-deprivation-mediated apoptosis of effector T cells. However, Tregs can block autoimmune disease even in IL-2-deficient mice and the importance of IL-2 consumption for Treg effector function is still a matter of debate.

Matters are complicated by the fact that IL-2 is important for the apoptosis of antigen-activated T cells. Hence, the lack of IL-2 or IL-2 signalling does not only result in Treg deficiency but also obliterates peripheral clonal deletion of receptor-activated T cells. Therefore, the clinical manifestations of the IL-2 deficiency syndrome cannot be attributed completely to the loss of Tregs.

Cytolysis. Tregs are cytotoxic to different cell types, including DCs, CD8⁺ T, NK and B cells. In different experimental systems, Treg cytotoxicity depended on granzyme B-, perforin- or Fas-FasL-dependent pathways. Treg-mediated DC death in lymph nodes has been demonstrated in vivo and limits the onset of CD8⁺ T-cell responses.

Modulation of DC maturation and function. Some of the in vitro experiments to assess the suppressive function of Tregs are performed by stimulating the responder T cells with plate-bound antibodies in the absence of antigen-presenting cells. Data from such experiments indicate that Tregs can act directly on responder T cells. In vivo, however, the modulation of DC/T interactions is also an important mechanism of Treg-mediated immunosuppression. Depletion of Treg cells in vivo results in increased DC maturation and elevated numbers of DC. Direct

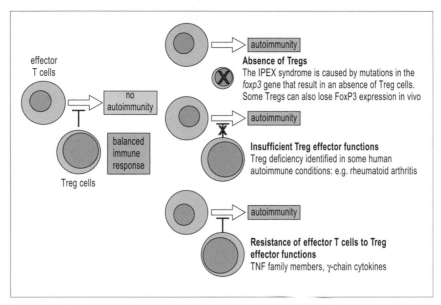

Fig. 11.11 Loss of Treg effector functions In the balanced steady state, Tregs prevent overshooting or unwanted immune responses. Mutations in the FoxP3 gene can result in a complete lack of Treg cells and lethal autoimmune disease. FoxP3 expression is unstable in iTregs and these cells can convert into effector T cells. Impaired Treg function could also contribute to the pathogenesis of autoimmune diseases. Effector T cells can become resistant to Treg-mediated suppression in response to TNF family and other activating cytokines. (Adapted from Buckner JH. Nat Rev Immunol 2010;10:849.)

interactions between Treg cells and DCs have also been observed by intravital microscopy. During these interactions, Treg cells can exert different effects on DC.

Direct cytolysis. In vivo studies have shown that Treg cells can induce the death of antigen-presenting DCs in lymph nodes in a perforin-dependent manner. This depletion of DCs limited the onset of CD8$^+$ T-cell responses.

Treg cells can also modulate maturation and function of DCs and can probably also modulate the function of mononuclear phagocytes. In vitro, Treg cells can downregulate the expression of co-stimulatory molecules, including CD80 and CD86, by DC. By averting co-stimulatory interactions between DC and effector T cells, the Treg cells can efficiently inhibit T-cell priming. CD152 (CTLA-4), which is expressed constitutively by Treg cells, plays an important role in reducing the DC's co-stimulatory capacity.

The effects of Treg cells on DC are severely reduced when blocking antibodies against CD152 are added or CD152-deficient Treg cells are used in these assays. Moreover, mice that lack CD152 expression selectively in Treg cells spontaneously develop systemic autoimmune disease. This latter finding clearly illustrates that CD152 is pivotal for Treg effector functions.

Clearly there is not one dominant molecular or cellular interaction by which Tregs exert their effector functions. Instead, Treg cells use different effector functions to prevent or suppress different innate or adaptive immune responses triggered by different stimuli at different anatomical locations. With few exceptions, the dramatic phenotype seen in scurfy mice or IPEX patients who lack FoxP3 does not develop when just one of the pathways mentioned in this section is absent. One such exception is the lack of CD152, which causes widespread

lymphocytic infiltration of multiple organs. Moreover, IL-10 deficiency and the IL-2 deficiency syndrome, which cause a similar dramatic phenotype, are not solely attributable to disturbed Treg function.

Can loss of Treg function explain autoimmune disease?
Several pathological mechanisms have been proposed to explain why autoimmunity occurs despite the presence of Tregs. Could Tregs, despite being present in normal or even enhanced numbers, have lost (some of) their effector functions? There is some evidence in mice that Tregs can lose their function or that effector T cells become resistant to their action.

However, except for the IPEX syndrome (Fig. 11.11), in which FoxP3$^+$ Tregs are completely absent, there is currently no convincing evidence that reduced numbers of Tregs would cause autoimmune disease. In contrast, Tregs are frequently found in increased numbers at the site of autoimmune lesions.

T-CELL ANERGY

T cells that cannot be completely activated upon recognition of their cognate antigen are called anergic. The phenomenon of **T-cell clonal anergy** was discovered in CD4$^+$ TH1 clones that failed to produce IL-2 and proliferate when stimulated in vitro with antigen in the absence of co-stimulatory signals. In such clones, the anergic state may be maintained for several weeks. Characteristically, full effector functions can be rescued in anergic T-cell clones by in vitro exposure to IL-2.

T cells with diminished proliferation and cytokine production can also be isolated ex vivo: e.g. after non-immunogenic peptide application, exposure to superantigens or prolonged exposure to antigen. This phenomenon is sometimes called

adaptive tolerance. T-cell clonal anergy induced in vitro differs from T-cell anergy, or adoptive tolerance, in vivo. Nevertheless, some of the major molecular pathways leading to anergy seem to be similar in vitro and in vivo. Mice deficient for molecules known to be important for anergy induction in vitro are resistant towards the induction of T-cell anergy in vivo.

One plausible explanation for the functional and molecular differences between clonal T-cell anergy in vitro and in vivo is that several different pathways can induce and enforce T-cell clonal anergy.

The induction of anergy is an active process. T cells in which protein synthesis is pharmacologically blocked cannot be rendered anergic. How, then, do T cells integrate signals received via the TCR, co-stimulatory receptors and cytokine receptors to respond with activation, differentiation or anergy? Anergy induction can be described as a series of molecular switches, all of which share three characteristics:

- they are present in naive T cells;
- they result in the suppression of IL-2 gene expression;
- their actions are antagonized by signals emanating from CD28 or the IL-2R.

The transcription factor NF-AT1 fulfils these criteria and is indeed central for anergy induction.

NF-AT1 is activated after T cells are stimulated via their TCR. However, full T-cell activation requires co-stimulation and activation of AP-1, which forms a transcription factor complex with NF-AT1 (see Fig. 7.w1). Cells lacking the dual activation signal become anergic.

In vitro, T-cell anergy can be overcome by the addition of exogenous IL-2. The fate of in vivo anergized T cells is less clear. It has been shown that anergic T cells can survive for several weeks in vivo. Currently it is unknown if such cells will ultimately be removed or if they can be reactivated.

T cells can be deleted in the periphery. T cells that have survived thymic selection can still be deleted in the periphery. When TCR transgenic T cells are adoptively transferred into recipient mice that express the antigen recognized by the transgenic TCR, the transferred T cells will undergo apoptosis in the recipient mice. The transferred T cells survive if they lack the pro-apoptotic protein Bim (Bcl2 interacting mediator of cell death) or if they over-express the anti-apoptotic protein Bcl2 (Bim antagonizes Bcl2). Peripheral deletion not only enforces self tolerance, it is also helps maintain lymphocyte homeostasis throughout life. At the height of the immune response against certain viruses, almost half of all CD8[+] T cells in the blood of the infected patients can be specific for one dominant virus-derived peptide. The majority of these cells must be removed once the virus has been cleared.

Cytokine withdrawal can induce apoptosis. One mechanism of peripheral deletion results from the lack of growth factors, particularly IL-2, for which all activated T cells compete. Cytokine withdrawal triggers an intrinsic pathway of apoptosis involving activation of the Bim factor. Regulatory T cells can accelerate or induce cytokine-withdrawal-induced apoptosis of effector T cells by consuming IL-2.

IL-2 is not only critically important for the proliferation and differentiation of naive T cells. When effector T cells are re-stimulated with large amounts of antigen, the addition of IL-2 induces apoptosis in the cycling T cells. This form of peripheral deletion has been called **activation-induced cell death** (AICD) or **re-stimulation-induced cell death** (RICD). Mice deficient in IL-2 or IL-2 signalling develop an autoimmune syndrome characterized by an abundance of activated T lymphocytes, multiple autoantibodies and lymphocytic infiltration of several organs. RICD is one explanation for the observation that the administration of high doses of antigen can induce tolerance. This phenomenon has been called **high-dose tolerance**.

Thus, IL-2 has contradictory effects at different phases of the T-cell response. During priming, IL-2 is critically required to support clonal expansion and differentiation and a lack of IL-2 at that stage will induce apoptosis. When already activated, an effector T cell simultaneously encountering high concentrations of antigen and IL-2 will undergo apoptosis. Therefore, IL-2 both initiates and terminates T-cell responses.

T cells can be killed by ligation of Fas. The death of T cells is also mediated by the pathway involving Fas (CD95) and its ligand (FasL or CD95L); engagement of the Fas receptor induces apoptosis. Since T cells express both Fas and its ligand on activation, the interaction between the two molecules can induce apoptosis. The importance of this mechanism for the maintenance of self tolerance is illustrated by the fact that patients with defective Fas have a severe autoimmune lymphoproliferative disease. A similar phenotype including the accumulation of chronically activated T lymphocytes and the development of autoimmunity is caused by a Fas mutation in lpr mice and by a FasL mutation in gld mice.

Some tissues, such as the anterior chamber of the eye, the CNS and the testes, normally express Fas ligand. Consequently, when CD95[+] effector T cells enter these tissues, they undergo apoptosis and cannot damage the tissue.

B-CELL TOLERANCE

B cells that produce antibodies that recognize self antigens (autoantibodies) can potentially cause autoimmune disease (see Chapter 20). The generation of B-cell receptors by random combinations of V, D and J gene segments (see Figs. 9.3 and 9.4) can produce autoreactive receptors. Indeed, a large percentage of immature B cells are autoreactive, creating a demand for immunological pathways that ensures tolerance induction and maintenance in B cells. How B-cell tolerance is achieved and maintained differs in several important ways from the immunological pathways to T-cell tolerance:

- First, B cells mature in the bone marrow and in mammals there is no B-cell equivalent of thymic repertoire selection in T cells.
- Second, mature B cells change their receptors by random mutation in a process called somatic hypermutation

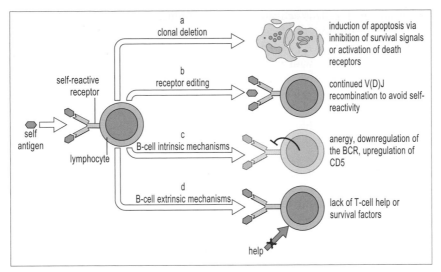

Fig. 11.12 B-cell tolerance mechanisms Autoreactive B cells can be controlled by clonal deletion *(a)*, receptor editing *(b)*, B-cell intrinsic mechanisms such as the induction of anergy *(c)* and the B-cell extrinsic mechanisms such as their dependence on T-cell help and growth factors *(d)*. (Adapted from Goodnow CC et al. Nature 2005;435:590.)

(see Fig. 9.17). While this process generates antibodies with increased affinity for harmful antigens, these mutations could also generate antibodies with high affinity for self antigens.

• Third, the production of high affinity, class-switched antibodies depends on T-cell help.

Several mechanisms establish B-cell tolerance to autoantigens, including clonal deletion, receptor editing, the induction of anergy and the B cells' dependence on T-cell help (Fig. 11.12).

B cells undergo negative selection in the bone marrow.

Clonal deletion of B lymphocytes was first directly demonstrated in mice that expressed a transgenic B-cell receptor (BCR) specific for a foreign antigen (hen egg lysozyme, HEL). These mice were bred with another strain of transgenic mice that expressed HEL. The F1 mice expressed both HEL and BCRs that recognized HEL. The HEL-specific B cells were deleted (negatively selected) in the bone marrow of the F1 mice. When HEL-specific mature B cells from mice that did not express the HEL transgene were adoptively transferred into mice that expressed HEL, these B cells were also deleted in the recipient mice. Apoptosis of mature germinal centre B cells occurs rapidly, within 4–8 hours of encountering the self antigen. When the BCR transgenic mice were also Bim-deficient, they survived in the recipient mice. Similar to T cells, the pro-apoptotic factor Bim is important for BCR-induced apoptosis. This is further illustrated by the fact that Bim-deficient mice spontaneously produce autoantibodies against DNA.

Receptor editing allows potentially self-reactive B cells to avoid negative selection.

Death by apoptosis is not the only possible outcome for immature B cells in the bone marrow when the strength of signals received through the BCR exceeds a certain threshold. Internalization of the BCR is an important early step in the BCR-induced apoptosis programme. This has a number of consequences relevant for BCR-induced apoptosis, including a reduced expression of receptors for the cytokine B-cell-activating factor (BAFF), which is necessary to sustain B-cell survival. In contrast, expression of the genes that encode the key enzymes for V(D)J recombination, RAG1 and RAG2, continues. This offers B cells the chance to rearrange their V_H or V_L regions to replace the autoreactive one. This process is called **BCR editing**. Approximately 2 days remain for the B cell to rearrange a less autoreactive receptor. If it fails to do so, it will undergo apoptosis, either in the bone marrow or upon arrival in the spleen. Single-cell PCR analyses reveal secondary rearrangements in roughly two-thirds of the immature B cells in the bone marrow. As the frequency of cells with secondary rearrangements is only about 50% of all B cells in the spleen, receptor editing does not always result in a useful, non-autoreactive BCR.

B-cell anergy can be induced by self antigens.

B cells can also become anergic upon recognizing a tolerizing self antigen. Anergic B cells lack the capacity to proliferate and to produce antibodies in response to BCR signalling. In anergic B cells, signalling via the BCR is uncoupled from NF-κB, thus preventing B-cell proliferation. At the same time, BCR signalling still prevents apoptosis. Similar to other immature and naive B cells, anergic B cells have a very limited life span if they do not receive appropriate signals. The anergic state can be reversed if the B cell receives signalling via the BCR simultaneously with synergistic signals from another receptor. Such simultaneous signalling is likely to occur when the B cell encounters microbial rather than self antigens. One example is signalling both via the BCR and TLRs. This would typically be the case when a B cell encounters a pathogen, e.g. Gram-negative bacteria possessing LPS, which triggers signalling via TLR4.

Another rescue pathway for anergic B cells is activation of phosphatidylinositol 3-kinase (PI3 kinase). Again, this would typically occur when the B cell encounters microbial antigens tagged with C3d, which promotes interaction with the B-cell coreceptor (see Fig. 9.7). The dual signalling results in the activation of PI-3 kinase and rescues the B cell from the anergic state.

The pool of autoreactive B cells is considerably reduced by the processes described above. Nevertheless, it has been estimated that up to 10% of peripheral B cells are potentially autoreactive.

Somatic hypermutation can generate autoreactive B cells.

Generation of the secondary antibody response occurs in germinal centres by interaction of B cells and T cells, in the presence of follicular dendritic cells. The process involves somatic hypermutation of the recombined antibody genes with the potential to generate autoreactive B cells. It is possible that some of the autoreactive germinal centre B cells enter from the initial pool of autoreactive B cells. However, most of them appear to arise by somatic hypermutation in the germinal centre and the question arises how these cells are controlled. There is no evidence for anergic B cells in germinal centres and receptor editing is unlikely to occur since the required RAG genes are not activated. There is limited evidence for cytotoxic killing of autoreactive B cells in germinal centres, but the most likely explanation for failure of autoreactive cells to develop is the lack of T-cell help, which is required for survival at this stage of B-cell differentiation.

B-cell tolerance because of lack of T-cell help.

Perhaps the main mechanism to ensure B-cell tolerance is the B cell's dependence on T-cell help for high-affinity isotype switched antibody production. BCR signalling results in changes in gene expression that facilitate antigen presentation to T cells:

- Enhanced CCR7 expression enables the B cells to migrate from the follicle towards the T-cell zone in the secondary lymphatic organs.
- Induction of CD86 increases the number of ligands for the co-stimulatory receptor CD28 on T cells.
- Productive antigen presentation to T cells results in the increased secretion of T-cell cytokines such as IL-4 and IL-21 that prevent B-cell apoptosis and support B-cell proliferation.

In vivo imaging studies have shown the formation of conjugates between T and B cells at the border between the follicle and the T-cell zone. Each of these contacts lasts for approximately 10–40 minutes and the B cells spend about 1.5 days in this perifollicular area. A T-cell subset, the T follicular helper (TFH) cells, express the chemokine receptors CXCR5 that enable them to migrate towards the B-cell follicles. It also produces cytokines such as IL-4 and IL-21 that support B-cell differentiation into antibody-secreting cells and it has the co-stimulatory receptor ICOS that enhances interactions with ICOSL$^+$ B cells. Dysregulation of TFH development or function has been associated with autoimmunity. For example, mice with a mutation of the TFH regulatory protein Roquin-1 have massively increased TFH numbers in their germinal centres and develop pathogenic autoantibodies.

The survival of germinal centre (GC) B cells also depends on repeated interactions between CD40 on B cells and its ligand CD154 on T cells. Injection of a blocking mAb against CD154 results in the dissolution of germinal centres within several days. To survive and to differentiate into antibody producing cells, naive B cells need to receive two signals:

- signal one upon antigen binding to the BCR; and
- signal two from TH cells.

Only those B cells that present antigen recognized by a TH cell will receive anti-apoptotic signals from that T cell. Since the T-cell repertoire has been largely purged of self-reactive receptors, a B cell recognizing and presenting a microbial antigen is much more likely to receive T-cell help than a B cell that recognizes a self antigen. Thus, both T-cell and B-cell tolerance must be overcome before high-affinity autoantibodies can be produced.

CRITICAL THINKING: IMMUNOLOGICAL TOLERANCE

See Critical thinking: Explanations, section 11

1. Figure 11.12 depicts four mechanisms to establish B-cell tolerance. Compare these with the mechanisms used to establish T-cell tolerance and explain similarities and differences.

2. The transcriptional regulator AIRE (autoimmune regulator) is considered to be critical for the establishment of self tolerance. Explain the experimental and clinical evidence on which this statement is based.

3. T-cell precursors undergo positive selection processes in the thymus. Explain 'positive selection'. There is no positive selection for B cells. Can you speculate why positive selection is required for T cells but not for B cells?

4. Explain how dendritic cells contribute to peripheral T-cell tolerance.

5. Pathogens with exclusively peripheral tissue tropism (such as papilloma-virus) can evade immune responses. Can you explain which tolerance mechanism is subverted by such pathogens?

6. Mice that express a transgene-encoded TCR, which is specific for a self antigen, usually do not develop autoimmune disease. How could you distinguish in an in vitro assay whether the transgenic T cells were ignorant or anergic?

7. Patients with autoimmune diseases often have increased numbers of regulatory T cells (Tregs) in diseased tissue. Speculate about possible explanations for this seemingly paradoxical finding.

FURTHER READING

Brink R, Giang Phan T. Self-reactive B cells in the germinal center reaction. Ann Revs Immunol 2018;36:339–357.

Germain RN. Special regulatory T-cell review: A rose by any other name: from suppressor T cells to Tregs, approbation to unbridled enthusiasm. Immunology 2008;123:20–27.

Hongo D, Tang X, Dutt S, Nador RG, Strober S. Interactions between NKT cells and Tregs are required for tolerance to combined bone marrow and organ transplants. Blood 2012;119:1581–1589.

Kamradt T, Mitchison NA. Tolerance and autoimmunity. N Engl J Med 2001;344:655–664.

Klein L, Hinterberger M, Wirnsberger G, Kyewski B. Antigen presentation in the thymus for positive selection and central tolerance induction. Nat Rev Immunol 2009;9:833–844.

Meredith M, Zemmour D, Mathis D, Benoist C. Aire controls gene expression in the thymic epithelium with ordered stochasticity. Nat Immunol 2015;16:942–949.

Panduro M, Benoist C, Mathis D. Tissue Tregs. Annu Rev Immunol 2016;34:609–633.

Pulendran B, Tang H, Manicassamy S. Programming dendritic cells to induce T(H)2 and tolerogenic responses. Nat Immunol 2010;11:647–655.

Saibil SD, Deenick EK, Ohashi PS. The sound of silence: modulating anergy in T lymphocytes. Curr Opin Immunol 2007;19:658–664.

Sakaguchi S, Wing K, Onishi Y, Prieto-Martin P, Yamaguchi T. Regulatory T cells: how do they suppress immune responses? Int Immunol 2009;(10):1105–1111.

Shevach EM. Mechanisms of fox3p+ T regulatory cell-mediated suppression. Immunity 2009;30:636–645.

von Boehmer H, Melchers F. Checkpoints in lymphocyte development and autoimmune disease. Nat Immunol 2010;11:14–20.

12

Regulation of the Immune Response

SUMMARY

- **Many factors govern the outcome of any immune response.** These include the antigen itself, its dose, its route of administration and the genetic background of the individual responding to antigenic challenge. A variety of control mechanisms restore the immune system to a resting state when the response to a given antigen is no longer required.
- **Antigen-presenting cells (APCs) and innate immune cells have important effects on the immune response** through their ability to provide co-stimulation to T cells and by the production of cytokines and chemokines that influence both the nature and make-up of the ensuing response. In addition, APC heterogeneity aids in the promotion of different modes of immune response.
- **T cells regulate the immune response.** Cytokine production by T cells influences the type of immune response elicited by antigen. CD4$^+$ T cells can differentiate into several effector phenotypes such as TH1, TH2, TH17 and TfH. These subsets play important roles in the protection of the host against a range of pathogen challenges. CD4$^+$ T cells can also differentiate into regulatory T cells (Treg), which play roles in maintaining tolerance to self antigen and provide a negative feedback mechanism to control inflammation.

These cells work through a variety of mechanisms: via cell-to-cell contact or by the production of anti-inflammatory cytokines.
- **Innate lymphoid cells (ILCs) produce cytokines to regulate the immune response.** ILC1 produce similar cytokines to TH1 cells, ILC2 produce similar cytokines to TH2 cells and ILC3 produce similar cytokines to TH17 cells. They are important for immune responses in tissue and respond more rapidly than T cells.
- **Immunoglobulins can influence the immune response.** They may act positively, through the formation of immune complexes, or negatively, by reducing antigenic challenge or by feedback inhibition of B cells. In addition, IL-10 produced by regulatory B cells can limit inflammation.
- **Metabolic reprogramming regulates T-cell activation.** Upon activation, naive T cells switch metabolism from oxidative phosphorylation to glycolysis, which regulates translation of IFNγ and IL-2.
- **The neuroendocrine system influences immune responses.** Cells from both systems share similar ligands and receptors, which permit cross-interactions between them. Corticosteroids in particular downregulate TH1 responses and macrophage activation.

Ideally, an immune response is mounted quickly to clear away a pathogenic challenge with the minimum of collateral damage and then the system is returned to a resting state. The immune response is therefore subject to a variety of control mechanisms. Additional mechanisms help regulate the levels of immunopathology that are often a necessary side effect of pathogen elimination. An insufficient immune response can result in an individual being overwhelmed by infection or the failure to clear cancerous cells (see Chapter 22). An inappropriate or over-vigorous immune response can lead to high levels of immunopathology or even autoimmunity (see Chapter 20). The balance between these two is therefore critical.

At its most basic, an effective immune response is an outcome of the interplay between antigen and a network of immunologically competent cells. This chapter provides an overview of how immune responses are regulated by:
- antigen dose and route of administration;
- co-stimulation, cytokine milieu and chemokine gradients;
- regulatory T cells and their suppression of unwanted immune responses;
- feedback control through immunoglobulin;
- apoptosis following the resolution of the immune response.

T-CELL AND B-CELL REGULATION BY ANTIGEN

T and B cells are activated by antigen after effective engagement of their antigen-specific receptors (often referred to as signal 1), together with appropriate co-stimulation (signal 2) (see Chapter 7). Repeated antigen exposure is required to maintain their proliferation and during an effective immune response there is a dramatic expansion of antigen-specific T and B cells. At the end of an immune response, reduced antigen exposure results in a reduction of T- and B-cell survival factors, leading to apoptosis of the antigen-specific cells. The majority of antigen-specific cells therefore die at the end of an immune response, leaving a small population of long-lived T and B cells to survive and to give rise to the memory population.

Different antigens elicit different kinds of immune response.
Intracellular organisms such as some bacteria, parasites or viruses induce a cell-mediated immune response. Cell-mediated immune responses are also induced by agents such as silica. In contrast, extracellular organisms and soluble antigens induce a humoral response, with the polysaccharide capsule antigens of bacteria generally inducing IgM responses.

In some situations, antigens (e.g. those of intracellular micro-organisms) may not be cleared effectively, leading to a sustained immune response. Chronic immune responses have several possible pathological consequences and can lead to autoimmunity and hypersensitivity (Chapters 20, 23–26)

Large doses of antigen can induce tolerance. Very large doses of antigen often result in specific T-cell and sometimes B-cell tolerance.

Administration of antigen to neonatal mice often results in tolerance to the antigen. It was once speculated that this might be the result of immaturity of the immune system. However, neonatal mice can develop efficient immune responses (Fig. 12.1) and their non-responsiveness may in some cases be attributable, not to the immaturity of T cells, but to immune deviation. In this case, a non-protective type 2 cytokine response would dominate a protective type 1 cytokine response. T-independent polysaccharide antigens have been shown to generate tolerance in B cells after administration in high doses. Tolerance and its underlying mechanisms are discussed in Chapter 11.

Recent work has shown that in experimental autoimmune encephalomyelitis (EAE, a model of multiple sclerosis), a dose

escalation strategy with peptides of myelin basic protein (MBP) revealed that immune responses can be switched from a destructive TH1 response to a type 1 regulatory cell IL-10-producing phenotype (Fig. 12.2). Here it is thought that IL-10 production emerges as a negative feedback mechanism to control the immune response. Thus, peptide therapy has potential promise for the treatment of autoimmune diseases where relevant antigens are known (see Chapter 20).

Antigen route of administration can determine whether an immune response occurs. The route of administration of antigen has been shown to influence the immune response:
- Antigens administered subcutaneously or intradermally evoke an active immune response.
- Antigens given intravenously, orally or as an aerosol may cause tolerance or an immune deviation from one type of CD4+ T-cell response to another.

For example, rodents that have been fed ovalbumin do not respond effectively to a subsequent challenge with the corresponding antigen. This phenomenon may have some therapeutic value in allergy. Studies have shown that oral administration of a T-cell epitope of the Der p1 allergen of house dust mite (*Dermatophagoides pteronyssinus*) could tolerize to the whole antigen.

As well as dose, routes of administration elicit different types of immune response. Studies in mice have shown that aerosol administration of an MBP-derived peptide inhibits the development of EAE that would normally be induced by a conventional (subcutaneous) administration of the peptide (Fig. 12.3). A clear example of how different routes of administration may regulate the outcome of the immune response is provided by studies of

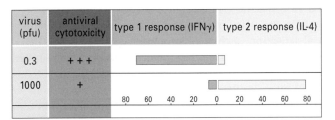

virus (pfu)	antiviral cytotoxicity	type 1 response (IFNγ)	type 2 response (IL-4)
0.3	+++		
1000	+		

Fig. 12.1 Effect of antigen dose on the immune response to murine leukaemia virus Newborn mice were infected with either 0.3 or 1000 plaque-forming units *(pfu)* of virus and the cytotoxic T-lymphocyte (CTL) response against virally infected targets was assessed together with the production of interferon-γ (IFNγ, a type 1 cytokine) or interleukin-4 (IL-4, a type 2 cytokine) in response to viral challenge. Mice infected with a low dose of virus make a type 1 response and are protected. The results are presented as arbitrary units.

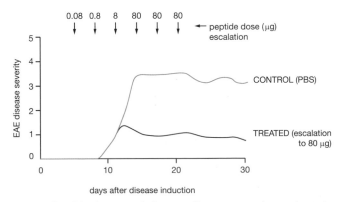

Fig. 12.2 Peptide dose escalation ameliorates experimental autoimmune encephalomyelitis *(EAE)* Mice were immunized to induce EAE. Control mice develop clinical symptoms around day 10. Treated mice received six injections of MBP peptide using a dose escalation protocol from 0.08 μg to 80 μg as shown by the *arrows*. The symptoms of EAE (weakness/paralysis) were significantly reduced in mice receiving an escalating dose of peptide.

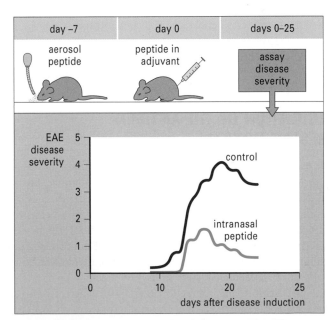

Fig. 12.3 Aerosol administration of antigen modifies the immune response Mice were treated with a single aerosol dose of either 100 μg peptide (residues 1–11 of myelin basic protein) or just the carrier. Seven days later the same peptide, this time in adjuvant, was administered subcutaneously. The subsequent development of experimental allergic encephalomyelitis *(EAE)* was significantly modified in animals that first received aerosolized peptide.

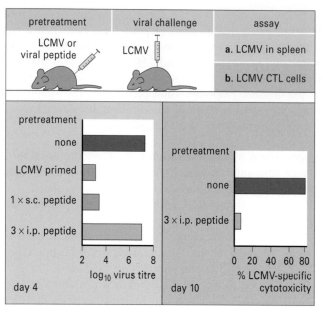

Fig. 12.4 Peptide-induced inactivation of LCMV-specific T cells Mice were either primed with lymphocytic choriomeningitis virus *(LCMV)* or injected with 100 µg LCMV peptide. The peptide was given either subcutaneously *(s.c.)* or three times intraperitoneally *(i.p.)* with incomplete Freund adjuvant. The animals were later infected with LCMV (day 0). The titre of virus in the spleen was measured on day 4. Animals that had been pretreated with subcutaneous peptide or with LCMV developed neutralizing antibody and protective immunity against the virus; animals pretreated with peptide i.p. did not develop immunity. Cytotoxic T-lymphocyte *(CTL)* activity was assessed in the mice on day 10. Mice that had received no pretreatment demonstrated CTLs specific for the LCMV peptide. Mice pretreated with peptide i.p. failed to show such activity.

infection with lymphocytic choriomeningitis virus (LCMV). Mice primed subcutaneously with peptide in incomplete Freund's adjuvant develop immunity to LCMV. However, if the same peptide is repeatedly injected intraperitoneally, the animal becomes tolerized and cannot clear the virus (Fig. 12.4). Therefore, both antigen dose and route of administration are critical factors to consider in vaccination strategies (see Chapter 17).

REGULATION BY THE ANTIGEN-PRESENTING CELL

The nature of the cell initially presenting the antigen may determine whether immune responsiveness or tolerance ensues. Effective activation of T cells requires the expression of co-stimulatory molecules on the surface of the antigen-presenting cell (APC). Therefore, presentation by dendritic cells or activated macrophages that express high levels of major histocompatibility complex (MHC) class II molecules, in addition to co-stimulatory molecules, results in highly effective T-cell activation. Furthermore, the interaction of CD40L on activated T cells with CD40 on dendritic cells is important for the high-level production of IL-12 necessary for the generation of an effective type 1 cytokine response.

If antigen is presented to T cells by a non-professional APC that is unable to provide co-stimulation, unresponsiveness or immune deviation results. For example, when naive T cells are exposed to antigen by resting B cells, they fail to

respond and become tolerized. Experimental observations illustrate this point.

Neonatal animals are more susceptible to tolerance induction: mice administered MBP in incomplete Freund adjuvant (an oil and water emulsion without bacterial components) during the neonatal period are resistant to the induction of EAE. This is a result of the development of a dominant type 2 response (see Fig. 12.1). The prior type 2 response to MBP prevents the development of the type 1/3 pathological response, which mediates EAE. This effect is not restricted to neonatal animals. Indeed, adult Lewis rats can be tolerized to the induction of EAE by similar administration of MBP in incomplete Freund's adjuvant.

Adjuvants may facilitate immune responses by inducing the expression of high levels of MHC and co-stimulatory molecules on APCs. Furthermore, their ability to activate Langerhans cells leads to the migration of these skin dendritic cells to the local draining lymph nodes where effective T-cell activation can occur.

The importance of dendritic cells in initiating a cytotoxic T-lymphocyte (CTL) response is illustrated by experiments showing that newborn female mice injected with male spleen cells fail to develop a CTL response to the male antigen, H-Y. However, if male dendritic cells are injected into female newborn mice, a good H-Y-specific CTL response develops.

APCs can also express important negative regulators of T-cell activation, such as programmed death-ligand 1 (PD-L1). Activated T cells express programmed death 1 (PD-1), which binds PD-L1 and attenuates T-cell activation and proliferation (see Chapter 7). PD-L1 can be upregulated on tumour cells (see Chapter 22), which may prevent effective tumour immunity. Therefore, blockade of PD-1 and PD-L1 interactions is a current target for immunotherapy in cancer.

T-CELL REGULATION OF THE IMMUNE RESPONSE

Differentiation into CD4⁺ TH subsets is an important step in selecting effector functions. Naive CD4⁺ T cells are able to differentiate into a variety of phenotypes, the best characterized and understood being the TH1, TH2 and TH17 phenotypes (Fig. 12.5), which are associated with type 1, type 2 and type 3 (which are sometimes also called type 17) cytokine responses, respectively. The differentiation fates of TH cells are crucial to the generation of effective immunity. Factors that may influence the differentiation of TH cells include:

- the sites of antigen presentation;
- co-stimulatory molecules involved in cognate cellular interactions;
- peptide density and binding affinity–high MHC class II peptide density favours TH1 or TH17, low densities favour TH2;
- APCs and the cytokines they produce;
- the cytokine profile and balance of cytokines evoked by antigen;
- receptors expressed on the T cell;
- activity of co-stimulatory molecules and hormones present in the local environment;

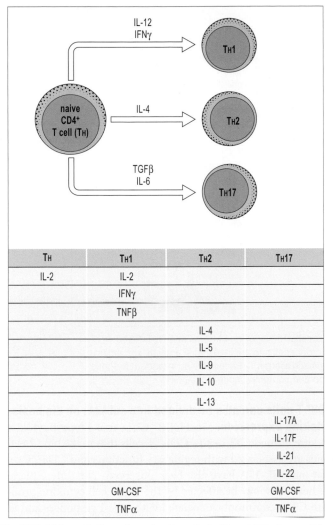

T_H	T_H1	T_H2	T_H17
IL-2	IL-2		
	IFNγ		
	TNFβ		
		IL-4	
		IL-5	
		IL-9	
		IL-10	
		IL-13	
			IL-17A
			IL-17F
			IL-21
			IL-22
	GM-CSF		GM-CSF
	TNFα		TNFα

Fig. 12.5 Differentiation of murine T_H cells IL-12 and IFNγ favour differentiation of T_H1 cells, and IL-4 favours differentiation of T_H2 cells. TGFβ and IL-6 drive T_H17-cell development. *GM-CSF*, Granulocyte–macrophage colony stimulating factor; *TNF*, tumour necrosis factor.

- host genetic background, for example some strains of mouse preferentially produce type 1 responses, while others tend to produce type 2 responses.

Cytokine balance is a major regulator of T-cell differentiation. Cytokines are part of an extracellular signalling network that controls every function of the innate and adaptive immune system, having:

- numerous effects on cell phenotypes; and
- the ability to regulate the type of immune response generated and its extent.

The local cytokine milieu is heavily influenced by cytokines derived from innate immune cells in the early stages of an immune response (see later). Cytokines and immune responses can be broadly classified as type 1 (T_H1), type 2 (T_H2) or type 3 (sometimes called T_H17).

IL-12 is a potent initial stimulus for IFNγ production by T cells and natural killer (NK) cells and therefore promotes a type

1 response and T_H1 differentiation. IFNα, a cytokine produced by virally infected cells early in infection, induces IL-12 and can also switch cells from a T_H2 to a T_H1 profile.

By contrast, early production of the type 2 cytokine IL-4 favours the generation of T_H2 cells. NK T cells, M2 macrophages (see Fig. 5.19), ILC2s and basophils have all been suggested to be early producers of IL-4. T_H17 cells in mice develop in the presence of TGFβ with IL-6 or IL-21 and share an interesting reciprocal developmental relationship with inducible Tregs, which is discussed in more detail later.

Cytokines from the various T_H subsets can cross-regulate each other's development:

- IFNγ secreted by T_H1 cells can inhibit the responsiveness of T_H2 cells.
- the type 3 cytokine IL-17A can inhibit the development of T_H1 responses (Fig. 12.6).
- IL-10 produced by T_H2 cells reduces B7 and IL-12 expression by APCs, which in turn inhibits T_H1 activation.

The T_H subset balance is modulated not only by the level of expression of cytokines such as IL-12 or IL-4 but also by expression of cytokine receptors. For instance, the high-affinity IL-12R is composed of two chains, β1 and β2, with both chains being constitutively expressed on T_H1 cells. T_H1, T_H2 and T_H17 cells express the β1 chain, but expression of the β2 chain is induced by IFNγ and inhibited by IL-4 (Fig. 12.7). Therefore cytokines reinforce the lineage decisions of the various T_H subsets at least in part by controlling the expression of lineage-specific receptors.

An immune response therefore tends to settle into a type 1, type 2 or type 3 mode of response, but immune responses are not always strongly polarized in this way, particularly in humans. Indeed, T_H subsets can exhibit functional plasticity, allowing deviation of the immune response.

T_H cell subsets determine the type of immune response. It is clear that:

- local patterns of cytokine and hormone expression help to select lymphocyte effector mechanism; and
- the polarized responses of CD4+ T_H cells are based on their profile of cytokine secretion.

Type 1 cytokines including IFNγ and IL-12, also promote:
- macrophage activation;
- antibody-dependent cell-mediated cytotoxicity; and
- delayed-type hypersensitivity.

T_H2 clones are typified by production of the type 2 cytokines IL-4, IL-5, IL-9, IL-10 and IL-13 (see Fig. 12.5). These cells provide optimal help for humoral immune responses biased towards:
- IgG1 and IgE isotype switching;
- mucosal immunity;
- stimulation of mast cells, eosinophil growth and differentiation; and
- IgA synthesis.

Type 3 cytokines produced by T_H17 cells include IL-17A, IL-17F, TNFα and IL-22. Since many stromal cells express receptors for these cytokines, the effects of T_H17 cells can promote inflammation. In addition:

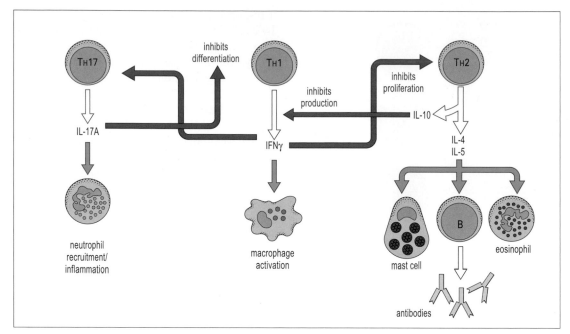

Fig. 12.6 Selection of effector mechanisms by Tн1 and Tн2 cells The cytokine patterns of Tн1, Tн2 and Tн17 cells drive different effector pathways. Tн1 cells activate macrophages and are involved in antiviral and inflammatory responses. Tн2 cells are involved in humoral responses and allergy. Tн17 cells are an important defence at mucosal barriers, recruiting neutrophils to sites of infection and tightening epithelial barriers.

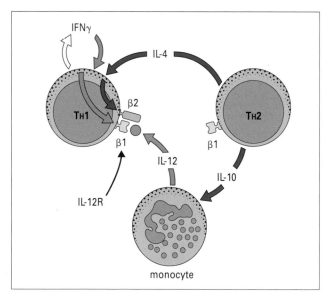

Fig. 12.7 Regulation of the Tн1 response by IL-12 The high-affinity IL-12R, consisting of the β1 and β2 chains, is constitutively expressed on Tн1 cells. IL-12 released by mononuclear phagocytes promotes the development and activation of Tн1 cells, but IL-12 production is inhibited by IL-10 released by Tн2 cells. IFNγ from Tн1 cells promotes production of the β2 chain and therefore production of the high-affinity IL-12R. However, this is inhibited by IL-4.

- IL-17A has been proposed to be important for the recruitment of neutrophils and induction of anti-microbial peptides from resident cells.
- IL-17A is important for host defence against *Klebsiella pneumoniae* and *Candida albicans*.

CD8+ T cells can also be divided into subsets on the basis of cytokine expression. Most CD8+ CTLs make type 1 cytokines and are termed CTL1 cells. CD8+ T cells that make type 2 cytokines are associated with regulatory functions and CD8+ T cells that make IL-17A have also been observed. The differentiation of these cells may be affected by the CD4+ cell cytokine profile, with CTLs commonly associated with type 1 responses and less commonly found when Tн2 cells are present. Thus:

- IFNγ and IL-12 may encourage CTL1 generation; and
- IL-4 may encourage CTL2 generation.

However, both CTL1 and CTL2 cells can be cytotoxic and kill mainly by a Ca^{2+}/perforin-dependent mechanism (see Fig. 8.11).

CD4+ T cells display some plasticity between Tн1, Tн2 and Tн17. Studies of Tн cells have revealed considerable developmental plasticity. In particular, Tн17 cells can be induced to produce IFNγ (a type 1 cytokine) and shut down production of IL-17A if they are stimulated in the presence of IL-12 (Fig. 12.8). Similarly, at least in vitro, Tн2 cells can be driven to a mixed Tн2/1 phenotype, in which cells co-express IL-4 and IFNγ, by culture with type I IFNs and IL-12. It is thought that such plasticity may enable rapid site-specific immune responses to infections to occur.

Innate lymphoid cells polarize the immune response by producing cytokines. The three types of immune response and their characteristic cytokines were originally described in the context of T-helper cells. However, recently, a new family of lymphocytes, called the innate lymphoid cells (ILCs), has been discovered (see Chapter 2).

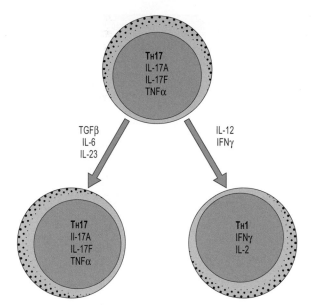

Fig. 12.8 TH17 cells exhibit plasticity in TH1 cytokine environments. TH17 cells can differentiate into TH1 cells in response to IL-12 and IFNγ signalling.

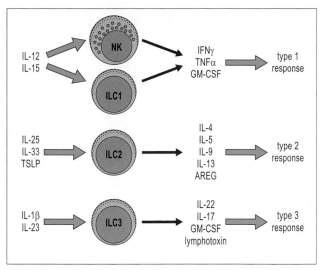

Fig 12.9 ILCs polarize the immune response. IL-12 and IL-15 promote the activity of NK cells and ILC1, both of which produce type 1 cytokines, particularly IFNγ. IL-25, IL-33 and thymic stromal lymphopoietin *(TSLP)* promote ILC2 production of type 2 cytokines, including IL-4 and IL-13 as well as amphiregulin *(AREG)*, which promotes epithelial cell growth during wound healing. IL-1β and IL-23 promote ILC3 activity and the production of type 3 cytokines, including IL-22 and IL-17. *NK*, Natural killer cells.

ILCs are cells of the lymphoid lineage but, unlike T and B cells, they lack highly variable antigen receptors generated by somatic recombination (see Chapters 6 and 9). They play key roles in innate immunity, tissue repair and homeostasis at barrier surfaces, including the skin, airways and gastrointestinal tract.

There are now considered to be five groups of ILCs, four of which can be thought of as innate counterparts to T cells:

- NK cells are the innate counterparts of cytotoxic T cells. Their main function is cytotoxicity (see Chapter 8) but they also produce the type 1 cytokine IFNγ
- ILC1 are innate counterparts of TH1 cells. They produce IFNγ, TNFα and GM-CSF in response to IL-12 and IL-15.
- ILC2 are innate counterparts of TH2 cells. They produce IL-4, IL-5, IL-9 and IL-13 in response to IL-25, IL-33 and thymic stromal lymphopoietin (TSLP).
- ILC3 are innate counterparts of TH17 cells. They produce IL-22 and IL-17 in response to IL-1β and IL-23 (Fig. 12.9)

The fifth group of ILCs is the lymphoid tissue inducer cells (LTis). These were originally considered to be a subset of ILC3 but are now thought of as a separate lineage. They have an important role in the formation of lymph nodes and Peyer's patches (see Chapter 2).

A subset of ILC that produces IL-10 in response to TGFβ has been described and it is possible that these are innate counterparts to Tregs. However, the development and function of this subset of ILCs is not yet well understood.

Because ILCs respond earlier than T cells, it is likely that they have a critical role in polarizing the immune response, with the cytokines that they produce feeding back on T cells as the adaptive response develops. It has also been argued that, since ILCs are generally tissue-resident and present earlier in development than T cells, they may have a role in initiating the characteristic cytokine milieus of the various tissues.

ILCs can affect the immune response via cell–cell interactions. Subsets of both ILC2 and ILC3 express MHC class II and are able to present antigen to CD4$^+$ T cells in vitro, although the co-stimulatory molecules that they express suggest that they are best suited to interacting with T cells that have already been activated (see Chapter 7).

Genetic deletion of MHC class II molecules specifically from ILC2 results in impaired T-cell responses, suggesting that ILC2 interactions enhance the T-cell response. Mice lacking MHC class II molecules on ILC3 display an impaired splenic T-cell response to systemic immunization but also have an inappropriate over-reaction to commensal bacteria, implying that the type and site of challenge may affect whether ILC3 promote or inhibit the immune response via antigen presentation.

ILC3 express high levels of TNF superfamily members, including CD252 and CD30L (CD153), whose ligands are expressed on activated T cells and are required for sustaining the immune response. Mice lacking CD252 and CD30L exhibit defects in memory response, indicating that ILC3 may play a role in promoting the development of memory T cells.

IMMUNE REGULATION BY SELECTIVE CELL MIGRATION

The spatial and temporal production of chemokines by different cell types is an important mechanism of immune regulation. There is good evidence to suggest that the recruitment of TH1, TH2 and TH17 cells is differentially controlled, thereby ensuring the maintenance of locally polarized immune responses.

The expression of different chemokine receptors on TH1 cells (CXCR3 and CCR5), TH2 cells (CCR3, CCR4, CCR8) and TH17 (CCR6) allows chemotactic signals to produce the differential

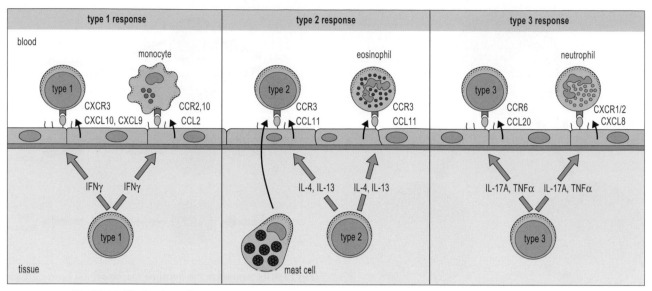

Fig. 12.10 Mechanisms for local reinforcement of different modes of immune response Activated TH1 cells release IFNγ, which induces the chemokines CXCL10 (IP10) and CXCL9 (Mig). These act on the chemokine receptors CXCR3, which are selectively expressed on TH1 cells, thereby reinforcing this type of response. Macrophage chemotactic protein-1 (MCP-1, CCL2), which attracts macrophages and monocytes, is also induced by IFNγ. Mast cells release CCL11 (eotaxin) when activated and endothelial cells and bronchial epithelium can also synthesize this chemokine in response to IL-4 and IL-13 from TH2 cells. Eotaxin acts on CCR3, which is selectively expressed on TH2 cells, thereby reinforcing the TH2 response. Eosinophils and basophils, which mediate allergic responses in airways, also express CCR3. TH17 cells express the chemokine receptor CCR6. IL-17A production by TH17 cells induces expression of CCL20, which acts on CCR6, thus recruiting TH17 cells to the site of infection. Chemokines can therefore potentiate both the initiation and effector phases of a specific type of immune response.

localization of T-cell subsets to sites of inflammation (see Fig. 3.11).

Chemokines can be induced by cytokines released at sites of inflammation, providing a mechanism for local reinforcement of particular types of response (Fig. 12.10). Once a response is established, the T cells can induce further migration of appropriate effector cells. This is clearly illustrated in type 1 responses where the secondary production of CCL2, CCL3, CXCL10 and CCL5 serves to attract mononuclear phagocytes to the area of inflammation. Production of IL-17A can drive the expression of CCL20, the ligand for CCR6, recruiting more TH17 cells to the site of inflammation. The ability of cytokines such as TGFβ, IL-12 and IL-4 to influence chemokine or chemokine receptor expression provides a further level of control on cell migration or recruitment.

T follicular helper (TFH) cells express the B-cell follicle homing receptor CXCR5, which allows them to regulate B-cell germinal centre formation. TfH cells express CD40L and secrete IL-21, which mediates the selection and survival of B cells as they undergo proliferation and antibody diversification.

Immune responses do not normally occur at certain sites in the body such as the anterior chamber of the eye and the testes. These sites are called **immune privileged** (see Chapter 13).

The failure to evoke immune responses in these sites is partly because of the presence of inhibitory cytokines such as TGFβ and IL-10, which inhibit inflammatory responses. The presence of migration inhibition factor (MIF) in the anterior chamber of the eye also inhibits NK-cell activity.

T-Cell expression of different molecules can regulate tissue localization. Most studies on the human immune system are performed on blood because of the ethical issues in obtaining tissues. However, only a small proportion of the lymphocyte pool circulates in the blood, most being resident in lymphoid or effector tissues.

The expression of molecules on T cells can mediate circulation through different tissues. Loss of the lymph node homing molecules CCR7 and CD62L on the surface of T cells prevents cells from circulating through lymphoid tissue. In this way, highly differentiated memory cells migrate to non-lymphoid sites where they can exert effector functions.

It has been suggested that there are two types of memory cell:
- **Central memory cells** express CCR7, home to lymphoid tissues, and do not have immediate effector function.
- **Effector memory cells** do not express CCR7, migrate to non-lymphoid tissues and produce effector cytokines. Effector cells in non-lymphoid tissues, such as the skin, can proliferate and senesce, which has a direct effect on the level of local immune responses.

REGULATORY T CELLS

Although T cells modulate the immune response in a positive sense by providing T-cell help as discussed above, T cells are also capable of downregulating immune responses.

A naturally occurring population of CD4$^+$CD25$^+$ regulatory T cells (Tregs) is generated in the thymus. Additionally, CD4$^+$

Tregs can be induced from non-regulatory T cells in the periphery.

Tregs maintain peripheral tolerance and have important roles in the prevention of autoimmune diseases such as type 1 diabetes. They are also thought to play critical roles in limiting the levels of immunopathology during an active immune response but are increasingly seen as a potential barrier to effective immune surveillance in cancer (see Chapter 22).

Treg differentiation is induced by Foxp3. The immunosuppressive functions of CD4$^+$ cells were initially observed by adoptively transferring T cells depleted of CD25$^+$ cells into immunodeficient mice. This resulted in multi-organ autoimmunity, suggesting that CD25$^+$ cells play an important role in preventing self reactivity. When the CD25$^+$ T cells were replaced, autoimmune disease was prevented.

Comparison of CD4$^+$CD25$^+$ Tregs with naive and activated CD4$^+$ T cells shows that regulatory T cells selectively express **Foxp3**, a member of the forkhead/winged helix transcription factors essential for the development and function of CD4$^+$CD25$^+$ Tregs. Mutations in the Foxp3 gene cause immune dysregulation, polyendocrinopathy enteropathy and X-linked syndrome (IPEX). Individuals with this disease have increased autoimmune and inflammatory diseases.

The importance of Foxp3 in the development of CD4$^+$CD25$^+$ Tregs was underlined following transfection of Foxp3 into naive T cells (which do not express Foxp3). This increased expression of CD25 and induced suppressor function.

A two-stage model for Treg development within the thymus has been proposed (Fig. 12.11). Strongly self-reactive CD4$^+$ T cells upregulate CD25 in response to strong and persistent T-cell receptor (TCR) signals. This then allows for IL-2-driven induction of Foxp3 expression, which represses T-cell IL-2 and IFNγ expression and imparts the suppressive Treg phenotype. Interestingly, differences in human HLA alleles have been suggested to affect risk of autoimmunity. For instance, HLA polymorphism can alter the relative abundance of self epitope-specific Treg cells that can lead to protection or increased risk of autoimmunity.

CD4$^+$CD25$^+$ Foxp3$^+$ Tregs constitute 5%–10% of peripheral CD4$^+$ T cells in both mice and humans and although athymic mice have severely reduced levels of Tregs, it is clear that Foxp3$^+$ Tregs can arise in the periphery. These so-called peripheral (p) Tregs have been extensively studied in vitro. If naive CD4$^+$ T cells are stimulated in the presence of TGFβ, then many cells start expressing Foxp3. The additional presence of retinoic acid is thought to accentuate the conversion of naive CD4$^+$ T cells into Foxp3$^+$ Tregs.

There is a Reciprocal Developmental Relationship Between Induced Tregs and TH17 Cells

Induced Treg populations and inflammatory TH17 cells are thought to share a reciprocal developmental pathway. In mice, both induced Treg and TH17 cells are dependent on TGFβ for their development. In the presence of TGFβ, naive CD4$^+$ T cells upregulate Foxp3 and develop into induced Tregs. However, in the additional presence of inflammatory cytokines such as IL-6 or IL-1β, naive T cells develop into inflammatory TH17 cells that secrete cytokines such as IL-17A, IL-17F and TNFα. This dichotomous relationship implies an important role for cytokines derived from the innate immune system in determining the outcome of an adaptive immune response (Fig. 12.12). Such induced Tregs have been seen to arise following allograft transplantation and also after oral administration of antigen. They are also thought to play important roles at mucosal surfaces within the gut. Studies of induced Treg have proven difficult because of a lack of methods to track new Foxp3 expressers during peripheral immune responses.

Tr1 are Induced by IL-10 and Do Not Express FoxP3

Another class of CD4$^+$ regulatory T cells, called Tr1 cells, can also be generated from naive TH cells in the periphery. These cells are generated in response to IL-10 and mediate suppression through IL-10 production (Fig 12.13). They do not express

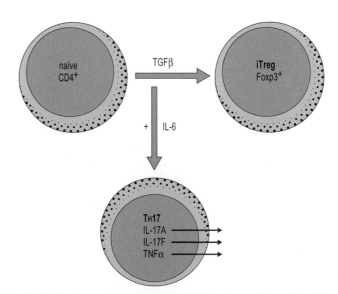

Fig. 12.12 Reciprocal development of TH17 cells and Tregs The differentiation of TH17 cells and Tregs is regulated by cytokines. In the presence of TGFβ, naive T cells express Foxp3. However, the presence of IL-6 in combination with TGFβ can drive the differentiation of TH17 cells.

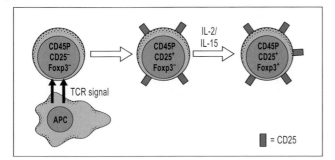

Fig. 12.11 A two-step differentiation process for thymic Foxp3$^+$ regulatory T cells. Strong T-cell receptor *(TCR)* signalling in response to presentation of self antigens within the thymus induces expression of CD25 on CD4 single-positive (SP) cells. IL-2 and/or IL-15 signalling then promotes Foxp3 expression and the development of CD25$^+$Foxp3$^+$ Treg cells. *APC*, Antigen-presenting cell.

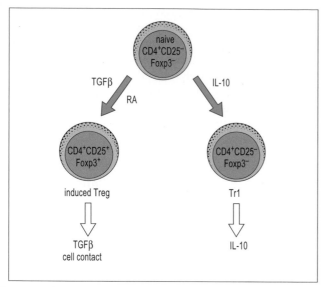

Fig. 12.13 Regulatory T cells can be generated in the periphery Naive CD4+ CD25– cells in the periphery can be stimulated to become suppressive. If TGFβ is present, cells upregulate Foxp3 and CD25. In the presence of IL-10, cells can become suppressive, but they do not express Foxp3 or CD25. *RA*, Retinoic acid.

CD25 or Foxp3 but are frequently identified through expression of CD49b and LAG3, which is a co-inhibitory receptor capable of binding MHC class II.

Tregs Suppress the Immune Response Using Multiple Mechanisms

Many mechanisms of Treg suppression have been proposed. For instance, initial studies suggested that natural Tregs require cell contact to suppress and induced Treg populations may suppress by the release of soluble factors. The vast majority of these studies have examined the behaviour of Tregs using in vitro culture systems. These highly controlled environments do not consider the need for regulatory T-cell populations to home to different locations in order to interact with target cells. Therefore, our knowledge of the exact functions of Tregs in vivo is less clear. This is further confounded by the different types of regulatory T cell and the exact contribution of natural and induced regulatory populations may differ depending on the antigenic challenges encountered. In spite of this, at least four mechanisms of Treg suppression have been proposed (Fig. 12.14). Upon activation Treg cells can upregulate an array of immunosuppressive molecules. A key molecule called CTLA-4 acts as an important negative regulator of T-cell activation. CTLA-4 binds the B7 molecules CD80 and CD86 and therefore reduces the co-stimulatory capacity of APCs such as DC. This pathway has been seen as a potential barrier to effective tumour immunity (see Chapter 22) and, like PD-1:PD-L1, is a target of current immunotherapies. In addition to CTLA-4 expression, Treg can release anti-inflammatory cytokines, such as IL-10, which dampen T-cell proliferation and cytokine production. They also express high levels of CD25, the high-affinity chain of the IL-2 receptor. This allows Treg to act as a sink for IL-2 and prevent effector T-cell proliferation. Some groups have also proposed that Treg may directly kill cells through the release of granzyme, in similar ways to CD8 T cells (see Fig. 12.14).

Tregs Prevent Immune-Mediated Pathology in Infection but Can also Dampen Protective T-Cell Responses

Although CD4+ Tregs play a vital role in the prevention of autoimmune diseases (see Chapter 20), their role in infections is less clear. CD4+ Tregs have a protective role against immune-mediated pathology and their ability to suppress is important in reducing inflammation. For example, lesions in the eye in stromal keratitis are less severe in the presence of CD4+ CD25+ Tregs.

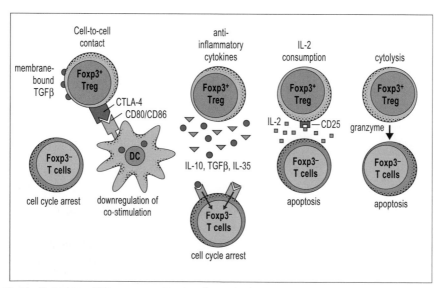

Fig. 12.14 Mechanisms of Treg suppression Tregs may suppress by a variety of mechanisms. (1) Via cell-to-cell contact (secreted or cell surface molecules such as CTLA-4 expression or membrane-bound TGFβ). (2) Release of suppressor cytokines such as IL-10, TGFβ and IL-35. (3) IL-2 consumption (Tregs can express high levels of CD25, the IL-2 receptor). (4) Cytolysis, akin to CD8+ T-cell killing. (Adapted from Shevach EM, Immunity 2009;30:636–645.)

CD4$^+$ Tregs can also suppress virus-specific responses. Many pathogens induce high levels of IL-10 and TGFβ, which promote the induction of CD4$^+$CD25$^+$ Tregs. In chronic viral infections, including HIV, cytomegalovirus (CMV) and herpes simplex virus (HSV) infections, increased numbers of Tregs are responsible for decreased antigen-specific responses by CD4$^+$ and CD8$^+$ T cells, which can lead to disease development.

NKT cells produce immunoregulatory cytokines and chemokines. NKT cells produce cytokines when their TCR engages glycolipids in association with CD1d. It has been suggested that these cells play an immunoregulatory role in the control of autoimmunity, parasite infection and tumour cell growth. They are capable of making type 1 (IFNγ), type 2 (IL-4) and type 3 (IL-17A) cytokines depending on the cytokines present in the microenvironment when they are activated (Fig. 12.15). These early sources of cytokine are important in influencing the nature of the T-cell response.

Deficiencies of NKT cells have also been reported in animal and human autoimmune diseases, highlighting their regulatory roles. For example, non-obese diabetic (NOD) mice have a deficit in NKT cells and injection of NKT cells into these mice prevents the spontaneous development of autoimmune diabetes. Human autoimmune diseases where NKT deficiencies may play a role include:

- rheumatoid arthritis;
- psoriasis;
- ulcerative colitis; and
- multiple sclerosis.

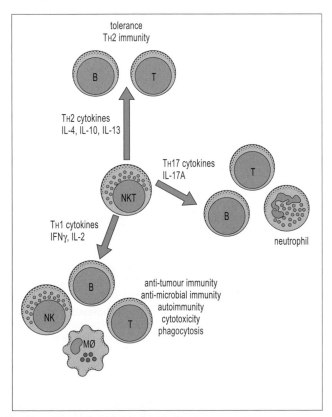

Fig. 12.15 Natural killer (NK) T cells produce type 1, type 2 and type 3 cytokines NKT cells exert effects on many cell types. They can produce cytokines of all three types and are involved in all aspects of the immune response.

REGULATION OF THE IMMUNE RESPONSE BY IMMUNOGLOBULINS

Antibody exerts feedback control on the immune response. Passive administration of IgM antibody with an antigen specifically enhances the immune response to that antigen, whereas IgG antibody suppresses the response. This was originally shown with polyclonal antibodies but has since been confirmed using monoclonal antibodies (Fig. 12.16).

The ability of passively administered antibody to enhance or to suppress the immune response has certain clinical consequences and applications:

- Certain vaccines (e.g. mumps and measles) are not generally given to infants before 1 year of age because levels of maternally derived IgG remain high for at least 6 months after birth and the presence of such passively acquired IgG at the time of vaccination would result in the development of an inadequate immune response in the baby.
- In cases of Rhesus (Rh) incompatibility, the administration of anti-RhD antibody to Rh$^-$ mothers prevents primary sensitization by fetally derived Rh$^+$ blood cells, presumably by removing the foreign antigen (fetal erythrocytes) from the maternal circulation (see Chapter 24).

IgM enhances the immune response to its antigen. The mechanisms by which IgM enhances the response to its antigen are not completely defined. The most likely explanation is that IgM-containing immune complexes are taken up by Fc or C3 receptors on APCs, including follicular dendritic cells, and are processed more efficiently than antigen alone.

IgG antibody can regulate specific IgG synthesis. IgG can suppress antibody responses in a number of ways:

- Passively administered antibody binds antigen in competition with B cells (antibody blocking) (Fig. 12.17). In this case, suppression is highly dependent on the concentration of the antibody and on its affinity for the antigen compared with the affinity of the B-cell receptors. Only high-affinity B cells compete successfully for the antigen. This mechanism is independent of the Fc portion of the antibody.

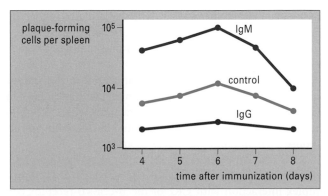

Fig. 12.16 Feedback control by antibody Mice received a monoclonal IgM anti-SRBC (sheep red blood cells), an IgG anti-SRBC or a medium alone (control). Two hours later all groups were immunized with SRBC. The antibody response measured over the following 8 days was enhanced by IgM and suppressed by IgG.

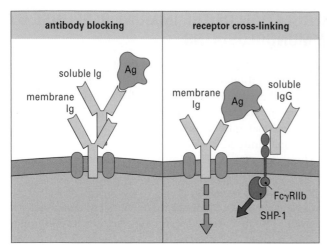

Fig. 12.17 Antibody-dependent B-cell suppression Antibody blocking: high doses of soluble immunoglobulin *(Ig)* block the interaction between an antigenic determinant (epitope) and membrane immunoglobulin on B cells. The B cell is then effectively unable to recognize the antigen *(Ag)*. This receptor-blocking mechanism also prevents B-cell priming, but only antibodies that bind to the same epitope to which the B cell's receptors bind can do this. Receptor cross-linking: low doses of antibody allow cross-linking by antigen of a B cell's Fc receptors and its antigen receptors. The FcγRIIb receptor associates with a tyrosine phosphatase (SHP-1), which interferes with cell activation by tyrosine kinases associated with the antigen receptor. This allows B-cell priming but inhibits antibody synthesis. Antibodies against different epitopes on the antigen can all act by this mechanism. *Ag*, antigen.

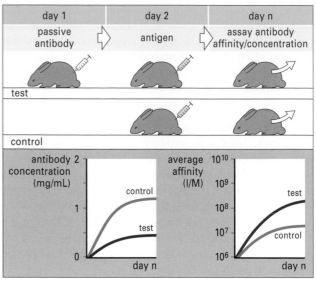

Fig. 12.18 Antibody feedback on affinity maturation The effect of passive antibody on the affinity and concentration of secreted antibody. One of two rabbits was injected with antibody (passive antibody) on day 1. Both rabbits were immunized with antigen on day 2 and the affinity and concentration of antibody raised to this antigen were assayed at a later time (day n). The antibody assay results show that passive antibody reduces the concentration but increases the affinity of antibody produced.

- Immunoglobulin can inhibit B-cell differentiation by cross-linking the antigen receptor (BCR) with the Fc receptor (FcγRIIb) on the same cell (see Fig. 12.17). In this case, the suppressive antibody and the B cell's receptor antibody may recognize different epitopes.
- Doses of IgG that are insufficient to inhibit the production of antibodies completely have the effect of increasing the average antibody affinity because only those B cells with high-affinity receptors can successfully compete with the passively acquired antibody for antigen. For this reason, antibody feedback is believed to be an important factor driving the process of affinity maturation (Fig. 12.18).

Immune complexes may enhance or suppress immune responses. One of the ways in which antibody (either IgM or IgG) might act to modulate the immune response involves an Fc-dependent mechanism and immune complex formation with antigen.

Immune complexes can inhibit or augment the immune response (Fig. 12.19). By activating complement, immune complexes may become localized via interactions with CR2 on follicular dendritic cells (FDCs). This could facilitate the immune response by maintaining a source of antigen.

CR2 is also expressed on B cells and, as co-ligation of CR2 with membrane IgM has been shown to activate B cells, immune complex interaction with CR2 of the B-cell–co-receptor complex and membrane Ig might lead to an enhanced specific immune response.

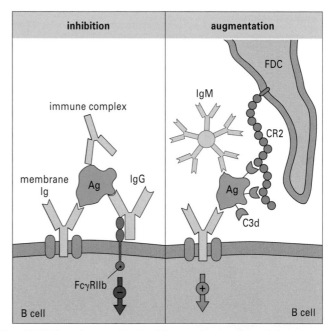

Fig. 12.19 Regulatory effects of immune complexes Immune complexes can act either to inhibit or to augment an immune response. Inhibition: when the Fc receptor of the B cell is cross-linked to its antigen *(Ag)* receptor by an antigen–antibody complex, a signal is delivered to the B cell, inhibiting it from entering the antibody production phase. Passive IgG may have this effect. Augmentation: antibodies encourage presentation of antigens to B cells when present on an antigen-presenting cell (APC), bound via Fc receptors or, in this case, complement receptors *(CR2)* on a follicular dendritic cell *(FDC)*. Passive IgM may have this effect. *Ag*, antigen.

Regulatory B Cells Produce IL-10

Recent work has highlighted the role that IL-10-producing B cells have in inhibiting excessive inflammation. Regulatory B cells (Bregs) may act primarily through the skewing of T-cell differentiation in favour of Treg development. In addition, Breg may also express TGFβ and IL-35, akin to Treg cells, which can modulate dendritic cell activation and Tн-cell responses. Bregs are probably a heterogeneous population of cells that arise during different stages of B-cell differentiation. No single transcription factor that controls Breg development has yet been identified, but their development has been linked to expression of the cytokines IL-1β and IL-6.

APOPTOSIS IN THE IMMUNE SYSTEM

Apoptosis is a cellular clearance mechanism through which homeostasis is maintained.

Unlike cell damage-induced death (i.e. **necrosis**), which can trigger immune responses, apoptosis maintains intracellular structures within the cell. Apoptotic cells undergo nuclear fragmentation and the condensation of cytoplasm, plasma membranes and organelles into apoptotic bodies. Apoptotic cells are rapidly phagocytosed by macrophages, which prevents the release of toxic cellular components into tissues, hence avoiding immune responses to the dead cells.

Apoptosis is:

- involved in clearing cells with a high avidity for antigen in the thymus and is an important mechanism of immunological tolerance (see Chapter 11);
- an important mechanism in maintaining homeostasis in the immune system.

At the End of an Immune Response, Antigen-Specific Cells Die by Apoptosis

Following resolution of an immune response, the majority of antigen-specific cells die by apoptosis. This ensures that no unwanted effector cells remain and also maintains a constant number of cells in the immune system.

Apoptosis is controlled by a number of factors in the cell and depends on expression of the death trigger molecule CD95 (Fas). Deficiencies in the FAS/ FASL pathway can give rise to lymphoproliferative disorders with autoimmune manifestations.

A small number of cells are prevented from undergoing apoptosis and enter the memory T-cell pool. Memory T cells generally express high levels of the anti-apoptotic molecule **Bcl-2**, which makes them more resistant to cell death. This may contribute to the rescue of memory populations from apoptosis.

METABOLIC REGULATION OF THE IMMUNE RESPONSE

Immune responses are bio-energetically expensive and it is becoming increasingly apparent that metabolic pathways regulate T-cell differentiation and effector functions in vivo. This is not surprising given that during T-cell and B-cell responses, the immune system must meet the energetic demands to synthesize macromolecules, such as proteins and DNA, whilst also producing ATP. It is notable that many lymph nodes are located within adipose tissue, where they have a ready access to precursors released by activation of the adipocytes by cytokines. Three major pathways regulate energy demands: glycolysis, the tricarboxylic acid (TCA) cycle and mitochondrial oxidative phosphorylation (OXPHOS).

T-CELL ACTIVATION INVOLVES A SWITCH FROM OXPHOS TO GLYCOLYSIS

Naive T-cell metabolic requirements are maintained principally through OXPHOS of glucose and fatty acids. IL-7 signalling in combination with TCR signalling maintains expression of the glucose transporter GLUT1 on naive T cells, allowing glucose to enter the cell (Fig. 12.20). However, T-cell activation induces considerable metabolic reprogramming. TCR signalling acts via ERK signalling pathways to promote uptake and breakdown of glutamine, which is an essential component to replenish TCA cycle intermediates for macromolecule synthesis. In addition, CD28 co-stimulation activates the PI3K/AKT pathway to induce further expression of GLUT1 and switch metabolism from OXPHOS to glycolysis. Interestingly, recent work has shown that activation of glycolysis may play a pivotal role in controlling expression of the cytokines IL-2 and IFNγ in T cells as a result of translational control. The glycolytic enzyme GAPDH binds to AU-rich motifs in the 3′ untranslated region (UTR) of *IFNG* and *IL-2* transcripts and represses their translation. Upon activation of glycolysis, GAPDH disengages these regions, thus permitting translation of these important cytokines.

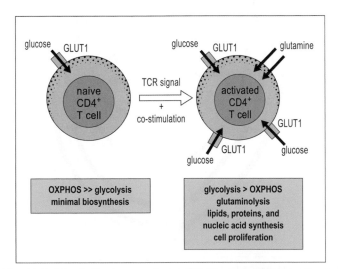

Fig. 12.20 Metabolic changes during T-cell activation In naive T cells, metabolic requirements are principally met through the oxidative phosphorylation (OXPHOS) of glucose. Upon T-cell receptor *(TCR)* signalling and co-stimulation, T cells increase uptake of glucose and switch metabolism to glycolysis. In addition, T cells increase uptake of glutamine and glutaminolysis. These changes support increases in lipid, protein and nucleic acid synthesis, which are required for cell growth and proliferation. *GLUT1*, glucose transporter 1.

NEUROENDOCRINE REGULATION OF IMMUNE RESPONSES

It is now widely accepted that there is extensive cross-talk between the neuroendocrine and immune systems. Both systems share similar ligands and receptors that permit intra- and inter-system communication. These networks of communication are deemed essential for normal physiological function and good health. For instance, they play important roles in modulating the body's response to stress, injury, disease and infection. The interconnections of the nervous, endocrine and immune systems are depicted in (Fig. 12.21).

There are several routes by which the central nervous system and immune system can interact:
- Most lymphoid tissues (e.g. spleen and lymph nodes) receive direct sympathetic innervation to the blood vessels passing through the tissues and directly to lymphocytes.

- The nervous system directly and indirectly controls the output of various hormones, in particular corticosteroids, growth hormone, prolactin, α-melanocyte-stimulating hormone, thyroxine and epinephrine (adrenaline).
- Immune-derived growth factors and cytokines can in turn feed back on the neural and endocrine systems, which probably have an important role in regulating the use of the body's resources.

Lymphocytes express receptors for many hormones, neurotransmitters and neuropeptides: expression and responsiveness vary between different lymphocyte and monocyte populations, such that the effect of different transmitters may vary in different circumstances.

Corticosteroids are immunosuppressive. Corticosteroids, endorphins and enkephalins, all of which may be released during stress, are immunosuppressive in vivo. Such hormones can have strong effects on lymphocyte proliferation and can bring about the reactivation of latent viral infections. The precise in vitro effects of endorphins vary depending on the system and on the doses used: some levels are suppressive and others enhance immune functions.

It is certain, however, that corticosteroids act as a major feedback control on immune responses. This can be harnessed clinically: for example, as part of immunosuppression after transplantation (see Chapter 21).

Lymphocytes can respond to corticotrophin-releasing factor to generate their own adrenocorticotrophic hormone (ACTH), which in turn induces corticosteroid release. Corticosteroids:
- inhibit TH1 cytokine production while sparing TH2 responses; and
- induce the production of TGFβ, which in turn may inhibit the immune response.

This interplay between the neuroendocrine system and the immune system is bidirectional. Cytokines, in particular IL-1 and IL-6 produced by T cells, neurons, glial cells and cells in the pituitary and adrenal glands, are potent stimulators of ACTH production through their effect on corticotrophin-releasing hormone (CRH).

Sex hormones affect immune cell function. Gender-based differences in immune responses also occur. Immune cells have been shown to express receptors for oestrogens and androgens and it is likely that circulating levels of these hormones can affect their function. It is noted that, during reproductive years, females demonstrate more pronounced humoral and cellular immunity than males.

Some autoimmune diseases also show a gender bias. The systemic autoimmune disease systemic lupus erythematosus (SLE) is 10 times more common in females than males. Additionally, in animal models of autoimmunity, female NOD mice develop a much higher incidence of diabetes than males (although this sex bias is not observed in humans) and male BXSB mice have a higher spontaneous incidence of an SLE-like syndrome compared with females. This provides some evidence for the effects of sex hormones on immune function.

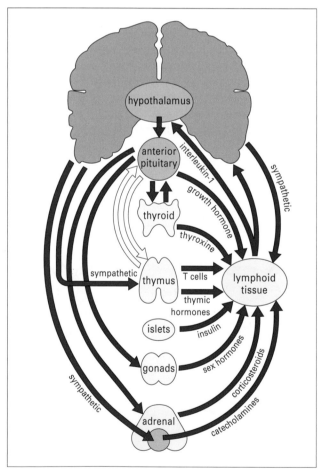

Fig. 12.21 Neuroendocrine interactions with the immune system The diagram indicates some of the potential connections between the endocrine, nervous and immune systems. *Blue arrows* indicate nervous connections, *red arrows* indicate hormonal interactions and *white arrows* indicate postulated connections for which the effector molecules have not been established.

CRITICAL THINKING: REGULATION OF THE IMMUNE RESPONSE
See Critical thinking: Explanations, section 12

A scientist is starting a project looking at EAE, a mouse model of MS in which a type 1 response dominates. She decides to test her protocol on mice of two strains: C57BL/6 and BALB/c. She mixes MBP with complete Freund's adjuvant (an emulsion of oil in water with heat-killed mycobacteria) and uses this to immunize the two strains of mice. Two days later, she treats the mice with pertussis toxin, which is thought to make the CNS more accessible to immune cells.

Over the course of a few weeks, the C57BL/6 mice develop limp tails, weak hind limbs and in some cases partial hind limb paralysis, but the BALB/c mice are unaffected.

1. Why do you think this might have occurred?
2. How could you test your hypothesis?

The scientist wonders whether the two strains of mice might differ in their responses to other diseases. She takes new cohorts of C57BL/6 and BALB/c mice and infects their footpads with *Leishmania*, an intracellular pathogen that infects macrophages.

3. What kind of immune response would you expect to be effective against *Leishmania*?

Looking at the lymph nodes draining the site of infection, the scientist observes a large number of *Leishmania* parasites in the BALB/c mice, but not in the C57BL/6 mice.

4. Why do you think this might have occurred?

The scientist notes that the draining lymph nodes of the C57BL/6 express high levels of IL-12 mRNA. In her next experiment, she injects recombinant IL-12 into the BALB/c mice at the same time as infecting them.

5. What do you predict will happen?

FURTHER READING

Cain DW, Cidlowski JA. Immune regulation by glucocorticoids. Nat Rev Immunol 2017;17:233–247.

Ganeshan K, Chawla A. Metabolic regulation of immune responses. Annu Rev Immunol 2014;32:609–634.

Hepworth MR, Sonnenberg GF. Regulation of the adaptive immune system by innate lymphoid cells. Curr Opin Immunol 2014;27:75–82.

Hjelm F, Carlsson F, Getahun A, Heyman B. Antibody-mediated regulation of the immune response. Scand J Immunol 2006;64(3):177–184.

Josefowicz SZ, Lu LF, Rudensky AY. Regulatory T cells: mechanisms of differentiation and function. Annu Rev Immunol 2012;30:531–564.

Korn T, Bettelli E, Oukka M, Kuchroo VK. IL-17 and TH17 cells. Annu Rev Immunol 2009;27:485–517.

Murphy KM, Stockinger B. Effector T cell plasticity: flexibility in the face of changing circumstances. Nat Immunol 2010;11:674–690.

Rosser EC, Mauri C. Regulatory B cells: origin, phenotype, and function. Immunity 2015;42(4):607–612.

Shevach EM. Mechanisms of Foxp3[b] T regulatory cell-mediated suppression. Immunity 2009;30:636–645.

Taub DD. Neuroendocrine interactions in the immune system. Cell Immunol 2008;252:1–10.

Vivier E, Artis D, Colonna M, et al. Innate lymphoid cells: 10 years on. Cell 2018;174:1054–1066.

13

Immune Responses in Tissues

SUMMARY

- **A tissue can influence local immune responses**, promoting some classes of immunity and suppressing others. Each tissue has distinctive sets of antigen-presenting cells and the vascular endothelium expresses chemokines and adhesion molecules that attract specific subsets of leukocytes.
- **Certain sites in the body are immunologically privileged** and fully allogeneic tissue can be transplanted into them without risk of rejection. These sites, which include the anterior chamber of the eye and the central nervous system (CNS), suppress immune responses that can do irreparable local damage.
- **The endothelium in the CNS has barrier properties, which exclude most serum proteins.** Direct cell–cell interactions and anti-inflammatory cytokines normally suppress immune responses. Acute inflammation in the CNS is characterized by TH1 cells, TH17 cells and mononuclear phagocytes.
- **Immune responses in gut and lung distinguish between pathogens and innocuous organisms and antigens.** The immune response in mucosal tissues tends to promote TH2-type responses with IgA production. Gut enterocytes influence the local immune response. Intra-epithelial lymphocytes (IELs) respond to stress induced class Ib molecules and produce many immunomodulatory cytokines. Regulatory T cells normally limit the level of inflammatory reactions.
- **T cells are present in normal skin and immune responses are characterized by T-cell infiltration.** The endothelium of the dermis attracts TH1 cells, which express cutaneous lymphocyte antigen (CLA) and receptors for IFNγ-induced chemokines.

TISSUE-SPECIFIC IMMUNE RESPONSES

What determines whether an immune response should consist of, for example, activated cytotoxic T lymphocytes (CTLs) or a particular class of antibodies? Although immune responses are primarily tailored to the pathogen, there is also a strong influence from the local tissue, where the immune response occurs (Fig. 13.1).

This chapter focuses on:

- the features of immune responses that are unique to individual tissues; and
- the mechanisms by which the tissues influence local and systemic characteristics.

There are several reasons why a particular organ may need to modify local immunity. For example, tissues such as liver or skin have substantial capacity for regeneration and a CTL response to kill virally infected cells is advantageous. In contrast, the capacity for regeneration of neurons in the central nervous system (CNS) is very limited and infected cells are often resistant to killing by CTLs: the infection is controlled but not eradicated. *Herpes simplex* and *Herpes zoster* have exploited this ecological niche and can remain latent in neurons for many years, sporadically reactivating to produce cold sores or shingles, respectively.

These observations suggest that the immune responses in tissues are modulated in order to be appropriate for that site and even within one tissue there may be micro-environments that have their own physiology and preferred immune reactivity. Consequently, tissues have evolved regulatory mechanisms that influence the immune response that occurs within them. Tissue-specific controls occur from the earliest stages of development, when mononuclear phagocytes populate tissues and differentiate into tissue-specific macrophages with distinctive phenotypes.

Some tissues are immunologically privileged. There are certain sites in the body where fully allogeneic tissue can be transplanted without risk of rejection. These include the anterior chamber of the eye, the brain and testes. Several factors may contribute to the **immunological privilege** of these sites, some of which affect the initiation of the immune response and some affect the effector phase.

The 'privileged sites' were long thought to be locations where adaptive immune responses are so dangerous that the immune system is not allowed entry, is destroyed upon arrival or is prevented from functioning. Recent evidence suggests that the concept of privileged sites may have been a misconception based on the limitations of the experimental systems. Once the experiments were expanded to include a wider variety of assays, it became apparent that privileged sites are not immunologically impaired. They are simply sites that are able to promote certain kinds of beneficial classes of immune responses while suppressing classes that can do irreparable local damage.

Locally produced cytokines and chemokines influence tissue-specific immune responses. A number of factors control the type of immune response occurring in each tissue:

- The vascular endothelium plays a major role in determining which leukocytes will enter the tissue by secretion of distinct blends of chemokines and expression of site-specific adhesion molecules.

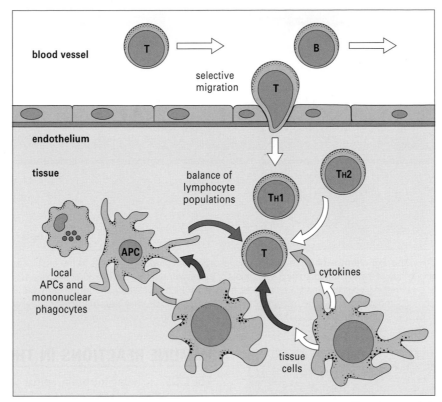

Fig. 13.1 Factors controlling the characteristic immune response of a tissue The characteristic immune response of a tissue is controlled both by the leukocyte populations present and by the direct and indirect signals from the endogenous cells of the tissue. The population of lymphocytes that enter a particular tissue is controlled by the vascular endothelium in that tissue. Antigen presentation within the tissue depends on the populations of antigen-presenting cells *(APCs)*, which include resident mononuclear phagocytes and dendritic cells. APCs and T cells are influenced directly by endogenous cells of the tissue and indirectly via cytokines.

- The local antigen-presenting cells, including the resident mononuclear phagocytes and dendritic cell populations, determine whether the tissue environment promotes or limits T-cell activation and what type of response occurs.
- Cells in the tissue can also exert their effects via cytokines/chemokines and by direct cell–cell interactions. In effect, cells of the tissue can signal infection damage or stress and modulate immune cell activation.

Endothelium controls which leukocytes enter a tissue.
Migration of leukocytes into different tissues of the body is dependent on the vascular endothelium in each tissue. For many years, it was thought that the endothelium in different tissues was essentially similar, with the possible exception of tissues such as the brain and retina, which have barrier properties (see later). However, it was also well known that inflammation in different tissues had different characteristics, even when the inducing agents were similar.

It is now clear that a major element controlling inflammation and the immune response is the vascular endothelium in each tissue, which has its own characteristics; different endothelia produce distinctive blends of chemokines (Table 13.1) and have their own sets of adhesion molecules to mediate leukocyte transmigration into the tissue. In addition, the endothelium can

TABLE 13.1 **Production of Chemokines by Endothelium Derived from Different Human Tissues**			
	ENDOTHELIUM		
	Lung	**Dermis**	**Brain**
CXCL8	++	++	+++
CXCL10	+	+	+++
CCL2	+++	++	+
CCL5	+	++	+

Brain endothelium produces high levels of CXCL8 and CXCL10 associated with a TH1-type immune response. Dermal endothelium produces high levels of CCL5 associated with T-cell migration, whereas lung endothelium produces high levels of CCL2, a chemokine that causes macrophage migration.

transport chemokines produced by cells in the tissue from the basal to the luminal surface by transcytosis or by surface diffusion in tissues that lack barrier properties (Fig. 13.2).

The surface (glycocalyx) of vascular endothelium also varies considerably between tissues and this affects which chemokines are retained on the luminal surface to signal to circulating leukocytes.

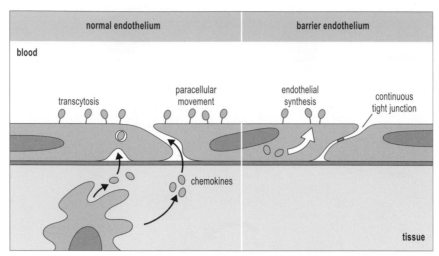

Fig. 13.2 Transport of chemokines In most tissues, chemokines produced by cells in the tissue can move to the lumenal surface of the endothelium by transcytosis or by movement through the paracellular junctions, to be held on the endothelial glycocalyx. In tissues such as the brain, which have a barrier endothelium, there is limited transcytosis and almost no paracellular movement of proteins such as chemokines. In these tissues, chemokine production by the endothelium is particularly important in controlling leukocyte migration.

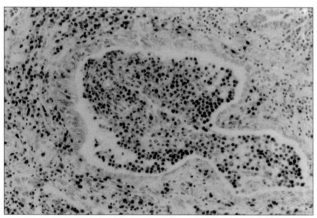

Fig. 13.3 Histological section of an airway from a case of fatal asthma The lumen of an alveolus of the lung is heavily infiltrated with inflammatory exudates, fibrin and cellular debris. Immunohistochemical staining with monoclonal antibody against EG2 indicates that the majority of cells are eosinophils. (Courtesy Arshad SH. Allergy: An Illustrated Colour Text. Philadelphia: Churchill Livingstone; 2002. With permission from Elsevier.)

Hence the different sets of leukocytes present in each tissue can be partly related to the chemokines synthesized by the local cells. For example, in normal lung there is a high level of macrophage migration, which relates to the high expression of CCL2 (macrophage chemotactic protein-1) by lung endothelium. In allergic asthma, the proportion of eosinophils increases, as a result of the production of IL-5 and CCL3 (eotaxin), which are characteristic of the TH2 response that predominates in mucosal tissues (Fig. 13.3). By contrast, in acute inflammation in the CNS TH1 cells and mononuclear phagocytes predominate. This can be related to the production of IFNγ-induced chemokines, such as CXCL10 by brain endothelium.

The following sections outline the distinctive features of immune responses in a selection of tissues.

IMMUNE REACTIONS IN THE CNS

The CNS, including the brain, spinal cord and retina of the eye, is substantially shielded from immune reactions. The peripheral nervous system is also partially protected. The low levels of immune reactivity in the brain are ascribed to a number of factors:

- The blood–brain barrier (endothelium plus astrocytes) prevents the movement of over 99% of large serum proteins into the brain tissue (IgG, complement, etc.); there are similar barriers in the eye (blood–retinal barrier).
- Low levels of major histocompatibility complex (MHC) molecule expression and co-stimulatory molecules result in inefficient antigen presentation. The brain lacks (leukocyte) dendritic cells and these molecules are normally at low levels on microglia, the brain's resident mononuclear phagocyte population.
- There are no conventional lymphatics in the CNS, although drainage can occur to cervical lymph nodes through the cribriform plate. The meninges do have lymphatics and immune reactions in meninges have different characteristics from those within the brain.
- Low levels of leukocyte traffic into the CNS compared with other tissues.
- Neurons have direct immunosuppressive actions on glial cells. Astrocytes, neurons and some glial cells produce immunosuppressive cytokines.
- Some neurons and glia are protected against CTLs because they express Fas-ligand and can induce apoptosis in the CTL, using one of the mechanisms normally used by CTLs.

The blood–brain barrier excludes most antibodies from the CNS. The blood–brain barrier is a composite structure formed by the specialized brain endothelium and the foot processes of astrocytes. Astrocytes are required to induce the special properties of brain endothelial cells, including continuous tight

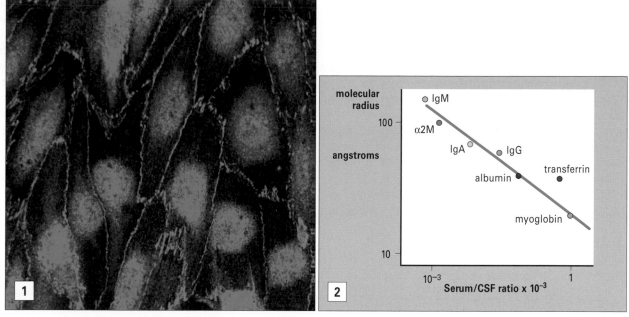

Fig. 13.4 **The blood–brain barrier** (**1**) Brain endothelial cells have a continuous ring of tight junctions, identified in this micrograph by the junctional marker ZO-1. The resulting permeability barrier excludes serum proteins from the brain tissue. (**2**) The graph shows the serum/cerebrospinal fluid *(CSF)* ratio for different proteins. There is an inverse relationship between molecular size and the level in CSF. Molecules such as transferrin, which are transported into the brain, are present at higher levels than would be expected from their size. Immunoglobulins are not transported.

junctions connecting them to neighbouring endothelial cells. The junctions prevent large hydrophilic molecules from moving through the extracellular space between blood and brain (Fig. 13.4). For example, the level of IgG found in the CNS is normally approximately 0.2% of the level found in serum. The level may rise during an immune reaction as the endothelial barrier becomes more permeable in response to inflammatory cytokines (IFNγ, TNFα). In some conditions, such as multiple sclerosis, there is often local synthesis of antibody within the CNS, which is reflected in abnormally high antibody levels in cerebrospinal fluid, even accounting for the increased leakage into the CNS. This finding demonstrates that some B cells have migrated into the CNS and plasma cells have been identified in the spaces surrounding the larger blood vessels in diseases such as multiple sclerosis. Macrophages also contribute to immune reactions in the CNS and they can synthesize some complement components locally (e.g. C3). However, the overall level of serum proteins, including antibodies and complement, rarely exceeds 2% of the levels in serum even in the most severe inflammatory reactions.

Neurons suppress immune reactivity in neighbouring glial cells. Healthy neurons are able to extend an immunosuppressive action to surrounding cells, an effect first observed in co-cultures that included neurons and astrocytes. Neurons in contact with the astrocytes suppressed the induction of MHC class I by IFNγ, but no effect was seen when the cells were not in contact, thereby excluding the possibility that suppression was a result of cytokines alone (Table 13.2). Subsequently, a similar effect was shown for induction of astrocyte MHC class II molecules.

TABLE 13.2 Immunosuppression by Neurons

INTERFERON-Υ	NEURONS IN CO-CULTURE WITH ASTROCYTES		
	Astrocytes alone	No contact	In contact
−	+	+	+
+	+++	+++	+

MHC, Major histocompatibility complex.
Expression of MHC class I molecules on astrocytes cultured alone or with neurons. Neurons in contact with the astrocytes suppress IFNγ-induced induction of MHC molecules.

Later work showed that the electrical activity of the neurons is important: neurons that are functioning normally can suppress their neighbouring glial cells (and downregulate their own MHC molecules), whereas damaged neurons lift the local immunosuppression to allow an immune response to develop. For example, severing the facial nerve in a model of neuro-inflammation causes leukocytes to enter the facial nucleus where the nerve bodies are located. These neurons are still alive, but they are able to signal via the glial cells and the endothelium that they are damaged.

Neurons can also act on microglia, which are resident mononuclear phagocytes of the CNS. The molecular mechanisms that underlie the suppressive activity of neurons include:
• Expression of CD200 and fractalkine (a cell surface chemokine CX3CL1) on the surface of neurons inhibits the activation of microglia by binding to CD200L and the chemokine receptor CX3CR1, respectively, on the microglia.

- Neuronal CD47 binds to a microglial signal regulatory protein (SIRP-1α), which inhibits phagocytosis and TNFα production by the microglia.

Immunosuppressive cytokines regulate immunity in the normal CNS. Observations of immune reactions in the CNS have led to the view that TH1-type immune responses with macrophage activation and IFNγ/TNFα production or TH17-type responses are most damaging. By comparison, TH2-type immune responses are less damaging and strains of animals that make strong antibody responses against CNS antigens are often less susceptible to CNS pathology than strains that make weaker antibody responses. Certainly, the production of IL-12, IL-23 and TNFα are associated with damaging responses in CNS (Fig 13.5). Interestingly, IFNγ appears to have a dual role, involved in the acute phase of CNS inflammation and necessary for the recovery phase. In some neuroinflammation models, deletion of the IFNγ receptor gene has not reduced the pathology, whereas deletion of IL-23 receptors does. Such observations have led to the view that **immune deviation** (the switching of an immune response from TH1 towards a TH2 type) can be protective in the CNS.

This view is supported by findings that cells of the normal CNS can produce cytokines associated with TH2 responses. For example, astrocytes produce TGFβ and microglia produce IL-10 when co-cultured with T cells and both astrocytes and neurons secrete prostaglandins, which inhibit lymphocyte activation. Additionally, several neuropeptides and transmitters (e.g. noradrenaline, vasoactive intestinal peptide and calcitonin gene-related peptide (CGRP)) are suppressive. Acute immune responses can develop in the CNS, particularly in susceptible strains, but the normal immunosuppressive controls usually reassert themselves within 1–2 weeks, causing remission. Such a relapsing–remitting pattern of disease occurs in multiple sclerosis and the animal model of CNS inflammation, CREAE (chronic relapsing experimental allergic encephalomyelitis) (Fig. 13.6).

Immune reactions in CNS damage oligodendrocytes. Oligodendrocytes are glial cells that produce the myelin sheaths, which act as electrical insulation around nerve axons. When immune reactions occur in the CNS, these cells appear to be particularly vulnerable (Fig. 13.7). For example, multiple sclerosis is characterized by focal areas of myelin loss called plaques, typically a few millimetres in diameter. Nerve transmission through these demyelinated areas is seriously impaired, which may cause disease symptoms such as weakness and loss of sensation. But it is only in the later stages of the disease that the neurons themselves are damaged.

The reason that oligodendrocytes are vulnerable in multiple sclerosis is less clear. It is possible that they are most readily damaged, because they normally maintain very large amounts of plasma membrane forming the myelin sheath. There is evidence that they can be targeted by autoantibodies that allow macrophages and activated microglia to recognize them and

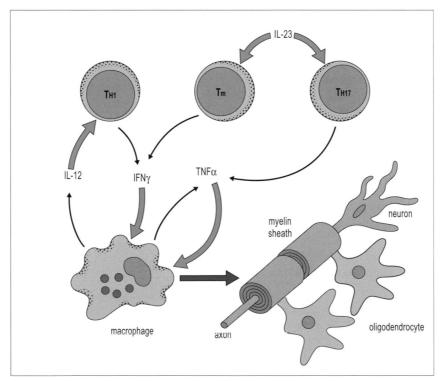

Fig. 13.5 Immune regulation in the central nervous system (CNS) In immune reactions in the CNS, the myelin sheath formed by oligodendrocytes around nerve axons is particularly susceptible to damage by activated macrophages. Macrophages are activated by IFNγ produced by TH1 cells and memory T cells *(Tm)* and IL-12 is important in promoting this type of immune response. Alternatively, TH17 cells induced by IL-23 and mononuclear phagocytes (macrophages and microglia) can also produce TNFα, which enhances macrophage activation and contributes to myelin damage. *Black arrows,* production; *green arrows,* activation.

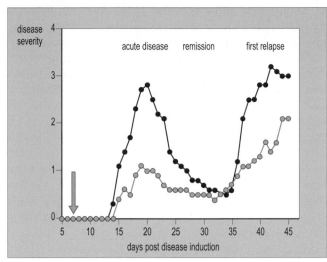

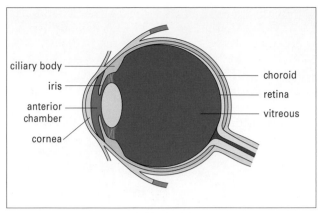

Fig. 13.6 Chronic relapsing experimental allergic encephalomyelitis (CREAE) The relapsing remitting disease course of CREAE in Biozzi Ab/H mice is shown in the days after immunization with myelin components on day 0 *(black)*. Animals that were treated at day 7 with a cell line expressing a soluble TNF receptor (to mop up TNFα in the brain) had a less serious acute disease and relapse. (Based on data of Croxford JL, Triantaphyllopoulos KA, Neve RM, et al. J Immunol 2000;164:2776–2781.)

Fig. 13.8 Anatomical and immunological basis of immune privilege in the eye The uvea, consisting of the iris, ciliary body and choroid, is highly vascularized but lacks draining lymphatic vessels. Tight junctions between the vessels in the iris and between non-pigmented ciliary epithelial cells maintain a blood–aqueous barrier. Similar junctions on the retinal pigment epithelium and the retinal endothelium maintain a blood–retinal barrier. The iris and ciliary body secrete immunomodulatory cytokines.

The eye has therefore evolved several major mechanisms to suppress cell-mediated responses actively.

- First, the epithelial cells lining the anterior chamber and the cornea express Fas ligand; corneal allografts that lack Fas ligand (in rats) are almost always rejected. This mechanism is thought to protect partly the cells of the eye from damage by CTLs, if they have become infected by virus. Observations that the expression of Fas ligand is associated with the resolution of anterior uveitis and limited angiogenesis support this view.
- Second, the fluid of the anterior chamber contains cytokines such as TGFβ and IL-10, which deviate the immune response towards the less-damaging Th2 type and promote development of regulatory T cells.
- Third, the cells of the iris and ciliary body secrete immunomodulatory cytokines, including TGFβ, vasoactive intestinal peptide (VIP), γ-melanocyte-stimulating hormone (γMSH) and CGRP.

These cytokine and molecular controls on immunity are underpinned by the cellular organization of the eye, which has barriers that limit the movement of molecules into the retina, anterior chamber and vitreous (Fig. 13.8). As with the CNS, the combination of immunosuppressive and tolerogenic mechanisms normally maintains immune privilege in the eye.

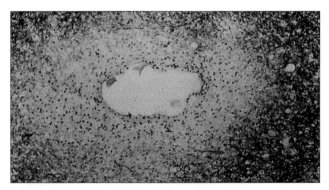

Fig. 13.7 Type IV hypersensitivity in central nervous system Myelin stain of cerebral cortex in a case of para-infectious encephalomyelitis shows demyelination in an extended area around a venule where lymphocyte infiltration has occurred. (Courtesy Dr N Woodroofe and Dr H Okazaki.)

that release of reactive oxygen and nitrogen intermediates from the phagocytes then damage the myelin.

IMMUNE REACTIONS IN THE EYE

The eye is a complex organ and subject to immune privilege. Indeed, the retina and optic nerve are extensions of the CNS with neurons, glia and a blood–retinal barrier, which is analogous to the blood–brain barrier. Also, like the CNS, the eye lacks a conventional lymphatic drainage system.

Allogeneic corneal grafting is usually successful as a result of immune privilege, although rejection may occur: the eye has very limited self-regenerative capacity and can be completely destroyed by a cell-mediated immune response with the concomitant local production of TNFα and IFNγ (Fig. 13.w1).

IMMUNE RESPONSES IN THE GUT AND LUNG

In contrast to the CNS, the gut and lung are examples of tissues that are continuously in contact with high levels of harmless commensal organisms and innocuous antigens as well as potential pathogens. It is essential that the immune system in the gut does not make strong immune responses against antigens in food or harmless commensal bacteria. (Note that food antigens are primarily present in the small intestine, whereas bacterial antigens predominate in the large intestine.) Similarly, many airborne antigens (e.g. pollen) are harmless and a strong

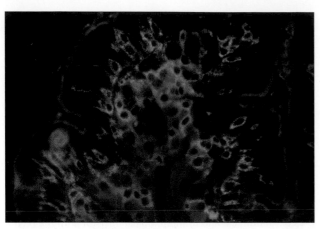

Fig. 13.9 IgA synthesis in the lamina propria Lymphoid cells in the epithelium and lamina propria fluoresce green using antibody to leukocyte common antigen (CD45). Red cytoplasmic staining is obtained with anti-IgA antibody, which detects plasma cells in the lamina propria and IgA in the mucus. (Courtesy Professor G Janossy.)

immune response in the lung is inappropriate: it would be considered hypersensitivity.

Nevertheless, antigens introduced orally can invoke an immune response that is appropriate for mucosal surfaces: namely, the production of local IgA and some systemic IgG (Fig. 13.9). However, there is generally little production of TH1 cells or CTLs and limited cell-mediated immune responses. The populations of tissue cells and leukocytes present in the gut are illustrated in Figure 13.10.

Gut enterocytes influence the local immune response. Intestinal epithelial cells (enterocytes) are the major cell type forming the epithelium of the gut. They have continuous tight junctions and thus form a barrier to prevent antigens from entering the body. They are polarized, so that microbial products such as lipopolysaccharide (LPS) on the basal membrane (tissue side) will activate them, but if in contact with the apical membrane (gut lumen) they do not. They can also detect pathogen invasion via intracellular receptors such as NOD-1. Enterocytes can package antigen fragments from partly digested gut contents in secreted vesicles called **tolerosomes** coated with αVβ6 integrin, which directs them to the local dendritic cells. Hence the enterocytes form a staging post in development of oral tolerance or immunity and influence the local immune response by secreting a variety of immunomodulatory factors such as TGFβ, VIP, IL-1, IL-6, IL-7, CXCL8 and CCL3.

Paneth cells are a specialized epithelial cell found at the bottoms of the crypts. These crypts produce several natural antibiotic peptides (Fig. 13.w2), which help prevent bacterial overgrowth in these sensitive sites of cellular differentiation. M cells are another specialized form of enterocyte that can transport intact antigens to the gut lymphoid tissues.

The gut immune system tolerates many antigens but reacts to pathogens. There are many examples where an individual encounters an antigen in food and subsequently becomes

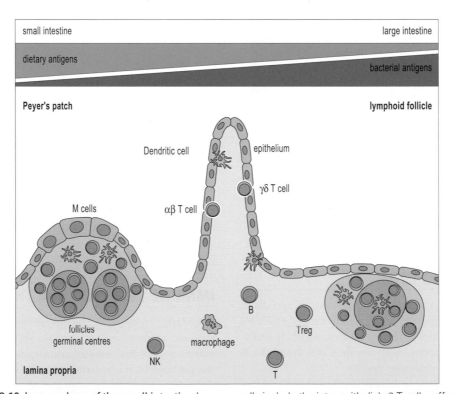

Fig. 13.10 Immunology of the small intestine Immune cells include the intra-epithelial γδ T cells, effector αβ T cells and dendritic cells found in the epithelial layer interact with epithelium via αEβ7 integrins. The lamina propria includes populations of macrophages, effector T cells and regulatory T cells (Tregs). IgA-producing B cells and associated T cells are found in the encapsulated lymphoid organs, including the Peyer's patches and the lymphoid follicles. Tregs are also found in T-cell areas of the lymphoid tissues.

tolerant to it. This phenomenon is called **oral tolerance** and it is related to **nasal tolerance** where antigen delivered to nasal mucosa as an aerosol inhibits subsequent immunization.

Oral tolerance illustrates two points:

- Tolerance can extend systemically to non-mucosal sites.
- It is transferable to naive individuals by CD4 (or occasionally CD8) T cells.

Oral tolerance is related to the development of Tregs in mesenteric lymph nodes during development. These cells express α4β7-integrin, which binds to the adhesion molecule MadCAM-1, expressed on the endothelium of the intestinal lamina propria. The induction of α4β7 and the chemokine receptor CCR9 depends on αEβ7 intestinal dendritic cells, a distinct population that differentiates in the mesenteric lymph nodes and promotes development and recirculation of the intestinal Tregs.

Tolerance is not the only form of immunity that arises from ingestion of antigens. **Oral vaccination** has been recognized since 1919 when Besredka noticed that rabbits were protected from fatal dysentery by oral immunization with killed shigella. The attenuated polio vaccine that was developed in the 1950s was also given as an oral vaccination. In both cases these vaccines are not viewed as harmless antigens by the immune system; the activation depends on antigen presentation and induction of co-stimulation:

- Shigella contain antigens that activate the intracellular PRR, NOD-1.
- The polio genome is ssRNA (recognized by TLR7 and TLR8) and it replicates using a dsRNA intermediate, which is recognized by TLR3.

Hence, the default state of the gut immune system is to tolerate the antigenic load from food and the commensal microbiome, but the balance is tipped towards immune activation if pathogens (PAMPs) or damage (DAMPs) are recognized.

Intra-epithelial lymphocytes produce many immunomodulatory cytokines. The IELs are a diverse but distinct population that express α4β7 integrins, which promote homing to the mucosal tissues; α4β7-integrin interacts with MadCaM on mucosal endothelium and αEβ7-integrin binds to E-cadherin, present on epithelium. Gut enterocytes express E-cadherin, and secrete TGFβ, which upregulates the expression of αEβ7, and thus they provide a signal for the selective accumulation and retention of IELs.

Tolerance to food antigens depends on a variety of overlapping mechanisms, including how antigen is presented, but the production of TGFβ and IL-10 from Tregs and TH2 cells also limits inflammatory reactions. For example, IL-10 knockout mice develop colitis if they contact appropriate triggering microorganisms and, in humans, IL-10 is a susceptibility locus for ulcerative colitis. TGFβ is an important TH2-promoting cytokine and it also induces FoxP3 in naive T cells, thus promoting development of regulatory T cells.

When immune responses develop in the gut, IELs can produce IL-1, lymphotoxin (LT), IFNγ and TNFα. Therefore, a switch in the balance of pro-inflammatory cytokines and regulatory cytokines in the epithelium and lamina propria occurs when damaging immune reactions develop in the gut.

Many IELs have an activated or memory phenotype and recognize the ancient conserved MHC class-I -like molecules **MICA** and **MICB**, which are upregulated by cellular stress. When activated by MICA and MICB, some of the mucosa-associated lymphocytes secrete epidermal growth factor (EGF) and may therefore induce repair and renewal of damaged intestinal epithelium.

Chronic Inflammation in the Gut

The most common types of chronic inflammatory disease of the gut are inflammatory bowel disease (IBD), including Crohn's disease, which may affect the entire intestinal tract, and ulcerative colitis affecting the large intestine. Both of these conditions are thought to occur because of an overreaction to intestinal bacteria; both have a strong genetic component and pattern recognition receptors (e.g. NOD2) are disease susceptibility loci.

In coeliac disease, the patient is sensitive to gluten in the food and susceptibility is strongly related to HLA haplotype and to loci for inflammatory cytokines and chemokines. In all three conditions, ulcerative colitis, coeliac disease and Crohn's disease, there is production of TNFα and IFNγ, dysregulation of the normal mucosal immune response and damage to tissue, including the epithelium responsible for absorbing nutrients. These chronic inflammatory diseases all appear to be a result of a reduction of the normal tolerogenic mechanisms in the gut, so that the immune response is tipped towards inflammation.

Immune Responses in the Lung

The lung is another example of a tissue that is in normal contact with external antigens and pathogens, including bacteria from the upper airways. Particles trapped in the trachea and on the bronchial mucosa are propelled upwards on the ciliary escalator, which considerably reduces the antigen load reaching the lung. Bronchioles and alveoli contain large numbers of pulmonary macrophages, while the lung tissue also contains lymphocytes and respiratory (plasmacytoid) dendritic cells (pDCs) (Fig. 13.11). The macrophages and pDCs are major sources of IFNα and IFNβ, which are particularly important in controlling the initial spread of viral infections.

Early recruitment of leukocytes to the lung is mediated by chemokines secreted by the macrophages, pDCs and the epithelial cells of the lung itself (pneumocytes). Neutrophils and natural killer (NK) cells are the first cells to appear after infection, while dendritic cells traffic to the local bronchus-associated lymphoid tissue (BALT). Migration of the dendritic cells normally occurs at a steady rate, but following infection there is an increase in movement of pDCs to the lymphoid tissues and they increase their expression of MHC class II and co-stimulatory molecules CD80/86 and CD40.

The structure of BALT resembles that of other encapsulated lymphoid tissues, with distinct T-cell and B-cell areas, and high endothelial venules and the migration of the pDCs to the local lymph nodes depends on signalling from CCL21 acting on CCR7, as in other tissues.

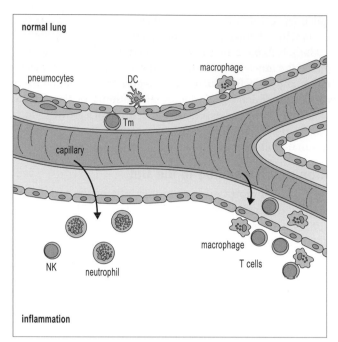

Fig. 13.11 Immune responses in the lung In the resting lung, memory T cells and macrophages are present in the alveolar air spaces and the lung tissue. Respiratory dendritic cells *(DCs)* are located below the respiratory epithelium, which consists of type I pneumocytes with a large surface area for gas exchange and type II pneumocytes, which secrete surfactants. In acute inflammation, natural killer *(NK)* cells and neutrophils enter the air spaces. How the inflammatory response develops depends on the initiating pathogen. Viral infections result in the accumulation of effector T cells and macrophages, whereas neutrophils persist in many bacterial infections.

In viral infections of the lung, the early recruitment of NK cells, which recognize virus-infected cells via NCR1, helps control the spread of the infection, until the later arrival of CD4[+] and CD8[+] effector T cells; CD8[+] CTLs recognize and destroy virally infected pneumocytes using Fas/FasL, and by releasing granzymes and perforin.

In bacterial infections, neutrophils and macrophages are prevalent in the bronchi (bronchitis) or the alveoli (pneumonia) and the smaller air spaces fill with a fluid exudate that leaks through the damaged pulmonary epithelium.

IMMUNE REACTIONS IN THE LIVER

The liver has an open circulation and receives blood from both the hepatic artery and the portal vein and therefore it is potentially in contact with any bacteria or bacterial products that have invaded the gut. It is estimated that 99% of LPS that enters the liver is removed during transit, thus protecting other tissues. Kupffer cells that line the liver sinusoids and constitute more than 90% of all tissue macrophages are a major element of the liver immune system. Like lung macrophages and microglia, they are initially derived from yolk-sac macrophages, but they can also differentiate from blood monocytes, expressing Ig receptors as well as TLRs and scavenger receptors. In addition to regular macrophage complement receptors CR1 and CR3, they express a complement

receptor of the immunoglobulin superfamily (CRIg), which can tether C3b-coated pathogens or debris under shear stress and thus can efficiently remove these particles. Potentially, Kupffer cells can act as antigen-presenting cells (APCs), as they express MHC class II and CD1d, which presents α-galactosylceramide to NKT cells (up to 25% of liver lymphocytes are NKT cells with a limited repertoire of TCRs; see Chapter 6). However, Kupffer cells normally lack co-stimulatory molecules and are not efficient in lymphocyte activation.

Sinusoidal liver endothelial cells also line the sinusoids and they may contribute to the low immune reactivity of the liver. They have low levels of MHC molecules and co-stimulatory molecules and express PD-L1, which binds to PD-1 on T cells to induce tolerance. They also constitutively express IL-10. Like the gut, the default status of the liver is to limit inflammatory reactions unless stimulated by PAMPs or DAMPs.

IMMUNE REACTIONS IN THE SKIN

The skin is the largest organ of the body and in humans there may be up to 10^6 T cells/cm^2, in the dermis, tissue macrophages and at least two major populations of dendritic cells, the Langerhans cells in the epidermis and the plasmacytoid dendritic cells, mostly in the dermis. T cells constitute the major cell type present both in normal skin and in immune reactions (Fig. 13.12). They are characterized by a skin-homing marker CLA (cutaneous lymphocyte antigen) and the chemokine receptors CCR4 and CCR6; CCR4 recognizes CCL5 (RANTES), which is strongly expressed by dermal endothelium (see Table 13.1). CLA is a sialylated molecule that binds to ELAM-1 (endothelial leukocyte adhesion molecule-1), a lectin-like molecule that is strongly expressed on endothelium in the skin. CLA[+] lymphocytes also express high levels of receptors for IL-12 and IL-2 and the chemokine receptor CXCR3, which recognizes IFNγ-induced chemokines. This can explain why active immune responses in skin are characterized by a T$_H$1-type immune response, with high expression of IFNγ and low IL-4. However,

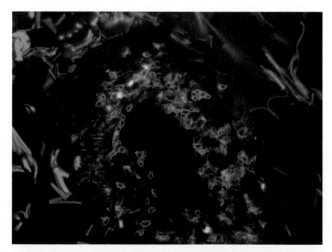

Fig. 13.12 Tregs in the skin A section of normal human skin (dermis) co-stained with antibody to CD3 *(red)* and FOXP3 *(green)* to identify regulatory T cells. T-cell infiltrates, including Tregs, are seen around a vessel. (Courtesy of Dr Rachael Clark. Blood 2007;109:194–202.)

as inflammation subsides, there is an increase in IL-4 production and a shift towards a TH2-type response. An outline of the initiation and effector phases of immune responses in the skin (type IV hypersensitivity) are shown in Figures 26.16–26.18. Immune reactions in skin are also seen in psoriasis and mycosis fungoides, both with strong T-cell infiltration.

The cells of the tissue also contribute to the development of the immune response. Keratinocytes, which form the epidermis, express high levels of IL-1, which may be released when the skin is damaged, to promote inflammation and repair. Fibroblasts in the dermis respond to TNFα by releasing IL-15, which activates effector T cells as an immune response develops and induces Tregs during the resolution phase.

CONCLUSIONS

The immune responses and inflammatory reactions that occur in each tissue are distinctive and are directed by interactions between the endothelial chemokines and adhesion molecules and the circulating leukocytes. The endothelium in each tissue synthesizes distinct sets of chemokines, and expresses specific adhesion molecules, which attracts distinct leukocyte subsets.

In the CNS and the skin, TH1-type immune responses are favoured, whereas TH2-type responses predominate in mucosal tissues. The type of immune response may switch within individual tissues as the reaction resolves, although this is very much dependent on the inducing antigen, and the immune status of the individual. In tissues with barrier properties, the endothelium also limits entrance of immunoglobulins and serum molecules and the movement of cytokines from cells in the tissue to the blood. Consequently, vascular endothelium and the resident cells of the tissue play a central role in determining the characteristics of the inflammatory response in each tissue.

CRITICAL THINKING: IMMUNE REACTIONS IN THE GUT

See Critical thinking: Explanations, section 13

Oyster poisoning occurs when an individual eats an oyster that contains concentrated bacteria or Protoctista from sea water. Often an individual who has eaten an infected oyster will then be unable to eat oysters again—even good oysters make them ill. Construct a logical explanation for this observation, based on your understanding of immune reactions in the gut.

FURTHER READING

Caspi R. A look at autoimmunity and inflammation in the eye. J Clin Invest 2010;120:3073–3083.

Engelhardt B, Ransohoff RM. The ins and outs of T-lymphocyte trafficking to the CNS: anatomical sites and molecular mechanisms. Trends Immunol 2005;26:485–495.

Fagarasan S, Kawamoto S, Kanagawa O. Adaptive immune regulation in the gut: T cell dependent and T cell independent IgA synthesis. Ann Rev Immunol 2010;28:243–273.

Galea I, Bechmann I, Perry VH. What is immune privilege? Trends Immunol 2007;28:12–18.

Izcue A, Coombes JL. Regulatory lymphocytes and intestinal inflammation. Ann Rev Immunol 2009;27:313–318.

Kubes P, Jenne C. Immune responses in the liver. Ann Rev Immunol 2018;36:247–277.

Male DK. Adaptive immune responses in the CNS. In: Woodroofe N, Amor S, eds. Neuroinflammation and CNS Disorders, Oxford: Wiley-Blackwell; 2014, pp 37–57.

Miron N, Cristea V. Enterocytes: active cells in tolerance to food and microbial antigens in the gut. Clin Exp Immunol 2011;167:405–412.

Ohnmacht C, Park JH, Cording S, Wing JB, Atarashi K, et al. The microbiota regulates type 2 immunity through RORγ+ T cells. Science 2015;349:989–993.

Panduro M, Benoist C, Mathis D. Tissue Tregs. Ann Rev Immunol 2016;34:609–633.

Richmond JM, Harris JE. Immunology and skin in health and disease. Cold Spring Harb Perspect Med 2014;4(12):a015339.

14

Immunity to Viruses

SUMMARY

- **Innate immune responses restrict the early stages of infection, delay spread of virus and promote the activation of adaptive responses**. Innate defences are triggered following recognition of molecular patterns characteristic of viral but not host components. Type I interferons (IFNs) exert direct antiviral activity and also activate other innate and adaptive responses. Natural killer (NK) cells kill virally infected cells. Macrophages act to destroy virus and virus-infected cells.
- **As a viral infection proceeds, the adaptive immune response unfolds.** T cells mediate viral immunity in several ways: CD8[+] T cells destroy virus-infected cells or cure them of infection; CD4[+] T cells promote antibody production and CD8[+] T-cell responses and are a major effector cell population in the

response to some viral infections. Antibodies and complement can limit viral spread or re-infection.
- **Viruses have evolved strategies to evade the immune response.** They may impair the host immune response at the induction and/or effector stages; avoid recognition by the immune response, e.g. via latency or antigenic variation; or resist control by immune effector mechanisms. Many viruses employ multiple strategies to prolong their replication in the host.
- **Responses induced during viral infections can have pathological consequences.** Damage can be mediated by antiviral responses (e.g. via the formation of immune complexes or T-cell–induced damage to host tissues) or by autoimmune responses triggered during the course of infection.

INNATE IMMUNE DEFENCES AGAINST VIRUSES

The early stage of a viral infection is often a race between the virus and the host's defence system, in which the virus tries to overcome host defences in order to establish an infection and then spread to other tissues.

The initial defence against virus invasion is the integrity of the body surface: for a virus to infect its host, it needs to overcome anatomical barriers such as acid pH, proteolytic enzymes, bile and mucous layers. Once these outer defences are breached, the presence of infection triggers activation of an inflammatory response with activation of local dendritic cells (DCs) and macrophages and production of a variety of cytokines, chemokines and antimicrobial peptides that establish a local antiviral state and guide immune cells to the site of infection.

The innate response plays a critical role in control of early virus replication and spread. Key innate antiviral effectors include type I interferons (IFNs), tumor necrosis factor (TNF) α, defensins, natural killer (NK) cells, neutrophils and macrophages. A second important role of the innate response is to promote the activation of adaptive responses to eliminate the infection and provide protection against re-infection.

Microbicidal peptides have broad-spectrum antiviral effects. The innate immune response to viruses involves complex interactions between soluble factors and cells. For example, during influenza viral infection mucins, gp 340 and

pentraxins compete with the virus for its receptor, sialic acid, and cause aggregation of virus particles. Respiratory secretions are also rich in the collectin surfactant proteins (SP)-A and SP-D. These molecules bind to carbohydrates on a range of pathogens, including influenza virus where they adhere to the haemagglutinin protein (HA), resulting in virus neutralization. Some strains of influenza virus fail to be recognized by collectins because of reduced levels of glycosylation of HA. An example of this was the H1N1 virus that caused the 1918 pandemic.

Other families of anti-microbial peptides with antiviral activity include the defensins and the related cathelicidins. Alpha-defensin and the cathelicidin LL37 are produced by epithelial cells and neutrophils in response to infection. They have broad-spectrum direct antiviral activity and also modulate the inflammatory response at sites of infection.

Interferons have critical antiviral and immunostimulatory roles. The activation of the IFN system is arguably the most important defence for containing the initial stages of viral infection. There are three major families of IFNs:
- type I (including multiple subtypes of IFNα, also IFNβ and IFNω);
- type II (IFNγ); and
- type III (IFNλ1, IFNλ2 and IFNλ3, also known as IL-29, IL-28a and IL-28b).

Other types of IFN exist, including IFNτ, -δ and -κ, some of which play a role during pregnancy. Here we will focus on the IFNs with antiviral activity. Of these, type I and type III IFNs are induced directly after viral infection, whereas IFNγ is produced by activated T cells and NK cells. Type III IFNs are less well characterized than type I IFNs. Their functions are thought to be similar, although type III interferons seem to act at fewer anatomical locations, with epithelial barriers being their main sites of activity.

Type I IFN production typically starts to be induced within the first few hours after viral infection. Type I IFNs can be produced by almost any cell type in the body if it becomes infected with a virus. There are also specialized interferon-producing cells, plasmacytoid DCs and a subset of inflammatory monocytes, which can be triggered to produce high levels of type I IFN following exposure to virus without themselves becoming infected. This is important because, as discussed later, many viruses have evolved strategies for impairing type I IFN production in the cells they infect. These specialized cells typically make at least half of the type I IFN produced during a viral infection.

Type I interferons are produced when PRRs detect viral PAMPs.
Type I IFN production is triggered following recognition of molecular patterns characteristic of viral but not host components (Fig. 14.1). Host pattern recognition receptors

(PRRs) involved in detecting the presence of viral infections include cytoplasmic PRRs expressed by almost all cells, such as:
- the retinoic acid-inducible gene I (RIG-I)-like receptors that sense viral RNA. RIG-I recognizes viral 5′-triphosphorylated ssRNA and dsRNA while melanoma differentiation factor 5 (MDA5) senses long dsRNAs (see Fig. 5.13); and
- cytoplasmic DNA sensors such as cyclic GMP-AMP (cGAMP) synthase (cGAS), which, after binding to DNA, catalyses production of cGAMP, a soluble mediator that can trigger type I IFN production in both the infected cell and neighbouring cells.

Another major family of PRRs involved in recognizing viral infection are the Toll-like receptors (TLRs), which are expressed on the cell membrane or within endosomes/lysosomes of immune system cells and certain non-immune cells located at common sites of pathogen entry, e.g. epithelial cells. TLR3, TLR7 and TLR9 recognize viral dsRNA, viral ssRNA and DNA containing CpG motifs, respectively.

Both the location and the specificity of PRRs help to ensure that they are triggered when infection occurs, but not by the nucleic acids normally present in host cells.

Triggering of PRRs initiates signalling along pathways that culminate in the activation of transcription factors, including IFN regulatory factor (IRF)3 and NF-κB, which translocate into the nucleus and activate the transcription of type I IFNs and inflammatory cytokines, respectively (see Fig. 14.1).

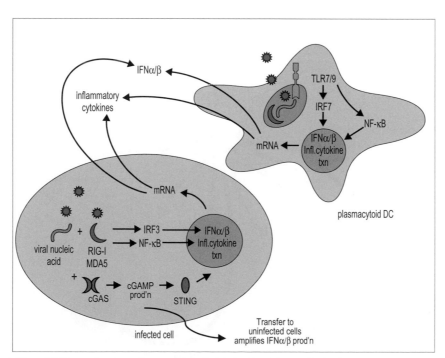

Fig. 14.1 Type I IFN production triggered by viral infection Most cells in the body express cytoplasmic pattern-recognition receptors such as RIG-I, MDA5 and cGAS. If the cell becomes infected, these detect the presence of viral nucleic acids in the cytoplasm and stimulate IRF3 and NF-κB activation, leading to transcription (txn) of type I IFN and inflammatory (Infl.) cytokine genes and production of these factors. Plasmacytoid dendritic cells *(DCs)* can detect the presence of virus and upregulate type I IFN production without becoming infected. Following virion uptake, viral nucleic acids are detected by Toll-like receptors *(TLRs)* 7 and 9 in endosomal compartments. This stimulates IRF7 and NF-κB activation, leading to production of type I IFNs and inflammatory cytokines.

Plasmacytoid DCs also have a unique signalling pathway for induction of type I IFN production in response to TLR7 or TLR9 ligation that involves the transcription factor IRF7.

Interferons act on cells to produce an antiviral state. The IFN released acts on both the cell producing it and neighbouring cells where it establishes an antiviral state, enabling them to resist viral infection (Fig. 14.2).

IFNs mediate their activity by upregulating the expression of a large number of genes known as IFN-stimulated genes (ISGs), some of which encode proteins that contribute to viral sensing and IFN production and/or mediate antiviral activity, whilst others downmodulate IFN signalling in the responding cell to control the response. Antiviral ISGs inhibit virus replication at many different stages of the viral life cycle. Depending on their mode of action, ISGs may exhibit broad-spectrum antiviral activity or limit infection with particular classes of viruses. For example:

- Interferon-induced transmembrane proteins (IFITMs) inhibit the entry of a number of viruses into cells.
- Mx proteins (MxA, an important inhibitor of viruses including influenza virus, and MxB, which acts on viruses including HIV-1) block early steps of the viral replication cycle.

- The dsRNA-dependent enzymes protein kinase R (PKR) and 2′,5′-oligoadenylate synthetase. 2′,5′-Oligoadenylate synthetase specifically activates a latent endonuclease (RNaseL) that targets the degradation of viral RNA. PKR disrupts viral infection by phosphorylating and inhibiting eukaryotic initiation factor (eIF)-2α, hence blocking the translation of viral mRNA and by initiating apoptosis via Bcl-2 and caspase-dependent mechanisms, killing the cell before the virus can be released.
- Tetherin inhibits the release of enveloped viruses from infected cells.
- Apolipoprotein B mRNA editing enzyme, catalytic polypeptide-like (APOBEC) proteins combat infection with retroviruses including HIV-1 by several mechanisms including introduction of mutations into viral DNA during replication, which impacts on the fitness of newly produced virions.

INTERFERONS ENHANCE THE ANTIVIRAL ACTIVITY OF MACROPHAGES AND NK CELLS

In addition to the direct inhibition of virus replication, IFNs also activate macrophages and NK cells and enhance their antiviral

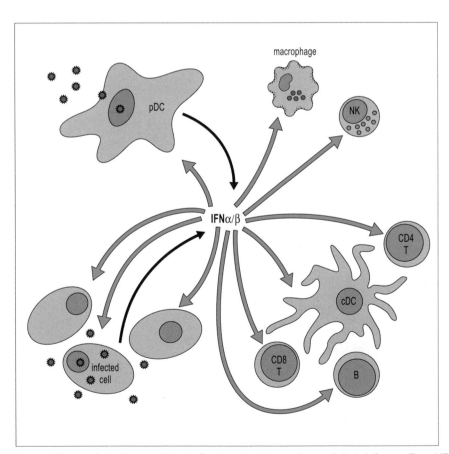

Fig. 14.2 Type I IFNs mediate direct antiviral effects and activate other antiviral defences Type I IFNs produced by infected cells and plasmacytoid dendritic cells *(pDCs)* detecting virion components upregulate the expression of antiviral genes in both infected and uninfected cells, thereby helping to eradicate infection and block its spread. Type I IFNs also activate cells participating in the innate response, including pDCs, conventional DCs *(cDCs)*, natural killer *(NK)* cells and macrophages (mØs) and promote the activation of adaptive responses not only via DC activation but also by acting directly on T and B cells.

activity (see Fig. 14.2). They also help to promote the activation of adaptive responses by acting on antigen-presenting cells, including conventional DCs, to stimulate increased expression of major histocompatibility complex (MHC) classes I and II, along with components of the antigen-processing machinery. They also act directly on T and B cells to promote an antiviral response (see Fig. 14.2).

The importance of type I IFNs in vivo is underlined by the increased susceptibility of mice lacking the IFNα/β receptor to viral infection. Similarly, depletion of IFNs by specific antibody treatment also increases viral infection.

NK cells kill virally infected cells. Activated NK cells can typically be detected within 2 days of viral infection. Since viruses require the replicative machinery of live cells to reproduce, NK cells act to combat virus replication directly by recognizing and killing infected cells (see Chapter 8). They also produce cytokines such as IFNγ and TNFα, and mediate important immunomodulatory effects, stimulating the activation of macrophages via IFNγ and regulating DC and T-cell responses.

NK cells are non-specifically activated by innate cytokines, including type I IFNs, IL-12, IL-15 and IL-18, but their activation state and effector activity are also regulated by signalling through multiple activating and inhibitory receptors.

- Inhibitory NK receptors typically recognize ligands expressed on normal host cells, such as MHC class I molecules. As discussed later, many viruses downregulate MHC class I expression on the cells they infect to limit recognition by CD8⁺ T cells, but this helps to trigger NK-cell activation.
- Activating NK receptors typically recognize host cell proteins that are upregulated in response to stress, or viral proteins. For example, the natural cytotoxicity receptors NKp44 and NKp46 recognize certain viral glycoproteins including the influenza virus HA. Mice deficient in NKp46 are highly susceptible to influenza viral infection.
- NK cells can also be activated via antibody coating of the target cell, which crosslinks the NK surface receptor FcγRIII, or CD16. NK cells are one of the principal mediators of antibody-dependent cell-mediated cytotoxicity (ADCC).

Macrophages act at three levels to destroy virus and virus-infected cells. Macrophages are ever present in the tissues of the body and act as a first line of defence against many pathogens. In viral infections they act via three mechanisms to destroy virus and virus-infected cells:
- phagocytosis of virus and virus-infected cells;
- killing of virus-infected cells; and
- production of antiviral molecules such as TNFα, nitric oxide and IFNα.

Phagocytosis of infected cells and virus complexes is part of the normal housekeeping role of macrophages at a site of infection. As for many pathogens, the phagolysosome represents a hostile environment for viruses in which oxygen-dependent and oxygen-independent destructive mechanisms prevail. The induction of nitric oxide synthetase and the generation of nitric oxide are potent inhibitors of herpes virus and poxvirus infection.

ADAPTIVE IMMUNE RESPONSES TO VIRAL INFECTION

The adaptive immune response typically begins a few days after innate responses are activated (Fig. 14.3). T cells start to appear at sites of infection around 4 days after the initiation of viral expansion. In many viral infections, it is the action of CD8⁺ T cells that plays a key role in the resolution of infection. Antibodies are frequently induced slightly later, around day 6 or 7, and contribute to recovery from infection.

A key feature of the adaptive immune response is the establishment of immunological memory, which forms the basis of a number of highly successful vaccines against viral infections.

Antibodies can neutralize the infectivity of viruses. Antibodies provide a major barrier to virus spread between cells and tissues and are particularly important in restricting virus spread in the blood stream. IgA production becomes focused at mucosal surfaces where it serves to prevent re-infection.

Antibodies may be generated against any viral protein in the infected cell, but only antibodies directed against virion surface components such as glycoproteins that are expressed on the virion envelope or viral proteins expressed on the infected cell membrane are of importance in controlling infection.

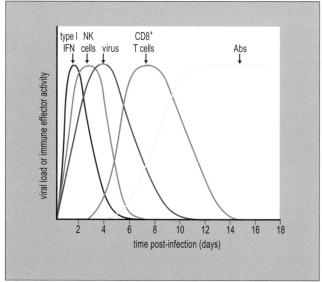

Fig. 14.3 Kinetics of host defences in response to a typical acute viral infection During an acute viral infection (e.g. with influenza or lymphocytic choriomeningitis virus), type I interferon *(IFN)* production is rapidly initiated in infected tissues and circulating levels of type I IFNs increase. Activated natural killer *(NK)* cells then start to be detected in the blood and at infection sites. Virus-specific T-cell responses are induced in local lymph nodes or the spleen and effector cells traffic to sites of viral infection. Expansion of virus-specific T-cell responses is followed by the appearance of neutralizing antibodies in serum. Virus-specific T cells decline in frequency after virus clearance has been mediated and activated T cells are no longer present by 2–3 weeks post-infection. However, high titres of neutralizing antibodies remain and T-cell memory is established and may last for many years.

TABLE 14.1	**Antiviral Effects of Antibody**	
Target	**Agent**	**Mechanism**
Free virus	Antibody alone	Blocks binding to cell
		Blocks entry into cell
		Blocks uncoating of virus
	Antibody + complement	Damage to virus envelope
		Blockade of virus receptor
Virus-infected cells	Antibody + complement	Damage of infected cell
		Opsonization of coated virus or infected cells for phagocytosis
	Antibody bound to infected cells	ADCVI by NK cells, macrophage and neutrophils

ADCVI, Antibody-dependent cell-mediated virus inhibition.

Defence against free virus particles involves neutralization of infectivity, which can occur in various ways (Table 14.1). Such mechanisms are likely to operate in vivo because injection of neutralizing monoclonal antibodies is highly effective at inhibiting virus replication. The presence of circulating virus-neutralizing antibodies is an important factor in the prevention of re-infection. Passively administered monoclonal antibodies have been used therapeutically to inhibit respiratory syncytial virus and influenza viral infections.

An important mechanism of IgA-mediated neutralization occurs intracellularly as IgA passes from the basal to the apical surface of the cell. During this transcytosis, vesicles containing IgA interact with those containing virus, leading to neutralization.

Complement is involved in the neutralization of some free viruses. Complement can also damage the virion envelope, a process known as virolysis, and some viruses can directly activate the classical and alternative complement pathways. Some herpes viruses and poxviruses carry viral homologues of complement regulatory proteins (CD46, CD55) that regulate complement activation and presumably these viruses would otherwise be susceptible to control by complement-dependent mechanisms. However, complement is not considered to be a major factor in the defence against viruses because individuals with complement deficiencies are not predisposed to severe viral infections.

Antibodies mobilize complement and/or effector cells to destroy virus-infected cells. Antibodies are also effective in mediating the destruction of virus-infected cells. This can occur by antibody-mediated activation of the complement system, leading to the assembly of the membrane attack complex and lysis of the infected cell (see Chapter 4). This process requires a high density of viral antigens on the membrane (about 5×10^6/cell) to be effective. In contrast, ADCC mediated by NK cells requires as few as 10^3 IgG molecules in order to activate NK-cell binding to and lysis of the infected cell. The IgG-coated target cells are bound using the NK cell's FcγRIII (CD16; see Fig. 10.15), and are rapidly destroyed by a perforin-dependent killing mechanism (see Fig. 8.11).

Just how important these mechanisms are for destroying virus-infected cells in vivo is difficult to resolve. The best evidence in favour of the importance of ADCC comes from studying the protective effect of non-neutralizing monoclonal antibodies in mice. Although these antibodies fail to neutralize virus in vivo, they can protect C5-deficient mice from a high-dose virus challenge. (C5-deficient mice were used in this study to eliminate the role of the late complement components.)

T cells mediate viral immunity in several ways. T cells exhibit a variety of functions in antiviral immunity:

- CD8$^+$ T cells are important effector cells that play a key role in the control of established viral infections.
- Most of the antibody response is T-cell dependent, requiring the presence of CD4$^+$ T follicular helper (CD4$^+$ Tfh) cells for class switching and affinity maturation.
- CD4$^+$ T cells also help in the induction of CD8$^+$ T-cell responses and in the recruitment and activation of macrophages at sites of viral infection.
- Memory CD8$^+$ T cells are effective in combatting re-infection with viruses such as influenza virus and respiratory syncytial virus. However, even memory T cells need time to develop a response when infection is re-encountered and antibodies typically assume a more dominant role in protection against secondary infection by neutralizing incoming virus, containing the infection and preventing spread to other tissues.

An absence of T cells renders the host highly susceptible to virus attack. For example, cutaneous infection of congenitally athymic 'nude' mice (which lack mature T cells) with herpes simplex virus (HSV) results in a spreading lesion and the virus eventually travels to the central nervous system, resulting in the death of the animal. The transfer of HSV-specific T cells shortly after infection is sufficient to protect the mice.

CD8$^+$ T cells target virus-infected cells. The principal T-cell surveillance system operating against viruses is highly efficient and selective. CD8$^+$ T cells identify virus-infected cells by recognizing MHC class I molecules presenting virus-derived peptides on the cell surface and are triggered to mediate effector functions that clear the infection.

CD8$^+$ T cells:
- kill infected cells through the release of perforin, granzymes and other cytolytic proteins;
- trigger the death of infected cells through binding of soluble factors they release (e.g. TNFα) or ligands they express (e.g. FasL) to cell surface receptors (such as Fas) that signal the cell to undergo apoptosis, i.e. effectively 'commit suicide' (see Fig. 8.9); and
- produce soluble factors such as IFNγ and/or TNFα that can 'cure' infection with some viruses (e.g. hepatitis B virus) without death of the cell. This can result in eradication of virus from not only the target cell with which the CD8$^+$ T cell is interacting but also from neighbouring cells.

Curative mechanisms are particularly important when infection is very widespread and it would be neither feasible for CD8$^+$ T cells to interact with and kill every infected cell, nor desirable for so many host cells to be destroyed.

Virtually all cells in the body express MHC class I molecules, making this an important mechanism for identifying and eliminating or curing virus-infected cells. Because of the central role played by MHC class I in targeting CD8+ T cells to infected cells, some viruses have evolved elaborate strategies to disrupt MHC class I expression, thereby interfering with T-cell recognition and favouring virus persistence (see later).

Almost any viral protein can be processed in the cytoplasm to generate peptides that are transported to the endoplasmic reticulum where they interact with MHC class I molecules. However, CD8+ T-cell responses targeting different viral proteins are not equally effective. For example, viral proteins expressed early in the replication cycle can be presented on infected cells relatively soon after they have been infected, enabling T-cell recognition to occur long before new viral progeny are produced. CD8+ T cell-mediated immunity against murine cytomegalovirus (MCMV) is mediated predominantly by T cells recognizing an epitope in the immediate early protein pp89 and immunization of mice with a recombinant vaccinia virus containing pp89 is sufficient to confer complete protection from MCMV-induced disease.

The importance of T cells in in vivo control of viral infections has been identified using various techniques.

In animals:

- the adoptive transfer of specific T-cell subpopulations or T-cell clones to infected animals;
- depletion of T-cell populations in vivo using monoclonal antibodies to CD4 or CD8; and
- creation of 'gene knockout' mice, in which genes encoding cell surface receptors (e.g. CD8, CD4), signal transduction molecules (e.g. signal transducer and activator of transcription (STAT)) or transcription factors (e.g. T-bet) are removed from the germline.

In humans:

- correlative studies addressing the relationship between the magnitude or functional efficacy of antigen-specific T-cell responses and the efficiency of control of virus replication in different infected individuals;
- assessment of control of virus replication in patients with defects in selected immune functions (e.g. DiGeorge syndrome patients lacking a thymus); and
- the finding that viruses have evolved strategies to escape recognition by host T cells (this would not happen unless T cells were exerting selective pressure on virus replication).

The ability of knockout mice that lack particular lymphocyte populations to mediate control of some viral infections illustrates the redundancy that can occur in the immune system. For example, in the absence of CD8+ T cells, CD4+ T cells, antibodies or other mechanisms, animals are sometimes able to compensate and still bring the infection under control.

CD4+ T cells are a major effector cell population in the response to some virus infections.

CD4+ T cells provide help for CD8+ T cells and antibody responses. In addition, CD4+ T cells have been identified as a major effector cell population in the immune response to some viral infections. A good example is in HSV-1 infection of epithelial surfaces. Here, CD4+ T cells

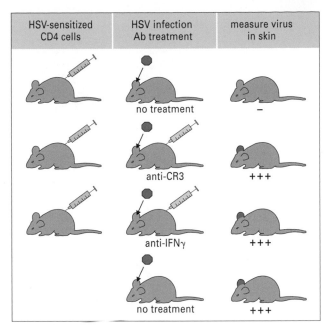

Fig. 14.4 Role of CD4+ T cells, macrophages and IFNγ in cutaneous HSV-1 infection CD4+ T cells were obtained from mice infected with HSV-1 8 days previously. The cells were transferred to syngeneic mice infected with HSV-1 in the skin. These mice were treated with anti-CR3 ($\alpha_M\beta_2$-integrin) to block macrophage migration to the site of infection or anti-IFNγ to block the activation of macrophages or were untreated. An additional control group was infected but did not receive CD4+ T cells. The amount of infectious virus remaining after 5 days was then determined. The results demonstrate that the protective effects of CD4+ T cells are mediated by macrophages and IFNγ.

participate in a delayed-type hypersensitivity response (see Chapter 26) that results in accelerated clearance of virus. They produce cytokines such as IFNγ and TNFα, which mediate direct antiviral effects and also help to activate macrophages at the site of infection. Macrophages play an important role in inhibiting viral infection, probably through the generation and action of nitric oxide (Fig. 14.4).

In measles and Epstein–Barr virus (EBV) infections, CD4+ CTLs are generated. These cells recognize and kill MHC class II-positive cells infected with the virus using the cytolytic mechanisms more often used by CD8+ CTLs. It is not clear whether MHC class II complexes presenting measles virus and EBV peptides are generated by normal pathways of class II antigen presentation (i.e. following phagocytosis and degradation, see Chapter 7) or by alternative pathways via which some measles proteins/peptides enter class II vesicles from the cytosol.

A summary of antiviral defence mechanisms is illustrated in Figure 14.5.

Host genetic variation affects antiviral immune defences.

Variation in human or animal populations in genes that encode components or modulators of innate or adaptive antiviral defences can affect the susceptibility of different individuals to acquisition of particular viral infections and their ability to control virus replication and/or likelihood of developing severe disease once they become infected. Identification of genetic

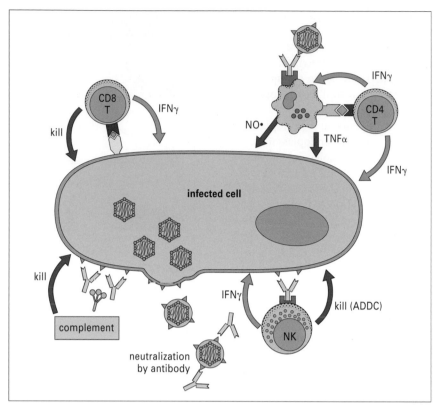

Fig. 14.5 Effector mechanisms combating virus replication CD8$^+$ T cells typically play a dominant role in control of established viral infections, mediating lysis of virus-infected cells and producing antiviral cytokines. CD4$^+$ T cells are important effectors in the control of certain viral infections, producing cytokines that mediate antiviral effects and activating macrophages to produce cytolytic and antiviral factors. They also help B cells to make antibodies, which are important in controlling free virus and can also target infected cells by activating complement-mediated lysis or triggering antibody-dependent cell-mediated cytotoxicity and virus inhibition (ADCC and ADCVI) by effector cells including natural killer (NK) cells and macrophages.

determinants of human susceptibility to viral infection and associated disease illuminates host factors involved in antiviral defence and can enable identification of particularly at-risk individuals to enable appropriate targeting with prophylactic or therapeutic measures. For example:

- A single nucleotide polymorphism in the gene encoding the IFN-induced protein IFITM3 (which is known to mediate antiviral activity against a number of viruses including influenza and HIV) has been shown to influence the severity of influenza viral infections and also to affect the outcome of certain other viral infections in human populations.
- A deletion in the promoter region of the gene encoding the chemokine receptor CCR5 (involved in chemotaxis of macrophages and T cells to sites of viral infections) affects the severity of West Nile virus (WNV) infection. Individuals homozygous for the deletion mutation (CCR5Δ32) have a greater risk of developing symptomatic WNV infection and succumbing to fatal central nervous system disease, demonstrating the importance of CCR5 in directing leukocyte trafficking to the brain to control WNV replication. Conversely, CCR5Δ32 homozygosity confers resistance to infection with HIV-1, because the majority of transmitted HIV-1 strains use the host CCR5 protein as a co-receptor that the virus needs to gain entry into host T cells and

macrophages where it replicates. The contrasting effects of this deletion mutation in these different infections help to illustrate why genetic variants that are detrimental in some infections are retained in the human population: variation at the population level is important to ensure that the species is capable of surviving infection with diverse pathogens.

- MHC genes are the most polymorphic (variable) genes in the human genome, which is necessary to maximize the chances of each individual inheriting a combination of diverse MHC class I and II genes that will be capable of presenting peptides from the many diverse pathogens that they may encounter. Particular MHC class I (and II) genes are known to be associated with beneficial or detrimental effects in a number of viral infections: e.g. in HIV-1 infection, MHC genes, including HLA-B27 and HLA-B57 (which efficiently present peptides derived from the conserved HIV-1 capsid protein (Gag), which is a good target for T-cell recognition), are associated with good control of viral replication and delayed disease progression, whereas other genes including certain HLA-B35 alleles are associated with rapid disease progression. Interestingly, HLA-B27 is associated with an enhanced risk of developing the arthritic disease ankylosing spondylitis, again illustrating how a particular gene variant can confer either beneficial or detrimental effects in different situations.

VIRUS STRATEGIES TO EVADE HOST IMMUNE RESPONSES

To promote their survival, viruses have evolved multiple strategies to evade control by the host immune response. Avoidance of immune clearance is essential for viruses that persist in their hosts for long periods. Even for viruses that cause acute infections, immune evasion strategies are important to prolong infection and to increase the opportunities for transmission to new hosts.

Viral immune evasion strategies can be categorized into mechanisms for:
- impairing the host response;
- avoiding recognition by the host immune defences; and
- resisting control by immune effector mechanisms.

Some viruses use multiple strategies in each category to promote their persistence in vivo: HIV-1 provides a particularly good example of this (Table 14.2).

Viruses can impair the host immune response. Viral infections can sometimes be associated with a profound widespread impairment of host immune functions, e.g. the generalized immune suppression associated with measles infection or the acquired immunodeficiency syndrome (AIDS) induced in the late stages of HIV-1 infection. Although induction of a state of generalized immune dysfunction impairs control of virus replication, it also impacts on host survival and is therefore not an ideal strategy for promoting virus persistence. Many viruses, instead, induce impairments in host immunity that are more localized, more limited and/or target virus-specific cellular or humoral responses.

The importance of type I IFNs in innate control of local virus replication and spread is illustrated by the fact that many different families of viruses have evolved strategies for blocking type I IFN production in the cells they infect. These include:

- mechanisms for hiding viral nucleic acids to prevent sensing of infection (e.g. incoming influenza virus RNA genomes are protected by the viral nucleocapsid from recognition by RIG-I as they traffic through the cytoplasm to the nucleus for replication);
- inhibition of cellular nucleic acid sensors (e.g. several herpes viruses encode proteins that interfere with the activity of cGAS or STING); and
- interference with downstream signalling events leading to type I IFN induction (e.g. multiple viruses inhibit IRF3 or IRF7 activity).

Some viruses also impair the recruitment of plasmacytoid DCs to sites of infection, reduce circulating plasmacytoid DC numbers or infect plasmacytoid DCs and impair their functions to reduce type I IFN production by these specialized IFN-producing cells.

Chemokines represent an important system for controlling immune cell migration and viruses have evolved elaborate strategies for disrupting the chemokine network. The herpes viruses encode:

- chemokine homologues (e.g. CCL3);
- chemokine receptor homologues; and
- chemokine-binding proteins, which have powerful effects on delaying or inhibiting cell migration during inflammation.

Viruses may also inhibit the induction of adaptive responses by infecting and interfering with the functions of key antigen-presenting cells such as DCs, or by producing cytokine homologues such as vIL-10 (herpes viruses) that inhibit the TH1 response, which combats these infections.

Given the critical role of T cells, particularly CD8$^+$ CTLs, in elimination of established viral infections, viruses that establish long-term persistent infections in their hosts frequently possess strategies for impairment of the virus-specific CD8$^+$ T-cell response.

TABLE 14.2 Strategies Used by HIV to Evade Immune Control

Host Defence Mechanism To Be Evaded	Impairment Strategies	Avoidance Strategies	Resistance Strategies
Type I IFN	In infected cells capsid shields genome from cytosolic PRR recognition pDCs make IFN in acute infection but are depleted in chronic infection	Latency (avoids control by all arms of the immune response)	Resistance to antiviral activity of some ISGs, e.g. HIV-1 Vif counteracts APOBECs and Vpu tetherin
NK cells	Decrease in NK cell numbers and decline in their functions in chronic infection	Expression of some MHC I alleles involved in NK inhibition retained on infected cells	Inhibition of TNF and Fas-mediated lysis of infected cells by HIV-1 Nef
CD8$^+$ T cells	Exhaustion of CD8$^+$ T-cell effector functions driven by persistent exposure to virus	Downregulation of MHC I expression Acquisition of escape mutations	Inhibition of TNF and Fas-mediated lysis of infected cells by HIV-1 Nef
CD4$^+$ T cells	Loss of CD4$^+$ T cells as a result of infection and lysis by HIV Impairment of CD4$^+$ Tfh function	Downregulation of MHC II expression	Inhibition of TNF and Fas-mediated lysis of infected cells by HIV-1 Nef
Antibodies	Delay in neutralizing Ab (nAb) production Conserved nAb epitopes made of glycans/lipids and Ab production to these key sites constrained by self-tolerance	Block of Ab binding to the virus by glycans Acquisition of escape mutations	Incorporation of CD59 into the virion envelope to block complement activation

APOBEC, Apolipoprotein B mRNA editing enzyme, catalytic polypeptide-like; IFN, interferon; ISG, interferon stimulated gene; MHC, major histocompatibility complex; nAb, neutralizing antibody; NK, natural killer; pDC, plasmacytoid dendritic cell; PRR, pattern recognition receptor; TNF, tumour necrosis factor.

- Some persistent viral infections are transmitted from mother to offspring in utero (e.g. lymphocytic choriomeningitis virus (LCMV) infection of mice and hepatitis B virus infection in humans). This can result in tolerization of virus-specific T cells as self tolerance is established in the developing host immune system, leading to failure to mount a virus-specific T-cell (or an effective antibody) response to the virus.
- Virus-specific CD8$^+$ T-cell responses in immunologically mature hosts may be impaired by a process termed 'exhaustion' during which virus-specific T cells exposed to high levels of antigenic stimulation in the face of ongoing virus replication upregulate expression of inhibitory receptors such as programmed cell death protein-1 (PD-1), develop transcriptional and metabolic abnormalities that render them increasingly functionally defective and may eventually be driven to undergo apoptosis. A similar process of T-cell exhaustion also occurs during cancer, and checkpoint blockade strategies now being used there to re-invigorate tumour-specific CD8$^+$ T cells (see Chapter 22) are also being considered for therapeutic use during chronic infection with viruses such as HIV-1 and HBV.

Viruses have strategies to avoid recognition by host immune defences. Strategies viruses use to avoid recognition by host immune defences include:

- latency;
- infection of immune privileged sites;
- rendering infected cells less visible to host effector cells; and
- antigenic variation.

Some viruses establish a latent infection within certain host cells, during which there is little or no production of viral proteins. Latently infected cells are thus essentially invisible to the host immune system. Cells such as HSV-infected neurons can persist for the life of the host in this form, although latency also needs to be accompanied by continuous or sporadic productive virus replication if the infection is to be spread to new hosts.

Another strategy that viruses use to avoid recognition by host immune defences is to replicate in immune privileged sites, i.e. parts of the body to which adaptive responses have limited access and where there may also be an immune-suppressive environment, such as in the brain (see Chapter 13).

Viruses avoid recognition by T cells by reducing MHC expression on infected cells. Other viruses try to render the cells they infect less visible to host's adaptive responses. The critical role played by CD8$^+$ T cells in elimination of viral infections is underlined by the plethora of strategies that viruses have evolved to reduce the level of MHC class I expression on the surface of infected cells.

MHC class I expression can be disrupted by:
- downregulating MHC class I synthesis (e.g. HIV-1);
- reducing the generation of epitope peptides in the cytoplasm (e.g. EBV);
- blocking peptide uptake into the endoplasmic reticulum (e.g. HSV-1);
- preventing maturation, assembly and migration of the trimolecular MHC class I complex (e.g. human cytomegalovirus (HCMV)); and/or

- recycling of MHC class I molecules from the cell surface (e.g. HIV-1).

Similar mechanisms apply for MHC class II molecules where some herpes viruses block transcription, whilst others induce premature targeting of MHC class II for degradation.

Downregulation of MHC class I may disrupt CD8$^+$ T-cell recognition, but NK cells are more efficient killers in the absence of MHC class I. Human and murine CMV have tried to redress the balance by encoding their own MHC class I homologues, which are expressed on infected cells and can inhibit NK-cell activation.

Mutation of viral target antigen allows escape from recognition by antibodies or T cells. Antigenic variation involves a virus acquiring sequence changes (mutations) in sites on proteins that are normally targeted by antibody or T cells so that these sites are no longer recognized. Antigenic variation can promote virus persistence within a given host: during HIV-1 infection, mutations are frequently selected for in and around the epitopes recognized by the initial T cell and neutralizing antibody responses, which confer escape from recognition by these responses and enable enhanced virus replication. It can also promote virus persistence at the population level, as exemplified by the antigenic shift and drift seen with influenza virus (Fig. 14.6). Humoral immunity to influenza virus provides protection against re-infection only until a new virus strain emerges, making effective long-lasting vaccines difficult to produce.

Viruses have evolved strategies to avoid control by a broad range of immune effector mechanisms. Viruses have evolved strategies for resisting control by many different immune effector mechanisms including:
- the antiviral activity of type I IFNs and other cytokines;

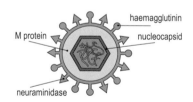

Pandemic	Date	Subtype	Deaths
Asiatic	1889–1890	? (H3N8 or H2N2)	~1 million
Spanish	1918–1919	H1N1	20–100 million
Asian	1957–1958	H2N2	1–1.5 million
Hong Kong	1968–1969	H3N2	0.75–1 million
Russian	1977–1978	H1N1	low
Global	2009–2010	H1N1/09	150–600 thousand

Fig. 14.6 Pandemic strains of influenza A virus The major surface antigens of influenza virus are haemagglutinin and neuraminidase. Haemagglutinin is involved in attachment to cells, and antibodies to haemagglutinin are protective. Antibodies to neuraminidase are much less effective. Influenza virus can change its antigenic properties slightly (antigenic drift) or radically (antigenic shift). Alterations in the structure of the haemagglutinin antigen render earlier antibodies ineffective and new virus epidemics therefore break out. The diagram shows the strains that have emerged by antigenic shift since 1890. The virus has changed by antigenic drift in most years between the arrival of new pandemic strains. The official influenza antigen nomenclature is based on the type of haemagglutinin (H$_1$, H$_2$, etc.) and neuraminidase (N$_1$, N$_2$, etc.) expressed on the surface of the virion. Note that, although new strains replace old strains, the internal antigens remain largely unchanged.

- the lytic mechanisms by which NK cells and CD8⁺ T cells destroy infected cells; and
- antibodies and complement.

In addition to impairing production of type I IFNs, viruses also have many strategies for resisting control by these important antiviral cytokines. This can be achieved via:
- production of soluble IFN receptors (e.g. poxviruses);
- interference with IFN signalling (e.g. WNV impairs expression of the type I IFN receptor, and multiple viruses block Jak/STAT signalling);
- impairment of transcription of ISGs (e.g. adenoviruses and hepatitis C virus);
- disruption or evasion of the activity of antiviral ISGs (e.g. lentiviruses induce degradation of key antiviral ISGs).

Viruses may also resist control by other antiviral cytokines: several poxviruses encode soluble receptors to interfere with TNF function. Other viral proteins produced in infected cells protect the cells from lysis by TNF: adenoviruses, herpes viruses and poxviruses all encode proteins with this function. HIV protects the cells it infects from lysis mediated not only via TNF but also via Fas.

As noted above, some viruses also possess strategies for resisting control by antibodies and complement. Some herpes viruses and poxviruses encode homologues for CD46 and CD55 (complement regulatory proteins that block C3 activation) and also for CD59, which blocks formation of the membrane attack complex. HIV makes use of cellular CD59, which is incorporated into the viral envelope, thereby blocking complement-mediated lysis of the virion.

Examples of virus-encoded homologues or mimics of the host defence system are shown in Table 14.3.

PATHOLOGICAL CONSEQUENCES OF IMMUNE RESPONSES INDUCED BY VIRAL INFECTIONS

Although the host immune response plays a vital role in combating viral infections, it can also have immunopathological consequences. These can result from inappropriate antiviral immune responses or from the induction of autoimmune responses during the course of a viral infection.

Excessive cytokine production and immune activation can be pathological. Cytokines and chemokines play a critical role in activation of immune responses following viral infection and recruitment of cells to the site of infection. However, excessive cytokine and chemokine production can have pathological consequences. For example:
- Infection with severe acute respiratory syndrome (SARS) virus and the highly pathogenic influenza viruses (H5N1), if not rapidly controlled by the early innate response, can be associated with hypercytokinaemia (cytokine storms), which drive an aggressive inflammatory response that can result in massive tissue damage (pneumonia), leading to death.

TABLE 14.3 Viral Homologues or Mimics of Host Proteins that Promote Viral Persistence

Many viruses with large DNA genomes encode proteins of this type

Host Defence Affected	Virus	Host Protein that Virus Encodes a Homologue or Mimic of	Mechanism of Action
Type 1 IFN	HHV-8	IRF homologue	Blocks type I IFN transcription
	Vaccinia	Type I IFN receptor homologue	Secreted and binds to IFNα/β
	Vaccinia	eIF-2α homologue	Prevents eIF-2α phosphorylation and inhibits PKR
Other cytokines	Multiple poxviruses	TNF receptor homologues	Secreted and bind to TNFα
	Vaccinia	IL-1β receptor mimic	Binds IL-1β and blocks the febrile response
	EBV, HCMV	IL-10 mimics	Mimic IL-10 activity and downregulate production of TH1 cytokines, e.g. IFNγ
Chemokines	MCMV, HCMV, HHV-6, 7 and 8, MHV-68	Chemokine receptor mimics	Secreted and bind CC and/or CXC chemokines, either enhancing or blocking their activity
	MCMV, HCMV, HHV-6, HHV-8	CC or CXC chemokine mimics	Attract monocytes for viral replication or attract TH2 cells
Complement	Vaccinia, smallpox, HSV-1 and 2, HVS, HHV-8, MHV-68	Homologues of complement-binding proteins, e.g. C4-binding protein, CR1, CD46 and CD55	Inhibit soluble complement factors
	HVS	CD59 homologue	Blocks formation of membrane-attack complex
Antibody	HSV-1 and 2, MCMV, coronavirus	Fc-receptor mimics	Bind IgG and inhibit Fc-dependent effector mechanisms
NK cells	HCMV, MCMV	MHC class I homologues	Inhibit NK recognition of infected cells
Destruction of infected cells	HHV-8, HVS, some poxviruses	FLIP mimics	Inhibit caspase activation, preventing death-receptor-mediated triggering of apoptosis
	HHV-8, HVS, adenovirus	Bcl 2 homologues	Block apoptosis

EBV, Epstein–Barr virus; *FLIP*, FLICE-like inhibitory protein; *HCMV*, human cytomegalovirus; *HHV*, human herpes virus; *HHV-8*, human herpesvirus-8 (Kaposi's sarcoma-associated herpes virus); *HSV*, herpes simplex virus; *HVS*, herpes virus saimiri; *IRF*, interferon regulatory factor; *MCMV*, murine cytomegalovirus; *MHV-68*, murine gamma herpes virus; *PKR*, protein kinase R.

- Activated CD4$^+$ T cells constitute the main cellular sites for HIV replication. The virus triggers an intense cytokine storm associated with extensive immune activation during acute infection, which helps to fuel virus replication by providing a large pool of activated CD4$^+$ target cells. A key difference between non-pathogenic simian immunodeficiency virus (SIV) infections of non-human primates and pathogenic SIV infection or HIV infection is that in non-pathogenic infections immune activation is rapidly downmodulated after the acute phase of infection and a constant state of immune activation is maintained in pathogenic infections. This helps to drive ongoing virus replication and CD4$^+$ T cell loss, ultimately leading to the development of AIDS.

Poorly neutralizing antibodies can enhance viral infectivity.

An unusual pathological consequence of some virus infections, where weakly neutralizing antibodies are produced is antibody-dependent enhancement (ADE) of viral infection. This involves Fc receptor-mediated uptake of antibody–virus complexes by macrophages and subsequent enhancement of virus infectivity. This is seen in many viral infections where virus replication occurs in macrophages. An example is dengue viral infection, where weakly cross-reactive antibodies induced during prior infections with different dengue virus subtypes can result in ADE with the initiation of:

- dengue haemorrhagic fever; and
- dengue shock syndrome, which results in excessive procoagulant release by monocytes.

Antiviral antibodies can form immune complexes that cause tissue damage.

Immune complexes may arise in body fluids or on cell surfaces and are most common during persistent or chronic infections (e.g. with hepatitis B virus). Antibodies are ineffective (non-neutralizing) in the presence of large amounts of the viral antigen; instead, immune complexes form and are deposited in the kidney or in blood vessels, where they evoke inflammatory responses leading to tissue damage (e.g. glomerulonephritis, see Fig. 25.1).

Virus-specific T-cell responses can cause severe tissue damage.

In any viral infection, some tissue damage is likely to arise from the activity of infiltrating T-cells. However, in some situations this damage may be considerable, resulting in the death of the host. A classic illustration of this is the CD8$^+$ T-cell response to LCMV in the central nervous system (Fig. 14.7). Removal of T cells protects LCMV-infected mice from death, indicating that they, rather than the virus, are mediating damage to the brain.

Viral infection may provoke autoimmunity.

Viruses may trigger autoimmune disease in a number of ways, including:

- **Virus-induced damage.** During the course of some viral infections, tissues become damaged, provoking an inflammatory response during which hidden antigens become exposed and can be processed and presented to the immune

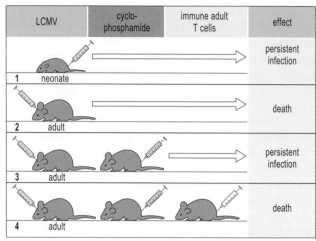

Fig. 14.7 Different outcomes of lymphocytic choriomeningitis virus infection The outcome of lymphocytic choriomeningitis virus (LCMV) infection of mice is related to differences in immune status. Infection of neonatal mice (1) results in virus persistence because virus-specific T cells are clonally deleted when self tolerance is established in the newborn animal. In the absence of T-cell help, non-neutralizing antibodies are produced and virus persistence is associated with immune complex disease, manifesting itself as glomerulonephritis and vasculitis. Intracerebral infection of adult mice (2) results in death from lymphocytic choriomeningitis. This is a result of the recruitment of virus-specific T cells to sites of virus replication in the brain. Suppression of immunity with cyclophosphamide (3) prevents death but leads to the establishment of a persistent infection. The protective effect produced by cyclophosphamide can be reversed by adoptive transfer of T cells from an LCMV-immune animal (4).

system. Examples of this include Theiler's virus (a murine picornavirus) and murine hepatitis viral infection of the nervous system, in which the constituents of myelin (the insulating material of axons) become targets for antibody and T cells, leading to development of a multiple sclerosis-like disease.

- **Molecular mimicry.** A sequence in a viral protein that is homologous to a self protein can be recognized, leading to a breakdown in immunological tolerance to cryptic self antigens in the consequent attack on host tissues by the immune system (see Chapter 11). A good example is coxsackie B virus-induced myocarditis. Patients with inflammatory cardiomyopathy have antibodies that cross-react with peptides derived from coxsackie B3 protein and with peptides derived from cellular adenine nucleotide translocator.

A number of other autoimmune conditions in humans are associated with preceding viral infections and it is implied that self tolerance is broken by molecular mimicry in some individuals who have an underlying genetic susceptibility. Examples are the association of narcolepsy with some strains of influenza A infection and the association of CMV and EBV infections with Guillain–Barré syndrome (see Fig 24.11). However, identifying the cross-reactive viral antigens that trigger autoimmunity is often problematic, because it depends on antigen presentation by MHC molecules, which vary between individuals. Hence different viruses can lead to the same autoimmune disease, depending on the genotype of the affected person.

CRITICAL THINKING: VIRUS–IMMUNE SYSTEM INTERACTIONS

See Critical thinking: Explanations, section 14

A scientist designs a vaccine that produces a series of IgG monoclonal antibodies against glycoprotein D of herpes simplex virus in mice. When she tests for virus neutralizing activity in vitro, the scientist can divide the antibodies into two groups: those capable of neutralizing virus infectivity and non-neutralizing antibodies. However, when she injects individual neutralizing or non-neutralizing antibodies into mice infected with herpes simplex virus, both sets of antibodies protect the animals from an overwhelming infection.

1. How do you explain the protection achieved by the non-neutralizing monoclonal antibodies?

2. What experiments would you propose to test some of your hypotheses? Another scientist in the same laboratory is working on a vaccine against HIV. He knows that CD8⁺ T cells play an important role in containing HIV replication and decides to focus his efforts on designing a vaccine that will elicit a strong HIV-specific CD8⁺ T-cell response.

3. Would T-cell responses directed against epitopes in any of the HIV proteins be likely to control viral replication equally well?

4. How could viral escape from vaccine-elicited T-cell responses be minimized?

FURTHER READING

Chen X, Liu S, Goraya MU, Maarouf M, Huang S, Chen JL. Host immune response to influenza A virus. Front Immunol 2018;9:320.

De Pelsmaeker S, Romero N, Vitale M, Favoreel HW. Herpesvirus evasion of natural killer cells. J Virol 2018;92:e02105–117.

Garcia-Sastre A. Ten strategies of interferon evasion by viruses. Cell Host Microbe 2016;22:176–184.

Haynes BF, Shaw GM, Korber B, et al. HIV–host interactions: implications for vaccine design. Cell Host Microbe 2016;19: 292–303.

 Klenerman P, Hill A. T cells and viral persistence: lessons from diverse infections. Nat Immunol 2005;6:873–879.

Schneider WM, Chevillotte MD, Rice CM. Interferon-stimulated genes: a complex web of host defenses. Annu Rev Immunol 2014;32:513–545.

Shin EC, Sung PS, Park SH. Immune responses and immunopathology in acute and chronic viral hepatitis infections. Nat Rev Immunol 2016;16:509–523.

Zehn D, Wherry EJ. Immune memory and exhaustion: clinically relevant mechanisms from the LCMV mouse model. Adv Exp Med Biol 2015;850:137–152.

15

Immunity to Bacteria and Fungi

SUMMARY

- **Mechanisms of protection from bacteria can be deduced from their structure and pathogenicity.** There are four main types of bacterial cell wall and pathogenicity varies between two extreme patterns. Non-specific, phylogenetically ancient recognition pathways for conserved bacterial structures trigger protective innate immune responses and guide the development of adaptive immunity.

- **Innate bacterial recognition pathways have several consequences.** Complement is activated via the alternative pathway. Release of pro-inflammatory cytokines and chemokines increases the adhesive properties of the vascular endothelium and promotes neutrophil and monocyte recruitment. Pathogen recognition generates signals that then engage a diverse set of innate lymphocytes, providing new pathways of phagocyte activation and recruitment before antigen-specific lymphocyte responses arise.

- **Antibody provides an antigen-specific protective mechanism.** A neutralizing antibody may be all that is needed for protection if the organism is pathogenic only because of a single toxin, adhesion molecule or capsule. Opsonizing antibody responses are particularly important for resistance to extracellular bacterial pathogens. Complement can kill some bacteria, particularly those with an exposed outer lipid bilayer, such as Gram-negative bacteria.

- **Ultimately, most bacteria are killed by phagocytes** after a multistage process of chemotaxis, attachment, uptake and killing. Macrophage killing can be enhanced on activation. Optimal activation of macrophages is dependent on T_H1 CD4 T cells, whereas neutrophil responses are promoted by T_H17 CD4 T cells. Persistent macrophage recruitment and activation can result in granuloma formation, which is a hallmark of cell-mediated immunity to intracellular bacteria.

- **Successful pathogens have evolved mechanisms to avoid phagocyte-mediated killing** and have evolved a startling diversity of mechanisms for avoiding other aspects of innate and adaptive immunity.

- **Infected cells can be killed by cytotoxic T lymphocytes (CTLs).** Other T-cell populations and some tissue cells can contribute to antibacterial immunity.

- **The response to bacteria can result in immunological tissue damage.** Excessive release of cytokines caused by microorganisms can result in immunopathological syndromes, such as endotoxin shock and the Schwartzman reaction.

- **Fungi can cause life-threatening infections.** Immunity to fungi is predominantly cell mediated and shares many similarities with immunity to bacteria.

INNATE RECOGNITION OF BACTERIAL COMPONENTS

Bacterial infections have had an enormous impact on human society and continue to be a major threat to public health despite the discovery of antibiotics.

Plague caused by *Yersinia pestis* is estimated to have killed one-quarter of the European population in the Middle Ages, whereas infection with *Mycobacterium tuberculosis* is currently a global health emergency. The development of resistance to commonly used antibiotics (anti-microbial resistance, AMR) makes understanding the function of immune defences against these organisms and how they can be leveraged for host protection, such as in vaccination, of even greater importance.

The immune defence mechanisms elicited against pathogenic bacteria are determined by their:
- surface chemistry;
- mechanism(s) of pathogenicity; and
- whether they are predominantly extracellular or also have the ability to survive inside mammalian cells.

There are four main types of bacterial cell wall. The four main types of bacterial cell wall (Fig. 15.1) belong to the following groups.

- Gram-positive bacteria;
- Gram-negative bacteria;
- mycobacteria;
- spirochaetes.

The outer lipid bilayer of Gram-negative organisms is of particular importance because it can be susceptible to lysis by complement. However, killing of most bacteria usually requires uptake by phagocytes. The outer surface of the bacterium may also contain fimbriae or flagella or it may be covered by a protective capsule. These can impede the functions of phagocytes or complement, but they also act as targets for the antibody response, the role of which is discussed later.

Pathogenicity varies between two extreme patterns. The two extreme patterns of pathogenicity are:
- toxicity without invasiveness; and
- invasiveness without toxicity (Fig. 15.2).

However, most bacteria are intermediate between these extremes, having some invasiveness assisted by some locally acting toxins and spreading factors (tissue-degrading enzymes).

Corynebacterium diphtheriae, *Clostridium tetani* and *Vibrio cholerae* are examples of organisms that are toxic, but not invasive. Because their pathogenicity depends almost entirely on toxin production, neutralizing antibody to the toxin is probably

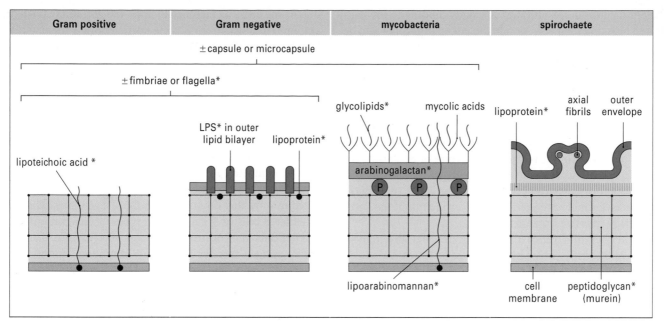

Fig. 15.1 Bacterial cell walls Different immunological mechanisms have evolved to destroy the cell wall structure of the different groups of bacteria. All types have an inner cell membrane and a peptidoglycan wall. Gram-negative bacteria also have an outer lipid bilayer in which lipopolysaccharide *(LPS)* is embedded. Lysosomal enzymes and lysozyme are active against the peptidoglycan layer, whereas cationic proteins and complement are effective against the outer lipid bilayer of the Gram-negative bacteria. The compound cell wall of mycobacteria is extremely resistant to breakdown and it is likely that this can be achieved only with the assistance of the bacterial enzymes working from within. Some bacteria also have fimbriae or flagella, which can provide targets for the antibody response. Others have an outer capsule, which renders the organisms more resistant to phagocytosis or to complement. The components indicated with an asterisk *(*)* are recognized by the innate immune system as a non-specific danger signal that selectively boosts some aspects of immune activity. (Gram staining is a method that exploits the fact that crystal violet and iodine form a complex that is more abundant on Gram-positive bacteria. The complex easily elutes from Gram-negative bacteria.)

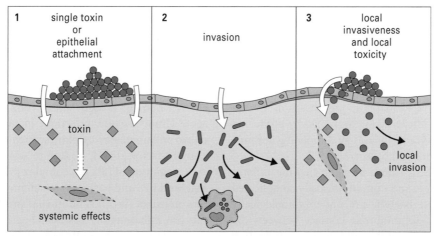

Fig. 15.2 Mechanisms of immunopathogenicity (**1**) Some bacteria cause disease as a result of only a single toxin (e.g. *Corynebacterium diphtheriae*, *Clostridium tetani*) or because of an ability to attach to epithelial surfaces (e.g. in group A streptococcal sore throat). Immunity to such organisms may require only antibody to neutralize this critical function. (**2**) At the other extreme there are organisms that are not toxic and cause disease by invasion of tissues and sometimes cells, where damage results mostly from the bulk of organisms or from immunopathology (e.g. lepromatous leprosy). Where organisms invade cells, they must be destroyed and degraded by the cell-mediated immune response. (**3**) Most organisms fall between the two extremes, with some local invasiveness assisted by local toxicity and enzymes that degrade extracellular matrix (e.g. *Staphylococcus aureus*, *Clostridium perfringens*). Antibody and cell-mediated responses are both involved in resistance and the latter is a major cause of antibiotic-induced colitis and diarrhoea.

sufficient for immunity, although antibody binding to the bacteria and blocking their adhesion to the epithelium could also be important.

In contrast, the pathogenicity of most invasive organisms does not rely heavily on a single toxin and immunity requires killing the organisms themselves.

The first lines of defence do not depend on antigen recognition.
The body's first line of defence against pathogenic bacteria consists of simple barriers to the entry or establishment of the infection. Thus, the skin and the mucosal epithelium lining the respiratory, gastrointestinal and urogenital tracts have non-specific or innate protective systems, which limit the entry of potentially invasive organisms.

The outer keratin layer of intact skin is impenetrable to most bacteria. Additionally, fatty acids produced by the skin are toxic to many organisms. Indeed, the pathogenicity of some strains correlates with their ability to survive on the skin. Epithelia release potent anti-microbial peptides known as defensins and cathelicidins, which act as endogenous antibiotics. Epithelial surfaces are also mechanically cleansed: for example, by ciliary action in the trachea or by flushing of the urinary tract.

Many bacteria are destroyed by pH changes in the stomach and vagina, both of which provide an acidic environment. In the vagina, the epithelium secretes glycogen, which is metabolized by particular species of commensal bacteria, producing lactic acid.

Commensals can limit pathogen invasion.
Commensal bacteria have co-evolved with us over millions of years, providing an essential protective function against more pathogenic species by occupying an ecological niche that would otherwise be occupied by something more unpleasant. In fact it has been estimated that the human body contains approximately 10 times more bacterial cells than human cells. This is mostly because of the gut microbiota, made up of perhaps thousands of different bacterial species many of which have not been cultured but identified more recently by high throughput sequencing technology of 16S ribosomal RNA sequences. The precise makeup of this microbiota is different between individuals, with a core of common species together with an additional set that is determined in part by the genetics of the host. The normal flora protect against pathogens by competing more efficiently for nutrients, by producing antibacterial proteins termed colicins and by stimulating immune responses, which act to limit pathogen entry.

Maintaining this protective flora without eliciting inflammatory reactions is a delicate and immunologically complicated process because even these bacteria are not immunologically inert. The host attempts to minimize contact between the bacteria and the epithelial cells of the gut lumen by production of mucins and by effector molecules, including anti-microbial peptides and secretory IgA. Nevertheless, some commensal bacteria do penetrate these barriers and are sampled by intestinal dendritic cells, inducing local (but not systemic) immune responses involving CD4$^+$ T cells and regulatory T cells.

When the normal flora is disturbed by antibiotics, infections by *Candida* spp. or *Clostridium difficile* can occur. Several studies suggest that the re-introduction of non-pathogenic probiotic organisms such as lactobacilli into the intestinal tract (or in extreme circumstances even the normal flora from an otherwise healthy person) can alleviate the symptoms, presumably by replacing those killed by the antibiotics.

In practice, only a minute proportion of the potentially pathogenic organisms around us ever succeed in gaining access to the tissues.

The second line of defence is mediated by recognition of bacterial components.
If organisms enter the tissues, they can be combated initially by further elements of the innate immune system. Numerous bacterial components are recognized in ways that do not rely on the antigen-specific receptors of either B cells or T cells. These types of recognition are phylogenetically ancient broad-spectrum mechanisms that evolved before antigen-specific T cells and immunoglobulins, allowing protective responses to be triggered by common microbial components bearing so-called **pathogen-associated molecular patterns (PAMPs)**, recognized by **pattern recognition molecules** of the innate immune system (see Chapter 3).

Many organisms, such as non-pathogenic cocci, are probably removed from the tissues as a consequence of these pathways, without the need for a specific adaptive immune reaction. Figure 15.3 shows some of the microbial components involved and the host responses that are triggered.

The immune system has selected these structures for recognition because they are not only characteristic of microbes but also are essential for their growth and cannot be easily mutated to evade discovery (although, as might be predicted, there are now many examples of pathogen strategies that subvert this process).

It is interesting to note that the Limulus assay, which is used to detect contaminating lipopolysaccharide (LPS) in preparations for use in humans, is based on one such recognition pathway found in an invertebrate species. In *Limulus polyphemus* (the horseshoe crab), tiny quantities of LPS trigger fibrin formation, which walls off the LPS-bearing infectious agent.

LPS is the dominant activator of innate immunity in Gram-negative bacterial infection.
Injection of pure LPS into mice or even humans is sufficient to mimic most of the features of acute Gram-negative infection, including massive production of pro-inflammatory cytokines, such as IL-1, IL-6 and tumour necrosis factor (TNF), leading to severe shock.

Recognition of LPS is a complex process involving molecules that bind LPS and pass it on to cell membrane-associated receptors on leukocytes and endothelial and other cells, which initiate this pro-inflammatory cascade (Fig. 15.4 and see Fig. 5.9).

Binding of LPS to TLR4 is a critical event in immune activation. TLR4 knockout mice are resistant to LPS-induced shock and there is some evidence that polymorphisms in human TLR4 may influence the course of infection with these bacteria. TLR4 activation also involves several co-factors, firstly LPS-binding protein (LBP), then MD2 (which binds Lipid-A) and CD14, which together are also involved in recognition of lipid-containing bacterial components from mycoplasmas, mycobacteria and spirochaetes.

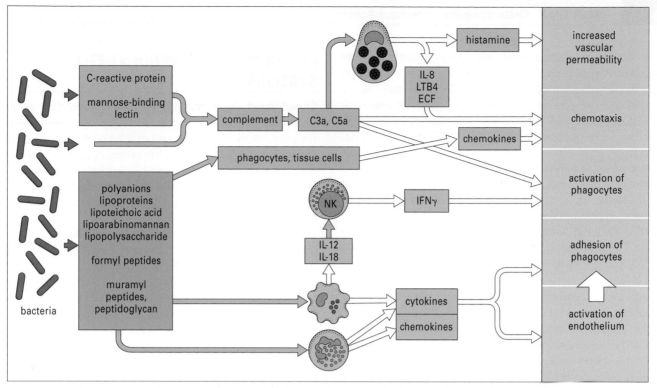

Fig. 15.3 Protective mechanisms not involving antigen-specific B or T cells Several common bacterial pathogen-associated molecular patterns are recognized by molecules present in serum and by receptors on cells. These recognition pathways result in activation of the alternative complement pathway (factors C3, B, D, P) with consequent release of C3a and C5a; activation of neutrophils, macrophages and natural killer *(NK)* cells; triggering of cytokine and chemokine release; mast cell degranulation, leading to increased blood flow in the local capillary network; and increased adhesion of cells and fibrin to endothelial cells. These mechanisms, plus tissue injury caused by the bacteria, may activate the clotting system and fibrin formation, which limit bacterial spread.

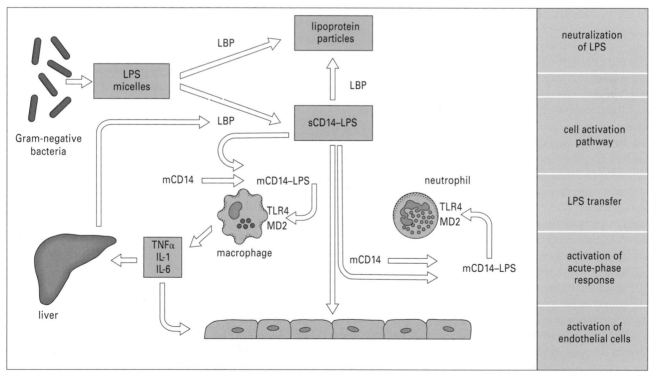

Fig. 15.4 Effects of lipopolysaccharide Lipopolysaccharide *(LPS)* released from Gram-negative bacteria becomes bound to LPS-binding protein *(LBP)*, which promotes transfer of LPS to either soluble CD14 (sCD14) or to a GPI-linked membrane form of the protein (mCD14) expressed on neutrophils and macrophages and to a lesser extent on epithelial and endothelial cells. LBP then dissociates and transfers LPS to the TLR4/MD2 complex, allowing TLR4 to transduce intracellular signals that increase release of many pro-inflammatory cytokines including TNFα and IL-6, as well as type I IFN and IL-1. These in turn activate endothelial cells, increasing adhesion molecule expression, and drive the acute-phase response in the liver. One product of the acute-phase response is further production of LBP and sCD14.

Other bacterial components are also potent immune activators. Gram-positive bacteria do not possess LPS yet still induce intense inflammatory responses and severe infection via the actions of other chemical structures such as peptidoglycans and lipoteichoic acids of their cell wall, which can be recognized by TLR2, TLR1/2 dimers and TLR2/6 dimers.

Most capsular polysaccharides are not potent activators of inflammation (although some can activate macrophages) but they shield the bacterium from host immune defences and, in particular, impair uptake by phagocytes.

Other bacterial molecules that trigger innate immunity include lipoproteins (via TLR 2/6), flagellin (via TLR5) and DNA (due to its distinct **CpG motifs**) via TLR9 (see Table 3.2).

Most pattern recognition receptors are expressed on the plasma membrane of cells, making contact with microbes during the process of binding and/or phagocytosis. These also include the scavenger receptors (see Fig. 5.10) and a family of C-type lectin receptors (dectin 1/2, Mincle and the mannose receptor, which bind microbial carbohydrates in a Ca^{2+}-dependent manner) (see Fig. 5.11). However, others are designed to detect intracellular pathogens and their products inside phagosomes (such as TLR9) or in the cytosol such as members of the NOD-like receptor family, which sense bacterial peptidoglycans (see Fig. 5.13) and the cytosolic DNA-sensing pathway involving STING and cGAS, which detect cytosolic bacterial DNA and cyclic dinucleotides in what is otherwise an abnormal location. TLR-mediated responses typically induce the production of pro-inflammatory cytokines such as TNF, IL-6 and (indirectly) IL-1, via signal transduction molecules such as MyD88 and NF-κB.

Epithelial cells of the gut and lung can have few TLRs on their luminal surface but may be triggered by pathogens that:
- actively invade the cell (such as *Listeria* spp.);
- inject their components (such as *Helicobacter pylori*); or
- actively reach the basolateral surface (e.g. *Salmonella* spp.).

This helps to explain why constant exposure to non-pathogenic microbes in the intestine and airways does not induce a chronic state of inflammation: the host waits until they move beyond the lumen, signifying the presence of a real pathogenic threat.

Finally, an important but more recent concept is the recognition of cellular damage as an activator of innate defences. Here the host responds to its own damage-associated molecular patterns (DAMPs), which include HMGB1. In most infections both DAMPs and PAMPs are present and these two pathways often work in cooperation.

The inflammasome is an important mediator of responses to more subtle cytosolic DAMPs such as the disruption of cell membranes by uric acid crystals, changes in K^+ ion fluxes and the presence of reactive oxygen species. The inflammasome is a complex multi-component aggregation of subunits that promotes generation of active caspase-1, which cleaves precursors of IL-1, IL-18 and IL-33 into biologically active mediators; this process does not occur for other cytokine or chemokine responses (see Fig. 5.13).

LYMPHOCYTE-INDEPENDENT EFFECTOR SYSTEMS

Complement is activated via the alternative pathway. Complement activation can result in the killing of some bacteria, particularly those with an outer lipid bilayer susceptible to the **lytic complex (C5b–9)**. However, clinical evidence from children with primary immunodeficiencies selectively affecting the membrane attack complex only show evidence of infection with *Neisseria* spp. indicating that lytic activity is redundant in most bacterial infections.

Perhaps more importantly, complement activation releases C5a, which attracts and activates neutrophils and causes degranulation of mast cells (see Chapter 3). The consequent release of **histamine** and **leukotriene (LTB4)** contributes to further increases in vascular permeability (see Fig. 15.3).

Opsonization of the bacteria, by attachment of **cleaved derivatives of C3**, is also critically important in subsequent interactions with phagocytes.

Release of pro-inflammatory cytokines increases the adhesive properties of the vascular endothelium. The rapid release of cytokines such as TNF and IL-1 (see Fig. 15.4) from resident tissue macrophages (and possibly also dendritic cells/tissue mast cells and epithelial cells) increases the adhesive properties of the local vascular endothelium and facilitates the passage of more phagocytes into inflamed tissue. Combined with the release of chemokines such as CCL2, CCL3 and CXCL8 (see Chapter 3), which locally decorate the endothelial lining of blood vessels, this directs the recruitment of different leukocyte populations from post-capillary venules into the infected tissues. In addition to simply providing more cells, the incoming cells are activated for improved microbicidal and inflammatory responses as they reach the site of infection.

IL-1, TNF and IL-6 also initiate the **acute-phase response**, increasing the production of complement components and other proteins involved in scavenging material released by tissue damage and, in the case of CRP, an opsonin for improving phagocytosis of bacteria.

Activation of innate lymphoid cells provides the next phase of phagocyte activation. To this point, the cytokines, which promote phagocyte recruitment, are all derived from the initial tissue sentinel cells and the first recruited phagocytes themselves. Some of these cytokines, in particular IL-12, IL-18 and IL-23, now activate an unusual range of cells with lymphoid morphology termed 'innate lymphoid cells' (ILCs). These provide the first sources of two critical new cytokines: IFNγ from NK cells and other ILC1 cells (for macrophage microbicidal activation) and IL-17 from γ/δ T cells and ILC3 cells (for further recruitment of neutrophils). For example, when NK cells are stimulated by **IL-12** and **IL-18**, they rapidly release large quantities of IFNγ. This response happens within the first day of infection, well before the clonal expansion of antigen-specific T cells and provides a rapid source of IFNγ to activate macrophages. This T-cell independent pathway helps to explain the considerable resistance of mice with SCID (severe combined immune deficiency, a defect in lymphocyte maturation) to infections such as with *Listeria monocytogenes*. CD1-restricted NK T cells can also secrete IFNγ and potentially help to activate further both NK cells and macrophages.

Pathogen recognition generates signals that regulate the antigen-specific lymphocyte-mediated response. The signals generated following the recognition of pathogens not only generate a cascade of innate immune events but also regulate the development of the appropriate B-cell and T-cell-mediated responses.

Dendritic cells (DCs) are crucial for the initial priming of naive T cells specific for bacterial antigens. Contact with bacteria in the periphery induces immature DCs to migrate to the draining lymph nodes and augments their antigen-presenting ability by increasing their:

- display of MHC molecule–peptide complexes;
- expression of co-stimulatory molecules (such as CD40, CD80 and CD86); and
- secretion of T-cell-differentiating cytokines.

Some of this DC activation occurs secondary to their production of cytokines such as type I IFN.

Activated macrophages also act as antigen-presenting cells (APCs) but probably function more at the site of infection, providing further activation of effector rather than naive T cells. Following initial T-cell activation by dendritic cells, B cells are also able to act as APCs during B-cell–T-cell cooperation and are essential for the protective action of polysaccharide-conjugate vaccines in children against encapsulated bacteria such as *Streptococcus pneumoniae* and *Haemophilus influenzae*.

Binding of bacterial components to pattern recognition receptors such as TLRs induces a local environment rich in IL-12 as well as IFNγ and IL-18, which promote T-cell differentiation down the TH1 rather than TH2 pathway.

Immunologists have made use of these effects for many decades (even without knowing their true molecular basis) in the use of **adjuvants** in vaccination. 'Adjuvant' is derived from the Latin *adjuvare*, to help. When given experimentally, soluble antigens evoke stronger T-cell and B-cell-mediated responses if they are mixed with bacterial components that act as adjuvants. Components with this property are indicated in Figure 15.1. This effect probably reflects that the antigen-specific immune response evolved in a tissue environment already contained these pharmacologically active bacterial components.

With the exception of proteins such as **flagellin**, which itself stimulates TLR5 and is also a strong T-cell immunogen, the response to pure bacterial antigens, injected without adjuvant-active bacterial components, is essentially an artificial situation that does not occur in nature.

The best known adjuvant in laboratory use, **complete Freund's adjuvant**, consists of killed mycobacteria suspended in oil, which is then emulsified with the aqueous antigen solution.

New-generation adjuvants based on bacterial components (and safe to use in humans, unlike Freund's adjuvant) include synthetic TLR activators such as CpG motifs and monophosphoryl lipid A (MPL). Other adjuvants target either only the DAMP pathway of innate immune activation such as oil in water emulsions (e.g. MF59) or both DAMP and PAMP pathways, such as AS04, which contains MPL plus Alum. Identifying the best adjuvant for inclusion in a vaccine is arguably as important as the choice of antigens and is dramatically illustrated in the RTS,S malaria vaccine—a product that was not effective until reformulated with a new MPL-based adjuvant.

ANTIBODY-DEPENDENT ANTIBACTERIAL DEFENCES

The relevance to protection of interactions of bacteria with antibody depends on the mechanism of pathogenicity. Antibodies clearly play a crucial role in dealing with bacterial toxins:

- they neutralize diphtheria toxin by blocking the attachment of the binding portion of the molecule to its target cells;
- similarly they may block locally acting toxins or extracellular matrix-degrading enzymes, which act as spreading factors.

Antibodies can also interfere with motility by binding to flagella.

An important function on external and mucosal surfaces, often performed by secretory IgA (sIgA, see Chapter 10), is to stop bacteria binding to epithelial cells. For instance, antibody to the M proteins of group A streptococci gives type-specific immunity to streptococcal sore throats.

It is likely that some antibodies to the bacterial surface can block functional requirements of the organism such as binding of iron-chelating compounds or intake of nutrients (Fig. 15.5).

An important role of antibodies in immunity to non-toxigenic bacteria is the more efficient targeting of complement.

Naturally occurring IgM antibodies, which bind to common bacterial structures such as phosphorylcholine, are important for protection against some bacteria (particularly streptococci) via their complement-fixing activity.

Specific, high-affinity IgG antibodies elicited in response to infection are most important. This is particularly true for anti-toxin responses where the antibody must compete against the affinity of the toxin receptor on host cells in vivo. Children with primary immune deficiencies in B-cell development or in T-cell help have increased susceptibility to extracellular rather than intracellular bacteria. These antibodies are also essential for resistance to encapsulated bacteria and underpin the huge public health success of polysaccharide-protein conjugate vaccines against *S. pneumoniae*, *Neisseria meningitidis* and *H. influenzae* type b. Binding of the polysaccharide-specific IgG overcomes the anti-phagocytic properties of the capsule and promotes uptake and killing by neutrophils and macrophages via FcγRs.

In addition, with the aid of antibodies, even organisms that resist the alternative (i.e. innate) complement pathway (see later) are damaged by complement or become coated with C3 products, which then enhance the binding and uptake by phagocytes (Figs. 15.6 and 15.7).

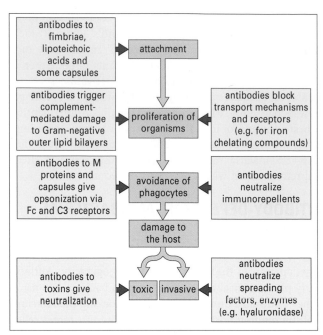

Fig. 15.5 The antibacterial roles of antibody This diagram lists the stages of bacterial invasion *(blue)* and indicates the antibacterial effects of antibody *(yellow)* that operate at the different stages. Antibodies to fimbriae, lipoteichoic acid and some capsules block attachment of the bacterium to the host cell membrane. Antibodies trigger complement-mediated damage to Gram-negative outer lipid bilayers. Antibodies directly block bacterial surface proteins that pick up useful molecules from the environment and transport them across the membrane. Antibodies to M proteins and capsules opsonize the bacteria via Fc and C3 receptors for phagocytosis. Bacterial factors that interfere with normal chemotaxis or phagocytosis are neutralized. Bacterial toxins may be neutralized by antibodies, as may bacterial spreading factors that facilitate invasion (e.g. by the destruction of connective tissue or fibrin).

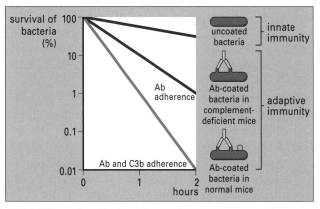

Fig. 15.6 Effect of antibody and complement on rate or clearance of virulent bacteria from the blood Uncoated bacteria are phagocytosed rather slowly (unless the alternative complement pathway is activated by the strain of bacterium); on coating with antibody *(Ab),* adherence to phagocytes is greatly increased. The adherence is somewhat less effective in animals temporarily depleted of complement.

The most efficient **complement-fixing antibodies** in humans are IgM, then IgG3 and to a lesser extent IgG1, whereas IgG1 and IgG3 are the subclasses with the highest affinity for Fc receptors.

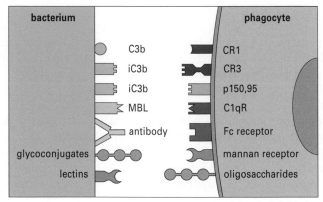

Fig. 15.7 The interaction between bacteria and phagocytic cells A variety of molecules facilitate the binding of the organisms to the phagocyte membrane. These are in addition to the Toll-like receptor (TLR) system (e.g. TLR4 for LPS, TLR5 for flagellin and TLR2 (plus TLR1/TLR6) for bacterial lipoproteins and peptidoglycans). The precise nature of the interaction will determine whether uptake occurs and whether cytokine secretion and appropriate killing mechanisms are triggered. Recognition invariably involves combinations of different receptor families. Note that apart from complement, antibody and mannose-binding lectin *(MBL),* which bind to the bacterial surface, the other components are constitutive bacterial molecules.

Pathogenic bacteria may avoid the effects of antibodies.

Neisseria gonorrhoeae is an example of a pathogenic bacterium that uses several immune evasion strategies (Fig. 15.8) and humans can be repeatedly infected with *N. gonorrhoeae* with no evidence of protective immunity.

Antibodies may also be important for effective immunity against some intracellular bacteria, such as *Legionella* and *Salmonella* spp., presumably acting either before cell entry or after release from dying cells in infected tissues.

Pathogenic bacteria can avoid the detrimental effects of complement.
Some bacterial capsules are very poor activators of the alternative pathway (Fig. 15.9).

For other bacteria, long side chains (O antigens) on their LPS may fix C3b at a distance from the otherwise vulnerable lipid bilayer. Similarly, smooth-surfaced Gram-negative organisms (*Escherichia coli, Salmonella* spp., *Pseudomonas* spp.) may fix but then rapidly shed the C5b–C9 membrane attack complex.

Other organisms exploit the physiological mechanisms that block destruction of host cells by complement. When C3b has attached to a surface it can interact with factor B, leading to further C3b amplification, or it can become inactivated by factors H and I. Capsules rich in sialic acid (as host cell membranes are) seem to promote the interaction with factors H and I. *N. meningitidis, E. coli* K1, and group B streptococci all resist complement attachment in this way.

The M protein of group A streptococci acts as an acceptor for factor H, thus potentiating C3bB dissociation. These bacteria also have a gene for a C5a protease.

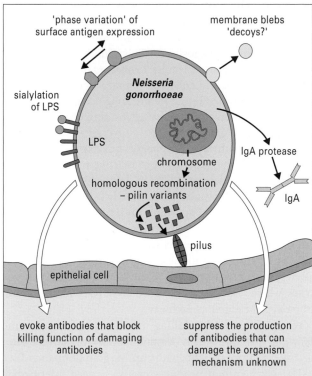

Fig. 15.8 Mechanisms used by *Neisseria gonorrhoeae* to avoid the effects of antibody *N. gonorrhoeae* is an example of a bacterium that uses several strategies to avoid the damaging effects of antibody. First, it fails to evoke a large antibody response and the antibody that does form tends to block the function of damaging antibodies. Second, the organism secretes an IgA protease to destroy antibody. Third, blebs of membrane are released and appear to adsorb and hence deplete local antibody levels. Finally, the organism uses three strategies to alter its antigenic composition: (i) the lipopolysaccharide *(LPS)* may be sialylated, so that it more closely resembles mammalian oligosaccharides and promotes rapid removal of complement; (ii) the organism can undergo phase variation, so that it expresses an alternative set of surface molecules; (iii) the gene encoding pilin, the subunits of the pilus, undergoes homologous recombination to generate variants. *N. gonorrhoeae* also impairs T-cell activation by engaging a co-inhibitory receptor CEACAM-1 on the lymphocyte surface by one of its opacity proteins (OPA).

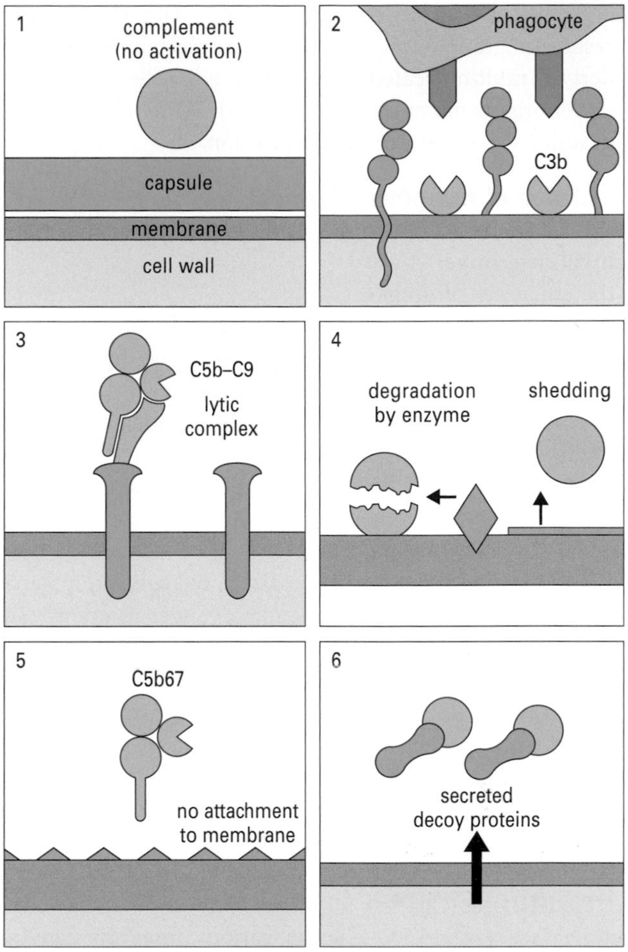

Fig. 15.9 Avoidance of complement-mediated damage Bacteria avoid complement-mediated damage by a variety of strategies. (**1**) An outer capsule or coat prevents complement activation. (**2**) An outer surface can be configured so that complement receptors on phagocytes cannot obtain access to fixed C3b. (**3**) Surface structures can be expressed that divert attachment of the lytic complex (MAC) from the cell membrane. (**4**) Membrane-bound enzyme can degrade fixed complement or cause it to be shed. (**5**) The outer membrane can resist the insertion of the lytic complex. (**6**) Secreted decoy proteins can cause complement to be deposited on them and not on the bacterium itself.

BACTERIAL KILLING BY PHAGOCYTES

A few, mostly Gram-negative, bacteria are directly killed by complement. However, immunity to most bacteria, whether considered as extracellular or intracellular pathogens, ultimately needs the killing activity of neutrophils and macrophages. This process involves several steps.

Bacterial components attract phagocytes by chemotaxis.

Unlike neutrophils, which in the uninfected host are found almost entirely in the blood, resident macrophages are constitutively present in tissues where exposure to pathogens first occurs (such as alveolar macrophages in the lung and Kupffer cells in the liver). These macrophages have some killing activity but invariably need to be supplemented by recruitment of neutrophils and/or monocytes across the blood vessel wall. Phagocytes are attracted by:

- bacterial components such as **f-Met-Leu-Phe**;
- complement products such as C5a;
- locally released chemokines and cytokines derived from resident macrophages and epithelial cells (see Chapter 3). This is followed by similar mediator release from the first arriving neutrophils and monocytes themselves, promoting further recruitment.
- IL-17 secreted by mucosa-resident γ/δ T cells and ILC3 cells (and later CD4$^+$ TH17 cells) also promotes neutrophil recruitment.

The cellular composition of this inflammatory response varies according to the pathogen and the time since infection. For instance:

- Acute infection with encapsulated bacteria such as *Streptococcus pyogenes* gives rise to tissue lesions rich in neutrophils (typical of so-called pyogenic or pus-forming infections).

- At the other extreme, chronic infections with *M. tuberculosis* result in granulomas rich in macrophages, macrophage-derived multinucleated giant cells and T cells.
- Other organisms, such as *Listeria* and *Salmonella* spp., result in lesions of more mixed composition.

The choice of receptors is critical. The choice of receptors used for attachment of the phagocyte to the organism is critical and will determine:
- the efficiency of uptake;
- whether killing mechanisms are triggered;
- whether the process favours the pathogen by subverting immunity.

The binding can be mediated by lectins on the organism (e.g. on the fimbriae of *E. coli*), but receptors on the phagocyte are the most important. These bind either directly to the bacterium or indirectly via host complement and antibody deposited on the bacterial surface (**opsonization**).
- Direct binding is mediated by pattern recognition molecules including Toll-like receptors and scavenger receptors (such as SRA, MARCO), mannose receptor and dectin-1.
- Opsonization is mediated through complement receptors such as CR1, CR3 and CR4, which recognize complement fragments deposited on the organism via the alternative or classic complement pathways.

Complement can also be fixed by MBL present in serum, which can itself bind to **C1q receptors** and CR1.

Additionally, Fc receptors on the phagocyte (**FcγRI, FcγRII** and **FcγRIII**, see Chapter 10) bind antibody that has coated bacteria (see Fig. 15.7), whereas various integrins can bind **fibronectin** and **vitronectin** opsonized particles.

Although experimentally single ligand–single receptor interactions are often described (e.g. LPS binding to TLR4), in infected tissues the host is presented simultaneously with multiple chemical structures on intact bacteria. Binding and activation are usually mediated by the combined, and often co-operative, actions of multiple receptors (such as TLR1, 2 and 6 and TLR2 together with dectin-1).

Uptake can be enhanced by macrophage-activating cytokines. The binding of an organism to a receptor on the macrophage membrane does not always lead to its uptake. For example, zymosan particles (derived from yeast) bind via the glucan-recognizing lectin-like site on the CR3 of the macrophage and are taken up, whereas erythrocytes coated with iC3b are not, even though the iC3b also binds to CR3. This can, however, be enhanced by macrophage-activating cytokines such as granulocyte–macrophage colony stimulating factor (GM-CSF).

Different membrane receptors vary in their efficiency at inducing a microbicidal response. Just as the binding of an organism to membrane receptors does not guarantee uptake, so different membrane receptors vary in their efficiency at inducing a microbicidal response. For example, mannose receptors and Fc receptors are particularly efficient at inducing the respiratory burst, but complement receptors are not, providing an evasion strategy for some organisms.

Phagocytic cells have many killing methods. Killing of bacteria and fungi occurs most efficiently when the organisms have been internalized by the phagocyte and are now within a host membrane-bound phagosome. This confinement helps to deliver anti-microbial molecules to the organism at high concentrations and reduces collateral damage to the host. Maturation of the phagosome into a killing zone occurs by acquisition of microbicidal mediators following fusion with other intracellular vesicles such as lysosomes.

The killing pathways of phagocytic cells can be oxygen dependent, with the generation of reactive oxygen intermediates, or oxygen independent (see Chapter 5). In neutrophils, the oxidative burst may also act indirectly by promoting the flux of K^+ ions into the phagosome and activating microbicidal proteases.

A second oxygen-dependent pathway involves the creation of nitric oxide (NO$^\bullet$) from the guanidino nitrogen of L-arginine. This in turn leads to further toxic substances such as the peroxynitrites, which result from interactions of NO$^\bullet$ with the products of the oxygen reduction pathway.

Oxygen-independent killing mechanisms may be more important than previously thought. Many organisms can be killed by cells from patients with chronic granulomatous disease (CGD), which cannot produce reactive oxygen intermediates, and from patients with myeloperoxidase (MPO) deficiency, which cannot produce hypohalous acids. Some of this killing may be caused by NO$^\bullet$, but many organisms can be killed anaerobically; therefore other mechanisms must exist. Some have been identified and are discussed later. Indeed, many innate immune factors have actually evolved to work optimally in the hypoxic environment of infected tissues. Under conditions of low oxygen tension and pH, phagocytes specifically upregulate genes that contain hypoxic-response elements, resulting in increased phagocytic activity, a longer life span and the production of anti-microbial molecules and inflammatory cytokines.

Some cationic proteins have antibiotic-like properties. The **defensins** (Fig. 15.10) are cysteine- and arginine-rich cationic peptides of 30–33 amino acids found in phagocytes such as neutrophils, where they comprise 30%–50% of the granule proteins. Defensins evolved early in evolution and similar molecules are found in insects. They act by integrating into microbial lipid membranes (in some cases forming ion-permeable channels) and disrupting membrane function and structure, resulting in lysis of the pathogen. Defensins can act both inside and outside of host cells and kill organisms as diverse as *Staphylococcus aureus*, *Pseudomonas aeruginosa*, and *E. coli*, as well as fungi such as *Cryptococcus neoformans*.

Defensins also have important immunostimulatory properties, including:
- promoting chemotaxis and phagocytosis;
- regulating cytokine production; and
- acting as adjuvants for adaptive immunity by promoting multiple facets of dendritic cell function, including antigen uptake, processing and presentation as well as their migration and maturation.

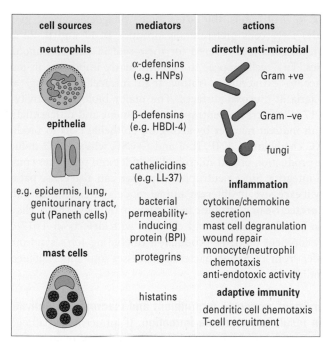

cell sources	mediators	actions
neutrophils	α-defensins (e.g. HNPs)	**directly anti-microbial**
		Gram +ve
	β-defensins (e.g. HBDI-4)	Gram −ve
epithelia		fungi
	cathelicidins (e.g. LL-37)	**inflammation**
e.g. epidermis, lung, genitourinary tract, gut (Paneth cells)	bacterial permeability-inducing protein (BPI)	cytokine/chemokine secretion mast cell degranulation wound repair monocyte/neutrophil chemotaxis anti-endotoxic activity
	protegrins	
mast cells	histatins	**adaptive immunity**
		dendritic cell chemotaxis T-cell recruitment

Fig. 15.10 Cationic host defence peptides in immunity to fungi and bacteria Numerous cationic host defence peptides are produced by neutrophils, monocytes, epithelia and mast cells. Their synthesis is usually constitutive but is also enhanced by pro-inflammatory cytokines such as TNF, IL-1, IL-22 and IFNγ generated following infection. Originally defined by their direct killing activity against pathogens, they are now known also to act on immune cells, having multiple immunomodulatory effects on inflammation and adaptive immunity. −ve, Negative; +ve, positive.

Other antibacterial peptides include the **cathelicidins** (which can kill *M. tuberculosis* under the regulation of vitamin D) and **protegrins** (which can bind LPS and form membrane pores).

There are also cationic proteins with different pH optima, including **cathepsin G** and **azurocidin**, both of which are related to elastase but have activity against Gram-negative bacteria, which is unrelated to their enzyme activity.

Neutrophils possess an extracellular mechanism of microbicidal activity by release of so-called neutrophil extracellular traps (NETs). This involves the release of chromatin, histones and anti-microbial proteins, which bind and kill bacteria and fungi as well as generating a barrier against the spread of infection.

Other anti-microbial mechanisms also play a role. Following lysosome fusion, there is a transient rise in pH before acidification of the phagolysosome takes place. This occurs within 10–15 minutes.

The acidification of phagosomes containing bacteria following their fusion with lysosomes is an important step in the killing process and is related to the low pH optima of lysosomal enzymes.

Certain Gram-positive organisms may be killed by **lysozyme**, which is active against their exposed peptidoglycan layer.

Restricting the access of intracellular bacteria to essential nutrients is a microbistatic strategy of host defence. Induction of indoleamine 2-3 dioxygenase (IDO) in macrophages by IFNγ depletes tryptophan, which is an essential amino acid for growth

of *Chlamydia*. The tryptophan starvation pathway also functions in endothelial cells and fibroblasts. NRAMP 1 (also known as SLC11A1) performs its microbistatic function by removing divalent cations from the phagosome; these are needed for bacterial metabolism and their evasion of the respiratory burst.

The availability of intracellular iron is another important factor in the interplay between host and pathogen. Iron is essential for the growth of many bacteria and also influences their expression of key virulence genes. Sequestration of iron can therefore be an effective anti-microbial strategy, particularly for intracellular bacteria.

Lactoferrin is a mammalian iron-binding protein released by degranulating neutrophils that sequesters iron from pathogens, inhibiting their growth and in the case of *P. aeruginosa* also reducing biofilm formation, a key event in the pathogenesis of infection in cystic fibrosis patients. **Lactoferricin**, an anti-microbial peptide derived from lactoferrin, kills other bacteria.

Iron is also required for many host immune functions, including the respiratory burst, the generation of NO· and the development of pathogen-specific T cells.

Both iron excess and iron deficiency can therefore have complex effects on the outcome of infection. For example, individuals with iron overload syndromes resulting from genetic defects (such as thalassaemia or haemochromatosis), nutritional excess or after iron or red cell supplementation (such as in the treatment of anaemias) have increased susceptibility to infection with *Yersinia* and *Salmonella* spp., and *M. tuberculosis*.

Finally, in addition to engaging pathogens on the cell surface via phagocytosis, neutrophils and particularly macrophages also deal with intracellular pathogens by an internal engulfment process termed autophagy. This is an adaptation of an ancient intracellular recycling pathway that degrades and reuses host cell constituents. In the context of infection, pathogens in the cytosol, in damaged vacuoles or not able to be killed in intact phagosomes are engulfed in a new double membrane—the autophagosome. Autophagy is promoted in times of cellular stress and in response to cytokines such as IFNγ and is an important additional microbicidal pathway for bacteria such as *M. tuberculosis* and *Listeria*. There is considerable interest in re-purposing drugs known to promote autophagy as host-directed therapies for treatment of infection.

Macrophage killing can be enhanced on activation. Unlike neutrophils, which have a short life span but are efficient killers even in their normal state, macrophages are long-lived cells that, without appropriate activation, can actually provide a haven for microbial growth. Indeed, most intracellular bacteria and fungi target the macrophage as a site of persistence and replication.

Macrophage activation occurs most effectively by the combination of exposure to cytokines (particularly IFNγ) and microbial products (through the receptors described earlier). Attempts to activate macrophages that have already been infected are often less effective.

Optimal activation of macrophages is dependent on TH1 cells. Microbial products can directly activate monocytes and resident macrophages to secrete pro-inflammatory cytokines and thus initiate the immune process. However, complete activation, including the ability to kill intracellular microbes, requires the action of IFNγ. IFNγ knockout mice are extremely susceptible to infection and children with deficiencies in either the IFNγ receptor or the cytokines necessary for its production (such as IL-12, IL-18 and IL-23) have increased susceptibility to intracellular bacteria such as *Salmonella* spp. and mycobacteria including bacillus Calmette–Guérin (BCG). Thus, although other cytokines are also involved in macrophage activation and function (such as the essential role of TNF in granuloma formation), no other cytokine is as important as IFNγ for macrophage microbicidal activity.

IFNγ is so potent because it enhances several different microbicidal pathways, including the respiratory burst, the generation of NO• and the induction of IDO.

NK cells (ILC1), NK T cells and mucosa-associated invariant T cells (MAIT) can produce IFNγ during the innate immune response. However, the additional actions of antigen-specific T cells are necessary for optimal cell-mediated immunity.

The most important source of IFNγ during the adaptive immune response to intracellular bacteria is from antigen-specific TH1 CD4+ T cells (Fig. 15.11).

Patients who have AIDS and a reduced CD4 T-cell number and function have dramatically increased susceptibility to *M. tuberculosis*, *Mycobacterium avium* and atypical salmonella.

Macrophages activated by IFNγ are primarily microbicidal and pro-inflammatory and are usually referred to as classically activated (as they were the first to be described) or M1 macrophages.

As mentioned previously, many bacterial components activate the TLR pattern recognition receptors, ensuring the preferential expression of TH1 rather than TH2 T-cell responses in most cases.

TH1 T cells provide both IFNγ for macrophage activation and B-cell help to produce IgG subclasses for opsonization of bacteria, rather than the eosinophilia and IgE responses typical of helminth infections.

There is mutual antagonism between the TH1 and TH2 pathways at the level of both T-cell differentiation and also directly on the macrophage:

- IFNγ upregulates induced NO• synthetase expression; whereas
- IL-4 and IL-13 promote the expression of arginase, which inhibits NO• production, reducing the macrophage killing potential and diverting it to a profibrotic phenotype. These cells are called alternatively activated (or M2) macrophages whose primary functions are repair, immune regulation and restoration of infected tissues to homeostasis.

Other cytokines such as GM-CSF and TNF can also contribute to macrophage activation.

Macrophage activation is also promoted by direct contact with CD4 T cells via **CD40–CD40L** interactions.

Thus, T-cell-mediated help for macrophages and B cells share the common themes of soluble and cell-contact-mediated activation by CD4 TH1 cells.

While this functional link between CD4 TH1 cells and macrophages has been known for many years, only recently have we discovered that a different T-cell subset (TH17 cells) mediate a link to neutrophils, the other major phagocyte group in the body. TH17 cells preferentially produce IL-17 and IL-22 and were originally discovered for their role in autoimmune diseases. TH17 cells appear to be particularly important in resistance to extracellular (rather than intracellular) fungi and bacteria at mucosal surfaces. The major biological activity of IL-17 is to increase neutrophil recruitment and differentiation in an indirect manner by acting on epithelial cells to produce CXC chemokines, TNF, IL-6 and G-CSF, whilst IL-22 induces the production of anti-microbial peptides and promotes epithelial integrity. Since neutrophil responses can also cause pathology if excessive, in different animal models TH17 cells can either be protective or contribute to immune pathology. These cells are also found in humans and children with defects in TH17-cell development or IL-17 production (including Job's syndrome) suffer from recurring bacterial abscesses and mucocutaneous candidiasis.

Persistent monocyte recruitment and macrophage activation can result in granuloma formation. If intracellular pathogens are not quickly eliminated, the persistent recruitment and activation of macrophages and T cells to an infected tissue can result in the formation of **granulomas**. These are generally associated with chronic bacterial infections such as tuberculosis and syphilis, but similar (although not identical) structures are also induced in parasitic diseases such as schistosomiasis and in response to non-infectious materials such as asbestos.

In the classic example of active tuberculosis, granulomas are composed of a central caseous necrotic core, surrounded by infected (and uninfected) macrophages, epithelioid cells and multinucleated giant cells (derived from the fusion of activated macrophages), and a peripheral accumulation of T cells. Neutrophils and dendritic cells can also be found in granulomas, along with fibroblasts and extracellular matrix components such as collagen. Within each granuloma there are complex mixtures of both M1 and M2 macrophages, but how the balance between these two cell types is regulated and what finally achieves sterilization of the granuloma is still not clear. The presence of activated macrophages and the fibrosis that ensues is believed to control bacterial growth and prevent dissemination to other organs but may also provide a niche for bacterial persistence and can be an obstacle to penetration of antibiotics. There is also experimental evidence that, at least initially, the TB bacillus actively induces the granulomatous response in order to have a source of naive macrophages in which to grow. Generating these new immunological structures is a highly complex event involving multiple adhesion molecules, chemokines and cytokines. Once formed, their continued existence also requires active immunological input. New intra-vital imaging techniques, where the movement of host cells in and out of the granuloma can be measured in real time, are now providing insights into just how dynamic these structures are in vivo.

AIDS and diabetes mellitus are important risk factors for loss of control of *M. tuberculosis*. TNF is also critical for granuloma maintenance—some patients given TNF-blocking antibodies to alleviate the symptoms of rheumatoid arthritis rapidly reactivate tuberculosis that had otherwise been controlled for many years.

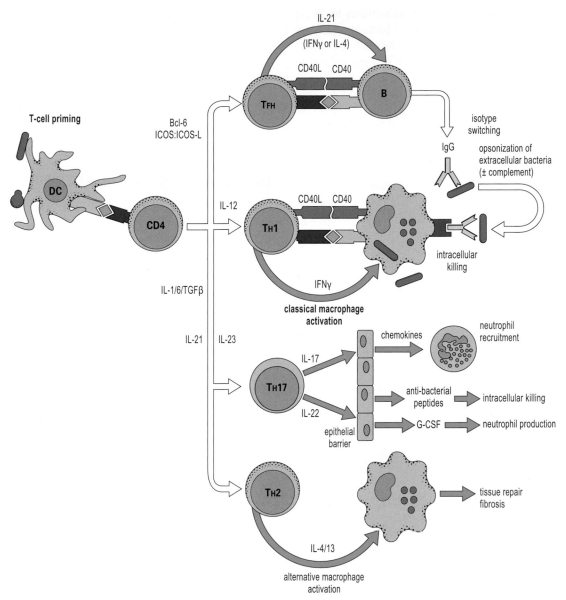

Fig. 15.11 Overview of CD4⁺ T-cell mediated immunity to bacteria and fungi Naive CD4⁺ T cells are stimulated by MHC class II positive antigen-bearing dendritic cells *(DCs)* via the T-cell receptor (TCR), in conjunction with co-stimulatory molecules such as CD80/86 and CD28, which induce T-cell activation and proliferation. Differentiation into TH1, TH17 or TH2 effector cells is strongly influenced by the cytokine environment during this interaction—microbial pattern recognition events that favour production of IL-12 promote TH1 development, low IL-12/presence of IL-4 favours TH2 responses, whereas combinations of IL-6, IL-1 TGFβ, IL-21 and IL-23 are required for development and maintenance of TH17 responses. IFNγ derived from TH1 cells induces so-called classically activated macrophages (because they were discovered first), which kill intracellular pathogens and are pro-inflammatory. TH17 cells mediate their biological activities via secretion of IL-17, which induces G-CSF and CXC family chemokines to enhance neutrophil production and recruitment, and of IL-22, which helps repair damaged epithelia. Both cytokines also induce anti-microbial peptides such as defensins and mucins. Optimal T-cell help for either B cells or classical macrophage activation responses involves T-cell-derived cytokines and direct cell contact. TH1 cells can promote opsonizing antibody production of high affinity, which complements their activation of phagocytes by IFNγ, but the main activators of antibody synthesis are CD4⁺ T-follicular helper cells *(T_FH)*, which are induced by strong TCR interactions with antigen-presenting dendritic cells inducing Bcl-6 and then by interaction with B cells via ICOS:ICOS-L. TH2 responses are not dominant or protective in most bacterial or fungal infections, although if present could promote tissue repair and fibrosis by secretion of IL-4/IL-13, resulting in alternatively activated macrophages. Although not shown here, conditions with high levels of IL-10 or TGFβ can induce regulatory T cells, rather than effector (i.e. TH1, TH2 or TH17) subsets.

Successful pathogens have evolved mechanisms to avoid phagocyte-mediated killing. Because most bacteria and fungi are ultimately killed by phagocytes, it is not surprising that successful pathogens have developed an array of mechanisms to counteract this risk (Fig. 15.12).

Intracellular pathogens may 'hide' in cells. Some organisms may thrive inside metabolically damaged host phagocytes or escape killing by moving out of phagosomes into the cytoplasm.

L. monocytogenes, *Shigella* spp. and *Burkholderia pseudomallei* achieve this by releasing enzymes that lyse the phagosome membrane and allow entry into the cytoplasm. However, all is not lost, because the host can still capture cytosolic bacteria into the lysosome system for destruction via the autophagy pathway, which these pathogens also actively attempt to evade. These organisms clearly illustrate the concept that bacteria are not just inert particles but have developed multiple strategies for taking control of functions of the host cell in order to avoid being killed and to obtain the nutrients they need for replication.

Other organisms, such as *Mycobacterium leprae* and salmonellae, cause themselves to be taken up by cells that are not normally considered phagocytic and have little antibacterial potential such as Schwann cells, hepatocytes and epithelial cells.

Before they can be taken up by activated phagocytes or exposed to other killing mechanisms, the organisms may need to be released from such cells.

DIRECT ANTIBACTERIAL ACTIONS OF T CELLS

Infected cells can be killed by CTLs. CD8+ cytotoxic T lymphocytes (CTLs) can release intracellular organisms by killing the infected cell. For example, mice become more susceptible to *M. tuberculosis* if class I MHC genes are knocked out so that antigen-specific CD8+ T cells do not develop and kill infected macrophages.

This is consistent with an important role for CTLs in resistance to intracellular bacteria and inducing these responses is now a primary goal of new vaccines against bacteria such as *M. tuberculosis* and other pathogens.

Tissue cells that are not components of the immune system can also harbour bacteria such as *M. leprae*, invasive *Shigella* and *Salmonella* spp. and *Rickettsia* and *Chlamydia* spp. These infected cells may also be sacrificed by CTLs.

Dendritic cells appear to be particularly important in the generation of strong CD8+ T-cell responses to bacteria such as *L. monocytogenes* and *Salmonella* spp.

Although antigen processing and presentation via the class I MHC pathway is most efficient for microbial antigens derived from the cytosol, CTLs are also induced by bacteria that do not always escape the phagosome such as *M. tuberculosis*, salmonellae and chlamydiae. This occurs by **cross-presentation** of antigens within the same cell (see Chapter 7) or where antigens are released from infected cells undergoing apoptosis and then transferred to nearby DCs for efficient presentation via the MHC class I pathway. Conversely, bacteria encountered in the cytosol can also induce MHC class I restricted CD4+ T cells via the autophagy pathway. Thus in most bacterial infections, regardless of their intracellular location, both CD4+ and CD8+ T-cell responses are induced, although their relative importance may vary. In some cases, lysis of infected host cells by CTLs can result in killing the organism inside. This can be a result of the action of **granulysin**—an antibacterial peptide stored in the cytotoxic granules and released during the cytotoxic process.

CTLs can also secrete IFNγ when they recognize infected targets, providing an additional pathway of macrophage activation and protective immunity (Fig. 15.13).

Other T-cell populations can contribute to antibacterial immunity. In addition to the classic MHC class I-mediated and MHC class II-mediated recognition of bacterial proteins by αβ CD4+ and CD8+ T cells, other non-conventional T-cell populations allow the host to respond rapidly to other microbial chemistries.

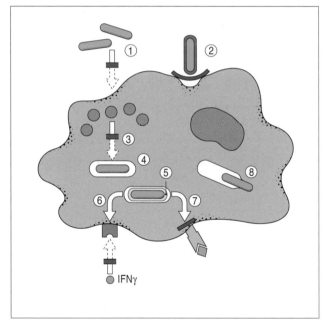

Fig. 15.12 Evasion mechanisms Bacteria (and some fungi), particularly those that are successful intracellular parasites, have evolved the ability to evade different aspects of phagocyte-mediated killing. *(1)* Some can secrete repellents or toxins that inhibit chemotaxis. *(2)* Others have capsules or outer coats that inhibit attachment by the phagocyte (e.g. *Streptococcus pneumoniae* or the yeast *Cryptococcus neoformans*). *(3)* Others permit uptake but release factors that block subsequent triggering of killing mechanisms. Once ingested, some, such as *Mycobacterium tuberculosis*, inhibit lysosome fusion with the phagosome. They also inhibit the proton pump that acidifies the phagosome, so that the pH does not fall. *(4)* They may also secrete catalase (e.g. staphylococci), which breaks down hydrogen peroxide. *(5)* Organisms such as *Mycobacterium leprae* have highly resistant outer coats. *M. leprae* surrounds itself with a phenolic glycolipid, which scavenges free radicals. *(6)* Mycobacteria also release a lipoarabinomannan, which blocks the ability of macrophages to respond to the activating effects of interferon-γ *(IFNγ)*. *(7)* Cells infected with *Salmonella enterica*, *M. tuberculosis* or *Chlamydia trachomatis* have impaired antigen-presenting function. *(8)* Several organisms (e.g. *Listeria* and *Shigella* spp.) can escape from the phagosome to multiply in the cytoplasm. Finally, the organism may kill the phagocyte via either necrosis (e.g. staphylococci) or induction of apoptosis (e.g. *Yersinia* spp.).

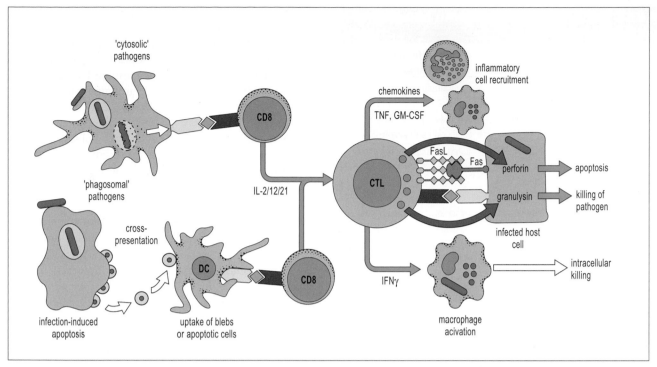

Fig. 15.13 Pathways of CD8 T-cell activation and function Naive CD8⁺ T cells are activated by peptides presented via major histocompatibility complex (MHC) class I molecules, primarily derived from microorganisms that reside in the cytoplasm, such as viruses and some intracellular bacteria that escape the phagosome such as *Listeria* spp. Other pathogens that do not escape the phagosome (such as *Mycobacterium tuberculosis*) can still induce CD8⁺ T-cell responses via cross-priming, in which infected and apoptotic host cells release antigenic fragments that are taken up by dendritic cells *(DCs)*. Effector CD8⁺ T cells *(CTLs)* provide protection by releasing pro-inflammatory and macrophage-activating cytokines and killing infected host cells via perforin release and ligation of Fas. In some cases, the release of granulysin from the CTL can also result in killing of the pathogen.

T cells bearing γδ (rather than αβ) receptors (see Chapter 2) proliferate in response to bacterial infection.

Some γδ T cells recognize small phospholigands derived from *M. tuberculosis* and possibly other bacteria, whereas others are triggered in an antigen-independent manner by the presence of pathogen-activated DCs expressing high levels of co-stimulatory molecules and IL-12.

NK T cells are a diverse group of T cells, some of which have an invariant T-cell antigen receptor. They recognize not proteins, but hydrophobic antigens, particularly microbial glycolipids such as the **lipoarabinomannan** from *M. tuberculosis*, presented via CD1 molecules.

Such γδ and NK T cells secrete multiple cytokines including IFNγ and IL-17 (depending on how they are stimulated) giving a potential role in host defence. Finally, mucosal-associated T cells (MAIT cells) are among the most recently described non-conventional T cells and recognize bacterial (and some fungal) antigens derived from precursors of riboflavin (vitamin B2). These are presented on MR-1 molecules, which are MHC class-I–like, but not polymorphic and have a narrower binding groove to bind these small structures rather than peptides or glycolipids. These cells are potentially cytotoxic but mostly secrete pro-inflammatory cytokines such as IFNγ and IL-17 to promote phagocyte-mediated immunity and are of particular interest in tuberculosis. In animal models of infection, these non-conventional T cells can be protective or

immunoregulatory, but their relative importance in human immunity is not resolved.

Examples to illustrate the relationship between the nature of an organism, the disease and immunopathology caused and the mechanism of immune response that leads to protection are given in Table 15.1.

IMMUNOPATHOLOGICAL REACTIONS INDUCED BY BACTERIA

The events described so far are generally beneficial to the host and critical for resistance against pathogenic bacteria. However, all immune responses designed to kill invading pathogens have the potential for causing collateral damage to the host.

Excessive cytokine release can lead to endotoxin shock. If cytokine release is sudden and massive, several acute tissue-damaging syndromes can result and are potentially fatal.

One of the most severe examples of this is **septic shock**, when there is massive production of cytokines (a so-called 'cytokine storm'), caused by bacterial products released during septicaemic episodes. Endotoxin (LPS) from Gram-negative bacteria is usually responsible, although Gram-positive septicaemia can cause a similar syndrome. There can be life-threatening fever, circulatory collapse, diffuse intravascular coagulation

TABLE 15.1 Immunity in Some Important Bacterial Infections

Infection	Pathogenesis	Major Defence Mechanisms
Corynebacterium diphtheriae	Non-invasive pharyngitis toxin	Neutralizing antibody
Vibrio cholerae	Non-invasive enteritis toxin	Neutralizing and adhesion-blocking antibodies
Neisseria meningitidis (Gram negative)	Nasopharynx →bacteraemia →meningitis →endotoxaemia	Killed by antibody and lytic complement; opsonized and phagocytosed
Staphylococcus aureus (Gram positive)	Locally invasive and toxic in skin, etc.	Opsonized by antibody and complement; killed by phagocytes
Mycobacterium tuberculosis	Invasive, evokes immunopathology	Macrophage activation by cytokines from T cells, CTLs
Mycobacterium leprae	Invasive, space-occupying and/or immunopathology	

This table provides examples of how knowledge of the organism and the mechanism of disease can lead to a prediction of the relevant protective mechanism.

and haemorrhagic necrosis, leading eventually to multiple organ failure (Fig. 15.14).

Individuals who recover from the initial life-threatening phase are also at increased risk of death by secondary infection some weeks later as a result of immune hyporesponsiveness. Here many innate and adaptive immune functions are perturbed, leading to increased apoptosis of DCs and NK cells, exhaustion of CD4$^+$ and CD8$^+$ T cells as well as abnormal induction of regulatory T cells and their cytokines. Management of sepsis is still very difficult because both inflammatory and anti-inflammatory processes are found together in a changing balance as sepsis occurs and recovery progresses.

The toxicity of superantigens results from massive cytokine release. Certain bacterial components called **superantigens** bind directly to the variable regions of β chains (Vβ) of antigen receptors on subsets of T cells and cross-link them to the MHC molecules of APCs, usually outside the normal antigen-binding groove (Fig. 15.15). Both staphylococci and streptococci have different superantigens and these molecules can also be found in other bacteria such as mycoplasmas. The full biological significance of this bacterial adaptation is not yet clear—it could

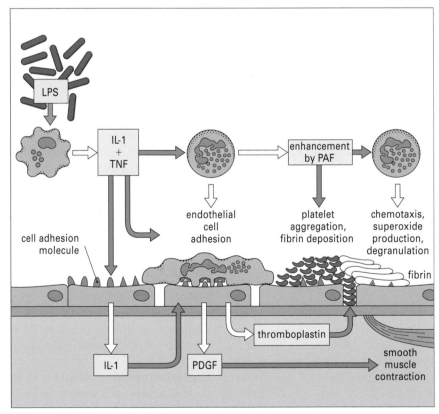

Fig. 15.14 Endotoxin shock Excessive release of cytokines, often triggered by the endotoxin (lipopolysaccharide; *LPS*) of Gram-negative bacteria, can lead to diffuse intravascular coagulation with consequent defective clotting, changes in vascular permeability, loss of fluid into the tissues, a fall in blood pressure, circulatory collapse, and haemorrhagic necrosis, particularly in the gut. This figure illustrates some important parts of this pathway at the cellular level. The cytokines tumour necrosis factor *(TNF)* and IL-1 cause endothelial cells to express cell adhesion molecules and tissue thromboplastin. These promote adhesion of circulating cells and deposition of fibrin, respectively. Platelet-activating factor *(PAF)* enhances these effects. In experimental models, shock can be blocked by neutralizing antibodies to TNF and greatly diminished by antibodies to tissue thromboplastin or by inhibitors of PAF or of nitric oxide production, but these have not been successful clinically. Gram-positive bacteria can induce shock:L for example, by massive release of cytokines mediated by superantigens. *PDGF*, Platelet-derived growth factor, produced by both platelets and endothelium.

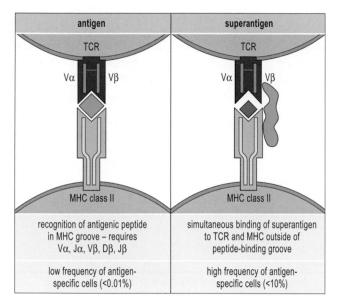

antigen	superantigen
TCR	TCR
Vα Vβ	Vα Vβ
MHC class II	MHC class II
recognition of antigenic peptide in MHC groove – requires Vα, Jα, Vβ, Dβ, Jβ	simultaneous binding of superantigen to TCR and MHC outside of peptide-binding groove
low frequency of antigen-specific cells (<0.01%)	high frequency of antigen-specific cells (<10%)

Fig 15.15 T-cell stimulation by superantigens Normally, antigenic peptides are processed and presented on major histocompatibility complex *(MHC)* molecules *(left)*. Superantigens, such as staphylococcal enterotoxins, are not processed but bind directly to MHC class II molecules and Vβ of the T-cell receptor *(TCR) (right)*. Each superantigen activates a distinct set of Vβ-expressing T cells.

be to the organism's advantage to exhaust or to deplete T cells that would otherwise be protective.

One certain effect is the toxicity of the massive release of pro-inflammatory cytokines (including IL-2, TNFα and TNFβ, together with IL-1β from activated macrophages) as a result of the simultaneous stimulation of up to 20% of the entire T-cell pool.

The staphylococcal toxins responsible for the **toxic shock syndrome** (toxic shock syndrome toxin-1 (TSST-1), etc.) operate in this way, although not all shock syndromes caused by staphylococci are the result of T-cell activation.

Recent evidence suggests that streptococcal M protein, a known virulence factor of *S. pyogenes*, forms a complex with fibrinogen, which then binds to β-integrins on neutrophils, causing the release of inflammatory mediators, which also result in massive vascular leakage and shock.

FUNGAL INFECTIONS

Fungi are eukaryotes with a rigid cell wall enriched in complex polysaccharides such as chitin, glucans and mannan.

Among the 70 000 or so species of fungi, only a small number are pathogenic for humans. However, because there are no approved vaccines and because antifungal drugs often have severe side effects, fungi can cause serious and sometimes life-threatening infections.

Fungi can exist as:
* single cells (yeasts), which reproduce by budding and are small enough to be ingested by host phagocytes; or
* long slender, branching hyphae (moulds), which reproduce by spore formation and may require extracellular killing processes.

Some pathogenic fungi are dimorphic, in that they switch from a hyphal form in the environment to a yeast form as they adapt to life in the host at 37°C. Both phases possess important virulence determinants and pose different problems to the immune system.

There are four categories of fungal infection. Although some fungi can cause disease in otherwise healthy individuals, severe fungal infections are a growing problem because of the markedly increased numbers of immunologically compromised hosts. Fungal infections are therefore regularly seen in:
* patients with untreated AIDS;
* patients with cancer and undergoing chemotherapy;
* patients with transplants on immunosuppressive agents; and
* some patients taking long-term corticosteroids.

These clinical findings point to the key roles of neutrophils and macrophages and the CD4 T-cell subsets that regulate their activity (i.e. TH1 and TH17) in antifungal immunity.

Human fungal infections fall into the following four major categories:
* **Superficial mycoses** are caused by fungi known as dermatophytes, usually restricted to the non-living keratinized components of skin, hair and nails, and include infection by *Trichophyton* and *Microsporum* spp. (which cause ringworm and athlete's foot) and *Malassezia* spp. (which causes pityriasis). Oral candidiasis is another example of a superficial fungal infection.
* **Subcutaneous mycoses** are a particular problem in tropical and subtropical regions, as a result of introduction by local trauma of saprophytic fungi, which cause chronic nodules or ulcers in subcutaneous tissues (e.g. chromoblastomyces, sporotrichosis and mycetoma) and may also lead to osteomyelitis. These are highly debilitating infections with significant public health impact, such that one, mycetoma, has now been listed by the WHO as a Neglected Tropical Disease.
* **Systemic mycoses** can be grouped according to whether they cause diseases as primary pathogens in otherwise healthy individuals or as opportunistic infections following loss of cell-mediated immune function (such as in neutropenia, AIDS, transplantation, etc.). *Histoplasma*, *Blastomyces*, *Coccidioides* and *Paracoccidioides* are soil saprophytes inhaled from the environment and can all cause primary disease in otherwise immunocompetent individuals. *Aspergillus* spp., *Pneumocystis jirovecii*, Zygomyces, *Penicillium marneffei* and *C. neoformans* act more as opportunists.
* **Candidiasis** is caused by *Candida albicans*, a ubiquitous commensal and the most common opportunistic fungal pathogen: disturbance of normal physiology by immunosuppressive drugs, of normal flora by antibiotics or of T-cell function (as in severe combined immune deficiency, thymic aplasia and AIDS) results in superficial infections of the skin and mucous membranes. Systemic disease can occur in intravenous drug users and patients with lymphoma or leukaemia.

Innate immune responses to fungi include defensins and phagocytes. The basic protective features of the skin and normal commensal flora against bacterial infections are also important in resistance to fungi.

Defensins have antifungal as well as antibacterial properties and collectins such as MBL and the surfactant proteins A and D can bind, aggregate and opsonize fungi for phagocytosis.

Phagocytes, particularly neutrophils (Fig. 15.16) and macrophages, are essential for killing fungi, either by:

- degranulation and release of toxic materials onto large indigestible hyphae; or
- ingestion of yeast or conidia.

The oxidative burst plays a crucial role in some antifungal responses, as seen in the susceptibility to severe aspergillosis by patients with CGD who have defects in the NADPH oxidase system. However, phagocytes from such patients with defective oxygen-reduction pathways nevertheless kill other yeast and hyphae with near-normal efficiency, thus demonstrating the role of other killing mechanisms (Table. 15.2). For instance, NO• and its derivatives are important for resistance to *C. neoformans*. The myeloperoxidase system is a major component of neutrophil granules and, in particular, kills *Candida*, *Aspergillus* hyphae and *Coccidioides*.

These responses rely on the recognition of PAMPs in the fungal cell wall by either soluble or cell-bound pattern recognition molecules. The TLR family again plays an important role in this process, along with the mannose receptor and complement receptors:

- TLR2 (which can cooperate with the β-glucan receptor dectin-1) recognizes fungal phospholipomannans, *C. albicans* yeasts and *Aspergillus fumigatus* hyphae and conidia;
- TLR4/CD14 recognizes *C. albicans*, *A. fumigatus* and the glucuronoxylomannan capsule of *C. neoformans*.

Dectin-1, a C-type lectin receptor is widely expressed on myeloid cells of the gut and airway mucosa. Recognition of fungi via this receptor promotes phagocytosis, triggers the respiratory burst and elicits inflammatory cytokine, chemokine and prostaglandin responses. TNF is one of these important cytokines in humans, because individuals given anti-TNF therapy have increased susceptibility to multiple fungal pathogens. Not all of these recognition events are to the host's advantage: for example, binding of *C. albicans* mannan via TLR4 induces

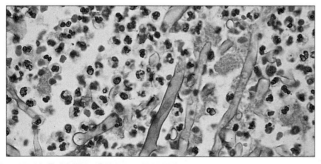

Fig. 15.16 Evidence for neutrophil-mediated immunity to mucormycosis This is a section from the lung of a patient suffering from mucormycosis – an opportunistic infection in an immunosuppressed subject. The inflammatory reaction consists almost entirely of neutrophil polymorphs around the fungal hyphae. The disease is particularly associated with neutropenia (lack of neutrophils). Silver stain. ×400. (Courtesy Professor RJ Hay.)

TABLE 15.2   Monocyte/Macrophage Killing of Fungi

Organism	SOURCE OF MONOCYTES/MACROPHAGES		
	Normal	CGD	MPO deficiency
Candida albicans	Killed	Sometimes killed	Sometimes killed
Candida parapsilosis	Killed	Not killed	Unknown
Cryptococcus neoformans	Killed	Unknown	Killed
Aspergillus fumigatus conidia	Killed	Sometimes killed	Killed
Aspergillus fumigatus hyphae	Killed	Killed	Killed

CGD, Chronic granulomatous disease; *MPO*, myeloperoxidase. Many fungi are killed by monocytes or macrophages. Individuals with CGD are highly susceptible to *Aspergillus* spp. infections, whereas MPO deficiency does not usually lead to opportunistic infection, suggesting that non-oxygen-dependent mechanisms are also important in host defence.

pro-inflammatory chemokine responses, whereas ligation of *Candida* phospholipomannan and glucans with TLR2/dectin-1 generates a strong IL-10 response, which may inhibit the relevant immune response.

T-Cell mediated immunity is critical for resistance to fungi.

Most fungi are highly immunogenic and induce strong antibody and T-cell-mediated immune responses, which can be detected by serology and delayed-type (type IV) hypersensitivity skin reactions (see Chapter 26).

Considerable evidence points to the dominant protective role of TH1 and TH17 cells as well as phagocyte activation, rather than antibody-mediated responses.

Patients with T-cell deficiencies, rather than defects in antibody production, are more at risk of disseminated fungal disease and antibody titres, although useful as an epidemiological tool to determine exposure, do not necessarily correlate with prognosis. Nevertheless, fungi can elicit both protective and non-protective antibodies and the protection afforded by some experimental vaccines can be adoptively transferred by immune sera.

Resistance to most pathogenic fungi (including dermatophytes and most systemic mycoses, including *C. neoformans*, *Histoplasma capsulatum*, etc., but not *Aspergillus* spp.), is clearly dependent upon T-cell-mediated immunity, particularly CD4+ TH1 cells secreting IFNγ and to a lesser extent CD8+ T cells (Fig. 15.17). As in the case of bacteria, dendritic cells are necessary for this response and produce IL-12 after engulfing fungi.

The clinical relevance of TH1 versus TH2 responses is also clear for some human mycoses, for example:

- individuals with mild paracoccidioidomycosis have TH1 biased immune responses; whereas
- individuals with severe, disseminated infection have high levels of TH2 cytokines such as IL-4 and IL-10 and eosinophilia.

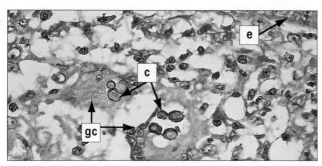

Fig. 15.17 Evidence for T-cell immunity in chromomycosis The pigmented fungal cells of chromomycosis (a subcutaneous mycosis) *(c)* are visible inside giant cells *(gc)* in the dermis of a patient. The area is surrounded by a predominantly mononuclear cell infiltrate. The basal layer of epidermis *(e)* is visible at the top of the frame. H&E stain. ×400. (Courtesy Professor RJ Hay.)

Children with the primary immunodeficiency hyper IgE syndrome have defects in the production of IFNγ, fail to develop TH17 cells and have increased susceptibility to fungal infections.

An increased level of IL-10 (with concomitant reductions in IFNγ) is also a marker of impaired immunity to systemic mycoses, *C. albicans*, and in neutropenia-associated aspergillosis. Regulatory T cells that secrete IL-10 and TGFβ are induced by many fungi and may promote fungal persistence, as in the case of *Candida*.

Fungi possess many evasion strategies to promote their survival.
Evasion strategies used by fungi to promote their survival include the following:

- *C. neoformans* produces a polysaccharide capsule, which inhibits phagocytosis (similar in principle to that of encapsulated bacteria), although this can be overcome by the opsonic effects of complement and antibodies.
- Similarly, *Candida* conceal the β-glucans of their cell wall, which would otherwise be efficiently recognized by host dectin-1, underneath an external coat of mannan, a molecule that is considerably less immunereactive. β-Glucans are also differentially expressed in the yeast versus filamentous forms of some fungi, contributing to the differences in immune response to these two distinct phases of infection.
- *H. capsulatum* is an obligate intracellular pathogen that evades macrophage killing by entering the cell via CR3 and then altering the normal pathways of phagosome maturation, in parallel to the strategies of intracellular bacteria such as *M. tuberculosis*.
- Dermatophytes suppress host T-cell responses to delay cell-mediated destruction.

Immune responses to fungi are therefore as complex and interesting as those against bacteria and for many infections (such as the subcutaneous mycoses) these responses remain poorly understood.

CRITICAL THINKING: IMMUNOENDOCRINE INTERACTIONS IN THE RESPONSE TO INFECTION
See Critical thinking: Explanations, section 15

Humans subclinically infected with tuberculosis (about one-third of the world's population) may harbour live organisms for the rest of their lives. Similarly, tuberculosis can establish a latent non-progressive infection in mice. If animals with such latent infection are subjected to a period of restraint stress (placed in a tube that limits movement) each day for several days, the infection may reactivate. This also happens if cattle with latent disease are transported in trucks. Similarly, tuberculosis increases in human populations in war zones, probably as a result of reactivation of latent disease.

1. What is the physiology of this reactivation?

When American military trainees were subjected to an extremely stressful training schedule, their serum IgE levels rose and they lost their previously positive delayed hypersensitivity skin-test responses. The levels of mRNA encoding IFNγ in the peripheral blood mononuclear cells of medical students were lower during the examination period than at other times of the year.

2. Do these observations suggest changes in cytokine profile? If so, why did it happen?

New immunological approaches are being developed to prevent and treat fungal infections.
Unlike many antibiotics, which are directly microbicidal, antifungal drugs need significant assistance from the immune system to be most effective.

Reducing the underlying immunosuppression that leads to susceptibility to fungi is an important goal and generic immunotherapies such as cytokine administration (using IFNγ in patients with CGD and G-CSF therapy to reduce neutropenia in patients with cancer) have had some success. Human antibodies specific for fungal antigens are being tested for their protective effects by passive transfer. In a clinical trial, administration of *Aspergillus*-specific donor CD4$^+$ T cells reduced the incidence of invasive aspergillosis in patients undergoing allogeneic bone marrow transplantation. Currently, there are no licensed vaccines against any human fungal pathogen; the number of clinical trials for new candidates is small and it is unclear whether they will be effective in the immunocompromised host. Polysaccharides that are either species specific (e.g. glucuronoxylomannan from *Cryptococcus*) or more broadly reactive (such as β-glucans) delivered as polysaccharide–protein conjugate vaccines, as well as fungi-specific proteins, are all being considered. There is also considerable interest in DC-based vaccine strategies to promote TH1-mediated immunity.

FURTHER READING

Anas A, van der Poll T, de Vos AF. Role of CD14 in lung inflammation and infection. Crit Care 2010;14:209.

Borghetti P, Saleri R, Mocchegiani E, et al. Infection, immunity and the neuroendocrine response. Vet Immunol Immunopathol 2009;130:141–162.

Borghi M, Renga G, Puccetti M, et al. Antifungal Th immunity: growing up in family. Front Immunol 2014;5:506.

Cerf-Bensussan N, Gaboriau-Routhiau V. The immune system and the gut microbiota: friends or foes? Nat Rev Immunol 2010; 10:735–744.

Cunha C, Romani L, Carvalho A. Cracking the Toll-like receptor code in fungal infections. Expert Rev Anti Infect Ther 2010;8:112.

Curtis MM, Way SS. Interleukin 17 in host defence against bacterial, mycobacterial and fungal pathogens. Immunology 2009;126:177–185.

Fletcher HA, Schrager L. TB vaccine development and the End TB Strategy: importance and current status. Trans R Soc Trop Med Hyg 2016;110:212–218.

Floyd K, Glaziou P, Zumla A, Raviglione M. The global tuberculosis epidemic and progress in care, prevention and research: an overview in year 3 of the End TB era. Lancet Resp Med 2018;6:299.

Hayward JA, Mathur A, Ngo C, Man SM. Cytosolic recognition of microbes and pathogens: inflammasomes in action. Microbiol Mol Biol Rev 2018;82(4). pii: e00015–18.

Hazlett L, Wu M. Defensins in innate immunity. Cell Tissue Res 2011;343:175–188.

Hooper LV, Macpherson AJ. Immune adaptations that maintain homeostasis with the intestinal microbiota. Nat Rev Immunol 2010;10:159–169.

Huang Lu, Russell David G. Protective immunity against tuberculosis: what does it look like and how do we find it? Curr Opin Immunol 2017;48:44.

Jorgensen I, Rayamajhi M, Miao EA. Programmed cell death as a defence against infection. Nat Rev Immunol 2017;17(3):151–164.

Levy M, Blacher E, Elinav E. Microbiome, metabolites and host immunity. Curr Opin Microbiol 2017 Feb;35:8–15.

Limper AH, Adenis A, Le T, Harrison TS. Fungal infections in HIV/AIDS. Lancet Infect Dis 2017;17(11):e334–e343.

McClean CM, Tobin DM. Macrophage form, function, and phenotype in mycobacterial infection: lessons from tuberculosis and other diseases. Pathog Dis 2016;74(7). pii: ftw068.

Paik S, Kim JK, Chung C, Jo EK. Autophagy: A new strategy for host-directed therapy of tuberculosis. Virulence 2018;15:1–12.

Radoshevich L, Dusserget O. Cytosolic innate immune sensing and signaling upon infection. Front Microbiol 2016;7:313.

Sansonetti PJ. To be or not to be a pathogen: that is the mucosally relevant question. Mucosal Immunol 2011;4:8–14.

Trottein F, Paget C. Natural killer T cells and mucosal-associated invariant T cells in lung infections. Front Immunol 2018;9(2):1750.

Zelante T, Pieraccini G, Scaringi L, Aversa F. Romani L Learning from other diseases: protection and pathology in chronic fungal infections. Semin Immunopathol 2016;38(2):239–248.

16

Immunity to Protozoa and Worms

SUMMARY

- **Parasites stimulate a variety of immune defence mechanisms.**
- **Parasitic infections are often chronic and affect many people.** They are generally host specific and most cause chronic infections. Many are spread by invertebrate vectors and have complicated life cycles. Their antigens are often stage specific.
- **Innate immune responses are the first line of immune defence.**
- **T and B cells are pivotal in the development of immunity.** Both CD4 and CD8 T cells are needed for protection from some parasites, and cytokines, chemokines and their receptors have important roles.
- **Effector cells such as macrophages, neutrophils, eosinophils and platelets can kill both protozoa and worms.** They secrete cytotoxic molecules such as reactive oxygen radicals and nitric oxide (NO$^{\bullet}$). All are more effective when activated by cytokines. Worm infections are usually associated

with an increase in eosinophil number and circulating IgE, which are characteristic of TH2 responses. TH2 cells are necessary for the elimination of intestinal worms.
- **Parasites have many different escape mechanisms to avoid being eliminated by the immune system.** Some exploit the host response for their own development.
- **Inflammatory responses can be a consequence of eliminating parasitic infections.**
- **Parasitic infections have immunopathological consequences.** Parasitic infections are associated with pathology, which can include autoimmunity, splenomegaly and hepatomegaly. Much immunopathology may be mediated by the adaptive immune response.
- **Vaccines against human parasites are not yet routinely available.**

PARASITE INFECTIONS

Parasitic infections typically stimulate a number of immune defence mechanisms, both antibody and cell mediated, and the responses that are most effective depend upon the particular parasite and the stage of infection. Some of the more important parasitic infections of humans (Fig. 16.1) affect the host in diverse ways. Parasitic protozoa may live:

- in the gut (e.g. amoebae);
- in the blood (e.g. African trypanosomes);
- within erythrocytes (e.g. *Plasmodium* spp.);
- in macrophages (e.g. *Leishmania* spp., *Toxoplasma gondii*);
- in liver and spleen (e.g. *Leishmania* spp.); or
- in muscle (e.g. *Trypanosoma cruzi*).

Parasitic worms that infect humans include trematodes or flukes (e.g. schistosomes), cestodes (e.g. tapeworms) and nematodes or roundworms (e.g. *Trichinella spiralis*, hookworms, pinworms, *Ascaris* spp. and the filarial worms).

Tapeworms and adult hookworms inhabit the gut, adult schistosomes live in blood vessels and some filarial worms live in the lymphatics (Fig. 16.2). It is clear that there is widespread potential for damaging pathological reactions.

Many parasitic worms pass through complicated life cycles, including migration through various parts of the host's body:

- Hookworms and schistosome larvae invade their hosts directly by penetrating the skin.
- Tapeworms, pinworms and roundworms are ingested.
- Filarial worms depend upon an intermediate insect host or vector to transmit them from person to person.

Most protozoa rely upon an insect vector, apart from *Toxoplasma* and *Giardia* spp. and amoebae, which are transmitted by ingestion. Thus:

- malarial parasites are spread by mosquitoes;
- trypanosomes by tsetse flies;
- *T. cruzi* by triatomine bugs; and
- *Leishmania* by sandflies.

IMMUNE DEFENCES AGAINST PARASITES

Host resistance to parasite infection may be genetic. The resistance of individual hosts to infection varies and may be controlled by a number of genes, which may be major histocompatibility complex (MHC) or non-MHC genes (Table 16.1).

It should not be assumed that host genetic background is the only reason determining the outcome of infection. There may be many factors involved. In most helminth infections, for example, a heavy worm burden occurs in comparatively few individuals but may cluster in families, implying a genetic basis. On the other hand, studies have shown that human behaviour can account for large variation in exposure between families.

Many parasitic infections are long-lived. It is not in the interest of a parasite to kill its host, at least not until transmission to another host has occurred. During the course of a chronic infection, the type of immune response may change and immunosuppression and immunopathological effects are common.

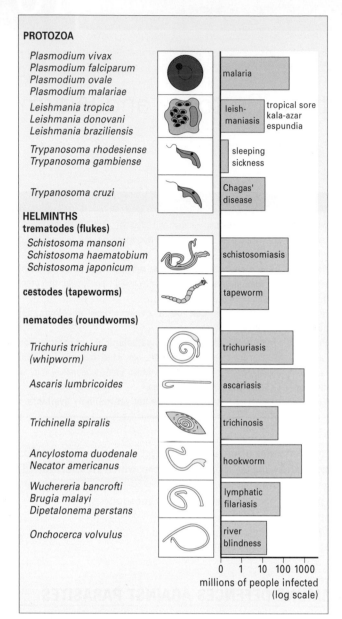

Fig. 16.1 Important parasitic infections of humans Important parasitic infections, including data from the World Health Organization (1993). Their sizes range from 1 m for the tapeworm to around 10^{-5} m for *Plasmodium* spp. (see Fig. 16.w1).

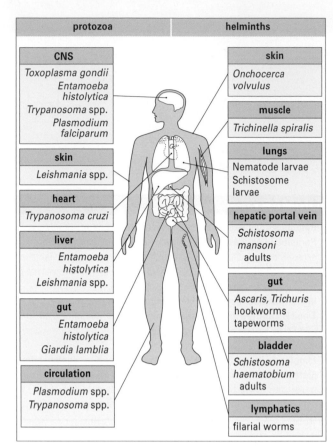

Fig. 16.2 Sites of infection of medically important parasites

TABLE 16.1 **Human Gene Polymorphisms that Affect the Outcome of Parasite Infection**	
Parasite	**Genetic Trait**
Plasmodium spp.	Sickle cell haemoglobin (HbS) protects from malaria
	Certain MHC genes common in West Africans, but rare in Caucasians, protect from malaria (e.g. HLA-B53)
	Duffy blood group antigen (Fy/Fy)-negative erythrocytes protect from *Plasmodium vivax*
Leishmania spp.	Polymorphisms in *Nramp1* govern susceptibility to macrophage invasion
Schistosoma spp.	Candidate polymorphic genes on chromosome 5q31-q33, a region that includes key cytokines IL-4 and IL-5
Ascaris spp.	Candidate polymorphic genes on chromosomes 1 and 13, a region that includes the TNF family of cytokines

Host defence depends on a number of immunological mechanisms. The development of immunity is a complex process arising from the activation of both adaptive and innate immune responses and the switching on of many different kinds of cell over a period of time. Effects are often local and many cell types secreting different mediators may be present at sites of immune rejection. Moreover, the processes involved in controlling the multiplication of a parasite within an infected individual may differ from those responsible for the ultimate development of resistance to further infection.

In some helminth infections, a process of concomitant immunity occurs, whereby an initial infection is not eliminated but becomes established and the host then acquires resistance to invasion by new parasites, mostly worms, of the same species.

In very general terms, humoral responses are important to eliminate extracellular parasites such as those that live in blood (Fig. 16.3), body fluids or the gut.

However, the type of response conferring most protection varies with the parasite. For example, antibodies, alone or with complement, can damage some extracellular parasites, but are more effective when acting with an effector cell.

As emphasized above, within a single infection different effector mechanisms act against different developmental stages of parasites. Thus, in malaria:

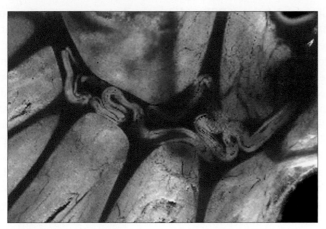

Fig. 16.3 Adult schistosome worm pairs in mesenteric blood vessels Although very exposed to immune effectors, adult schistosomes are highly resistant and can persist for an average of 3–5 years. (Courtesy Dr Alison Agnew.)

- antibodies against extracellular forms block their capacity to invade new cells;
- cell-mediated responses prevent the development of the liver stage within hepatocytes.

INNATE IMMUNE RESPONSES

The innate and adaptive immune responses are co-evolving to allow mammals to identify and to eliminate parasites. The innate immune system provides the first line of immune defence by detecting the immediate presence and nature of infection. Many different cells are involved in generating innate responses, including phagocytic cells and natural killer (NK) cells. It is also becoming clear that early recognition of parasites by antigen-presenting cells (APCs), for example dendritic cells, determines the phenotype of the adaptive response (Fig. 16.4).

Innate immune recognition relies on pattern recognition receptors (PRRs) that have evolved to recognize pathogen-associated molecular patterns (PAMPs) (see Chapters 3 and 5). A unifying feature of these targets is their highly conserved structures, which are invariant between parasites of a given class.

Although many parasites are known to activate the immune system in a non-specific manner shortly after infection, it is only recently that attention has been given to the mechanisms involved.

While major advances are being achieved in the area of microbial recognition by PRRs, a small but growing number of studies show that parasites also possess specific molecular patterns capable of engaging PRRs. Examples of some parasite PAMPs along with their receptors are given in Table 16.2.

Toll-like receptors recognize parasite molecules. The discovery of the Toll-like receptor (TLR) family, an evolutionarily conserved group of mammalian PRRs involved in antimicrobial immunity, has enriched our understanding of how innate and adaptive immunity are mutually dependent.

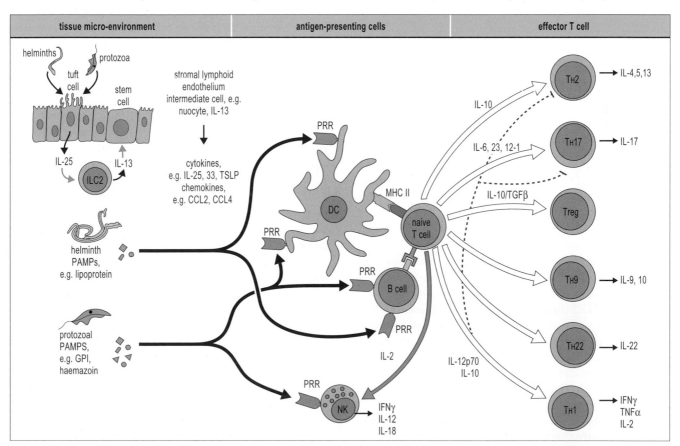

Fig. 16.4 Cytokines secreted by the different subsets of leukocytes The cytokines secreted by the different subsets of T cells are shown. Note the importance of antigen-presenting cells, e.g. dendritic cells (*DCs*) and B cells in driving maturation of different TH cell subsets. ILC2 cells promote stem cell division to maintain epithelial integrity. *NK*, Natural killer; *PAMPs*, pathogen-associated molecular patterns; *PRR*, pattern recognition receptor.

TABLE 16.2   Innate Immune Receptors Involved in Parasite Recognition

Family	Member	Parasite Ligand(s)
Collectins (see Fig. 3.w2)	MBL	Mannose-rich sugars from numerous protozoans and helminths
Pentraxins	CRP	Phospholipids and phosphosugars *Leishmania* spp. LPG
C-type lectins (see Fig. 5.11)	Macrophage mannose receptor, DC-SIGN; Mincle	*Trypanosoma cruzi* *Schistosoma* spp. (Lewis X and/or Omega-1) *Leishmania* spp.
Scavenger receptors (see Fig. 5.10)	SR-B (CD36)	*Plasmodium falciparum* (PfEMP1)
Complement receptors	CR1/CR3	*Leishmania* spp. LPG *Necator* NIF *Plasmodium* PfEMP1
Toll-like receptors (see Table 3.2)	TLR2 (with TLR1/TLR6)	GPI anchors from many protozoa
		Lyso-PS from *Schistosoma* spp.
	TLR3	Double-stranded RNA from *Schistosoma* spp.
	TLR2/6	Diacetylated lipoprotein from the filarial endosymbiont *Wolbachia* spp.
	TLR9	Protozoal DNA Malarial pigment haemazoin

CRP, C-reactive protein; *GPI*, glycosylphosphatidylinositol; *LPG*, lipophosphoglycan; *lyso-PS*, lysophosphatidylserine; *MBL*, mannose-binding lectin; *NIF*, neutrophil inhibition factor; *PfEMP1*, *P. falciparum* erythrocyte membrane protein-1.

A few studies have examined the role of TLRs in immunity to parasites. For example:

- *T. gondii* binds TLR11 via profilin and associates with TLR3, TLR7 and TLR9 via the endoplasmic reticulum protein UNC93B1.
- TLR9 mediates innate immune activation by the malaria pigment haemazoin.
- Lysophosphatidylserine (lyso-PS) from *Schistosoma mansoni*, glycophosphatidylinositol (GPI) anchors and Tc52 from *T. cruzi* are capable of signalling through TLR2.

Interestingly, TLR2 triggering by these diverse parasite patterns leads to different immune outcomes: for *S. mansoni*, triggering leads to the development of fully mature dendritic cells capable of inducing a Treg response, characterized by elevated IL-10 levels; for *T. cruzi*, mature dendritic cells induce a TH1 response with raised levels of IL-12. This dichotomous response could, in part, be explained by the cooperation between TLR2 and other TLRs. However, there has been difficulty in assigning definitive contributions of TLRs to activation by specific parasite proteins since samples are easily contaminated, e.g. with bacterial PAMPs.

Classical human PRRs also contribute to recognition of parasites. Classical PRRs also play important roles in the innate response to parasite infection (see Table. 16.2) and include collectins (e.g. MBL), pentraxins (e.g. CRP), C-type lectins (e.g. macrophage mannose receptor) and scavenger receptors (e.g. CD36) (see Chapters 3 and 5). For example, MBL binds mannose-rich lipophosphoglycan (LPG) from *Leishmania*, *Plasmodium*, trypanosomes and schistosomes; and polymorphisms in the MBL gene are associated with increased susceptibility to severe malaria. More recently, *Leishmania* parasites have been shown to use Mincle (CLEC-4E) to target an inhibitory immunoreceptor tyrosine-based activation motif (ITAM) signalling pathway in dendritic cells that dampens adaptive immunity to infection.

Complement receptors are archetypal PRRs. Complement receptors, in particular CR3, are archetypal PRRs involved in innate immune responses (see Table 16.2). They are truly multifunctional, being involved in phagocyte adhesion, recognition, migration, activation and microbe elimination.

Why then is CR3, a linchpin of phagocyte responses, the favoured portal of entry for diverse intracellular parasites, including *Leishmania* via LPG?

- CR3 offers a multiplicity of binding sites, enabling opsonic or non-opsonic binding.
- Phagocytosis by CR3 alone does not generate an oxidative burst in phagocytic cells.
- Binding of CR3 suppresses the secretion of IL-12.

In isolation, CR3 is not an activating receptor. It requires co-operation from other receptors, most notably Fc receptors, for pathogen killing. Helminths have also exploited this chink in the immune armoury. Hookworm NIF has been shown to bind a domain in the α subunit of CR3, presumably to downregulate cell-mediated immunity.

ADAPTIVE IMMUNE RESPONSES TO PARASITES

T and B cells are pivotal in the development of immunity. In most parasitic infections, protection can be conferred experimentally on normal animals by the transfer of spleen cells, especially T cells, from immune animals.

The T-cell requirement is also demonstrable because nude (athymic) or T-deprived mice fail to clear otherwise non-lethal infections of protozoa such as *T. cruzi* or *Plasmodium yoelii*, and T-cell-deprived rats fail to expel the intestinal worm *Nippostrongylus brasiliensis* (Fig. 16.5).

Counterintuitively, many parasites require signals from immune cells to thrive; for example, schistosomes fail to develop in the absence of hepatic CD4+ lymphocytes.

B cells also play key roles in regulating and controlling immunity to parasites. For example:

- B cells and antibodies are required for resistance to the parasitic gastrointestinal nematode *Trichuris muris*; and
- passive transfer of IgG can protect people from malaria.

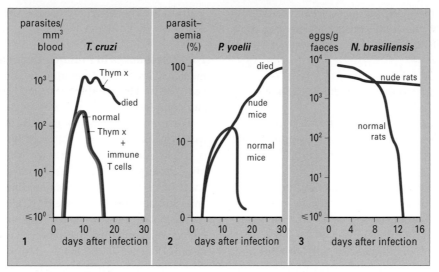

Fig. 16.5 Parasitic infections in T-cell-deprived mice The first two graphs plot the increase in number of blood-borne protozoa (parasitaemia) following infection. (**1**) *Trypanosoma cruzi* multiplies faster (and gives fatal parasitaemia) in mice that have been thymectomized and irradiated to destroy T cells *(Thym x)*. In normal mice, parasites are cleared from the blood by day 16. Reconstitution of T-cell-deprived mice with T cells from immune mice restores their ability to control the parasitaemia. In these experiments, both thymectomized groups were given fetal liver cells to restore vital haematopoietic function. (**2**) *Plasmodium yoelii* causes a self-limiting infection in normal mice and the parasites are cleared from the blood by day 20. In nude mice, the parasites continue to multiply, killing the mice after about 30 days. (**3**) This graph illustrates the time course of the elimination of the intestinal nematode *Nippostrongylus brasiliensis* from the gut of rats. In normal rats, the worms are all expelled by day 13, as determined by the number of worm eggs present in the rats' faeces. T cells are necessary for this expulsion to occur, as shown by the establishment of a chronic infection in the gut of nude rats.

Both CD4 and CD8 T Cells are needed for protection from some parasites. The type of T cell responsible for controlling an infection varies with the parasite and the stage of in4fection and depends upon the kinds of cytokine they produce. For example, CD4$^+$ and CD8$^+$ T cells protect against different phases of *Plasmodium* infection:

- CD4$^+$ T cells mediate immunity against blood-stage *P. yoelii;*
- CD8$^+$ T cells protect against the liver stage of *Plasmodium berghei.*

The action of CD8$^+$ T cells is twofold; they secrete IFNγ, which inhibits the multiplication of parasites within hepatocytes and they are able to kill infected hepatocytes, but not infected erythrocytes.

The immune response against *T. cruzi* depends not only upon CD4$^+$ and CD8$^+$ T cells but also on NK cells and antibody production. It is also true for the immune response against *T. gondii.*

CD8$^+$ T cells confer protection in mice depleted of CD4$^+$ T cells, both through their production of IFNγ and because they are cytotoxic for infected macrophages.

NK cells, stimulated by IL-12 secreted by the macrophages, are another source of IFNγ: chronic infections are associated with reduced production of IFNγ.

These observations probably underlie the high incidence of toxoplasmosis in patients with AIDS, who are deficient in CD4$^+$ T cells.

CD4$^+$ T cells are critical for the expulsion of intestinal nematodes and because immunity to *T. muris* can be transferred to a SCID (severe combined immune deficiency) mouse by the transfer of CD4$^+$ T cells alone, there is no evidence for a role of CD8$^+$ T cells.

The cytokines produced by CD4$^+$ T cells can be important in determining the outcome of infection. As TH1 and TH2 cells have contrasting and cross-regulating cytokine profiles, the roles of TH1 or TH2 cells in determining the outcome of parasitic infections have been extensively investigated.

As a result of early studies, predominantly in mouse infections, certain dogmas have arisen suggesting that:

- TH1 responses mediate killing of intracellular pathogens; and
- TH2 responses eliminate extracellular ones.

However, this is very much an oversimplification of the true picture and based on work in animal models that may not fully reflect the human immune system.

Although the TH1/TH2 paradigm may be a useful tool in some situations, it is probably more realistic in humans to consider that TH1 and TH2 phenotypes represent the extremes of a continuum of cytokine profiles and that perhaps it may be more accurate to look at the role of the cytokines themselves in the resolution of infectious disease, particularly as new TH subsets are being elucidated, e.g. TH17, TH22 and TH9, and their roles in immunity to parasites investigated.

Regulatory T cells are able to modulate the extremes of both TH2 and TH1 responses.

Cytokines, chemokines and their receptors have important roles. Cytokines not only act on effector cells to enhance their cytotoxic or cytostatic capabilities, but also act as growth factors to increase cell numbers, while chemokines attract cells to the sites of infection. Thus, in malaria, the characteristic enlargement of the spleen is caused by an enormous increase in cell numbers.

Other examples include:

- the accumulation of macrophages in the granulomas that develop in the liver in schistosomiasis;
- the eosinophilia characteristic of helminth infections; and
- the recruitment of eosinophils and mast cells into the gut mucosa that occurs in worm infections of the gastrointestinal tract.

Mucosal mast cells and eosinophils are both important in determining the outcome of some helminth infections and proliferate in response to the products of T cells – IL-3 and GM-CSF, and IL-5, respectively.

However, an increase in cell number can itself harm the host. Thus, administration of IL-3 to mice infected with *Leishmania major* can exacerbate the local infection and increase the dissemination of the parasites, probably through the proliferation of bone marrow precursors of the cells inhabited by the parasites.

IL-10 and transforming growth factor-β (TGFβ), the regulatory cytokines (see Chapter 12), downregulate the pro-inflammatory response and thus minimize pathological damage.

Chemokines are key molecules in recruiting immune cells by chemotaxis, but also act in leukocyte activation, haematopoiesis, inflammation and anti-parasite immunity.

Protozoan parasites have been most studied in the context of chemokines and their diverse roles in the parasite–host relationship. For example, *T. gondii* possesses cyclophilin-18, which binds to the chemokine receptor CCR5 and induces IL-12 production by dendritic cells.

T-Cell Responses to Protozoa Depend on the Species.
T-cell-mediated immunity operating to control protozoan parasites depends on the species of animal infected and the location and complexity of the parasite life cycle within the host.

For example, in mouse models, the induction of TH1 cells with concomitant upregulation of IFNγ and nitric oxide (NO) is crucial for protection of mice from *Leishmania*. Strains of mice driving TH2 responses on infection, manifested by high levels of IL-4, IL-13, IL-10 and antibodies, develop progressive and ultimately lethal disease (Fig. 16.6).

The polarization of TH-cell responses in murine models does not conveniently translate to humans, where both TH1 and TH2 responses appear to be involved in protection.

The importance of TH1 cells for protection from toxoplasmosis is also evident in murine models.

For malaria, the TH1/TH2 paradigm is less helpful in understanding immunity, because the type of immune response mounted and the ensuing risk of pathology depends on whether the first exposure to the parasite occurs during infancy or adulthood. As a consequence, immunity to malaria is best thought of in the context of regulated TH1 responses. Thus, in endemic populations, primary malaria infections in infants induce low levels of IFNγ and TNFα via an innate pathway (potentially involving NK cells), which leads to T-cell priming.

The infection induces minimal pathology and the parasites can be cleared, either immunologically via maternal antibody or because parasites fail to thrive in fetal haemoglobin.

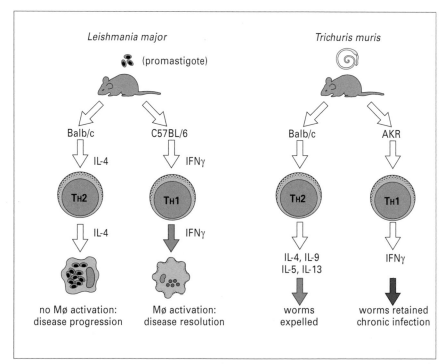

Fig. 16.6 Development of the immune response to *Leishmania major* and *Trichuris muris* infection The cytokines secreted by the different subsets of T cells and their effect on the resolution of the disease are shown. Note that resolution of infection is dependent on mouse strain. *Mø*, Macrophage.

On re-infection, the malaria-primed T cells produce massive amounts of IFNγ and TNFα, leading to an increased risk of unwanted pathology, including cerebral malaria.

Further infections induce effective anti-parasite immunity principally through the development of an individual's own repertoire of high-affinity antibodies, which inhibit parasite development. This change in immune environment ultimately leads to a switch in T-cell phenotype from TH1 to a regulatory T-cell phenotype in which raised levels of IL-10 and TGFβ can be detected.

By contrast, non-immune individuals who contract malaria for the first time in adulthood are unable to control their infections and are more likely to develop severe pathology. This is believed to arise from cross-reactively primed T cells generated against other microbes that appear to contribute to the development of severe disease.

The immune response to worms depends upon TH2-secreted cytokines.

IgE and eosinophilia are the hallmarks of the immune response to worm infections and depend upon cytokines secreted by TH2 cells (see Fig. 16.6).

In humans, schistosomiasis and infection with gastrointestinal nematodes, resistance to re-infection after drug treatment is correlated with the production of IgE and high pre-treatment levels of TH2 cytokines such as IL-4, IL-5 and IL-13.

The primary stimuli for TH2 development in schistosomiasis are egg antigens. Similarly, the excretory and secretory products of nematodes have been shown to polarize cells towards TH2 responses. Again, the control of T-cell phenotype seems to be exerted by the dendritic cell after exposure to these substances.

The mechanisms of induction of TH2 responses are less well understood than TH1 responses. One hypothesis, the default hypothesis, suggests that unless the triggers for TH1 responses are received (including high IL-12), TH2 responses occur. More recent evidence, however, suggests that specific signals induce the T cell to make TH2 cytokines, probably including cell–cell interactions.

The pattern of cytokine production in infected hosts may be different from that in vaccinated hosts. For example:

- In mice infected with *S. mansoni*, IL-5-producing TH2 cells predominate.
- In mice that have been immunized, IgE levels and eosinophil numbers are low: TH1 cells predominate and IFNγ activates effector cells that destroy lung stage larvae via the production of NO.

However, when adult worms start to produce eggs, a soluble egg antigen is released that has an effect only in susceptible mice. The antigen reduces levels of IFNγ and increases production of IL-5.

TH2 cytokines induce effector mechanisms, which are important for control of intestinal worm infections. Perhaps the example that demonstrates this most clearly is *T. muris* infection in mice:

- Animals normally resistant to infection develop persistent infections in IL-4 and/or IL-13 knockout mice.

- Conversely, susceptible mice expel the worms if IL-4 activity is promoted by administration of neutralizing antibody against IFNγ.

IL-9 is another TH2 cytokine that seems to be important in resistance to intestinal nematode infection and is involved in the production of mucosal mast-cell responses and the production of IgE. IL-9 transgenic mice that produce higher levels of this cytokine have enhanced expulsion of *T. muris*.

It is clear from a number of studies that there is no single mechanism by which a TH2 response mediates expulsion of all intestinal worms. The species of worm, its anatomical position within the gut and the immune status of the host are all factors likely to influence whether a particular immune mechanism will be effective at promoting worm loss.

Some worm infections deviate the immune response.

The role of IFNγ in promoting chronic infection is again shown by the administration of IL-12 to mice soon after infection with the intestinal worm *N. brasiliensis* (Fig. 16.w2).

N. brasiliensis stimulates IFNγ production, which delays expulsion of the worms.

IL-12 acts by inhibiting the production of TH2 cytokines, in particular IL-4 and IL-5, thereby preventing the production of IgE, eosinophilia and mast-cell hypertrophy.

The host may isolate the parasite with inflammatory cells.

In some parasitic infections, the immune system cannot completely eliminate the parasite but reacts by isolating the organism with inflammatory cells. The host reacts to locally released antigen, which stimulates the production of cytokines that recruit cells to the region. An example of this has been shown in mice vaccinated with radiation-attenuated schistosome cercariae. Infiltrating cells, which are mostly TH1-type lymphocytes, surround the lung-stage larvae as early as 24 hours after intravenous challenge infection. This prevents subsequent migration to the site necessary for development into the adult parasite.

The schistosome egg granuloma in the liver is another example of the host reacting by 'walling off' the parasite. This reaction is a chronic cell-mediated response to soluble antigens released by eggs that have become trapped in the liver. Macrophages accumulate and release fibrogenic factors, which stimulate the formation of granulomatous tissue and, ultimately, fibrosis. Although this reaction may benefit the host in that it insulates the liver cells from toxins secreted by the worm eggs, it is also the major source of pathology, causing irreversible changes in the liver and the loss of liver function. In the absence of T cells, there is no granuloma formation and no subsequent fibrous encapsulation. Different mechanisms may affect:

- worms that inhabit different anatomical sites, such as the gut (e.g. *Trichuris trichiura*) or the tissues (e.g. *Onchocerca volvulus*); and
- different stages of the life cycle (e.g. schistosome larvae in the lungs and adult worms in the veins).

Parasites induce non-specific and specific antibody production. Many parasitic infections provoke a non-specific hypergammaglobulinaemia, much of which is probably caused by substances released from the parasites acting as B-cell mitogens.

Levels of total immunoglobulins are raised:
- IgM in trypanosomiasis and malaria;
- IgG in malaria and visceral leishmaniasis.

The relative importance of antibody-dependent and antibody-independent responses varies with the infection and host (Fig. 16.7).

The mechanisms by which specific antibody can control parasitic infections and its effects are summarized in Figure 16.8. Antibodies:
- can act directly on protozoa to damage them, either alone or by activating the complement system (Fig. 16.9);
- can neutralize a parasite directly by blocking its attachment to a new host cell, as with *Plasmodium* spp., whose merozoites enter red blood cells through a special receptor; their entry is inhibited by specific antibody (Fig. 16.w3);

- may prevent spread (e.g. in the acute phase of infection by *T. cruzi*);
- can enhance phagocytosis by macrophages – phagocytosis is increased even more by the addition of complement; these effects are mediated by Fc and C3 receptors on macrophages, which may increase in number as a result of macrophage activation;
- are involved in antibody-dependent cell-mediated cytotoxicity (ADCC), for example in infections caused by *Plasmodium*,

T. cruzi, *T. spiralis*, *S. mansoni* and filarial worms; NK cells inhibit *Plasmodium falciparum* growth in red blood cells and cytotoxic cells such as macrophages, neutrophils and eosinophils adhere to antibody-coated worms by means of their Fc and C3 receptors and degranulate, spilling their toxic contents onto the worm (see Fig. 16.11).

Different antibody isotypes may have different effects. In individuals infected with schistosomes, parasite-specific IgE and IgA are associated with resistance to infection and there is an inverse relationship between the amount of IgE in the blood and re-infection.

IgG4 appears to block the action of IgE; re-infection is more likely in children who have high levels of IgG4 and infection rates are highest in 10–14 year olds when IgG4 levels are also at their highest. Class switching to IgG4 appears to occur in the context of a modified TH2 response involving the induction of Tregs.

In many infections, it is difficult to distinguish between cell-mediated and antibody-mediated responses because both can act in concert against the parasite. This is illustrated in Figure 16.10, which summarizes the immune reaction that can be mounted against schistosome larvae.

IMMUNE EFFECTOR CELLS

Macrophages, neutrophils, eosinophils, mast cells and platelets can all damage parasites. Antibody and cytokines produced specifically in response to parasite antigens enhance the anti-parasitic activities of all these effector cells, although tissue

parasite and habitat		antibody-dependent			antibody-independent	
		importance	mechanism	means of evasion	importance	mechanism
T. brucei free in blood	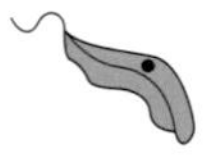	+ + + +	lysis with complement, which also opsonizes for phagocytosis	antigenic variation	–	
Plasmodium spp. inside red cell	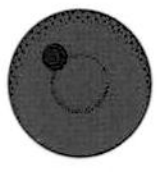	+ + +	blocks invasion, opsonizes for phagocytosis, ADCC	intracellular; antigenic variation	liver stage + + + blood stage + + +	cytokines / macrophage activation
T. cruzi inside macrophage	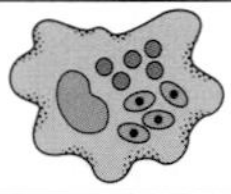	+ +	limits spread in acute infection, sensitizes for ADCC	intracellular	+ + + (chronic phase)	macrophage activation by IFNγ and TNFα, and killing by NO• and metabolites of O$_2$
Leishmania spp. inside macrophage	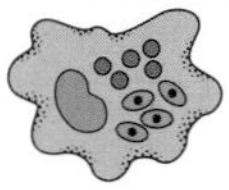	+	limits spread	intracellular	+ + + +	

Fig. 16.7 Relative importance of antibody-dependent and antibody-independent responses in protozoal infections This table summarizes the relative importance of the two immune responses, the mechanisms involved and, for antibodies, the means by which the protozoon can evade damage by antibodies. Antibodies are the most important part of the immune response against those parasites that live in the blood stream, such as African trypanosomes and malarial parasites, whereas cell-mediated immunity is active against those like *Leishmania* that live in the tissues. Antibody can damage parasites directly, enhance their clearance by phagocytosis, activate complement, or block their entry into their host cell and so limit the spread of infection. Once inside the cell, the parasite is safe from the effects of antibodies. *Trypanosoma cruzi* and *Leishmania* spp. are both susceptible to the action of oxygen metabolites released by the respiratory burst of macrophages and to NO•. Treating macrophages with cytokines enhances release of these products and diminishes the entry and survival of the parasites. *ADCC*, Antibody-dependent cell-mediated cytotoxicity.

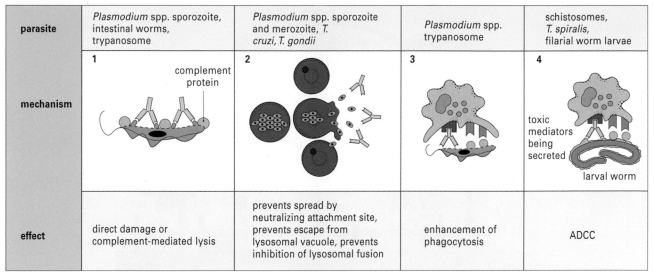

parasite	*Plasmodium* spp. sporozoite, intestinal worms, trypanosome	*Plasmodium* spp. sporozoite and merozoite, *T. cruzi, T. gondii*	*Plasmodium* spp. trypanosome	schistosomes, *T. spiralis,* filarial worm larvae
mechanism	1	2	3	4
effect	direct damage or complement-mediated lysis	prevents spread by neutralizing attachment site, prevents escape from lysosomal vacuole, prevents inhibition of lysosomal fusion	enhancement of phagocytosis	ADCC

Fig. 16.8 Mechanisms by which specific antibody controls some parasitic infections (1) Direct damage. Antibody activates the classical complement pathway, causing damage to the parasite membrane and increasing susceptibility to other mediators. **(2)** Neutralization. Parasites such as *Plasmodium* spp. spread to new cells by specific receptor attachment; blocking the merozoite-binding site with antibody prevents attachment to the receptors on the erythrocyte surface and prevents further multiplication. **(3)** Enhancement of phagocytosis. Complement C3b deposited on the parasite membrane opsonizes it for phagocytosis by cells with C3b receptors (e.g. macrophages). Macrophages also have Fc receptors. **(4)** Eosinophils, neutrophils, platelets and macrophages may be cytotoxic for some parasites when they recognize the parasite via specific antibody (ADCC). The reaction is enhanced by complement. *ADCC,* Antibody-dependent cell-mediated cytotoxicity.

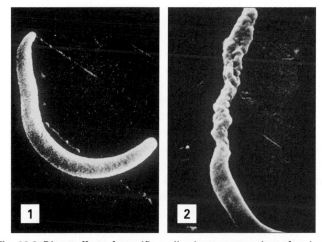

Fig. 16.9 Direct effect of specific antibody on sporozoites of malaria parasites These scanning electron micrographs show a sporozoite of *Plasmodium berghei*, which causes malaria in rodents, before (**1**) and after (**2**) incubation in immune serum. The surface of the sporozoite is damaged by the antibody, which perturbs the outer membrane, causing leakage of fluid. Specific antibodies protect against infection with *Plasmodium* spp. at several of the extracellular stages of the life cycle. The antibody is stage specific in each case. (Courtesy Dr R Nussenzweig.)

macrophages, monocytes and granulocytes have some intrinsic activity before enhancement. The point of entry of the parasite is obviously important. For example:

• The cercariae of *S. mansoni* enter through the skin: experimental depletion of macrophages, neutrophils and eosinophils from the skin of mice increases their susceptibility to infection.

• Trypanosomes and malarial parasites entering the blood are removed from the circulation by phagocytic cells in the skin, spleen and liver.

• Comparison of strains of mice with various immunological defects for their resistance to infection by *Trypanosoma rhodesiense* shows that the African trypanosomes are destroyed by macrophages and later, in infection, when opsonized with antibodies and complement C3b, they are taken up by macrophages in the liver even more quickly.

Before acting as APCs initiating an immune response, macrophages act as effector cells to inhibit the multiplication of parasites or even to destroy them. They also secrete molecules that regulate the inflammatory response:

• Some of these molecules, IL-1, IL-12, TNFα and the colony stimulating factors (CSFs), enhance immunity by activating other cells or stimulating their proliferation.

• Others, such as IL-10, prostaglandins and TGFβ, may be anti-inflammatory and immunosuppressive.

Macrophages can kill extracellular parasites. Phagocytosis by macrophages provides an important defence against the smaller parasites. Macrophages also secrete many cytotoxic factors, enabling them to kill parasites without ingesting them.

When activated by cytokines, macrophages can kill both relatively small extracellular parasites, such as the erythrocytic stages of malaria, and also larger parasites, such as the larval stages of the schistosome. Macrophages also:

• act as killer cells through ADCC – specific IgG and IgE, for instance, enhance their ability to kill schistosomules;

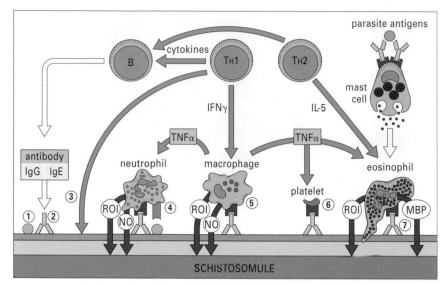

Fig. 16.10 Possible effector responses to schistosomules The various effector mechanisms damaging schistosomes in vitro are shown. Complement alone damages worms (**1**) and does so in combination with antibody (**2**). TH1 cells may act directly, reducing the number of larvae in the lungs (**3**). Antibodies sensitize neutrophils (**4**), macrophages (**5**), platelets (**6**) and eosinophils (**7**) for antibody-dependent cell-mediated cytotoxicity (ADCC). Neutrophils and macrophages probably act by releasing toxic oxygen and nitrogen metabolites, whereas eosinophils damage the worm tegument by the release of major basic protein *(MBP)* plus reactive oxygen intermediates *(ROI)*. The response is potentiated by cytokines (e.g. TNFα). IgE antibody is important in sensitizing both eosinophils and local mast cells, which release a variety of mediators, including those that activate the eosinophils.

- secrete cytokines, such as TNFα and IL-1, which interact with other types of cell, for example rendering hepatocytes resistant to malarial parasites.

Reactive oxygen intermediates (ROIs) are generated by macrophages and granulocytes following phagocytosis of *T. cruzi*, *T. gondii*, *Leishmania* spp. and malarial parasites; filarial worms and schistosomes also stimulate the respiratory burst.

When activated by cytokines, macrophages release more superoxide and hydrogen peroxide than normal resident macrophages and their oxygen-independent killing mechanisms are similarly enhanced.

Nitric oxide (NO), a product of L-arginine metabolism, is another potent toxin. Its synthesis by macrophages in mouse experimental systems is induced by the cytokines IFNγ and TNFα and is greatly increased when they act synergistically. NO˙ can also be produced by endothelial cells. It contributes to host resistance in leishmaniasis, schistosomiasis and malaria and is probably important in the control of most parasitic infections. For instance, the innate resistance to infection by *T. gondii* that is lost in immunocompromised individuals appears to be caused by the inhibition of parasite multiplication by such an oxygen-independent mechanism.

Activation of macrophages is a feature of early infection. All macrophage effector functions are enhanced soon after infection. Although their specific activation is by cytokines secreted by T cells (e.g. IFNγ, GM-CSF, IL-3 and IL-4), they can also be activated by T-cell-independent mechanisms. For example:

- NK cells secrete IFNγ when stimulated by IL-12 produced by macrophages;
- macrophages secrete TNFα in response to some parasite products (e.g. phospholipid-containing antigens of malarial parasites and some *Trypanosoma brucei* antigens); this TNFα then activates other macrophages.

Although TNFα may be secreted by several other cell types, activated macrophages are the most important source of TNFα, which is necessary for protective responses to several species of protozoa (e.g. *Leishmania* spp.) and helminths. Thus, TNFα activates macrophages, eosinophils and platelets to kill the larval form of *S. mansoni,* its effects being enhanced by IFNγ.

TNFα may be harmful as well as beneficial to the infected host, depending upon the amount produced and whether it is free in the circulation or locally confined. Serum concentrations of TNFα in cerebral malaria (*P. falciparum*) correlate with the severity of the disease. Because TNFα induces adhesion molecules on brain endothelium, it can promote adhesion of infected erythrocytes and also contribute to breakdown of the blood–brain barrier. Both of these actions potentially contribute to the disease pathology. In mice, administration of TNFα cures a susceptible strain infected with *Plasmodium chabaudi* but kills a genetically resistant strain. These observations suggest that TNFα is required for resistance but too much causes immunopathology.

Neutrophils can kill large and small parasites. The effector properties displayed by macrophages are also seen in neutrophils. Neutrophils are phagocytic and can kill by both oxygen-dependent and oxygen-independent mechanisms, including NO˙. They produce a more intense respiratory burst than macrophages and their secretory granules contain highly cytotoxic proteins.

Neutrophils can be activated by cytokines, such as IL-8, IFNγ, TNFα and GM-CSF.

Extracellular destruction by neutrophils is mediated by hydrogen peroxide, whereas granular components are involved in the intracellular destruction of ingested organisms.

Neutrophils are present in parasite-infected inflammatory lesions and probably act to clear parasites from bursting cells through neutrophil extracellular traps (NETs). These web-like structures of highly modified chromatin and anti-microbial peptides are released by activated neutrophils on contact with parasites and can also cause pathology in cerebral malaria.

Like macrophages, neutrophils bear Fc and complement receptors and can participate in antibody-dependent cytotoxic reactions to kill the larvae of *S. mansoni*, for example. In this mode, they can be more destructive than eosinophils against several species of nematode, including *T. spiralis*, although the relative effectiveness of the two types of cell may depend upon the isotype and specificity of antibody present.

Eosinophils are characteristically associated with worm infections.
It has been suggested that:
* the eosinophil evolved specifically as a defence against the tissue stages of parasites that are too large to be phagocytosed;
* the IgE-dependent mast-cell reaction has evolved primarily to localize eosinophils near the parasite and to enhance their anti-parasitic functions.

The importance of eosinophils in vivo has been shown by experiments using antiserum against eosinophils. Mice infected with *T. spiralis* and treated with the antiserum develop more cysts in their muscles than the controls. Without the protection offered by eosinophils, the mice cannot eliminate the worms and therefore encyst the parasites to minimize damage.

However, recent work has shown that although eosinophils can help the host to control a worm infection, particularly by limiting migration through the tissues, they do not always do so. For instance, their removal does not abolish the immunity of mice infected with *S. mansoni*; nor does it increase the parasite load in a tapeworm infection.

Removal of IL-5, which is important in the generation and activation of eosinophils, did not change the outcome of *T. spiralis* or *T. muris* infection. In contrast, the infectivity of *Strongyloides venezuelensis* is enhanced in IL-5-deficient mice. Although *T. spiralis* worm burdens were not affected in a primary infection of IL-5 deleted mice, the worm numbers were significantly higher after challenge infection.

The role of IL-5 and therefore eosinophils has also been suggested from human epidemiological studies on gastrointestinal nematode infections where, after drug treatment, low re-infection worm burdens were associated with high pre-treatment levels of IL-5.

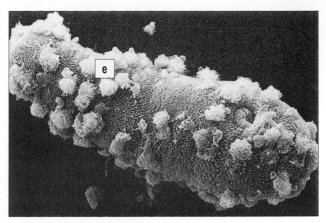

Fig. 16.11 Eosinophil adhesion and degranulation A schistosomule being killed by eosinophils from mouse bone marrow, cultured in the presence of IL-5. The larval helminth has been treated with IgG and the eosinophils adhere by means of their Fcγ receptors. (Courtesy Dr C Sanderson.)

Elevated eosinophilia is often associated with high levels of IgE, both of which are hallmarks of infection with parasites. Although eosinophils express FcεRI, most of the protein is confined to the cytoplasm, and there is little evidence for IgE-dependent function.

Eosinophils can kill helminths by oxygen-dependent and independent mechanisms.
Eosinophils are less phagocytic than neutrophils. They degranulate in response to perturbation of their surface membrane and their activities are enhanced by cytokines such as TNFα and GM-CSF. Most of their activities, however, are controlled by antigen-specific mechanisms. Thus, their binding in vitro to the larvae of worms (e.g. *S. mansoni* and *T. spiralis*) increases the release of their granular contents onto the surface of the worms (Fig. 16.11).

Damage to schistosomules can be caused by the major basic protein (MBP) of the eosinophil crystalloid core. MBP is not specific for any particular target but because it is confined to a small space between the eosinophil and the schistosome, there is little damage to nearby host cells.

Eosinophils and mast cells can act together.
The killing of *S. mansoni* larvae by eosinophils is enhanced by mast-cell products and when studied in vitro, eosinophils from patients with schistosomiasis are found to be more effective than those from normal subjects. The antigens released cause local IgE-dependent degranulation of mast cells and the release of mediators. These selectively attract eosinophils to the site and further enhance their activity. Other products of eosinophils later block the mast-cell reactions. These effector mechanisms may function in vivo, as has been shown in monkeys, where schistosome killing is associated with eosinophil accumulation.

Mast cells control gastrointestinal helminths.
In the case of *T. spiralis* and *Heligmosomoides polygyrus*, there is good evidence to suggest the recruitment of mucosal mast cells (Fig. 16.12). After mast-cell activation, the mast-cell contents are released, resulting in changes to the permeability of the

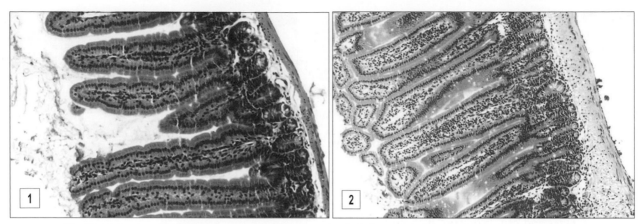

Fig. 16.12 Section through the gut of a mouse infected with *Heligmosomoides polygyrus* (**1**) Gut of an uninfected mouse. (**2**) Gut of an infected mouse. The crypts have shortened and a large influx of mast cells can be clearly seen.

intestinal epithelium and ultimately an environment that appears hostile for continued *T. spiralis* survival. By contrast, expulsion of *N. brasiliensis* and *T. muris* still proceeds normally following depression of mastocytosis, suggesting that the mast cell is not the major effector cell type for these infections.

Therefore, although TH2 cytokines are critical for the elimination of worms from the gut, the exact effector mechanism may vary depending on the species.

Platelets can kill many types of parasite. Potential targets for platelets include the larval stage of flukes, *T. gondii*, *Plasmodium* and *T. cruzi*. Like other effector cells, the cytotoxic activity of platelets is enhanced by treatment with cytokines (e.g. IFNγ and TNFα). In rats infected with *S. mansoni*, platelets become larvicidal when acute-phase reactants appear in the serum but before antibody can be detected. Incubation of normal platelets in such serum can cause their activation.

Platelets, like macrophages and the other effector cells, also bear Fcε and Fcγ receptors, by which they mediate antibody-dependent cytotoxicity.

PARASITE ESCAPE MECHANISMS

It is a necessary characteristic of all successful parasitic infections that they can evade the full effects of their host's immune response. Parasites have developed many different ways of doing this. Some even exploit cells and molecules of the immune system to their own advantage. For example, despite their protective role in the immune response to many different parasites:
- host TNFα actually stimulates egg production by adult worms of *S. mansoni*; and
- IFN is used as a growth factor by *T. brucei*.

Parasites can resist destruction by complement. In the case of *Leishmania*, resistance correlates with virulence:
- *Leishmania tropica*, which is easily killed by complement, causes a localized self-healing infection in the skin; whereas

- *Leishmania donovani*, which is 10 times more resistant to complement, becomes disseminated throughout the viscera, causing a disease that is often fatal.

The mechanisms whereby parasites can resist the effect of complement differ:
- The LPG surface coat of *Leishmania major* activates complement, but the complex is then shed, so the parasite avoids lysis.
- The trypomastigotes of *T. cruzi* bear a surface glycoprotein with activity resembling the decay-accelerating factor (DAF) that limits the complement reaction. The resistance that schistosomules acquire as they mature is also correlated with the appearance of a surface molecule similar to DAF.

Intracellular parasites can avoid being killed by oxygen metabolites and lysosomal enzymes. Intracellular parasites that live inside macrophages have evolved different ways of avoiding being killed by oxygen metabolites and lysosomal enzymes (Fig. 16.13):
- *T. gondii* penetrates the macrophage by a non-phagocytic pathway and avoids triggering the oxidative burst.
- *Leishmania* spp. use complement receptors to gain entry into macrophages, thus avoiding triggering the oxidative burst and cytotoxic ROIs.
- *Leishmania* also possess enzymes such as superoxide dismutase, which protects them against the action of oxygen radicals.

It has been demonstrated that *Leishmania* can survive in lysosomal vacuoles (Fig. 16.14), because the parasites have evolved mechanisms that protect against enzymatic attack. The LPG surface coat acts as a scavenger of oxygen metabolites and affords protection against enzymatic attack, but a glycoprotein, Gp63 (Fig. 16.w4), inhibits the action of the macrophage's lysosomal enzymes.

Leishmania spp. can also downregulate the expression of MHC class II molecules on the macrophages they inhabit, thus reducing their capacity to stimulate TH cells.

These escape mechanisms, however, are less efficient in the immune host.

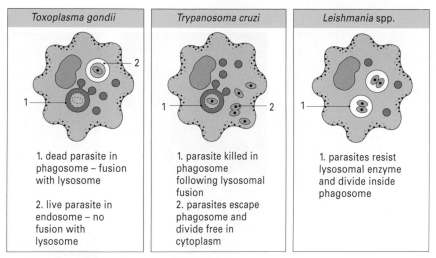

Fig. 16.13 Different ways by which protozoa multiply within macrophages avoid intracellular killing *T. gondii*: live parasites enter the cell actively into a membrane-bound vacuole. They are not attacked by enzymes because lysosomes do not fuse with this vacuole. Dead parasites, however, are taken up by normal phagocytosis into a phagosome (by interaction with the Fc receptors on the macrophage if they are coated with antibody) and are then destroyed by the enzymes of the lysosomes that fuse with it. *T. cruzi*: survival of these parasites depends upon their stage of development; trypomastigotes escape from the phagosome and divide in the cytoplasm, whereas epimastigotes do not escape and are killed. The proportion of parasites found in the cytoplasm is decreased if the macrophages are activated. *Leishmania* spp.: These parasites multiply within the phagosome and the presence of a surface protease helps them resist digestion. If the macrophages are first activated by cytokines, the number of parasites entering the cell and the number that replicate diminish.

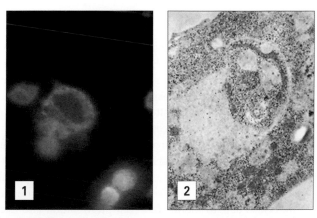

Fig. 16.14 The leishmania vacuole is lysosomal (**1**) Immunofluorescence of *Leishmania mexicana*-infected murine macrophages probed with a rhodamine-conjugated anti-tubulin antibody to illustrate the parasite (stained yellow/red) and a fluorescein-conjugated monoclonal antibody, which reacts with the late endosomal/lysosomal marker LAMP-1 (stained green). (**2**) Immunoelectron micrograph of *L. mexicana*-infected murine macrophage probed with gold-labelled anti-cathepsin D demonstrating the lysosomal aspartic proteinase in the leishmania vacuole. (Courtesy Dr David Russell.)

Parasites can disguise themselves. Parasites that are vulnerable to specific antibodies have evolved different methods of evading its effects.

African trypanosomes and malaria undergo antigenic variation. The molecule that forms the surface coat of the African trypanosome, the variable surface glycoprotein (VSG), changes to protect the underlying surface membrane from the host's defence mechanisms. New populations of parasites are antigenically distinct from previous ones (Fig. 16.15).

Several antigens of malarial parasites also undergo antigenic variation.

For example, the *P. falciparum* erythrocyte membrane protein-1 (PfEMP1) is extremely polymorphic and variable between different strains of the parasite because it is perpetually exposed to the immune system by its location on the red cell membrane. PfEMP1 can bind numerous host immune proteins, but particularly scavenger receptors, e.g. CD36, and scavenging antibodies that eliminate apoptotic or damaged cells, e.g. natural IgM (see Fig. 16.17).

Other parasites acquire a surface layer of host antigens. Schistosomes acquire a surface layer of host antigens so that the host does not distinguish them from self. Schistosomules cultured in medium containing human serum and red blood cells can acquire surface molecules containing A, B and H blood group determinants. They can also acquire MHC molecules and immunoglobulins. However, schistosomules maintained in a medium devoid of host molecules also become resistant to attack by antibody and complement, as mentioned earlier.

Some extracellular parasites hide from or resist immune attack. Some species of protozoa (e.g. *Entamoeba histolytica*) and helminths (e.g. *T. spiralis*) form protective cysts, while adult worms of *O. volvulus* in the skin induce the host to surround them with collagenous nodules.

Intestinal nematodes and tapeworms are preserved from many host responses simply because they live in the gut.

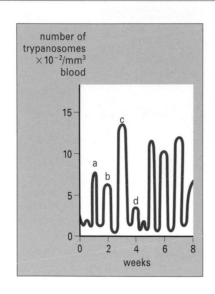
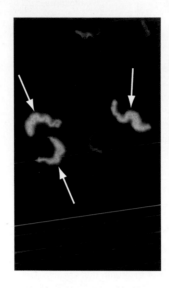
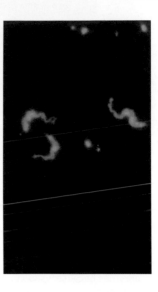

Fig. 16.15 Antigenic variation in trypanosomes Trypanosome infections may run for several months giving rise to successive waves of parasitaemia. The graph shows a chart of the fluctuation in parasitaemia in a patient with sleeping sickness. Although infection was initiated by a single parasite, each wave is caused by an immunologically distinct population of parasites (a, b, c, d); protection is not afforded by antibodies against any of the preceding variants. There is a strong tendency for new variants to appear in the same order in different hosts. The micrographs show immunofluorescent labelling of trypanosomes *(arrows)* with a variant antigen-type specific monoclonal antibody *(left panel)*. The panel on the *right* shows the same field but with the nuclei and kinetoplasts of all the parasites stained with a dye that binds to DNA. Only some of the parasites express a given antigen variant. (Courtesy Dr Mike Turner.)

There are numerous examples of simple, physical, protective strategies in parasites:

- Nematodes have a thick extracellular cuticle, which protects them from the toxic effects of an immune response.
- The tegument of schistosomes thickens during maturation to offer similar protection.
- The loose surface coat of many nematodes may slough off under immune attack.
- Tapeworms prevent attack by secreting an elastase inhibitor, which stops them attracting neutrophils.

Many parasitic worms have evolved methods of resisting the oxidative burst. For instance, schistosomes have surface-associated glutathione S-transferases and *Onchocerca* spp. can secrete superoxide dismutase.

Some nematodes and trematodes have evolved an elegant method of disabling antibodies by secreting proteases, which cleave immunoglobulins, removing the Fc portion and preventing their interaction with Fc receptors on phagocytic cells; for example, schistosomes can cleave IgE.

Most parasites interfere with immune responses for their benefit

Parasites produce molecules that interfere with host immune function. Parasites produce molecules that can affect the phenotype of the adaptive response, which may be to their own advantage (Table 16.3 and Fig. 16.16).

In leishmaniasis, T cells from patients infected with *L. donovani* when cultured with specific antigen do not secrete IL-2 or IFNγ. Their production of IL-1 and expression of MHC class II molecules is also decreased, whereas secretion of prostaglandins is increased. IL-2, characteristic of TH1 responses, is also deficient in other protozoal infections, including malaria, African trypanosomiasis and Chagas disease. In mice infected with *T. cruzi*, a parasite product appears to interfere with expression of the IL-2 receptor.

Filarial worms secrete a protease inhibitor that has been shown to affect the proteases critical in the processing of antigens to peptides, resulting in the reduction of class II molecule presentation in filariasis. One such protease inhibitor, onchocystatin, is also able to modulate T-cell proliferation and elicit the upregulation of IL-10 expression and is therefore able to modulate the T-cell phenotype. Prostaglandins (PGs) produced by helminth parasites may also perform a similar role by modulating APC function. PGE_2 is produced by filarial parasites and tapeworms and blocks the production of IL-12 by dendritic cells and thus may direct responses towards TH2.

Phosphorylcholine (PC)-containing molecules are commonly found in infectious organisms and experiments using a nematode PC-bearing glycoconjugate, ES-62, have been shown to desensitize APCs to subsequent exposure to LPS and may therefore also skew against a TH1 response (LPS is a classical inducer of TH1 responses). ES-62 is able to inhibit proliferation of T cells and B cells and inhibit IgE-mediated mast-cell responses.

Parasites also produce cytokine-like molecules that mimic TGFβ, migration inhibitory factor (MIF) and a histamine-releasing factor.

Genes encoding possible cytokine homologues are being found as part of the genome-sequencing projects that are under way for

TABLE 16.3   Some Mechanisms by Which Parasites Avoid Host Immunity

A summary of the various methods that parasites have evolved to avoid host defence mechanisms

Parasite	Habitat	Main Host Effector Mechanism	Method of Avoidance
Trypanosoma brucei	Blood stream	Antibody + complement	Antigenic variation
Plasmodium spp.	Hepatocyte blood stream	T cells, antibody	Antigenic variation, sequestration
Toxoplasma gondii	Macrophage	ROI, NO•, lysosomal enzymes	Suppresses IL-12, inhibits fusion of lysozymes
Trypanosoma cruzi	Many cells	ROI, NO•, lysosomal enzymes	Escapes to cytoplasm, so avoiding digestion
Leishmania spp.	Macrophage	ROI, NO•, lysosomal enzymes	Induction of Tregs, resists digestion by phagolysosome
Schistosoma spp.	Skin, blood, lungs, portal veins	Myeloid cells' antibody + complement	Acquisition of host antigens (e.g. IgG), proteolytic cleavage of immune proteins, inhibition of dendritic cell maturation
Filariasis	Lymphatics	Myeloid cells	Induction of Tregs, secretion of cytokine mimics, interference with antigen processing

NO•, Nitric oxide; *ROI*, reactive oxygen intermediates.

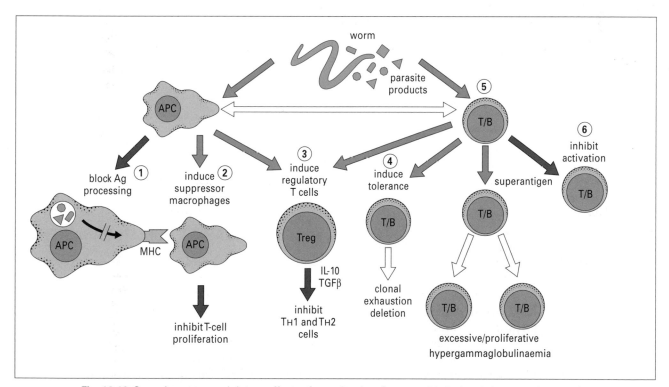

Fig. 16.16 Some immunomodulatory effects of parasites Interference with the host's immune response by molecules released by protozoa or worms. Parasite products act via the antigen-presenting cell *(APC) (1)* to interfere with antigen processing or presentation (e.g. protease inhibitors from filarial parasites interfere with proteases in the major histocompatibility complex *(MHC)* signalling pathway and block antigen presentation); *(2)* to induce suppressor macrophages, which can inhibit T-cell proliferation; *(3)* to induce regulatory T cells (e.g. lyso-PS from schistosomes acts via TLR2 on dendritic cells to induce T cells that secrete IL-10, which inhibits the inflammatory response). Parasite products may also affect lymphocytes *(3)* to make them become regulatory; *(4)* to induce T-cell or B-cell tolerance by clonal exhaustion or by the induction of anergy; *(5)* to cause polyclonal activation (many parasite products are mitogenic to T or B cells and the high serum concentrations of non-specific IgM (and IgG) commonly found in parasitic infections probably result from this polyclonal stimulation – its continuation is believed to lead to impairment of B-cell function, the progressive depletion of antigen-reactive B cells and thus immunosuppression); *(6)* to inhibit directly the activation of T or B cells (e.g. ES-62, a secreted product of a filarial parasite, is able to inhibit the proliferation of both T and B cells).

many parasites. Although the sequences are related to cytokines or cytokine receptors, their functions are still to be established.

Soluble parasite antigens released in huge quantities may impair the host's response by a process termed 'immune distraction'. Thus, the soluble antigens (S or heat-stable antigens) of *P. falciparum* are thought to mop up circulating antibody, providing a smokescreen and diverting the antibody from the body of the parasite.

Many of the surface antigens that are shed are soluble forms of molecules inserted into the parasite membrane by a GPI anchor, including the VSG of *T. brucei*, the LPG or excreted factor of *Leishmania* (see Fig. 16.w4) and several surface antigens of schistosomules. These proteins are released by endogenous phosphatidylinositol-specific phospholipases.

The hypergammaglobulinaemic immunoglobulins induced by malaria parasites can bind to FcγRIIB, which may benefit the parasite.

Some parasites suppress inflammation or immune responses. Immunosuppression is a common feature of chronic helminth infections, both parasite-specific and generalized. For example, patients with schistosomiasis and filariasis have diminished responsiveness to antigens from the infecting parasite. Studies have also shown diminished responses to bystander infections and vaccinations. This spillover suppression may be beneficial to the host in some situations. For example, reduced inflammatory responses have been observed in *Helicobacter pylori* infection with malaria.

Parasites have co-evolved with humans over millions of years and until recently it was normal for people to carry worms, a fact that argues for their importance in the **hygiene hypothesis**, which proposes that the rise in allergies and autoimmune illness is a result of cleaner living conditions and the almost complete elimination of parasitic infections in Westernized societies.

The ability of parasites to suppress hyperactive immune responses is believed to be because of the induction of regulatory T cells (see Fig. 16.16) and is an area of intensive research. The dendritic cell possibly polarizes the T cell towards a regulator phenotype after exposure to parasite extracts.

IMMUNOPATHOLOGICAL CONSEQUENCES OF PARASITE INFECTIONS

Apart from the directly destructive effects of some parasites and their products on host tissues, many immune responses themselves have pathological effects.

In malaria, African trypanosomiasis and visceral leishmaniasis, the increased number and heightened activity of macrophages and lymphocytes in the liver and spleen lead to enlargement of those organs. In schistosomiasis, much of the pathology results from the T-cell-dependent granulomas forming around eggs in the liver. The gross changes in individuals with elephantiasis are probably caused by immunopathological responses to adult filariae in the lymphatics.

The formation of immune complexes is common: they may be deposited in the kidney, as in the nephrotic syndrome of quartan malaria, and may give rise to many other pathological changes. For example, tissue-bound immunoglobulins have been found in the muscles of mice infected with African trypanosomes and in the choroid plexus of mice with malaria.

The IgE of worm infections can have severe effects on the host as a result of the release of mast-cell mediators. Anaphylactic shock may occur when a hydatid cyst ruptures. Asthma-like reactions occur in *Toxocara canis* infections and in tropical pulmonary eosinophilia when filarial worms migrate through the lungs.

Autoantibodies, which probably arise as a result of polyclonal activation, have been detected against red blood cells, lymphocytes and DNA (e.g. in trypanosomiasis and in malaria).

Antibodies against the parasite may cross-react with host tissues. For example, the chronic cardiomyopathy, enlarged oesophagus and megacolon that occur in Chagas disease are thought to result from the autoimmune effects on nerve ganglia of antibody and Tc cells that cross-react with *T. cruzi*. Similarly, *O. volvulus*, the cause of river blindness, possesses an antigen that cross-reacts with a protein in the retina.

Excessive production of cytokines may contribute to some of the manifestations of disease. Thus, the fever, anaemia, diarrhoea and pulmonary changes of acute malaria closely resemble the symptoms of endotoxaemia and are probably caused by TNFα. The severe wasting of cattle with trypanosomiasis may also be mediated by TNFα.

A single parasite protein may produce multiple pathological effects, as seen with PfEMP1, coded by the *var* genes, and expressed on the surface of infected erythrocytes (Fig. 16.17).

Lastly, the non-specific immunosuppression that is so widespread probably explains why people with parasitic infections are especially susceptible to bacterial and viral infections (e.g. measles). It may also account for the association of Burkitt's lymphoma with malaria because malaria-infected individuals are less able to control infection with the Epstein–Barr virus that causes Burkitt's lymphoma.

VACCINES AGAINST HUMAN PARASITES

Some vaccines composed of attenuated living parasites have proved successful in veterinary practice. However, so far there is none in use against human parasites, although much effort has been directed towards the development of subunit vaccines against malarial parasites and schistosomes in particular. Some clinical trials of vaccines against malaria, based on combinations of putatively protective antigens, are in progress (see Chapter 17). There is an urgent need to identify the key antigens involved and develop non-toxic adjuvants for their effective delivery to the immune system.

Parasite genome sequencing ventures and analysis of whole parasite proteomes are highlighting novel targets for both drug and vaccine design. These modern technologies are providing startling insights into how parasite and host immune systems interact. For example, the malaria protein PfEMP1 encoded by var genes, known to be expressed in the red blood cell stage within the human host and implicated in immune evasion, has been identified in the mosquito sporozoite stage, indicating that it may have several alternative functions (see Fig. 16.17).

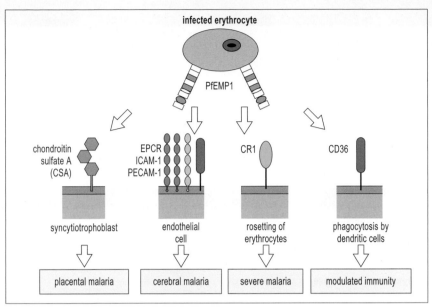

Fig. 16.17 Malarial pathology resulting from interactions with PfEMP1 Malaria-infected erythrocytes cause disease through many mechanisms involving the interaction between *Plasmodium falciparum* erythrocyte membrane protein-1 *(PfEMP1)* and diverse host receptors.

CRITICAL THINKING: IMMUNITY TO PROTOZOA AND HELMINTHS

See Critical thinking: Explanations section 16

1. In general, protozoa and helminths adopt different strategies for survival and for transmission to the subsequent host. How do they differ?
2. Many parasites have evolved to live in host cells. Consider the advantages and disadvantages to this mode of existence. Consider the different cell types and how parasites have to adapt this environment to their advantage. In particular,

T. gondii, T. cruzi and *Leishmania* spp. have adapted to live in the macrophage and can escape destruction by lysosomal enzymes, but the way in which they do this differs. How have these adaptations helped parasite survival?

3. Extracellular parasites have evolved sophisticated mechanisms to avoid the immune response. Give some examples of how they do this.

FURTHER READING

Anthony RM, Rutitzky LI, Urban JF Jr, et al. Protective immune mechanisms in helminth infection. Nat Rev Immunol 2007;7:975–987.

Arora G, Hart GT, Manzella-Lapeira J, et al. NK cells inhibit *Plasmodium falciparum* growth in red blood cells via antibody-dependent cellular cytotoxicity. Elife 2018; https://doi.org/10.7554/eLife.36806.002.

Boeltz S, Munoz LE, Fuchs TA, Herrmann M. Neutrophil extracellular traps open the Pandora's box in severe malaria. Front Immunol 2017;8:874.

Cowman AF, Healer J, Marapana D, March K. Malaria: biology and disease. Cell 2016;167:610–624.

Iborra S, Martınez-Lopez M, Cueto FJ, et al. Leishmania uses Mincle to target an inhibitory ITAM signaling pathway in dendritic cells that dampens adaptive immunity to infection. Immunity 2016;45:788–801.

Martinez FO, Helming L, Gordon S. Alternative activation of macrophages: an immunologic functional perspective. Annu Rev Immunol 2009;27:451–483.

Paul WE, Zhu J. How are T(H)2-type immune responses initiated and amplified? Nat Rev Immunol 2010;10:225–235.

Pleass RJ, Moore SC, Stevenson L, Hviid L. Immunoglobulin M: restrainer of inflammation and mediator of immune evasion by *Plasmodium falciparum* malaria. Trends Parasitol 2016;32:108–119.

Sorobetea D, Svensson-Frej M, Grencis R. Immunity to gastrointestinal nematode infections. Mucosal Immunol 2018;11:301–315.

Voehringer D. The role of basophils in helminth infection. Trends Parasitol 2009;25:551–556.

17

Vaccination

SUMMARY

- **Vaccination applies immunological principles to human health.** Adaptive immunity and the ability of lymphocytes to develop memory for a pathogen's antigens underlie vaccination. Active immunization is known as vaccination.
- **A wide range of antigen preparations are in use as vaccines,** from whole organisms to simple peptides and polysaccharides. Living and non-living vaccines have important differences, living vaccines being generally more effective.
- **Adjuvants enhance antibody production** and are usually required with non-living vaccines. They concentrate antigen at appropriate sites or induce cytokines.
- **Most vaccines are still given by injection,** but other routes are being investigated.
- **Vaccine efficacy needs to be reviewed from time to time.**
- **Vaccine safety is an overriding consideration.** When immunization frequencies fall, the population as a whole is not protected. Fears over the safety

of the MMR vaccine resulted in measles epidemics and increases in incidence of rubella.
- **Vaccines in general use have variable success rates.** Some vaccines are reserved for special groups only and vaccines for parasites and some other infections are only experimental.
- **Passive immunization can be life-saving.** The direct administration of antibodies still has a role to play in certain circumstance: for example, when tetanus toxin is already in the circulation.
- **Non-specific immunotherapy can boost immune activity.** Non-specific immunization, for example by cytokines, may be of use in selected conditions.
- **Immunization against a variety of non-infectious conditions is being investigated.**
- **Recombinant DNA technology will be the basis for the next generation of vaccines.** Most future vaccines will be recombinant subunit vaccines incorporated into viral or bacterial vectors. This should provide enhanced efficacy and safety.

VACCINATION

Vaccines apply immunological principles to human health.

Vaccination is the best known and most successful application of immunological principles to human health. It exploits the property of immunological memory to provide long-lasting protection against infectious disease.

The first vaccine was named after vaccinia, the cowpox virus. Jenner pioneered its use 200 years ago. It was the first deliberate scientific attempt to prevent an infectious disease and was based on the notion that infection with a mild disease (cowpox) might protect against infection with a similar but much more serious one (smallpox), although it was done in complete ignorance of viruses (or indeed any kind of microbe) and immunology.

It was not until the work of Pasteur 100 years later that the general principle governing vaccination emerged – altered preparations of microbes could be used to generate enhanced immunity against the fully virulent organism. Thus, Pasteur's dried rabies-infected rabbit spinal cords and heated anthrax bacilli were the true forerunners of today's vaccines, whereas, until very recently, Jenner's animal-derived (i.e. heterologous) vaccinia virus had no real successors.

Even Pasteur did not have a proper understanding of immunological memory or the functions of the lymphocyte, which had to wait another half century.

Finally, with Burnet's clonal selection theory (1957) and the discovery of T and B lymphocytes (1965), the key mechanism became clear.

In any immune response, antigens induce clonal expansion in specific T and/or B cells, leaving behind a population of memory cells. These enable the next encounter with the same antigen(s) to induce a secondary response, which is more rapid and effective than the normal primary response.

While for many infections the primary response may be too slow to prevent serious disease, if the individual has been exposed to antigens from the organism in a vaccine before encountering the pathogen, the expanded population of memory cells and raised levels of specific antibody are able to protect against disease. The principles of vaccination can be summarized as:

- priming of specific lymphocytes to expand the pool of memory cells;
- use of harmless forms of immunogen – attenuated organisms, subcellular fragments, toxoids or vectors;
- use of adjuvants to enhance immune responses; and
- production of safe, affordable vaccines to promote herd immunity.

Vaccines can protect populations as well as individuals.

Vaccines protect individuals against disease and if there are sufficient immune individuals in a population, transmission of the infection is prevented. This is known as **herd immunity**.

The proportion of the population that needs to be immune to prevent epidemics occurring depends on the nature of the infection:

- If the organism is highly infectious so that one individual can rapidly infect several non-immune individuals, as is the case for measles, a high proportion of the population must be immune to maintain herd immunity.
- If the infection is less readily transmitted, immunity in a lower proportion of the population may be sufficient to prevent disease transmission.

Effective vaccines must be safe to administer, induce the correct type of immunity and be affordable by the population at which they are aimed. During the middle of the 20th century, this was achieved with brilliant success for many of the world's major infectious diseases, culminating in the official eradication of smallpox in 1980. Beyond this era, progress was much slower and fears over vaccine safety made development more lengthy and costly. However, the advent of recombinant DNA technology has led to a number of significant advances in the first decade of the 21st century and a number of new, safe and effective vaccines have come onto the market during this period. Despite these successes, for many diseases development of an effective vaccine has remained elusive, in particular, parasitic diseases and HIV, although a vaccine candidate for the latter has shown extreme promise in the last year and will now enter a phase IIb trial.

Nevertheless, with the availability of new technologies and a greater understanding of the immunological principles that underlie effective vaccines, the future for new vaccine development looks brighter than it has for some years.

ANTIGEN PREPARATIONS USED IN VACCINES

A wide variety of preparations are used as vaccines (Table 17.1). In general, the more antigens of the microbe retained in the vaccine, the better, and living organisms tend to be more effective than killed organisms. Exceptions to this rule are:

- diseases where a toxin is responsible for the pathology – in this case the vaccine can be based on the toxin alone;
- a vaccine in which the genes for microbial antigens are inserted into a vector and expressed in a host cell.

Live vaccines can be natural or attenuated organisms.

Natural live vaccines have rarely been used. Apart from vaccinia, no other completely natural organism has ever come into standard use. However:

- bovine and simian rotaviruses have been tried in children;
- the vole tubercle bacillus was once popular against tuberculosis; and
- in the Middle East and Russia *Leishmania* infection from mild cases is reputed to induce immunity.

Although it is possible that another good heterologous vaccine will be found, safety problems with this approach remain considerable. Nevertheless, the ability to genetically manipulate heterologous organisms can increase safety (for example, by removing genes responsible for virulence) and allow the

TABLE 17.1 Antigenic Preparations

Type of Antigen		Vaccine Examples
Living organisms	Natural	Vaccinia (for smallpox) Vole bacillus (for tuberculosis; historical)
	Attenuated	Polio (Sabin; oral polio vaccine)*, measles*, mumps*, rubella*, yellow fever 17D, varicella-zoster (human herpes virus 3), BCG (for tuberculosis)*
Intact but non-living organisms	Viruses	Polio (Salk)*, rabies, influenza, hepatitis A, typhus
	Bacteria	*Pertussis, typhoid, cholera, plague
Subcellular fragments	Capsular polysaccharides	Pneumococcus, meningococcus, *Haemophilus influenzae*
	Surface antigen	Hepatitis B*
Toxoids		Tetanus*, diphtheria*
Recombinant DNA-based	Gene cloned and expressed	Hepatitis B (yeast-derived)*, human papilloma virus*, meningococcus serotype B
	Genes expressed in vectors	Ebola candidate vaccines
	Naked DNA	Experimental

A wide range of antigenic preparations are used as vaccines.
*Standard in most countries.

creation of hybrid organisms capable of eliciting a strong immune response to the natural human pathogen. A recent example of the successful application of this approach is in the development of new rotavirus vaccines (Fig 17.w1).

The vaccines provide high levels of protection against rotavirus gastroenteritis and have proven to be very useful in developing countries where infantile diarrhoea is a major cause of mortality. However, their use in in Europe and the USA has been more limited, owing to both vaccines carrying a slightly increased risk of a rare complication of the gut known as intussusception.

Attenuated live vaccines have been highly successful. Historically, the preferred strategy for vaccine development has been to attenuate a human pathogen, with the aim of diminishing its virulence while retaining the desired antigens.

This was first done successfully by Calmette and Guérin with a bovine strain (*Mycobacterium bovis*) of *Mycobacterium tuberculosis* which, during 13 years (1908–1921) of culture in vitro, changed to the much less virulent form now known as BCG (bacillus Calmette–Guérin), which has at least some protective effect against tuberculosis.

The real successes were with viruses, starting with the 17D strain of yellow fever virus obtained by passage in mice and chicken embryos (1937), and followed by a roughly similar approach with polio, measles, mumps and rubella (Table 17.2).

Just how successful the vaccines for polio, measles, mumps and rubella are is shown by the decline in these four diseases between 1950 and 1980 (Fig. 17.1). The effect of introducing

TABLE 17.2   Live Attenuated Vaccines

	Disease	Remarks
Viruses	Polio	Types 2 and 3 may revert; also killed vaccine
	Measles	80% effective
	Mumps	
	Rubella	Now given to both sexes
	Rotavirus	New genetic reassortant
	Yellow fever	Stable since 1937
	Varicella-zoster	Mainly in leukaemia
	Hepatitis A	Also killed vaccine
Bacteria	Tuberculosis	Stable since 1921; also some protection against leprosy

Attenuated vaccines are available for many, but not all, infections. In general, it has proved easier to attenuate viruses than bacteria.

the vaccines that make up the UK 5in1 is similarly striking (Table 17.w1).

Attenuated microorganisms are less able to cause disease in their natural host. Attenuation changes microorganisms to make them less able to grow and to cause disease in their natural host. In early attenuated organisms, 'changed' meant a purely random set of mutations induced by adverse conditions of growth. Vaccine candidates were selected by constantly monitoring for retention of antigenicity and loss of virulence – a tedious process.

When viral gene sequencing became possible, it emerged that the results of attenuation were widely divergent. An example is the divergence between the three types of live (Sabin) polio vaccine:

- Type 1 polio has 57 mutations and has almost never reverted to wild type.
- Types 2 and 3 vaccines depend for their safety and virulence on only two key mutations – frequent reversion to wild type has occurred, in some cases leading to outbreaks of paralytic poliomyelitis.

Those genes not essential for replication of the virus are mostly concerned with evasion of host responses and **virulence**, which is the ability to replicate efficiently and to disseminate widely within the body, with pathological consequences. Many pathogenic viruses contain virulence genes that mimic or interfere with cytokine and chemokine function. Some of these have sequence homology to their mammalian counterparts and others do not.

Killed vaccines are intact but non-living organisms. Killed vaccines are the successors of Pasteur's killed vaccines mentioned earlier:

- some are very effective (rabies and the Salk polio vaccine);
- some are moderately effective (typhoid, cholera and influenza);
- some are of debatable value (plague and typhus); and
- some are controversial on the grounds of toxicity (pertussis).

Table 17.3 lists the main killed vaccines in use today. These are gradually being replaced by attenuated or subunit vaccines. However, in the case of polio, some countries are reverting to the use of killed vaccine, which is safer than the attenuated vaccine, even though it is less effective. This choice only becomes relevant when the risk of contracting the disease is low in comparison with the risk of developing adverse reactions to the vaccine.

TABLE 17.3   Killed (Whole Organism) Vaccines

	Disease	Remarks
Viruses	Polio	Preferred in Scandinavia; safe in immunocompromised
	Rabies	Can be given post-exposure, with passive antiserum
	Influenza	Strain-specific
	Hepatitis A	Also attenuated vaccine
Bacteria	Pertussis	Discontinued owing to safety concerns replaced by safe acellular vaccine
	Typhoid	About 70% protection
	Cholera	Combined with recombinant modified toxin
	Plague	Short-term protection only
	Q fever	Good protection

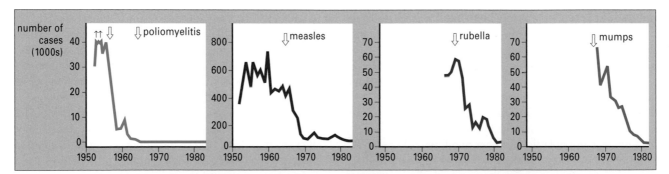

Fig. 17.1 Effect of vaccination on the incidence of viral disease The effect of vaccination on the incidence of various viral diseases in the USA has been that most infections have shown a dramatic downward trend since the introduction of a vaccine *(arrows)*.

TABLE 17.4 The Principal Toxin-Based Vaccines

Organism	Vaccine	Remarks
Clostridium tetani	Inactivated toxin (formalin)	Three doses, alum-precipitated; boost every 10 years
Corynebacterium diphtheriae		Usually given with tetanus
Vibrio cholerae	Recombinant modified toxin	Combined with whole killed organism
Clostridium perfringens	Inactivated toxin (formalin)	For newborn lambs

Note that there are no vaccines against the numerous staphylococcal and streptococcal exotoxins or against bacterial endotoxins such as lipopolysaccharides.

Inactivated toxins and toxoids are the most successful bacterial vaccines. The most successful of all bacterial vaccines, tetanus and diphtheria, are based on inactivated exotoxins (Table 17.4) and in principle the same approach can be used for several other infections. An inactive, mutant form of diphtheria toxin (CRM$_{197}$) has been used as the basis for a number of more recently generated conjugate vaccines (see later).

Subunit vaccines and carriers. Aside from the toxin-based vaccines, which are subunits of their respective microorganisms, a number of other vaccines are in use that use antigens either purified from microorganisms or produced by recombinant DNA technology (Table 17.5). For example, a recombinant hepatitis B surface antigen synthesized in baker's yeast has been in use since 1986.

Acellular pertussis vaccine consisting of a small number of proteins purified from the bacterium has been available for some years now and has been shown to be effective, safer and less toxic than the killed (whole organism) vaccine. It is usually administered as part of a DTaP (diphtheria, tetanus, pertussis) combination vaccine routinely given to infants.

TABLE 17.5 Subunit Vaccines

	Organism	Remarks
Virus	Hepatitis B virus	Surface antigen can be purified from blood of carriers or produced in yeast by recombinant DNA technology
Bacteria	Neisseria meningitidis	Capsular polysaccharide conjugates of groups A, C, W and Y are effective, B is non-immunogenic
	Streptococcus pneumoniae	84 serotypes; capsular polysaccharide vaccines contain 23 serotypes; conjugates with 13 bacterial serotypes now available
	Haemophilus influenzae B	Good conjugate vaccines now in use

Conjugate vaccines are replacing pure polysaccharides. N. meningitidis type B is non-immunogenic in humans because the capsular polysaccharide cross-reacts with self carbohydrates towards which the host is immunologically tolerant.

Conjugate vaccines are effective at inducing antibodies to carbohydrate antigens. Although protein antigens such as hepatitis B surface antigen are immunogenic when given with alum adjuvant (see later), for many types of bacteria, virulence is determined by the bacterial capsular polysaccharide, prime examples being *Neisseria meningitidis*, *Streptococcus pneumoniae* and *Haemophilus influenzae* type B. Such carbohydrate antigens, although they can be isolated and have been used for vaccination, are poorly immunogenic, particularly in infants under 2 years, and often do not induce IgG responses or long-lasting protection. Attempts to boost immunity by repeat administration of these vaccines can actually compromise immunity by depleting the pool of antibody-producing B cells.

A major advance in the efficacy of subunit vaccines has been obtained by conjugating the purified polysaccharides to carrier proteins such as tetanus or diphtheria toxoid. These protein carriers, which can now be produced in highly purified form by recombinant DNA techniques, are presumed to recruit TH2 cells and the conjugates induce IgG antibody responses and more effective long-lasting protection.

Starting with *H. influenzae* type B (Hib) in the early 1990s, conjugate vaccines for *N. meningitidis* strains A, C, Y and W-135 are also now in widespread usage. In the UK, until 1992 when the vaccine was introduced, Hib was the major cause of infantile meningitis leading to many hundreds of cases per year. The introduction of the vaccine led to a very rapid decline, making Hib meningitis a very rare occurrence (Fig. 17.2(1)).

Conjugate meningitis vaccines. The serogroup C meningococcal vaccine was first introduced in the UK in 1999 and has resulted in a reduction of >80% in the incidence of infection (Fig. 17.2(2)). Indeed, increased levels of immunity against MenC may have been instrumental in a recent rise in the cases of MenW in the UK, following the appearance of a new more virulent strain. The MenC vaccine has also been used successfully in Australia, Canada and Europe. Since 2005, a highly successful tetravalent combination conjugate vaccine active against strains A, C, Y and W-135 has been available across the developed world and a specially produced MenA vaccine produced for use in Africa.

Antigens can be expressed from vectors. Many antigens can now be produced in recombinant form by cloning their genes into a suitable expression vector. This approach has been highly successful with the hepatitis B surface (HBsAg) antigen cloned into yeast and this replaced the first-generation HBsAg vaccine, which was laboriously purified from the blood of hepatitis B carriers; it also brought down the cost of the vaccine.

The most spectacular success with this approach to date has been the development of the vaccines against human papilloma virus (HPV) infection. HPV has been established as the causative agent in cervical carcinoma and over 70% of cases are accounted for by the serotypes 16 and 18. Two new vaccines (Gardasil and Cervarix) have been developed using recombinant expression vectors that produce the viral surface protein L1. Aggregates of L1 spontaneously assemble into virus-like particles

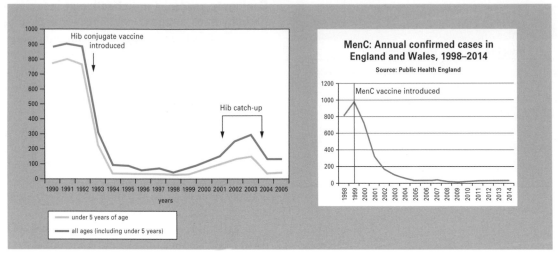

Fig. 17.2 Annual incidence of *Haemophilus* and meningitis C in the UK Introduction of the *Haemophilus influenzae* type-B *(Hib)* vaccine led to a rapid decline in meningitis in children in England and Wales (1990–2004). Vaccination was initiated in 1992. There was an upsurge in cases after 1999, possibly because the vaccine was less effective when used in combination with other vaccines, but this was controlled with a further campaign, initiated in 2003. The incidence of meningitis type C declined sharply after introduction of the MenC vaccine in 1999. (Based on data from the Health Protection Agency and Public Health England.)

(VLP) that are highly immunogenic. Because these particles contain no nucleic acid, the vaccine cannot lead to HPV infection and is very safe. Trials suggested that very high levels of protection against HPV infection and cervical carcinoma were reached with these vaccines and, in 2008, they were introduced to protect against cervical carcinoma.

Over 100 countries worldwide have offered the vaccination to adolescent girls and many have implemented mass vaccination programmes. In the UK, routine HPV immunization has been offered as part of the national immunization programme to girls aged 12–13 years. Uptake in the UK has been high (>80% in England and >90% in Scotland) and similarly across Northern Europe, but significantly lower in countries such as the USA where immunization is not usually provided free of charge.

Efficacy of the vaccines against HPV strains 16 and 18 now seems unequivocal. A recent and extensive meta-analysis of trials has clearly demonstrated that, in young women who are HPV negative, the vaccines provide complete protection from these HPV strains and the cellular abnormalities associated with early cervical carcinoma. Gardasil, a quadrivalent vaccine, has shown similarly effective results against HPV 6 and 11, the major causes of genital warts.

Long-term follow-up has shown that both vaccines offer lasting protection both in terms of serum antibody levels and levels of neutralizing antibody. Evidence of good induction of B-memory cells and T-cell responses, even against a background of reducing levels of circulating antibody (in the case of HPV 18) has also been observed. The longest studies have followed immunized individuals for more than 9 years. Owing to the long incubation period, however, it is still not possible to demonstrate a reduction in the number of cervical carcinoma cases.

Vaccination programmes in many countries have now been instigated for boys, as well as girls, to protect against anogenital cancers and reduce rates of HPV infection. There is some evidence that the vaccine has even greater immunogenicity in boys.

A new nonavalent vaccine, Gardasil 9, has recently been developed by Merck to replace Gardasil and should provide protection against HPV strains 31, 33, 45, 52 and 58 in addition to strains 6, 11, 16 and 18 targeted by the original vaccine. It is based on similar preparations of VLPs formed by purified L1 surface protein of the HPV and the safety profile seems very similar. A number of countries have now licensed this vaccine, including the USA and the UK.

The use of recombinant DNA technology lends itself well to interfacing with bioinformatics-based methodologies to identify potential target antigens for immunization – called reverse vaccinology.

The development of the 4CMenB vaccine to combat *N. meningitidis* infection with serogroup B has proven a major triumph for vaccine development using this approach. The strategy used to produce the extremely successful conjugate vaccine to combat MenC (and now the quadrivalent MenACWY) were, unfortunately, not an option for MenB owing to the similarity of the capsular carbohydrate with naturally occurring human cellular polysaccharides. In the case of MenB, a bioinformatic search of the whole *Neisseria* genome was undertaken to identify proteins most likely to be expressed on the bacterial surface and therefore accessible to antibodies. Three bacterial proteins were identified and used in recombinant form by *Novartis* (in combination with an outer membrane vesicle preparation, referred to as virosomes, containing the surface protein *PorA*) to create the 4CMenB vaccine. In 2015, the UK became the first country in the world to add this vaccine to their routine infant immunization programme. It is hoped that the vaccine will also confer protection against serotype W.

ADJUVANTS ENHANCE ANTIBODY PRODUCTION

The increasing use of purified or recombinant antigens has refocused attention on the requirement to boost immune responses through the use of adjuvants. These are often necessary as the antigens by themselves are insufficiently immunogenic.

Work in the 1920s on the production of animal sera for human therapy discovered that certain substances, notably aluminium salts (alum), added to or emulsified with an antigen, greatly enhance antibody production, i.e. they act as adjuvants. Aluminium hydroxide is still widely used with, for example, diphtheria and tetanus toxoids. A list of the adjuvants in general usage is shown in Table 17.6.

The difficulty with adjuvants is that they mediate their effect through stimulating the inflammatory response, generally necessary to produce a good immune response to antigen. Unfortunately, the inflammatory response is often responsible for the side effects of immunization, such as pain and swelling at the injection site, and can lead to greater malaise, elevated temperature and/or flu-like symptoms. These are often impediments to vaccine uptake, especially when the distress is caused in small infants who are the most common vaccine recipients.

With modern understanding of the processes leading to lymphocyte triggering and the development of immunological memory, it is hoped that better adjuvants can be developed. Considerable efforts have been made to produce better adjuvants, particularly for TH1-mediated responses; one recent innovation is monophosphoryl lipid A (MPL), a detoxified form of LPS, which acts on Toll-like receptors (TLRs; see later).

Adjuvants concentrate antigen at appropriate sites or induce cytokines. It appears that the effect of adjuvants is mainly the result of two activities:

- the concentration of antigen in a site where lymphocytes are exposed to it (the 'depot' effect); and
- the induction of cytokines that regulate lymphocyte function.

Aluminium salts have a depot function, inducing small granulomas in which antigen is retained, but their effect seems more complex, including activation of inflammasomes, stimulation of IL-1, cell necrosis and activation of pathogen-related receptors (PRRs). Cell death may actually play an important role in the action of metal salt adjuvants.

Despite the fact that alum adjuvants have proven remarkably effective and are generally well tolerated, fears remain over their long-term safety for some individuals. Aluminium-adjuvanted vaccines have been suspected to be associated with a condition known as macrophagic myofasciitis (MFF), the symptoms of which are similar to chronic fatigue syndrome. However, the WHO Global Advisory Committee on Vaccine Safety has questioned this concern.

Particulate antigens such as virus-like particles (polymers of viral capsid proteins containing no viral DNA or RNA) can be highly immunogenic and have the useful property that they may also induce cross-priming (i.e. enter the MHC class I processing pathway although not synthesized within the APC, see Chapter 7).

TLR-stimulating molecules as adjuvants. Activation of an innate immune response seems to be an important step in the generation of long-lasting immunity possibly through stimulation of a TH1 response. Ligation of PRRs can help to bias the response towards a balanced TH1/TH2 cytokine production, unlike alum adjuvants, which stimulate a strong TH2 response.

A new generation of adjuvants with more predictable and less toxic properties is now being actively researched. For example, MPL was developed by chemical degradation of lipopolysaccharide (LPS), the major component of the cell wall of Gram-negative bacteria. Unlike LPS, MPL has low toxicity but retains potent adjuvant activity via agonist activity towards TLR4. This compound is combined with alum in an adjuvant product AS04 and was used in HPV (Cervarix) and HepB (Fendrix) vaccines.

Other potential TLR agonists are CpG oligonucleotides, which stimulate TLR9, and flagellin, which interacts with TLR5. Both have shown promise in animal models but inevitably activate the transcription factor NF-κB, a central player in activation of the inflammatory response, resulting in greater reactogenicity. The balancing act needed from improved adjuvants is

TABLE 17.6 Adjuvants

Adjuvant Type	Routinely Used in Humans	Experimental* or too Toxic for Human Use[†]
Inorganic salts	Aluminium hydroxide (alhydrogel), aluminium phosphate, calcium phosphate	Beryllium hydroxide
TLR agonists	Monophosphoryl lipid A	
Oil emulsion	Squalene derivatives: MF59, AS02, AS03	
Delivery systems		Liposomes* ISCOMs* Block polymers Slow-release formulations*
Bacterial products	*Bordetella pertussis* (with diphtheria, tetanus toxoids)	BCG *Mycobacterium bovis* and oil[†] (complete Freund adjuvant), muramyl dipeptide (MDP)[†]
Natural mediators (cytokines)		IL-1 IL-2 IL-12 IFNγ

A variety of foreign and endogenous substances can act as adjuvants, but only aluminium and calcium salts and pertussis are routinely used in clinical practice.

to be able to induce enhanced immunity without generating too much inflammation. Thus far, this is still proving somewhat elusive. However, this may be a property of a promising polysaccharide adjuvant known as delta inulin, which has been well tolerated in human trials.

VACCINE ADMINISTRATION

Most vaccines are delivered by injection. Administration by injection presents some risks, particularly in developing countries, where re-use of needles and syringes may transmit disease, particularly HIV. Alternatives to needle delivery do exist, however, and can be beneficial for use in mass vaccination programmes and for improving compliance in those with needle phobia. Mass vaccination, for many years, made use of multiuse jet injectors that fire a high-velocity liquid stream, which is very effective. Unfortunately, the possibility of cross-contamination from the re-usable design has, in more recent years, limited their application. Efforts are now being made to develop disposable single-use cartridges for such injectors, but inevitably at greater cost per vaccination.

Jet injectors can deliver vaccine intramuscularly, as with a needle, but they can also be used for cutaneous delivery, which should help to reduce the discomfort and potential for distress in infants. Cutaneous delivery is a highly effective method for vaccination; the skin harbours many Langerhans cells, which are very active in antigen presentation to T cells in lymph nodes, to which they migrate when activated by exposure to antigen. They also help to initiate an inflammatory response through release of cytokines and chemical mediators, all of which can potentiate the vaccine.

The main difficulty with cutaneous delivery is penetrating below the outer, cornified layer of the skin. Techniques to improve this, such as the uses of microneedle arrays (Fig. 17.3), are under development and may one day allow vaccination using skin patches, similar to those used currently for delivering (small-molecule) drugs, such as contraceptives.

Mucosal immunization is a logical alternative approach. Because most organisms enter via mucosal surfaces, mucosal immunization makes logical sense. The success of the oral polio vaccine, the newly formulated rotavirus vaccine and an effective cholera vaccine indicates that it can be made to work. However, although live attenuated vaccines can be effective when delivered orally, most killed vaccines are not.

Similar problems relate to nasal immunization, usually tried against upper respiratory infections such as influenza or respiratory syncytial viruses (RSV). With the exception described later, no nasal vaccine has entered *routine* use because of:

- difficulties in balancing attenuation against immunogenicity in the case of live RSV vaccine strains;
- the need for an adjuvant for an inactivated nasal influenza virus; and
- safety worries because of the proximity of the nasal mucosa to the brain through the cribriform plate.

A nasally delivered trivalent influenza vaccine using live attenuated virus has been licensed since 2003 in the USA and has been found to be safe and well tolerated, even in infants. Exceptionally perhaps, the success of this vaccine is partly a result of the extra safety provided by the inability of the vaccine strain to replicate in cells other than those of the nasopharyngeal epithelium. Conversely, an inactivated nasal flu vaccine originally developed in Switzerland was withdrawn over safety concerns relating to its associated adjuvant.

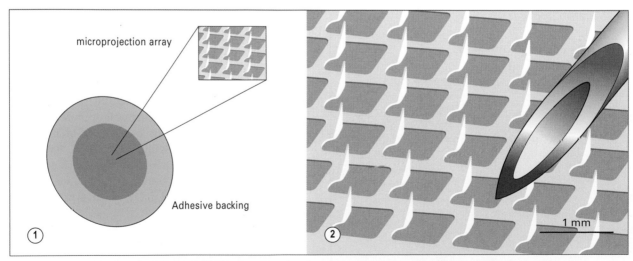

Fig. 17.3 Microneedle array (1) The size of an experimental microneedle array is shown. **(2)** Representation of a microprojection needle array, which is coated with vaccine suspension and used to deliver antigen to the skin subcutaneously. A 25-gauge needle is shown *(right)* for size comparison. (Figure redrawn courtesy J. Matriano (ALZA Corporation) with kind permission of Springer Science and Business Media.)

VACCINE EFFICACY AND SAFETY

To be introduced and approved, a vaccine must obviously be effective and the efficacy of all vaccines is reviewed from time to time. Many factors affect it.

An effective vaccine must induce the right sort of immunity:

- antibody for toxins and extracellular organisms such as *Streptococcus pneumoniae*;
- cell-mediated immunity for intracellular organisms such as the tubercle bacillus.

Where the ideal type of response is not clear (as in malaria, for instance), designing an effective vaccine becomes correspondingly more difficult. An effective vaccine must also:

- be stable on storage – particularly important for living vaccines, which normally require to be kept cold (i.e. a complete 'cold chain' from manufacturer to clinic), which is not always easy to maintain.
- have sufficient immunogenicity – with non-living vaccines it is often necessary to boost their immunogenicity with an adjuvant.

Live vaccines are generally more effective than killed vaccines.

Induction of appropriate immunity depends on the properties of the antigen. Living vaccines have the great advantage of providing an increasing antigenic challenge that lasts days or weeks and inducing it in the right site, which in practice is most important where mucosal immunity is concerned (Fig. 17.4).

Live vaccines are likely to contain the greatest number of microbial antigens, but safety is an issue in a time of increasing concern about the side effects of vaccines. The new Rotavirus vaccines, RotaTeq/Rotarix for example, seem to carry with them a slightly enhanced risk of gut intussusception.

Vaccines made from whole killed organisms have been used, but because a killed organism no longer has the advantage of producing a prolonged antigenic stimulus, killed vaccines have been frequently replaced by subunit vaccines. These can be associated with several problems:

- purified subunits may be relatively poorly immunogenic and require adjuvants;
- the smaller the antigen, the more major histocompatibility complex (MHC) restriction may be a problem (see Chapters 6 and 7); and
- purified polysaccharides are typically thymus independent – they do not bind to MHC and therefore do not immunize T cells.

These problems have been overcome in vaccines that are routinely used in humans by the use of adjuvants and by coupling polysaccharides either:

- to a standard protein carrier such as tetanus or diphtheria toxoid; or
- to a protein from the immunizing organism such as the outer membrane protein of pneumococci.

However, immunization even with the newer conjugate vaccines, especially when used in infants under 12 months, has shown that antibody levels wane after a number of years. For Hib this has indicated that a booster is required, generally given at around school age, although ironically

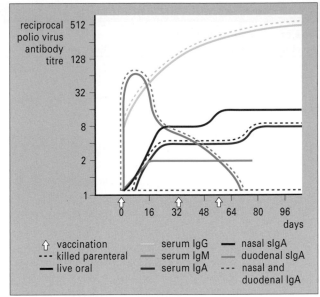

Fig. 17.4 Antibody responses to live and killed polio vaccine The antibody response to orally administered live attenuated polio vaccine *(solid lines)* and intramuscularly administered killed polio vaccine *(broken lines)*. The live vaccine induces the production of secretory IgA *(sIgA)* in addition to serum antibodies, whereas the killed vaccine induces no nasal or duodenal sIgA. Because sIgA is the immunoglobulin of the mucosa-associated lymphoid tissue (MALT) system (see Chapter 2), the live vaccine confers protection at the portal of entry of the virus, the gastrointestinal mucosa. (Courtesy Professor JR Pattison, Vaccines, in Brostoff J. et al. ed. Clinical Immunology. London: Mosby; 1991.)

the tendency for meningococci to colonize healthy individuals can provide a boost to immunity in those who are immunized. This latter effect may become less common in the future with improved herd immunity and, therefore, a reduced frequency of carriage.

MHC restriction is probably more of a hypothetical than real difficulty because most candidate vaccines are large enough to contain several MHC-binding epitopes. Nevertheless, even the most effective vaccines often fail to immunize every individual. For example, about 5% of individuals fail to seroconvert after the full course of hepatitis B vaccine.

Most of the vaccines in routine use in humans depend on the induction of protective antibody. However, for many important infections, particularly of intracellular organisms (e.g. tuberculosis, malaria and HIV infection), cellular immune responses are important protective mechanisms.

Vaccine safety is an overriding consideration. Vaccine safety is of course a relative term, with minor local pain or swelling at the injection site and even mild fever being generally acceptable. More serious complications may stem from the vaccine or from the patient (Table 17.7):

- Vaccines may be contaminated with unwanted proteins or toxins or even live viruses.
- Supposedly killed vaccines may not have been properly killed.
- Attenuated vaccines may revert to the wild type.
- The patient may be hypersensitive to minute amounts of contaminating protein, or immunocompromised, in which case any living vaccine is usually contraindicated.

TABLE 17.7   Safety Problems With Vaccines

Type of Vaccine	Potential Safety Problems	Examples
Attenuated vaccines	Reversion to wild type	Especially polio types 2 and 3
	Severe disease in immunodeficient patients	Vaccinia, BCG, measles
	Persistent infection	Varicella-zoster
	Hypersensitivity to viral antigens	Measles
	Hypersensitivity to egg antigens	Measles, mumps
Killed vaccines	Vaccine not killed	Polio accidents in the past
	Yeast contaminant	Hepatitis B
	Contamination with animal viruses	Polio
	Contamination with endotoxin	Pertussis
	Autoimmunity	Swine flu vaccine induced narcolepsy

The potential safety problems encountered with vaccines emphasize the need for continuous monitoring of both production and administration.

- In rare cases, autoimmune reactions are triggered by immunization. This was observed in a programme of influenza-A immunization in Scandinavia, which was associated with an increase in the incidence of narcolepsy, a condition caused by damage to hypocretin-secreting neurons in the CNS. The problem was associated with a particular formulation of the vaccine that was immediately withdrawn once the association was identified.

Although serious complications are very rare, vaccine safety has now become an overriding consideration, in part because of the very success of vaccines:

- Because many childhood infectious diseases have become uncommon in developed countries, the populations of these countries are no longer aware of the potentially devastating effects of infectious diseases.
- Unlike most drugs, vaccinations are given to people who have previously been perfectly well.
- Mass vaccination programmes always produce safety concerns owing to non-causal, temporal associations of medical conditions with vaccine administration.

MMR controversy resulted in measles epidemics. Anti-vaccine movements in the UK are essentially as old as vaccination itself, dating back to a few years after the introduction of smallpox vaccination by Jenner in 1796. In the modern era, difficulties concerning vaccine safety are well illustrated by the controversy over MMR (measles, mumps and rubella triple vaccine).

In 1998, a paper was published that received wide publicity in the UK media, purporting to support an association between MMR vaccination and the development of autism and chronic bowel disease. Although a large amount of subsequent work totally discredited these findings and the original paper was retracted, the take-up of MMR in the UK and Ireland declined over several years and epidemics of measles occurred because of declining herd immunity (Fig. 17.5). Even some 20 years later, Europe is experiencing a new measles epidemic owing to continued poor MMR uptake in some countries and in the UK amongst young adults who were not immunized as children.

In 2004, the introduction of a new 5-valent (now '6-in-1' with the addition of hepatitis B) vaccine containing diphtheria and tetanus toxoids, acellular pertussis, *H. influenzae* type B and

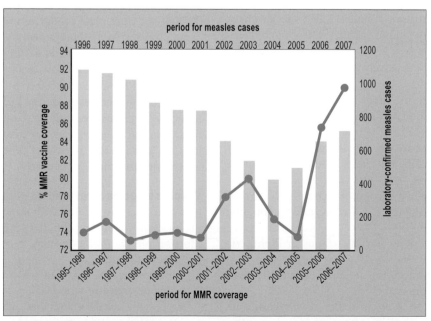

Fig. 17.5 The MMR controversy resulted in measles epidemics The fall in uptake of the MMR vaccine in the UK to a low point in 2003, resulted in an upsurge in cases of measles (green line). (Data McIntyre P, Leaske J. Improving uptake of MMR vaccine. BMJ 2008;336:729.)

inactivated polio virus threatened to result in decreased take-up in the UK, although the vaccine was shown to be safe and effective. It was argued that giving five immunogens simultaneously was 'too much' for the delicate immune system of infants. This argument is spurious, as most of the vaccines within it are subunits (except for inactivated polio). The whole vaccine therefore actually contains fewer antigens than the live bacteria and other organisms that infants encounter every day. Fortunately, the vaccine take-up has remained high.

The vaccines against HPV are some of the first developed using molecular techniques. The safety of the vaccines is demonstrably good, as would be expected where no infectious material is associated with the vaccine. Worldwide, over 200 million doses of the vaccines have now been administered. Adverse effects reports have, overwhelmingly, consisted of transient effects, immediately after immunization, such as pain and swelling at the injection site. However, as with all mass vaccination programmes, adverse effects were reported at or around the time of vaccination. Conditions such a postural orthostatic tachycardia syndrome (POTS), fibromyalgia and autoimmune post-viral fatigue syndromes have all been the subject of investigation, but no evidence in support of a causal link has been found. Fears about safety still linger and some doubt has been cast over the potential toxicity of the adjuvants used in these preparations. The possibility that individuals with a rare genetic susceptibility are at greater risk (see later) is always hard to rule out.

VACCINES IN GENERAL USE HAVE VARIABLE SUCCESS RATES

The vaccines in standard use worldwide are listed in Table 17.8. Four of them – polio, measles, mumps and rubella – are so successful that these diseases are earmarked for eradication early in the 21st century. In 2017, after 3 successive years free of outbreak, measles was declared eradicated from the UK by the

WHO. However, 2018 has seen a resurgence in cases, owing to poor European-wide herd immunity and a UK cohort of unimmunized young adults (see earlier). If these diseases can be eradicated, it will be an extraordinary achievement, because mathematical modelling suggests that they are all more difficult targets for eradication than smallpox was.

In the case of polio, where reversion to virulence of types 2 and 3 can occur, it has been necessary to switch to the use of killed virus vaccine for some years, so that virulent virus shed by live virus-vaccinated individuals is no longer produced.

For a number of reasons, other vaccines are less likely to lead to eradication of disease. These include:
- **The carrier state**: eradication of hepatitis B would be a major triumph, but it will require the breaking of the carrier state, especially in the Far East, where mother-to-child is the normal route of infection.
- **Suboptimal effectiveness**: effectiveness of BCG varies markedly between countries, possibly because of variation in environmental mycobacterial species (tuberculosis is increasing, especially in patients with immune deficiency or AIDS) and the pertussis vaccine is only about 70%–80% effective.
- **Safety fears**: especially when the risk of infection is low, these fears often lead to reduced levels of uptake. In the UK, the spurious association of the MMR vaccine with autism has continued to affect the public's willingness to be vaccinated.
- **Free-living forms and animal hosts**: the free-living form of tetanus will presumably survive indefinitely and it will not be possible to eradicate diseases that also have an animal host, such as yellow fever.

One of the future problems is maintaining awareness of the need for vaccination against diseases that seem to be disappearing, while, as the reservoir of infection diminishes, cases tend to occur at a later age, which with measles and rubella could actually lead to worse clinical consequences.

Some vaccines are reserved for special groups. In the developed world, BCG and hepatitis B fall into this category, but some vaccines will probably always be confined to selected populations, such as travellers, nurses, the elderly, etc. (Table 17.9). In some cases, this is because of:
- geographical restrictions (e.g. yellow fever);
- the rarity of exposure (e.g. rabies);
- problems in producing sufficient vaccine in time to meet the demand (e.g. each influenza epidemic is caused by a different strain, requiring a new vaccine).

Flu pandemics caused by emergence of totally novel influenza strains occur periodically, often caused by the acquisition of genetic material from strains of flu that normally infect animals, such as equine or avian influenza.

In the recent past, major pandemic scares have surfaced in relation to avian and swine flu. Intensive efforts have been made to improve vaccine production methods so that sufficient vaccine is available to deal with such outbreaks. This has involved production of virus in cell culture rather than, conventionally, in chicken eggs, and the application of new immunogens based on VLPs consisting of recombinant antigen mixtures, not inactivated virus. Virosomes produced from purified, solubilized virus complexed with lipid vesicles have also been used and possess enhanced

TABLE 17.8	**Vaccines in General Use**	
Disease	**Vaccine**	**Remarks**
Tetanus	Toxoid	Given together in three doses
Diphtheria	Toxoid	Between 2 and 6 months
Pertussis	Killed whole	Tetanus and diphtheria boosted
Polio (DTPP)	Killed (Salk) or attenuated (Sabin)	Every 10 years
Hib	Conjugate	Hib boosted at 1year
HepB (6in1)	Subunit	
MenB	Recombinant proteins	2 and 4 months, boosted at 1 year
Pneumococcal		
Pneumonia	Conjugate	2 and 4 months
Measles Mumps Rubella	Attenuated	Given together (MMR) at 12–18 months
MenACWY	Conjugate	Targeted at teenagers

Vaccines that are currently given, as far as is possible, to all individuals.

TABLE 17.9 Vaccines Restricted to Certain Groups

Disease	Vaccine	Eligible Groups
Tuberculosis	BCG	Tropics: at birth; UK: 10–14 years; USA: at risk only
Hepatitis B	Surface antigen	At risk (medical, nursing staff, etc.); drug addicts; male homosexuals; known contacts of carriers
	Monovalent	Babies of infected mothers
Rabies	Killed	At risk (animal workers); post-exposure
Meningitis	Polysaccharide	Travellers
Yellow fever	Attenuated	
Typhoid, cholera	Killed or mutant	
Hepatitis A	Killed or attenuated	
Influenza	Killed	At risk; elderly
Pneumococcal pneumonia	Polysaccharide	Elderly
Varicella-zoster	Attenuated	Leukaemic children

immunogenicity compared with conventional vaccines. Virosomal vaccine has proven highly effective in elderly patients and virosomes form part of the very effective MenB vaccine.

Both the haemagglutinin and neuraminidase antigens, which together make up the outer layer of the influenza virus and are the antigens of importance in the vaccine, are, however, subject to extensive variation. A vaccine effective against all strains of influenza would therefore be of tremendous value.

Vaccines for parasitic and some other infections are only experimental. Some of the most intensively researched vaccines are those for the major tropical protozoal and worm infections (see Chapter 16). However, none has come into standard use and some have argued that none will, because none of these diseases induces effective immunity and 'you cannot improve on nature'.

Nevertheless, extensive work in laboratory animals has shown that vaccines against malaria, leishmaniasis and schistosomiasis are perfectly feasible. In cattle, an irradiated vaccine against lungworm has been in veterinary use for decades.

It remains possible, however, that the parasitic diseases of humans are significantly more difficult to treat, possibly because of the polymorphic and rapidly changing nature of many parasitic antigens. For example:

- None of the small animal models of malaria shows such extensive antigenic variation as *Plasmodium falciparum*, the protozoon causing malignant tertian malaria in humans.
- Similarly, rats appear to be much easier to immunize against schistosomiasis than other animals, including possibly humans.

Part of the problem is that in the laboratory these parasites are usually not propagated in their natural host.

A vaccine against *Plasmodium falciparum* has been one of the most sought after for over a generation, as the burden of disease and death in endemic malarial regions in Africa is huge. Malaria is unusual in that its life cycle offers a variety of possible targets for vaccination. Over the years, several trials of clinical malaria vaccine have been published, using antigens derived from either the liver or the blood stage, with only very moderate success (Fig. 17.w2).

However, a realistic candidate vaccine has now emerged from a partnership begun in the early 1980s between the pharmaceutical company GlaxoSmithKline (GSK) and the US Walter Reed Army Institute of Research (WRAIS). The vaccine known as RS,S is based on a genetically engineered version of the circumsporozoite (CS) protein that is expressed on sporozoites and liver stage schizonts. Recombinant CS protein is expressed in yeast cells as a fusion protein with the hepatitis B surface antigen (HBsAg), the basis of the successful recombinant HepB vaccine. Co-expression of the fusion protein with unmodified HBsAg allows the formation of VLP-type aggregates of the antigens. To make this preparation sufficiently immunogenic, it required combination with the proprietary GSK adjuvant AS01.

Phase III trials in Africa have shown a significant protective effect on both infection rate and clinical malaria development; 15 459 children in 11 centres across seven African countries were enrolled in the trial. RTS,S/AS01 vaccination is estimated to have prevented 829 clinical malaria episodes per 1000 children over 18 months of study follow-up. A phase IV trial is now projected and should the initial promise be realized, the first licensed antimalarial vaccine may become available by 2020.

Our understanding of how the RS,S vaccine elicits a protective immune response unfortunately remains poor and the degree of protection provided is limited, but it is hoped that further research will result in an even more effective second-generation vaccine in the future.

A problem with these chronic parasitic diseases is that of immunopathology. For example, the symptoms of *Trypanosoma cruzi* infection (Chagas disease) are largely the result of the immune system (i.e. autoimmunity). A bacterial parallel is leprosy, where the symptoms are caused by the (apparent) over-reactivity of T_H1 or T_H2 cells. A vaccine that boosted immunity without clearing the pathogen could make these conditions worse.

Another example of this unpleasant possibility is dengue, where certain antibodies enhance the infection by allowing the virus to enter cells via Fc receptors.

Similarly, a historical HIV vaccine trial, although initially promising in inducing a cell-mediated response, was aborted because the risk of HIV infection in the vaccinated subjects was increased compared with the unvaccinated controls.

Other viral and bacterial vaccines that are also experimental are:

- attenuated shigella;
- Epstein–Barr virus surface glycoprotein;
- respiratory syncytial virus (RSV);
- group B *Streptococcus agalactiae*.

For Many Diseases There is no Vaccine Available

No vaccine is currently available for many serious infectious diseases, including staphylococci and streptococci, syphilis, chlamydia, leprosy and fungal infections. The predominant problem is often the lack of understanding of how to induce effective immunity. HIV infection heads this list of diseases (see Chapter 19), which represent the major challenge for research and development in the coming decade (Table 17.w2).

PASSIVE IMMUNIZATION

Driven from use by the advent of antibiotics, the idea of injecting preformed antibody to treat infection is still valid for certain situations (Table 17.10). It can be life-saving when:

- toxins are already circulating (e.g. in tetanus, diphtheria, and snake-bite);
- high-titre specific antibody is required, generally made in horses, but occasionally obtained from recovered patients.

At the opposite end of the scale, normal pooled human immunoglobulin contains enough antibody against common infections for a dose of 100–400 mg IgG to protect hypergammaglobulinaemic patients for a month. Over 1000 donors are used for each pool and the sera must be screened for HIV and hepatitis B and C.

In the light of this, it is still somewhat surprising that the use of specific monoclonal antibodies, although theoretically highly attractive, has not yet proved to be an improvement on traditional methods and their chief application to infectious disease at present remains in diagnosis.

One exception to this rule has been the monoclonal antibody palivizumab, launched in 1998, which has been used in prophylaxis against respiratory syncytial virus (RSV) infection, where the development of a vaccine has remained elusive. Palivizumab has proven effective in protecting high-risk individuals, such as premature infants.

Antibody genes can now be engineered to form Fab, single-chain Fv or V_H fragments (see Chapter 10). Libraries of these can be expressed in recombinant phages and screened against antigens of interest. Selected antibody fragments can be produced in bulk in bacteria, yeasts or mammalian cells, for use in vitro or in vivo. This technology has helped in the production of human and humanized mouse monoclonal antibodies for therapeutic application.

TABLE 17.10 Passive Immunization

Condition	Source of Antibody	Indication
Diphtheria, tetanus	Human, horse	Prophylaxis, treatment
Varicella-zoster	Human	Treatment in immunodeficiencies
Gas gangrene, botulism, snake bite, scorpion sting	Horse	Post-exposure
Rabies	Human	Post-exposure (plus vaccine)
Hepatitis B	Human	Post-exposure
Hepatitis A, measles	Pooled human immunoglobulin	Prophylaxis (travel), post-exposure

Although not as commonly used as 50 years ago, injections of specific antibody can still be a life-saving treatment in specific clinical conditions.

IMMUNIZATION AGAINST NON-INFECTIOUS CONDITIONS

The success of vaccine strategies against infectious disease has sparked renewed interest in the possibility of immunizing against non-communicable diseases, many of which are now the major sources of morbidity and mortality.

The most obvious candidate would be cancers, which are known to sometimes be spontaneously rejected as if they were foreign grafts (see Chapter 22). Much research is now directed at trying to induce autoimmune rejection of tumours, mainly utilizing genetic modification approaches to increase immunogenicity for the host.

The most successful application of this technology has been the development of chimeric antigen receptor (CAR) technology. This approach uses a chimeric molecule that is essentially an antibody at its N-terminus coupled to a T-cell receptor at its C-terminus. The construct is transfected into a patient's T cells in vitro, which are amplified and re-infused into the patient. A CAR-based approach to therapy in juvenile acute lymphatic leukaemia, using an anti-CD19 antibody region to target B cells, has met with excellent success in clinical trials thus far. Further experience with the use of the therapy will provide a better picture of its overall efficacy and safety. It is hoped, nevertheless, that the technique may also be applicable in therapy of solid tumours.

Other potential uses of immunization that are being explored include:

- treatment of autoimmune disease;
- the treatment of drug dependency, because it is possible to neutralize the effect of a drug by pre-immunization with the drug coupled to a suitable carrier (the hapten-carrier effect);
- reducing blood pressure to treat essential hypertension;
- lowering cholesterol by neutralizing lipid-binding proteins; and
- preventing Alzheimer's disease by immunizing against components of amyloid plaque.

So far these vaccines are largely experimental; however, given the success of antibody-based therapies, the possibility of long-term treatment by immunization remains an attractive possibility.

FUTURE VACCINES

Without doubt the future generation of new, improved and safer vaccines lies in the exploitation of recombinant DNA technology and genetic engineering of pathogenic organisms and their antigens. A development of the ability to clone genes is the possibility of using a benign, non-pathogenic virus as a vector to display antigens to the immune system in a way that mimics their natural exposure but is without the risks associated with attenuated pathogens. The gene(s) encoding the desired antigen(s) is(are) incorporated into the genetic material of the vector, which can then express the gene and produce the antigen in situ. The vector can then be injected into the patient and in some cases also allowed to replicate.

Many viruses, such as adenovirus, vesicular stomatitis virus (VSV), polio and measles have been exploited as potential vaccine vectors. Both VSV and adenovirus, for example, have been used to display antigens from the Ebola virus and used in recent clinical trials (Fig 17.w3).

The results of the limited field trials showed that the New Link ZEBOV candidate vaccine was effective in protecting individuals from Ebola infection. The viral spread was effectively controlled by a ring-fencing approach: first-degree contacts of infected individuals and health workers received the immunization to prevent transmission of the virus to the surrounding population.

Although results thus far have been positive, there are still issues surrounding the adoption of the NewLink vaccine candidate. It has yet to be established whether the vaccine provides lasting protection for immunized individuals. This may be less problematic if the vaccine is primarily to be deployed to limit outbreaks in the manner described above. More serious is the fact that the vaccine candidate, a replication-competent form of VSV, is infectious and can therefore spread, with unknown consequences.

Although, VSV infection is not thought to be a major safety concern, the virus is not completely without pathology in humans, often causing a flu-like illness. Several reports have also emerged of an inflammatory arthritic condition amongst the immunized individuals. Data from further trials will need to be evaluated before we have a complete picture of the safety of this vaccine.

The experience so far clearly demonstrates the potential this recombinant virus approach holds for new vaccine development. The design sidesteps many of the problems associated with producing vaccines to highly pathogenic microbes. The resulting vaccines lack the safety issues that surround the use of crippled strains and are likely to be significantly more immunogenic than killed/inactivated organisms. Unlike purified microbial components, the antigen can present multiple epitopes in their native configuration, including their post-translational modifications, such as glycosylation. Indeed, in the case of Ebola, the neutralizing antibodies found in survivors targeted the sugar moieties on the envelope glycoprotein.

As an alternative to viral vectors, attenuated bacteria have the advantage that they have large genomes and may therefore be used as polyvalent immunogens. The emergence of the powerful gene-editing technology CRISPR, used in combination with the now extensive bioinformatics data on microbial genomes, has opened up major possibilities for identification and mutation of genes responsible for virulence. The generation of new attenuated strains produced by such recombinant DNA technology could lead to a whole new generation of bacterial vaccines.

'Naked' DNA can be transfected into host cells. One of the most intriguing possibilities for future development remains the use of DNA for vaccination. Cells that take up the DNA express the encoded protein. The potential advantages of this approach are a long-term exposure to the antigen and the possibility of stimulating both an antibody and a cellular immune response. Uptake and expression of the DNA in APCs has been shown to induce long-lasting cellular and humoral immunity in experimental animals, but despite extensive research, DNA vaccines in humans have not fulfilled the promise they have shown in animal model systems.

CRITICAL THINKING: VACCINATION

See Critical thinking: Explanations, section 17

1. Why have attenuated vaccines not been developed for all viruses and bacteria?
2. 'A vaccine cannot improve on nature'. Is this unduly pessimistic?
3. 'The smallpox success story is unlikely to be repeated.' Is this true?
4. Will vaccines eventually replace antibiotics?
5. BCG: vaccine, adjuvant, or non-specific stimulant?
6. Why could an anti-worm vaccine do more harm than good?
7. By what means, other than their reaction with antibodies, might you identify antigens that could be used as vaccines?

FURTHER READING

Almond JW. Vaccine renaissance. Nat Rev Microbiol 2007;5:478–481.

Bidmos FA, Siris S, Gladstone CA, Langford PR. Bacterial vaccine antigen discovery in the reverse vaccinology 2.0 era: progress and challenges. Front Immunol. 2018;9:2315.

Green LR. et al. Approach to the discovery, development, and evaluation of a novel *Neisseria meningitidis* serogroup B vaccine. In: Thomas S, ed. Vaccine Design. Methods in Molecular Biology, vol 1403. New York: Humana Press; 2016.

Kusters I, Almond JW. Vaccine strategies. In: Mahy DWJ, van Regenmortel MHV, eds. Desk Encyclopedia of General Virology, Oxford: Academic Press; 2010, pp. 235–243.

Pollard AJ, Perret KP, Beverly PC. Maintaining protection against invasive bacteria with polysaccharide conjugate vaccines. Nat Rev Immunol 2009;9:213–220.

Rauch S, Jasny E, Schmidt KE, Petsch B. New vaccine technologies to combat outbreak situations. Front Immunol. 2018;9:1963.

Primary Immunodeficiencies

SUMMARY

- **Primary immunodeficiency diseases** result from defects of innate and adaptive immunity.
- **Defects in B-cell function** result in recurrent pyogenic infections. Defective antibody responses may be intrinsic to B cells, as occurs in X-linked agammaglobulinaemia, or secondary to ineffective T-cell signals to B cells, as occurs in CD40 ligand (CD40L) deficiency.
- **Defects in T-cell development and/or function** result in broad susceptibility to infections. Immune dysregulation with autoimmunity or lymphoproliferation is also frequently observed.
- **Hereditary complement component defects** cause various clinical phenotypes; the most common defect (C1 inhibitor deficiency) causes hereditary angioedema (HAE). Deficiencies of the terminal complement components (C5, C6, C7 and C8) and the alternative pathway proteins (factor H, factor I and properdin) lead to increased susceptibility to infections caused by *Neisseria gonorrhoeae* and *Neisseria meningitidis*.
- **Phagocyte defects**, resulting from reduced numbers or impaired function, can cause overwhelming bacterial and fungal infections. Failure to kill bacteria and persistence of bacterial products in phagocytes lead to abscesses or granulomas, depending on the pathogen.
- **Leukocyte adhesion deficiency (LAD)** is associated with a persistent leukocytosis because phagocytic cells cannot migrate into the tissues.

Primary immunodeficiency diseases (PIDs) are a heterogeneous group of disorders characterized by defects in development and/or function of the immune system. The classification of PIDs is based on the nature of the underlying immunological defect.

- **Antibody deficiencies** reflect impaired function of B lymphocytes as a result of intrinsic B-cell abnormalities or of defects in T lymphocytes that affect activation and terminal maturation of B lymphocytes.
- **Combined immunodeficiencies** are characterized by impaired development and/or function of T lymphocytes and functional B-cell abnormalities.
- **Phagocytic cell disorders** include defects in development and/or function of myeloid cells (granulocytes, macrophages).
- **Complement deficiencies** are represented by genetically determined defects of functional or regulatory components of the complement system.
- **Disorders of immune regulation** include diseases characterized by abnormalities in the mechanisms that control autoimmunity, apoptosis or extinction of immune responses.
- **Immunodeficiency syndromes** represent a heterogeneous group of PIDs in which defects of one or more components of the immune system are associated with extra-immune manifestations.

PIDs cause increased susceptibility to infections, consistent with the role played by the immune system in surveillance against pathogens. However, several forms of PID are also characterized by increased frequency of autoimmunity and malignancies, reflecting disturbances of immune regulation and of tumour surveillance.

Consistent with the role of different elements of the immune responses, PIDs are characterized by a distinct pattern of susceptibility to infections. In particular:

- Patients with antibody deficiencies are highly susceptible to recurrent **pyogenic infections** sustained by encapsulated bacteria (*Haemophilus influenzae*, *Streptococcus pneumoniae*, *Moraxella catarrhalis*, *Staphylococcus aureus*).
- Combined immunodeficiencies are characterized by broad susceptibility to infections that includes not only bacteria but also viruses and **opportunistic pathogens** (i.e. ubiquitous germs that do not pose significant harm to immunocompetent individuals).
- Patients with disorders of neutrophils are prone to bacterial and fungal infections.
- Defects of macrophages result in increased susceptibility to mycobacterial disease.
- Defects of signalling through Toll-like receptors (TLRs) that act as microbial sensors cause selective susceptibility to specific types of pathogens.
- Defects of complement may lead to increased risk of pyogenic infections and autoimmunity, consistent with the role played by complement in removal of immune complexes.

B-LYMPHOCYTE DEFICIENCIES

B-cell defects result in impaired antibody production. Patients affected with these disorders present with recurrent infections, which involve the upper and lower respiratory tract, particularly pneumonia and sinusitis as well as the ear (otitis media). Recurrent pneumonia may cause irreversible lung damage (bronchiectasis) and obstructive lung disease.

However, infections may also involve other tracts, such as the gut (in particular, infection by *Giardia lamblia* and norovirus), the skin and, less frequently, other organs.

Congenital agammaglobulinaemia results from defects of early B-cell development.

B lymphocytes develop in the bone marrow from the haematopoietic stem cell (HSC), through various stages of maturation during which time they rearrange their immunoglobulin genes to generate the pre-B-cell receptor (BCR). Defects in the expression and/or signalling through the pre-BCR cause congenital agammaglobulinaemia with lack of circulating B cells (Fig. 18.1).

X-linked agammaglobulinaemia (XLA) is the prototype of these disorders and was described by Dr Bruton in 1952. Affected males suffer from recurrent pyogenic infections. They lack serum IgA, IgM, IgD and IgE, and IgG levels are extremely low, usually <100 mg/dL.

Circulating B lymphocytes are absent or markedly reduced (<1% of peripheral lymphocytes). Tonsils are absent and lymph nodes are unusually small. XLA is caused by mutations of the Bruton tyrosine kinase (*BTK*) gene, which encodes an enzyme involved in signalling through the pre-BCR and the BCR (see Fig. 18.1). *BTK* mutations cause an incomplete, but severe, block at the pre-B-cell stage in the bone marrow. The BTK protein is also expressed by other cells (including monocytes and megakaryocytes), but its defect does not affect development of these cell types.

For the first 4–6 months of life, males with XLA are often protected by the maternally derived IgG that has crossed the placenta (see Fig. 10.13), but once this supply of IgG is exhausted, they develop recurrent bacterial infections. Patients with XLA are also at risk of enteroviral infections (such as echovirus) that may cause encephalitis. If immunized with attenuated poliovirus vaccine, they may develop paralytic poliomyelitis. Norovirus infection can cause severe watery diarrhoea and weight loss. Treatment of XLA is based on regular administration of immunoglobulins (IgG).

More rarely, congenital agammaglobulinaemia is inherited as an autosomal recessive trait, as a result of mutations of other genes that encode for components of the pre-BCR or of the adaptor molecule BLNK (see Fig. 18.1). In all of these cases, there is a severe block in B-cell development at the pre-B cell stage in the bone marrow. The clinical phenotype is virtually identical to that of XLA.

Defects in terminal differentiation of B cells produces selective antibody deficiencies.

Terminal maturation of B lymphocytes is marked by their differentiation into antibody-secreting plasma cells. Generation of plasma cells is markedly reduced in patients with **common variable immunodeficiency (CVID)**, who typically develop progressive hypogammaglobulinaemia in the second and third decades of life. CVID is the most common primary immunodeficiency (1:10 000 affected individuals in the general population), and is characterized by extensive clinical and immunological heterogeneity. Some patients have a reduced number of circulating B cells and especially of CD27[+] memory B lymphocytes; others show impaired function of T lymphocytes. CVID is usually sporadic and the underlying molecular defect remains unknown in most cases. However, in some families CVID is inherited as an autosomal dominant or an autosomal recessive trait. A minority of CVID patients carry mutations in genes that play a key role in T–B-cell interaction and B-cell signalling (Fig. 18.2).

Genetic defects in CVID. Approximately 15% of the patients with CVID carry genetic variants in the transmembrane activator and calcium modulator and cyclophilin ligand interactor (TACI), a member of the TNF receptor family (see Fig. 18.2). TACI is expressed on the cell membrane of B lymphocytes and interacts with two ligands: the B-cell activating factor (BAFF) and APRIL (see Fig. 9.13). In particular, a proliferation-inducing ligand (APRIL):TACI interaction promotes B-cell activation and class-switch recombination (CSR). Importantly, TACI mutations have also been identified in healthy individuals, although at lower frequency compared with CVID. Therefore, TACI mutations are considered to confer disease susceptibility, rather than being disease-causing. BAFF promotes B-cell survival;

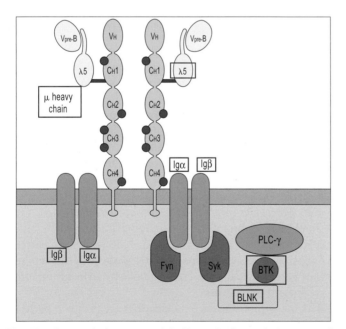

Fig. 18.1 Congenital agammaglobulinaemia Congenital agammaglobulinaemia results from defects of proteins that participate at signalling through the pre-B cell receptor (pre-BRC). This is composed of the µ heavy chain, the surrogate light chains V-preB and λ5, and the signal transducing molecules Igα and Igβ. Signalling through the pre-BCR triggers activation of tyrosine kinases such as Fyn, Syk and BTK, and involves the adaptor molecule BLNK. Ultimately, these signals converge on activation of the phospholipase C-γ (*PLC-γ*) and induction of calcium flux. The proteins whose mutations result in a known form of congenital agammaglobulinaemia in humans are in *red boxes*.

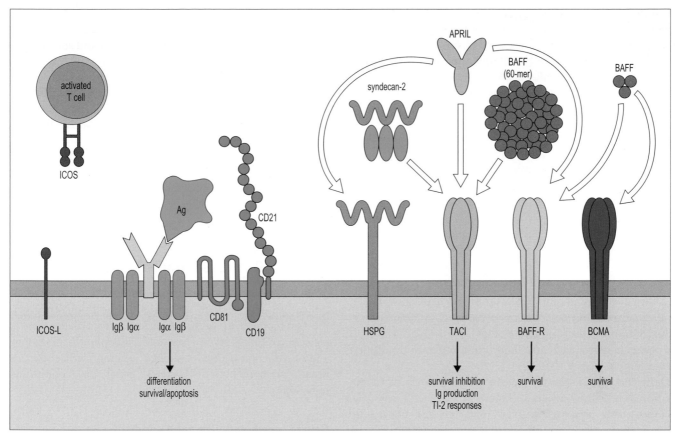

Fig. 18.2 Mutations associated with common variable immunodeficiency (CVID) CVID may be associated with mutations of proteins involved in B-cell activation. These include co-stimulatory components of the B-cell receptor (CD19, CD81, CD21), ICOS transmembrane activator and calcium modulator and cyclophilin ligand interactor *(TACI)* and the B-cell activating factor receptor *(BAFF-R)*. These molecules deliver survival, activation and differentiation signals in mature B lymphocytes. *APRIL*, A proliferation-inducing ligand; *BCMA*, B-cell maturation antigen; *HSPG*, heparan sulfate proteoglycan.

it binds not only to TACI but also to BAFF receptor (BAFF-R), which is mutated in few cases of CVID. Some patients with CVID are mutated in the *CD19*, *CD20*, *CD21* or in the *CD81* genes; the CD19 molecule forms a complex with CD21, CD81 and CD225 on the surface of B lymphocytes and lowers the threshold of BCR-mediated activation (see Fig. 9.7). Autosomal dominant mutations of the *IKZF1* gene, encoding the transcription factor IKAROS, cause hypogammaglobulinaemia; the number of circulating B cells often decreases with age. Autosomal dominant mutations of the *NFKB1* and *NFKB2* genes also cause hypogammaglobulinaemia and recurrent infections. Because NFKB2 is also involved in mechanisms of immune tolerance, patients with this defect also manifest autoimmunity and endocrinopathies.

CVID is characterized by reduced levels of specific antibody isotypes.
Individuals with CVID have impaired antibody production in response to immunization or to natural infections and there is a virtual absence of plasma cells in lymphoid tissues and in the bone marrow. They suffer from recurrent infections of the respiratory tract (sinusitis, otitis, bronchitis and pneumonia) sustained by common bacteria (non-typeable *H. influenzae*, *S. pneumoniae*, etc.); lack of mucosal antibodies results in increased risk of gastrointestinal infection due to *G. lamblia* (Fig. 18.3). They are also highly prone to autoimmune

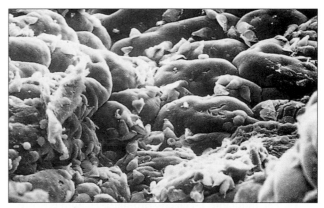

Fig. 18.3 *Giardia lamblia* infection Numerous *G. lamblia* parasites can be seen swarming over the mucosa of the jejunum of a patient with common variable immunodeficiency (CVID).

manifestations (cytopenias, inflammatory bowel disease), granulomatous lesions, lymphoid hyperplasia and tumours (especially lymphomas). Treatment is based on immunoglobulin replacement therapy and antibiotics. Immunosuppressive and anti-inflammatory drugs may be needed in patients with autoimmune or inflammatory complications.

Gain-of-function (GOF) mutations of the *PIK3CD* gene, encoding for the p110δ catalytic subunit of the PI3-kinase, cause hypogammaglobulinaemia associated with lymphoproliferation and increased risk of EBV-driven lymphoma. A similar phenotype is also observed in patients with certain mutations in the regulatory p85α subunit of PI3-K that cause dysregulated activation of p110δ.

IgA deficiency is relatively common. IgA deficiency (IgAD) is common in the general population (1:600 individuals) but remains asymptomatic in the majority of cases. However, recurrent infections, autoimmunity and allergy are possible, especially when IgAD is associated with a defect of IgG2 and IgG4 subclasses. The molecular basis of IgAD remains unknown; occurrence of both CVID and IgAD has been reported in some families.

Defects of Class-Switch Recombination

Class-switch recombination (CSR) is the mechanism by which the μ chain of immunoglobulins is replaced by other heavy chains, resulting in the production of IgG, IgA and IgE. The process occurs in germinal centres and is accompanied by affinity maturation (see Figs 9.17–9.19).

Deficiency of CD40L (X-linked) or more rarely of **CD40** (autosomal recessive) results in failure of CSR, with very low or undetectable levels of IgG, IgA and IgE and normal to increased levels of serum IgM. In the past, this condition was also known as '**hyper-IgM syndrome**'. In the lymph nodes, primary follicles are present, but germinal centres are absent. Binding of CD40L to CD40 is also important to promote interaction between activated T cells and dendritic cells or monocytes/macrophages. This promotes T-cell priming, production of interferon-γ (IFNγ) and activation of macrophages, which are important in the immune defence against intracellular pathogens. Consistent with this, the clinical phenotype of CD40L and of CD40 deficiency is characterized not only by recurrent bacterial infections but also by increased risk of early-onset opportunistic infections (*Pneumocystis jiroveci* pneumonia, cytomegalovirus infection, protracted and watery diarrhoea caused by *Cryptosporidium*). Neutropenia and severe liver disease are frequent. Therefore, CD40L and CD40 deficiency are not pure antibody deficiencies, but rather represent examples of combined immunodeficiency. Treatment of these disorders is based on administration of immunoglobulins and antibiotics, but often requires haematopoietic stem cell transplantation (HSCT). The inducible T-cell co-stimulator (ICOS) is expressed by activated T cells and interacts with ICOS-ligand (ICOS-L) expressed by B lymphocytes, promoting B-cell activation and antibody production. ICOS mutations also result in a combined immunodeficiency with hypogammaglobulinaemia and recurrent infections.

In B cells, signalling through CD40 promotes transcription of the gene encoding for **activation-induced cytidine deaminase** (AID), a DNA-editing enzyme that replaces deoxycytidine residues with deoxyuracil in the DNA of the immunoglobulin heavy chain-switch regions. The resulting mismatch in the DNA is recognized by the enzyme uracil N-glycosylase

(UNG) that removes the deoxyuracil residues, leaving abasic sites that are resolved by means of DNA repair mechanisms. These DNA modifications trigger both CSR and somatic hypermutation. Both AID and UNG mutations cause severe deficiency of IgG, IgA and IgE production; furthermore, the IgM antibodies produced by these patients have low affinity for the antigen. Clinically, these immunodeficiency diseases are characterized by recurrent bacterial infections. Tonsil and lymph node enlargement (reflecting expansion of germinal centres) and lack of susceptibility to opportunistic infections distinguish hyper-IgM syndrome caused by AID and UNG mutations from the forms caused by defects of CD40L or CD40. Treatment of AID and UNG deficiency is based on administration of immunoglobulins.

T-LYMPHOCYTE DEFICIENCIES

T lymphocytes play a critical role in the defence against intracellular pathogens, such as viruses. In addition, they permit the development of antibody responses to T-dependent antigens. Accordingly, severe defects of T-lymphocyte development and/or function cause combined immunodeficiencies, with broad susceptibility to bacterial, viral and opportunistic infections.

Severe combined immunodeficiency can be caused by many different genetic defects. Severe combined immunodeficiency (SCID) includes a heterogeneous group of genetic disorders that affect various stages of T-cell development or function (Fig. 18.4). Conditions in which the T-cell defect is present, but less pronounced than in SCID, are also referred to as combined immune deficiencies (CID). The main pathophysiology mechanisms of SCID and CID are:

- impaired survival of thymocytes and T lymphocytes (reticular dysgenesis, adenosine deaminase deficiency, purine nucleoside phosphorylase deficiency);
- defective cytokine-mediated expansion of lymphoid progenitors (X-linked SCID, JAK3 deficiency, interleukin-7 receptor deficiency) (Fig. 18.5);
- defective expression of the pre-T-cell receptor (deficiency of RAG1, RAG2, and of other components of the V(D)J recombination machinery);
- defective signalling through the pre-T-cell receptor (deficiency of CD3 chains; CD45 deficiency; defects of LAT, LCK, RHOH, STK4; deficiencies of MALT1, BCL10, CARD11);
- impaired positive selection of CD4$^+$ or of CD8$^+$ lymphocytes (HLA class II deficiency and ZAP-70 deficiency, respectively);
- defective egress of T lymphocytes from the thymus (coronin-1A deficiency);
- impairment of calcium flux and of T lymphocyte activation (STIM1 and ORAI1 deficiencies).

While severe T-cell abnormalities are a hallmark of all forms of SCID, some of these diseases also involve abnormalities of B and/or natural killer (NK) cells. In particular, some forms of

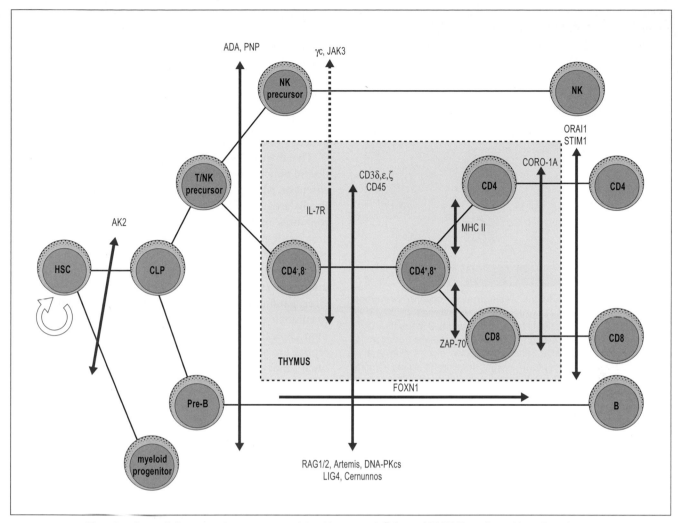

Fig. 18.4 Gene defects causing severe combined immunodeficiency (SCID) There is a wide range of gene defects that affect T-cell development or maturation and cause SCID in humans. Some of these defects also affect B-cell and/or NK-cell development. The diagram indicates the main stages affected by each deficiency. *γc*, Common γ chain; *ADA*, adenosine deaminase; *AK2*, adenylate kinase 2 (causing reticular dysgenesis); *CORO-1A*, coronin-1A; *DNA-PKcs*, DNA-protein kinase catalytic subunit; *IL-7R*, interleukin 7 receptor; *JAK3*, Janus-associated kinase 3; *LIG4*, DNA ligase IV; *MHC II*, major histocompatibility complex class II antigens; *NK*, natural killer; *PNP*, purine nucleoside phosphorylase; *RAG*, recombinase-activating gene; *STIM1*, stromal interaction molecule 1.

SCID are characterized by the absence of T cells, but presence of B cells (T⁻B⁺ SCID), whereas others show absence of both T and B cells (T⁻B⁻ SCID). Both of these groups of SCID include forms with or without NK cells.

SCID has a prevalence of approximately 1:50 000 live births and is more common in males, reflecting the existence of X-linked SCID (X-SCID), the most common form of SCID in humans. This disease is caused by mutation of the gene encoding for the common gamma chain (γc), shared by several cytokine receptors, namely those for IL-2, IL-4, IL-7, IL-9, IL-15 and IL-21. Since IL-7 is required for T-cell maturation and IL-15 is required for NK-cell development, patients with X-SCID have a T⁻ B⁺ NK⁻ phenotype.

Among the autosomal recessive forms of SCID in humans, the most common are represented by defects of RAG1 or RAG2 and by adenosine deaminase (ADA) deficiency. The recombinase-activating genes (*RAG*) 1 and 2 are lymphoid-specific genes that initiate the process of V(D)J recombination, which is required for both T- and B-lymphocyte development. Therefore, mutations of *RAG1* and *RAG2* genes cause T⁻ B⁻ NK⁺ SCID.

ADA is a ubiquitously expressed enzyme involved in purine metabolism. Lack of ADA results in accumulation of adenosine, deoxyadenosine and their phosphorylated derivatives. Among them, dATP is particularly toxic; it inhibits the enzyme ribonucleotide reductase, which is required for DNA synthesis and hence for cell replication (Fig. 18.6). Purine nucleoside phosphorylase (PNP) is another enzyme involved in related metabolic pathways.

Lymphopenia (typically, less than 300 T lymphocytes/µL), and marked reduction of the T-cell count in particular, is a hallmark of SCID. However, some infants with SCID have circulating T cells, occasionally even in normal numbers. This may reflect the presence of genetic defects that are permissive for T-cell development (as in late defects in T-cell development

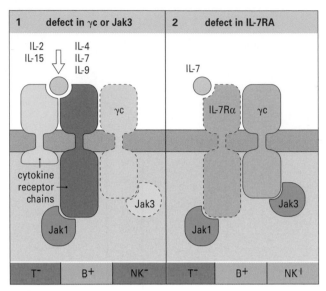

Fig. 18.5 Mutation of cytokine receptors in severe combined immunodeficiency (SCID) (**1**) A defect in the common chain (γc) of the cytokine receptors for IL-2, IL-15, IL-4, IL-7 and IL-9 leads to a SCID with loss of both T and NK cells. A similar deficiency results from a mutation in the janus kinase (Jak3), which transduces signals from the γc chain. Note IL-2 and IL-15 receptors have three chains in their high-affinity receptors, whereas IL-4, IL-7 and IL-9 have only two chains. (**2**) Absence of the specific IL-7R chain also produces a SCID that primarily affects T-cell development.

or in patients with hypomorphic mutations in SCID-causing genes), but more often is a result of engraftment of maternal T cells. Transplacental passage of maternally derived T cells is common in pregnancy, but these cells are rejected by the immune system of the fetus. In contrast, maternally derived T cells persist and expand in infants with SCID and may cause tissue damage (graft-versus-host disease, GvHD) upon recognition of paternally derived HLA alloantigens expressed by the patient's cells.

The thymus of SCID infants is very small and typically devoid of lymphoid elements (Fig. 18.7); lymph nodes are often absent or, when present, contain mostly stromal cells. Although B cells are normally present in some forms of SCID, antibody responses are profoundly impaired and immunoglobulin levels are usually reduced.

Clinically, SCID is apparent in the first months of life. Interstitial pneumonia (caused by *Pneumocystis jiroveci* or viral infections: cytomegalovirus, respiratory syncytial virus, adenovirus, parainfluenza virus type 3), protracted diarrhoea leading to failure to grow and persistent candidiasis (Fig. 18.8) are common clinical findings. However, other infections (meningitis, sepsis) are also possible. Use of live vaccines in SCID infants often leads to severe consequences and should be strictly

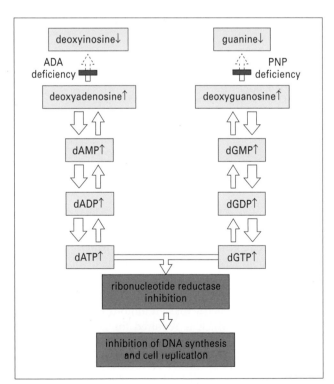

Fig. 18.6 Pathophysiology of severe combined immunodeficiency due to adenosine deaminase and purine nucleoside phosphorylase deficiency It is thought that deficiencies of adenosine deaminase (*ADA*) and purine nucleoside phosphorylase (*PNP*) lead to accumulations of dATP and dGTP, respectively. Both of these metabolites are powerful inhibitors of ribonucleotide reductase, which is an essential enzyme for DNA synthesis.

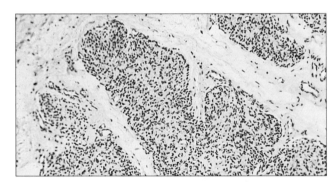

Fig. 18.7 Thymus of severe combined immunodeficiency Note that the thymic stroma has not been invaded by lymphoid cells and no Hassall corpuscle is seen. The gland has a fetal appearance.

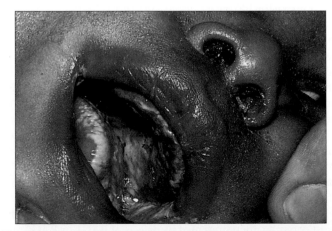

Fig. 18.8 *Candida albicans* in the mouth of a patient with severe combined immunodeficiency (SCID) *C. albicans* grows luxuriantly in the mouth and on the skin of patients with SCID.

avoided; in particular, administration of rotavirus vaccine may cause intractable diarrhoea, and immunization with BCG may lead to disseminated infection.

Omenn's syndrome represents a peculiar form of SCID and is characterized by generalized erythroderma, lymphadenopathy, hepatosplenomegaly, chronic diarrhoea, associated with eosinophilia, elevated serum IgE, and the presence of autologous, oligoclonal and activated T cells that infiltrate and damage target organs. In most cases, Omenn's syndrome is a result of hypomorphic mutations of the *RAG* genes. An Omenn-like phenotype is also observed in a proportion of infants with SCID and maternal T-cell engraftment causing GvHD.

Newborn screening for SCID and related disorders is currently available in the USA and in some other countries and is based on enumeration of T-cell-receptor excision circles (TRECs) (see Fig. 6.16), a by-product of T-cell receptor-α rearrangements, in DNA extracted from dried blood spots collected at birth. TRECs persist in T cells that are exported from the thymus to the periphery and dilute out as T cells undergo proliferation. Therefore, levels of TRECs correlate with the production of T cells in the thymus. Infants with low TREC levels at birth are evaluated for T-cell count and distribution of naive and memory T cells, which, if abnormal, should prompt genetic testing, which may reveal a diagnosis of SCID. With newborn screening, infants with SCID can be diagnosed at birth, before they develop serious infections; this early diagnosis also translates into a lower risk of complications and improved outcome of haematopoietic stem cell transplantation (HSCT).

Treatment of SCID. Infants with SCID must receive antimicrobial prophylaxis and immunoglobulin administration to reduce the risk of infections. However, unless immune reconstitution is attained, SCID is inevitably fatal within the first 2 years of life. Definitive treatment is mainly based on HSCT. The objective of HSCT for SCID is to obtain robust and stable engraftment of donor-derived T cells. This may also happen if no chemotherapy is used, because most forms of SCID are characterized by the inability to reject donor cells, even when one of the parents (who are both HLA-haploidentical to their affected child) is selected as the donor. However, engraftment of donor B cells (which may allow better reconstitution of antibody production) is more often obtained when chemotherapy is used. Currently, more than 85% of SCID babies can be permanently cured by HSCT. Factors associated with even better outcome (>90% survival) include:
- transplantation from an HLA-identical family donor;
- age less than 3.5 months at HSCT;
- lack of infections at the time of transplantation.

ADA deficiency may be treated by intramuscular injection of a pegylated form of recombinant ADA; however, this procedure must be repeated weekly for life. SCID has also represented the first example of the successful application of **gene therapy** in humans, in infants with X-SCID and with ADA deficiency. Use of first-generation retroviral vectors was associated with development of leukaemia in some patients who received gene therapy for X-linked SCID. This serious adverse event was caused by the insertion of the retroviral vector next to or within a proto-oncogene, followed by induction of deregulated expression of the oncogene (a phenomenon known as **insertional mutagenesis**). However, no leukaemic proliferations have been observed upon development of self-inactivating retroviral and lentiviral vectors.

TH-cell deficiency results from HLA class II deficiency. The failure to express class II HLA molecules on antigen-presenting cells is inherited as an autosomal recessive trait, which is not linked to the HLA locus. Rather, HLA class II deficiency results from defects in transcription factors that bind to the promoter region of the HLA class II genes, and induce HLA class II molecule expression. Affected infants have recurrent infections, particularly of the respiratory and gastrointestinal tracts.

Because the development of CD4$^+$ helper T cells (TH) depends on positive selection by HLA class II molecules in the thymus (see Fig. 2.26), HLA class II molecule-deficient infants have a deficiency of CD4$^+$ T cells. This lack of TH cells leads to a deficiency in antibodies.

DiGeorge's anomaly arises from a defect in thymus embryogenesis. The thymic epithelium is derived from the third and fourth pharyngeal pouches by the sixth week of human gestation. Subsequently, the endodermal anlage is invaded by lymphoid stem cells, which undergo development into T cells.

A congenital defect in the organs derived from the third and fourth pharyngeal pouches results in **DiGeorge's anomaly**. The T-cell deficiency is variable, depending on how badly the thymus is affected; in only <1% of the patients, the T-cell deficiency is so severe that it causes SCID. Infants with DiGeorge's anomaly have distinctive facial features (Fig. 18.9). They also have congenital malformations of the heart or aortic arch and neonatal tetany caused by hypocalcaemia resulting from the hypoplasia or aplasia of the parathyroid glands.

The majority of patients with DiGeorge's anomaly have partial monosomy of 22q11.2. Patients with DiGeorge's anomaly who present with a SCID phenotype may be treated by thymus transplantation. Thymic tissues from unrelated infant donors at the time of heart surgery are treated to remove all lymphoid cells

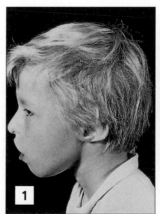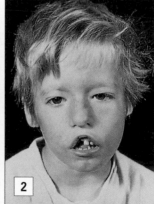

Fig. 18.9 DiGeorge's anomaly Note the wide-set eyes, low-set ears and shortened philtrum of upper lip.

(to avoid GvHD) and are implanted into muscular tissue of the affected patients. In spite of the complete HLA mismatch, lymphoid progenitors derived from haematopoietic stem cells of the patients colonize the transplanted thymic tissue, mature there and are then exported to the periphery.

DISORDERS OF IMMUNE REGULATION

Self–non-self discrimination is an essential function of the adaptive immune system. Failure to recognize non-self antigens leads to increased susceptibility to infections, as observed in patients with congenital defects of T-cell and/or B-cell-mediated immunity. In contrast, defects in recognition and tolerance of self antigens are associated with autoimmunity. Finally, modulation of immune responses is important to maintain homeostasis. In some forms of primary immunodeficiency, the inability to clear pathogens results in persistent inflammatory reactions and may cause severe tissue damage.

Defective function of regulatory T (Treg) cells causes severe autoimmunity. Regulatory T cells (Foxp3$^+$) normally suppress immune responses to self antigens in the periphery. Mutations of the *FOXP3* gene cause immune dysregulation-polyendocrinopathy-enteropathy-X-linked (IPEX) syndrome, a severe X-linked form of autoimmunity. Males with IPEX syndrome present in the first months of life with intractable diarrhoea, insulin-dependent diabetes and skin rash. Severe infections may follow because of breakage of the cutaneous and mucosal barriers. There is a lack of functional CD4$^+$ CD25$^+$ Foxp3$^+$ Treg lymphocytes. Activated, self-reactive T lymphocytes infiltrate target organs (Fig. 18.10) and there are high levels of autoantibodies against insulin, other pancreatic antigens and enterocytes. In typical cases, the disease evolves rapidly. Treatment with immunosuppressive drugs is required to control autoimmune manifestations; however, stem cell therapy is the only curative approach.

CD25 and STATB deficiency are IPEX-like conditions in which the genetic defect affects Treg function; in addition, STAT5B-deficient patients manifest short stature because STAT5 is required for signalling in response to growth hormone.

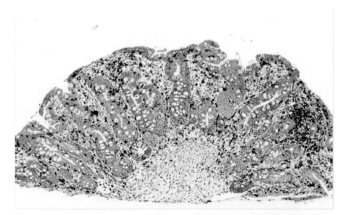

Fig. 18.10 Gut mucosa of a patient with IPEX The gut mucosa shows villous atrophy and severe infiltration by T cells, identified by staining for CD3.

CTLA-4 is a molecule expressed by Treg cells and by activated T cells; in the latter, it competes with CD28 for binding to CD80 and CD86 expressed by antigen-presenting cells, delivering an inhibitory signal that restrains T-cell activation. On the other hand, CTLA-4 engagement promotes Treg suppressive activity. CTLA-4 haploinsufficiency causes impaired Treg function and manifests with autoimmunity (cytopenias, enteropathy, interstitial lung disease). A similar phenotype is observed in patients with autosomal recessive LRBA deficiency. LRBA is a molecule involved in recycling the CTLA-4 molecule; in the absence of LRBA, upon internalization, CTLA-4 is targeted to the lysosomal compartment and degraded.

Impaired apoptosis of self-reactive lymphocytes causes autoimmune lymphoproliferative syndrome. Apoptosis of autoreactive lymphocytes is important to preserve immune homeostasis. Interaction between FAS ligand (FasL), expressed by activated lymphocytes, and FAS (CD95) triggers intracellular signalling that ultimately results in activation of caspases and cell death. Mutations of FAS are the predominant cause of autoimmune lymphoproliferative syndrome (ALPS), with lymphadenopathy, hepatosplenomegaly and autoimmune cytopenia. There is an increased risk of malignancies (especially B-cell lymphomas), which occur in 10% of the patients with FAS mutations. Patients with ALPS have an increased number of double-negative T lymphocytes that express the αβ form of the TCR but do not express CD4 or CD8 molecules. ALPS is most often inherited as an autosomal dominant trait and is caused by dominant-negative mutations that interfere with the signal-transducing activity of FAS trimeric complexes. A rare variant of ALPS is due to FasL mutations. In a few patients, mutations of caspase-8, caspase-10 and FADD have been also identified. Treatment is based on the use of immunosuppressive drugs.

Congenital defects of lymphocyte cytotoxicity result in persistent inflammation and severe tissue damage. The cytotoxic activity of T cells and NK cells depends on the expression of cytolytic proteins that are assembled into granules and transported through microtubules to the lytic synapse, which is formed upon contact with target cells (see Fig. 8.9). **Haemophagocytic lymphohistiocytosis** (HLH) includes a group of disorders characterized by impairment of the mechanisms of transport, docking or release of the lytic granules. Deficiency of perforin and MUNC13-4 is the most common genetic causes of HLH. In these diseases, persistence of the pathogen (most often a virus) causes expansion of CD8$^+$ T cells, which, while unable to mount a cytotoxic response, secrete increased amounts of TH1 cytokines, including IFNγ. Excessive amounts of IFNγ trigger macrophage activation, causing phagocytosis of blood elements and tissue damage. The disease is usually fatal and treatment is based on immunosuppressive drugs (to reduce immune activation) and HSCT.

Similarly, **X-linked proliferative syndrome type 1 (XLP1)** results from a failure to control the normal proliferation of

CD8$^+$ T cells following an infection with Epstein–Barr virus (EBV), which causes infectious mononucleosis.

Affected males appear healthy until they are infected with EBV, when they develop either:
- fatal infectious mononucleosis;
- hypogammaglobulinaemia (often with preserved levels of IgM);
- lymphoma; or
- aplastic anaemia.

The defective gene on the X chromosome encodes an adapter protein of T and B cells called **SAP** or the **SLAM-associated protein**. SLAM is expressed on the surface of T and B cells. Its intracellular tail interacts with the adapter protein SAP, which is required for cytolytic activity of T and NK cells. Furthermore, SAP is important also for the function of follicular helper T cells (T$_{FH}$), which govern trafficking of B lymphocytes to the germinal centres. Defective function of T$_{FH}$ cells accounts for the hypergammaglobulinaemia of XLP. Treatment is based on HSCT.

X-linked lymphoproliferative syndrome type 2 (XLP2) is caused by mutations of the X-linked inhibitor of apoptosis (*XIAP*) gene; in addition to HLH, these patients often manifest inflammatory bowel disease.

Besides XLP1, several other genetic defects (CD27, CD70, ITK and MAGT1 deficiencies) are associated with impaired control of the EBV by T cells and in some cases NK cells; consequently, these patients are at high risk of EBV-driven lymphoma.

IMMUNODEFICIENCY SYNDROMES

Immunodeficiency syndromes include a heterogeneous group of disorders characterized by immune and extra-immune manifestations. The immunological abnormalities associated with these diseases may involve both adaptive and innate immunity.

Chromosomal breaks occur in TCR and immunoglobulin genes in hereditary ataxia telangiectasia.
Hereditary ataxia telangiectasia (AT) is inherited as an autosomal recessive trait. Affected infants develop a wobbly gait (ataxia) at about 18 months and ultimately are confined to a wheelchair. Dilated capillaries (telangiectasia) appear in the eyes and on the skin by 6 years of age (Fig. 18.11). AT is accompanied by a variable T-cell deficiency. About 70% of patients with AT are also IgA deficient and some also have IgG2 and IgG4 deficiency.

Because the number and function of circulating T cells are greatly diminished, cell-mediated immunity is also depressed and patients develop severe sinus and lung infections. Their cells exhibit chromosomal breaks, usually in chromosome 7 and chromosome 14, at the sites of the T-cell receptor (TCR) genes and the genes encoding the heavy chains of immunoglobulins.

The cells of patients with AT are very susceptible to ionizing irradiation because the defective gene in AT encodes a protein involved in the repair of double-strand breaks in DNA. This

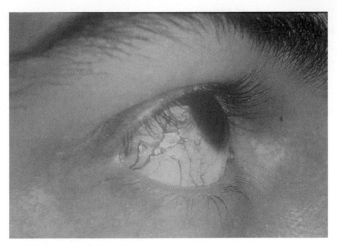

Fig. 18.11 Ocular telangiectasias

defect leads to increased risk of malignancies, especially lymphoma and leukaemia. Double-stranded DNA breaks are produced during the somatic gene recombination that takes place during the formation of the functional TCR and BCR genes as well as during class-switching recombination (see Chapters 6 and 9). Absence of the AT protein, which is required to resolve these breaks, explains why the defect is associated with immunodeficiency.

T-cell defects and abnormal immunoglobulin levels occur in Wiskott–Aldrich syndrome.
The **Wiskott–Aldrich syndrome (WAS)** is an X-linked immunodeficiency disease. Affected males with WAS:
- have a low number of platelets (thrombocytopenia) that are also unusually small in size;
- develop severe eczema as well as pyogenic and opportunistic infections;
- often have increased amounts of serum IgA and IgE, normal levels of IgG and decreased amounts of IgM;
- have T cells with defective function.

The malfunction of cell-mediated immunity gets progressively worse. The T cells have a uniquely abnormal appearance, as shown by scanning electron microscopy, reflecting a cytoskeletal defect. They have fewer microvilli on the cell surface than normal T cells. Similar defects of cytoskeleton reorganization are observed in the patients' monocytes and dendritic cells, with severe impairment of filopodia formation and of migration in response to chemokines. Patients with WAS have also a severe defect of NK cytolytic activity, which accounts for the higher rate of herpes virus infections.

The Wiskott–Aldrich syndrome protein (WASp) plays a critical role in cytoskeleton reorganization. In T and NK cells, it participates at formation of the immunological synapse, favouring tight interaction of T lymphocytes with dendritic cells and B cells and of NK cells with target cells.

Because of the severity of the disease and because expression of the *WAS* gene is restricted to the haematopoietic system, definitive treatment is based on HSCT.

Deficiency of STAT3 causes impaired development and function of Th17 cells in hyper-IgE syndrome. Hyper-IgE syndrome (HIES) can be inherited as an autosomal dominant or recessive trait; however, the clinical and immunological features of these forms are distinct. Autosomal dominant HIES is a result of heterozygous mutations of the **signal transducer and activator of transcription 3** *(STAT3)* gene. This is a transcription factor that is activated in response to activation of the JAK-STAT signalling pathway through cytokine and growth factor receptors that contain the gp130 protein. Biological responses to IL-6 and IL-10 are depressed and development of Th17 cells is impaired, resulting in poor secretion of IL-17 and IL-22. This causes impairment in immune defence against bacterial and fungal infections; in addition, production of antibacterial molecules (e.g. defensins) by epithelial cells is also affected. The clinical phenotype includes eczema, cutaneous and pulmonary infections sustained by *S. aureus* (with formation of pneumatoceles) and *Candida* spp. Patients with STAT3 deficiency also show defective shedding of primary teeth, scoliosis, higher risk of bone fractures, joint hyperextensibility and characteristic facial traits. By contrast, GOF mutations of STAT3 lead to a very different phenotype, with autoimmunity, short stature, lymphoproliferation and recurrent infections.

Autosomal recessive HIES syndrome is most often caused by mutations of the **dedicator of cytokinesis 8** *(DOCK8)* gene that encodes for a protein involved in cytoskeleton reorganization. Patients with DOCK8 deficiency suffer from severe infections from early life. Viral infections resulting from CMV, HPV and HSV and allergies are particularly common. There is also an increased risk of malignancies. In vitro proliferation of T cells to mitogens is markedly reduced. Immunoglobulin levels are variable, but IgG is often increased, whereas IgM is low. The clinical and immunological phenotype of DOCK8 deficiency indicates that this is a combined immunodeficiency.

GENETIC DEFECTS OF PHAGOCYTES

Phagocytic cells (polymorphs and mononuclear phagocytes) are important in host defence against pyogenic bacteria and other intracellular microorganisms.

A severe deficiency of neutrophils (**neutropenia**) can result in overwhelming bacterial infection. **Severe congenital neutropenia** (SCN) is defined as a neutrophil count that is persistently less than 0.5×10^9 cells/L. A variety of genetic defects may cause SCN in humans. The majority of these patients have a severe block in myeloid development in the bone marrow. The most common form of SCN is caused by mutation of the *ELA2* gene, encoding neutrophil elastase. In some cases, *ELA2* mutations cause cyclic neutropenia, with oscillations in the neutrophil count that reaches a nadir approximately every 21 days, resulting in periodicity of the infections.

Two groups of genetic defects affect phagocyte function without altering their development:
- chronic granulomatous disease (CGD); and
- leukocyte adhesion deficiency (LAD).

These disorders are clinically important in that they result in susceptibility to severe infections and are often fatal.

Chronic granulomatous disease results from a defect in the oxygen-reduction pathway. Patients with CGD have defective **NADPH oxidase**, which catalyses the reduction of O_2 to $\bullet O_2^-$ by the reaction:

$$NADPH + 2O_2 \rightarrow NADP^+ + 2O_2^- + H^+$$

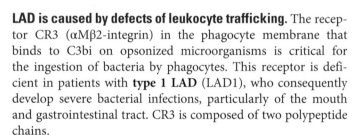

They are therefore incapable of forming superoxide anions (O_2^-) and hydrogen peroxide in their phagocytes following the ingestion of microorganisms. As a result, microorganisms remain alive in phagocytes of patients with CGD, particularly microbes that can produce catalase. This gives rise to a cell-mediated response to persistent intracellular microbial antigens, with formation of granulomas.

Children with CGD develop pneumonia, infections in the lymph nodes (lymphadenitis), and abscesses in the skin, liver and other viscera. Bacterial infections due to *S. aureus*, *Klebsiella pneumoniae*, *Serratia marcescens* and *Burkholderia cepacia* are particularly common. These catalase-positive bacteria are capable of breaking down the hydrogen peroxide that phagocytes use to fight infections. Patients with CGD are also uniquely prone to fungal (in particular *Aspergillus* and *Candida*) and mycobacterial infections. Treatment of CGD requires regular use of antibacterial and antifungal prophylaxis and aggressive management of infections. HSCT may provide a definitive cure.

LAD is caused by defects of leukocyte trafficking. The receptor CR3 ($\alpha M \beta 2$-integrin) in the phagocyte membrane that binds to C3bi on opsonized microorganisms is critical for the ingestion of bacteria by phagocytes. This receptor is deficient in patients with **type 1 LAD** (LAD1), who consequently develop severe bacterial infections, particularly of the mouth and gastrointestinal tract. CR3 is composed of two polypeptide chains.

In LAD1, there is a genetic defect of the β chain, encoded by a gene on chromosome 21.

Two other integrin proteins share the same β chain as CR3 – namely, lymphocyte functional antigen (LFA-1) and CR4 (also know as p150,95) (see Table 3.w1); these proteins are also defective in LAD1.

LFA-1 is important in cell adhesion and interacts with intercellular adhesion molecule-1 (ICAM-1) on endothelial cell surfaces and other cell membranes. Because of the defect in LFA-1, phagocytes from patients with LAD1 cannot adhere to vascular endothelium and cannot therefore migrate out of blood vessels into areas of infection. As a result, patients with LAD1 cannot form pus efficiently and this allows the rapid spread of bacterial invaders.

When leukocytes in the circulation enter an area of inflammation, their speed of movement is greatly retarded by the interaction of **selectins** with their ligands. E-selectin interacts with Sialyl Lewis X (SLeX), a fucosylated molecule that is expressed on the surface of neutrophils and monocytes. In **LAD2**, a genetic defect of intracellular fucose transporter prevents fucosylation of membrane glycoproteins, including SLeX. Consequently, the leukocytes of patients with LAD2 cannot roll on the endothelium and fail to extravasate and reach inflamed tissues. Since fucose metabolism is important in the central nervous system, patients with LAD2 also show mental retardation and dysmorphisms in addition to infections.

A third form of LAD (**LAD3**) is a result of impaired integrin signalling that also involves platelets. These patients suffer from severe infections and increased bleeding. All forms of LAD are characterized by marked elevation of the leukocyte count in peripheral blood (leukocytosis); this reflects the response of the bone marrow to inflammatory stimuli (with increased production of myeloid cells) and inability of the leukocytes to leave the circulation and reach peripheral tissues.

IMMUNODEFICIENCIES WITH SELECTIVE SUSCEPTIBILITY TO INFECTIONS

Most forms of primary immunodeficiency disease (PID) are characterized by broad susceptibility to infections, such as bacterial infections in patients with antibody deficiency, defects of neutrophils or complement, and infections of viral, fungal or bacterial origin in patients with combined immunodeficiency. In contrast, some forms of PID are characterized by susceptibility to some specific pathogens. The study of these patients has shown the critical role played by some components of the immune system in the response to these pathogens.

Macrophage microbicidal activity is impaired by defects in IFNγ signalling. The destruction of intracellular microorganisms that flourish in macrophages depends on the activation of microbicidal activity in macrophages by IFNγ. When microorganisms are taken up by macrophages, the macrophages secrete IL-12, which then binds to the IL-12 receptor on T cells and induces secretion of IFNγ.

Children with genetic defects in the genes encoding IL-12, the IL-12 receptor (IL-12R) or the IFNγ receptor suffer from recurrent infection with non-pathogenic mycobacteria and, to a lesser extent, with salmonella. These various defects are inherited as autosomal recessive or autosomal dominant traits. Treatment with recombinant IFNγ is beneficial in patients with IL-12 and IL-12R mutations, whereas HSCT is the treatment of choice for patients with mutations in IFNγ receptor.

Defects of TLR-signalling cause susceptibility to pyogenic infections. Toll-like receptors (TLRs) are a series of molecules that are expressed at the cell surface or at the membrane of endosomes and mediate recognition of pathogen-associated molecular patterns, such as lipopolysaccharide, glycolipids and single- or double-stranded RNA. The classical pathway of TLR activation involves the adapter molecules MyD88 and the intracellular kinases IRAK-4 and IRAK-1. Activation of this pathway upon binding of TLRs to their ligands, results in the induction of NF-κB and production of inflammatory cytokines (IL-1, IL-6, TNFα, IL-12). Mutations of **IRAK-4** and **MyD88** cause severe and invasive pyogenic infections early in life, often without significant inflammatory response. Infections tend to become less frequent later in life, when the adaptive immune system has matured.

TLR3, -7, -8 and -9 can activate an alternative pathway that involves the adapter molecule UNC-93B, resulting in the induction of type I interferons (IFNα and -β). Mutations of **TLR3**, **UNC-93B** and other components of the TLR3

signalling pathway (TRAF3, TRIF, TBK1) cause selective susceptibility to herpes simplex encephalitis as a result of infection by HSV-1. Severe viral infections are also observed in patients with complete deficiency of signal transducer and activator of transcription 1 (STAT1), a transcription factor that is activated following binding of type I interferon to the specific receptor, resulting in expression of IFN-dependent genes. By contrast, autosomal dominant partial STAT1 deficiency manifests with increased susceptibility to mycobacterial and viral infections, along with autoimmunity.

Primary immune deficiencies with increased susceptibility to fungal infections. IL-17 and IL-22 play an important role in the defence against *Candida* and are produced by TH17 cells. GOF mutations of *STAT1* cause defective development of TH17 cells and manifest with chronic mucocutaneous candidiasis (CMC), associated with immune dysregulation and susceptibility to recurrent and severe fungal, bacterial and viral infections.

Other genetic forms of CMC include autosomal recessive *IL-17RA* and *IL-17RC* mutations, and autosomal dominant *IL-17F* mutations. Mutations of the *RORC* gene, encoding for ROR-γT (the master transcription factor involved in TH17 cell development) are another cause of CMC, but also of mycobacterial infections.

Finally, invasive fungal infections are seen in patients with CARD9 deficiency.

GENETIC DEFICIENCIES OF COMPLEMENT PROTEINS

The proteins of the complement system and their interactions with the immune system are discussed in Chapter 4. Genetic deficiencies of almost all the complement proteins have been found in humans (Table 18.1) and these deficiencies reveal

TABLE 18.1 Genetic Deficiencies of Human Complement

Group	Type	Deficiency	AR	AD	XL
I	Immune complex disease	C1q	•		
		C1s or C1r + C1s	•		
		C2	•		
		C4	•		
II	Angioedema	C1 inhibitor		•	
III	Recurrent pyogenic infections	C3	•		
		Factor H	•		
		Factor I	•		
IV	Recurrent *Neisseria* infections	C5	•		
		C6	•		
		C7	•		
		C8	•		
		Properdin			•
		Factor D	•		
V	Asymptomatic	C9	•		

AD, Autosomal dominant; *AR*, phenotypically autosomal recessive; *XL*, X-linked recessive.

much about the normal function of the complement system (see Fig. 4.13).

Immune complex clearance, inflammation, phagocytosis and bacteriolysis can be affected by complement deficiencies.

Deficiencies of the classical pathway components, C1q, C1r, C1s, C4 or C2, result in a propensity to develop immune complex diseases such as systemic lupus erythematosus.

Deficiencies of C3, factor H or factor I result in increased susceptibility to pyogenic infections, which correlates with the important role of C3 in the opsonization of pyogenic bacteria.

Deficiencies of the terminal components C5, C6, C7 and C8, and of the alternative pathway components, factor D and properdin, result in remarkable susceptibility to infection with the two pathogenic species of the *Neisseria* genus: *N. gonorrhoeae* and *N. meningitidis*. This clearly demonstrates the importance of the alternative pathway and the macromolecular attack complex in the bacteriolysis of this genus of bacteria.

All of these genetically determined deficiencies of complement components are inherited as autosomal recessive traits, except:

- properdin deficiency, which is inherited as an X-linked recessive; and
- C1 inhibitor deficiency, which is inherited as an autosomal dominant.

Hereditary angioneurotic oedema results from C1 inhibitor deficiency.

The C1 inhibitor (C1INH) is responsible for dissociation of activated C1 by binding to C1r2C1s2. Deficiency of C1INH results in hereditary angioneurotic oedema (HAE) (see Fig. 4.14), which is inherited as an autosomal dominant trait. Patients have recurrent episodes of swelling of various parts of the body (angioedema):

- when the oedema involves the intestine, excruciating abdominal pains and cramps result, with severe vomiting;

- when the oedema involves the upper airway, the patients may choke to death from respiratory obstruction: angioedema of the upper airway therefore presents a medical emergency, which requires rapid action to restore normal breathing.

C1INH inhibits not only the classical pathway of complement but also elements of the kinin, plasmin and clotting systems.

The oedema is mediated by two peptides generated by uninhibited activation of the complement and surface contact systems (see Fig. 4.w1):

- a peptide derived from the activation of C2, called C2 kinin; and
- bradykinin derived from the activation of the contact system.

The effect of these peptides is on the post-capillary venule, where they cause endothelial cells to retract, forming gaps that allow leakage of plasma.

There are two genetically determined forms of HAE:

- in type I, the *C1INH* gene is defective and no transcripts are formed; and
- in type II, there are point mutations in the *C1INH* gene, resulting in the synthesis of defective molecules.

The distinction between type I and type II C1INH deficiency is important because the diagnosis of type II disease cannot be made by quantitative measurement of serum C1 inhibitor alone. Simultaneous measurements of C4 must also be made. C4 is always decreased in the serum of patients with HAE because of its destruction by uninhibited activated C1.

C1INH deficiency is not always genetically determined but may be acquired later in life. In particular, patients with autoimmune diseases or with B-cell lymphoproliferative disorders (chronic lymphocytic leukaemia, multiple myeloma or B-cell lymphoma) may produce autoantibodies to C1INH. C1INH brands are available for intravenous use to treat or to prevent acute attacks of angioedema. In addition, bradykinin receptor antagonists are also available for HAE treatment.

CRITICAL THINKING: HYPER-IGM IMMUNODEFICIENCY

See Critical thinking: Explanations, section 18

A 3-year-old girl was brought to the emergency room because of fever and rapid respiration. She had had pneumonia once before at age 25 months. She had also had otitis media on 10 different occasions, each time successfully treated with antibiotics. She had also suffered repeated episodes of tonsil and lymph node enlargement. A chest radiograph resulted in the diagnosis of left lower lobe pneumonia. Blood and sputum cultures contained *Streptococcus pneumoniae*. The white blood count was 13 500/mL of which 81% were neutrophils and 14% lymphocytes. Serum IgM was 470 mg/dL, IgG 40 mg/dL and IgA and IgE were undetectable. Antibody to tetanus toxoid was undetectable. Blood typing was A positive, anti-B 1:320. The distribution of T, B and NK cells was normal, with

72% CD3$^+$ T cells, 47% CD4$^+$, 23% CD8$^+$, 17% CD19$^+$ and 11% CD16$^+$ lymphocytes.

1. Which clinical and laboratory tests lead to the suspicion that this child has hyper-IgM (HIgM) immunodeficiency and how do you conclude that it is not caused by a mutation in CD40 ligand?
2. What is the most likely diagnosis in this case?
3. How do you explain that this child had no response to tetanus immunization and yet has a high titre for her age of antibody to blood group substance B?
4. Which treatment would you recommend to the parents for this child and what would you say is her prognosis?

FURTHER READING

Bonilla FA, Barlan I, Chapel H, et al. International Consensus Document (ICON): Common Variable Immunodeficiency Disorders. J Allergy Clin Immunol Pract 2016;4:38–59.

Candotti F. Clinical manifestations and pathophysiological mechanisms of the Wiskott-Aldrich syndrome. J Clin Immunol 2018;38:13–27.

Casanova JL. Severe infectious diseases of childhood as monogenic inborn errors of immunity. Proc Natl Acad Sci U S A 2015;112: E7128–E7137.

Conley ME, Dobbs AK, Farmer DM, et al. Primary B cell immunodeficiencies: comparisons and contrasts. Annu Rev Immunol 2009;27:199–227.

Dinauer MC. Primary immune deficiencies with defects in neutrophil function. Hematology Am Soc Hematol Educ Program 2016;2016:43–50.

Fischer A, LeDeist F, Hacein-Bey-Abina S, et al. Severe combined immunodeficiency: a model disease for molecular immunology and therapy. Immunol Rev 2005;203:98–109.

Frazer-Abel A, Sepiashvili L, Mbughuni MM, Willrich MA. Overview of laboratory testing and clinical presentations of complement deficiencies and Dysregulation. Adv Clin Chem 2016;77:1–75.

Notarangelo LD, Fleisher TA. Targeted strategies directed at the molecular defect: toward precision medicine for select primary immunodeficiency disorders. J Allergy Clin Immunol 2017;139:715–723.

Picard C, Bobby Gaspar H, Al-Herz W, et al. International Union of Immunological Societies: 2017 Primary Immunodeficiency Diseases Committee Report on Inborn Errors of Immunity. J Clin Immunol 2018;38:96–128.

Sepulveda FE, de Saint Basile G. Hemophagocytic syndrome: primary forms and predisposing conditions. Curr Opin Immunol 2017;49:20–26.

AIDS, Secondary Immunodeficiency and Immunosuppression

SUMMARY

- **Nutrient deficiencies often lead to impaired immune responses.** Malnutrition increases the risk of infant mortality from infection through reduction in cell-mediated immunity, including reduced numbers and function of CD4+ helper cells and a reduction in levels of secretory IgA. Trace elements of iron, selenium, copper and zinc are also important in immunity. Lack of these elements can lead to diminished neutrophil killing of bacteria and fungi, susceptibility to viral infections and diminished antibody responses. Vitamins A, B6, C, E and folic acid are likewise important in overall resistance to infection. Proper diet and nutrition, therefore, reduce morbidity and mortality caused by infection.
- **Some drugs selectively alter immune function.** Immunomodulatory drugs can severely depress immune functions. These drugs are often necessary to treat solid organ transplant, stem cell transplant patients and patients with an autoimmune or autoinflammatory disease. Although necessary in such settings, these drugs often act widely, thereby increasing

patients' susceptibility to a broad array of opportunistic infections caused by viruses, bacteria and fungi. Increasingly, therapies are targeted against specific cytokines, immune receptors or signal transduction molecules.
- **HIV is a significant worldwide cause of immunodeficiency.** HIV is a retrovirus that predominantly targets CD4+ T cells. Acute infection depletes CD4+ T-cell subsets and transiently suppresses circulating CD4+ T-cell numbers before the immune system establishes partial control of the virus and the chronic phase of infection begins. Although patients can remain in the chronic phase for an average of 10 years, without anti-retroviral drug treatment, CD4+ T-cell levels gradually fall, resulting in loss of cell-mediated immunity and susceptibility to life-threatening opportunistic infections. This final stage, AIDS, is marked by low CD4+ T-cell counts, high HIV plasma levels, reactivation of other latent infections and, often, virus-associated malignancies such as Kaposi's sarcoma and non-Hodgkin's lymphoma.

OVERVIEW

Secondary, or acquired, immunodeficiencies cause changes in the development or function of an otherwise normal immune system. Unlike primary immunodeficiencies, which are the result of genetic abnormalities and often present as part of a recognized syndrome, secondary defects are both more common and more heterogeneous. Therapeutic approaches for secondary immune deficiencies usually involve treating the primary extrinsic stressor, combined with increased vigilance for infection, as well as pharmacologic intervention or prophylaxis to address active or potential infections. Major causes of secondary immunodeficiency include:

- malnutrition;
- viral infection (e.g. HIV);
- iatrogenic immune suppression (e.g. post-solid organ or stem cell transplant, or secondary to therapy for autoimmune or immune deficiency/dysregulation);
- cancer metastases or leukaemias, especially those involving bone marrow;
- cancer treatments such as chemotherapy or irradiation;
- surgery or trauma (e.g. thymic removal during cardiac surgery);
- chronic disease;
- advanced age.

NUTRIENT DEFICIENCIES

Globally, malnutrition is the most common cause of immunodeficiency and affects both innate and cell-mediated immunity. The connection between nutrition and immunity has a long historic record with periods of famine preceding periods of pestilence. As a primary diagnosis, malnutrition is a treatable problem that can range from severe protein–energy malnutrition (PEM) to marginal deficiencies in a single micronutrient. Immune responses are significantly impaired when calories, macronutrients or any key micronutrients are in limited supply, leaving the undernourished at increased risk for infection. Undernourishment as a child is a risk factor for obesity in later life and excess energy intake can be associated with micronutrient deficiency in adults who are overweight. Furthermore, the state of overnutrition can lead to low-level chronic inflammation, which also affects immune function.

Infection and malnutrition can exacerbate each other. Malnutrition and infection act synergistically to depress immunity and increase morbidity and mortality. Presence of infection often exacerbates the malnourished state by:
- increasing metabolic demands;
- decreasing appetite, thereby lowering intake of nutrients; and
- decreasing nutrient absorption, as a result of gastrointestinal infection.

Once this cycle begins, it is self-propagating as infection compromises immunity, which then leads to more infection and morbidity (Fig. 19.1). Infection intensifies the immune response, which in turn increases energy demands. At a population level, this may lead to decreased productivity, further

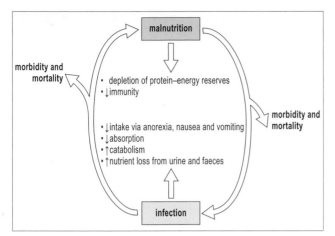

Fig. 19.1 Malnutrition and infection exacerbate each other in a vicious circle

decreasing economic and food resources and, again, driving the malnutrition and immune deficiency loop.

Risk factors for malnutrition include poverty, food scarcity, illiteracy and chronic debilitation. The impacts of malnutrition are seen globally. The World Health Organization (WHO) estimates worldwide 45%–50% of childhood deaths under the age of 5 are a result of malnutrition, many in developing nations. Malnourished children have a higher risk of death from infections. However, malnutrition is not just a problem of the poorest countries. In the USA, it is estimated that less than 50% of the elderly are adequately nourished and even within populations that consume adequate calories, poor dietary nutrient intake can cause marginal nutrient deficiencies with a significant detrimental impact on morbidity and mortality.

Protein–energy malnutrition and lymphocyte dysfunction. Maternal nutrition plays an important role in initial immune development by conferring epigenetic changes to the fetus. In addition, breastfeeding provides essential nutrients and immune components, such as IgA. Lymphoid atrophy is a prominent morphological feature of malnutrition and can be detected at birth in undernourished infants. The thymus, in particular, is a sensitive barometer in young children and the profound reduction in weight and size of the organ effectively results in **nutritional thymectomy**. This is reversible with nutritional repletion. Atrophy is evident in the thymus-dependent peri-arteriolar areas of the spleen and in the paracortical section of the lymph nodes. Decreases in the thymic hormones, thymulin and thymopoietin, accompany this loss in cellularity. Histologically:
- the lobular architecture is ill defined;
- there is increased connective tissue;
- there is a loss of corticomedullary demarcation;
- there are fewer lymphoid cells; and
- Hassall corpuscles are enlarged and degenerate – some may be calcified.

Studies have been conflicting about the effect of nutrition on numbers of circulating T cells. When assessed by flow cytometry, the number of CD3$^+$ and CD4$^+$ T cells appears to be normal in uninfected children who are undernourished. However, their T cells exhibit decreased mitogen and antigen proliferation.

Mechanistically, PEM may contribute to lymphocyte functional deficits because of limited availability of the amino acid glutamine, required for both nucleotide synthesis and cytokine production, and because of the increase in oxidative stress. PEM additionally causes imbalances in the neuroendocrine signals affecting lymphocyte survival. Glucocorticoids, released during stress, are increased with PEM, while leptin levels are decreased. Leptin, a hormone released from adipose tissues can act on receptors in the hypothalamus and on leukocytes. In mice it seems to protect thymocytes from glucocorticoid-induced apoptosis.

Humoral responses are also affected, in that B-cell numbers tend to be reduced. Although serum antibody levels are usually normal, serum IgA can be elevated, as can IgE. Studies are conflicting in terms of vaccine responses, but these may be decreased in children who are malnourished.

Nutrition also affects innate mechanisms of immunity. Poor nutrition also causes deficits in innate immune defences. For example,
- epithelial barriers are compromised;
- rashes may lead to increased ability of pathogens to cross the skin barrier;
- those with severe malnourishment may have decreased secretory IgA;
- wound healing is impaired;
- the production of certain inflammatory cytokines, such as IL-2 and TNFα, is decreased;
- there is an increase in cytokines associated with T$_H$2 responses;
- opsonization is decreased, largely because of a reduction in levels of various complement components – C3, C5 and factor B. This may be related to decreased production but also to increased consumption related to increased infection frequency.

Deficiencies in trace elements impact immunity. Zinc is one of several trace elements essential for optimal immune system function. WHO estimates that about one-third of the world's population is affected by some level of zinc deficiency. Populations with plant-based diets are at particular risk because fibre and phytate in plant foods inhibit zinc absorption. Similar to protein deficiencies, **zinc deprivation** can cause involution of the thymus, with significant, rapid reduction in thymic weight, primarily as a result of cortical region loss. Zinc is a structural element both in the peptide hormone thymulin and in many transcription factors. Thus, reduction in the activity of thymulin contributes to thymic and lymphoid atrophy and decreased activity of factors such as NF-κB prevents adequate IL-2 and IFNγ production impairing cell-mediated immune responses. NK-cell lytic activity and macrophage and neutrophil function are also diminished with zinc deficiency.

Iron deficiency results in a reduced ability of neutrophils to phagocytose or kill bacteria and fungi because of reduced myeloperoxidase activity. T-cell proliferation is iron dependent and the availability of iron influences CD4$^+$ T-cell differentiation. T_H1-cell differentiation seems to be particularly sensitive to iron deficiency and, therefore, IFNγ-dependent functions are affected. This in turn affects NK and macrophage activity. In addition, lymphocyte responses to mitogens and antigens are decreased. However, iron is a double-edged sword because iron-dependent enzymes have crucial roles in lymphocyte and phagocyte function and iron bioavailability favours growth of many microorganisms.

Selenium, incorporated as the amino acid selenocysteine, is an important component of the antioxidants catalase and glutathione peroxidase. It seems to have important antiviral effects, both in terms of viral replication and the host response to the viral infection. It has been found to promote viral vaccine responses (notably with polio virus) and may promote a T_H1 response. In vitro, selenium deficiency leads to decreased T-cell responses, decreased NK-cell function, decreased macrophage function and altered cytokine production. Selenium has been implicated as an important micronutrient in HIV infection; deficiency has been associated with disease progression. It is also important in *Mycobacterium tuberculosis* infection and is notably associated with the pulmonary form of this disease.

Vitamin deficiencies and immune function. Singular deficiencies in **vitamins B$_1$, B$_6$ and B$_{12}$** are rare; however, as with all nutrients, severe deficits impact immune responses. In vivo studies examining the effects of vitamin B deficiencies, both in humans and animal models, typically show impairment of thymic and lymphoid cellularity, decreased proliferative responses and decreased antibody production. Folate is also important in immune function; folate deficiency is associated with decreased circulating T cells and decreased ability to proliferate. Interestingly, in a small study, NK function appeared to be negatively impacted by high levels of unmetabolized folate. **Vitamin C** and **vitamin E** have known antioxidant functions. Serum vitamin C levels quickly diminish with stress or infection as it is scavenged to mitigate oxidative stress. Deficiency affects neutrophil chemotaxis and T-cell proliferation. Treatment of dendritic cells (DCs) in vitro with vitamin C can mediate p38 and NF-κB activation, augmenting IL-12 secretion. Vitamin E treatment of macrophages, via its antioxidant role, can decrease production of PGE$_2$. Vitamin E supplementation has been shown to have a broad variety of immune effects, including increasing T-cell proliferation in response to mitogens, NK cytotoxicity and increasing IL-2 production.

Other work has likewise documented the immunoregulatory effects of **vitamin A** on immune function. Vitamin A deficiency, which is endemic in developing nations, impairs epithelial and mucosal barriers, leading to hyperplasia, loss of mucus-producing cells and susceptibility to gastrointestinal and respiratory infections. It can negatively affect macrophages' ability to phagocytose and kill intracellular bacteria and decreases NK cell numbers and function. Moreover, it favours T_H1 responses by increasing production of IL-12 and TNFα, which suppresses T_H2 responses, thus impairing antibody responses. Multiple studies in vitamin A-deficient animals have shown that supplementation of vitamin A or its metabolites enhances immune responses to vaccination and production of antibodies to both T-dependent and polysaccharide antigens.

Until the advent of antibiotics, cod liver oil and sunlight, both sources of **vitamin D**, were used as primary treatments for TB. Vitamin D is very important for bone health but is also a powerful immunomodulator and deficiency has been associated with higher rates of infection. There is a high concentration of vitamin D receptors in thymic tissue and on developing T cells and mature CD8 cells. Many cell types express the vitamin D receptor (VDR) and while vitamin D metabolites may modulate adaptive immune responses, they can also enhance innate immunity. Notably, it has been shown to promote monocyte differentiation to macrophages. Importantly, particularly for TB, signalling via the VDR may enhance both cathelicidin and defensin expression, thus boosting macrophage anti-microbial activity (Chapter 5).

Finally, it is important to note that malnutrition due to insufficient intake or absorption is rarely one-dimensional. Thus, interpretation of any studies where individual micronutrients are supplemented must take into account that other nutrient deficiencies may remain.

Obesity is associated with altered immune responses.

Although the mechanisms remain unclear, obesity increases susceptibility to both nosocomial and post-surgical infections and increases the risk of serious complications from common infections. Obese subjects and animals show changes in various immune responses, including:

- a higher total leukocyte count;
- reduced NK activity; and
- increased oxidative burst of monocytes and granulocytes.

Altered levels of some micronutrients, lipids and hormones may explain these immunological changes. Leptin is one of the key hormones implicated in obesity and can communicate directly with the immune system via leukocyte leptin receptors. Leptin secretion is suppressed in obese individuals, which may lead to decreased immune responses.

IMMUNODEFICIENCY SECONDARY TO DRUG THERAPIES

Several classes of drugs suppress immune function, either intentionally for therapeutic effect or as an unwanted side effect. For example, patients undergoing solid organ transplantation or haematopoietic stem cell transplantation receive a variety of immunosuppressants to prevent rejection of the donor organ and graft-versus-host disease (GvHD), respectively (discussed in Chapter 21). Likewise, patients presenting with severe inflammatory, allergic or autoimmune reactions often require therapeutic immunosuppression (Chapter 20). Pharmacological treatments that suppress immunity as a side effect include cancer treatments such as cytotoxic or anti-metabolite reagents, which can also severely depress bone marrow haematopoiesis. Later, we will examine the different classes of immunosuppressive drugs commonly used and their impact on immune function.

Iatrogenic immune suppression post-organ transplantation.
Because genetic differences can cause the immune system to perceive donor organs as foreign, recipients of both organ and stem cell transplants receive immunosuppressive regimens, often long term. Essentially, the goal of these treatments is to prevent an immune response against either the host or donor tissues while minimizing toxic side effects and susceptibility of the patient to infection. The primary effectors for both donor organ rejection and GvHD are T lymphocytes. Therefore, both prophylactic and therapeutic immunosuppressant drugs target the T-cell branch of the immune system. We briefly summarize the mechanism of drugs that help prevent rejection and GvHD below (see also Chapter 21).

Approaches to suppress T-cell-mediated damage include interfering with:

- T-cell-receptor signalling and activation;
- cytokine secretion;
- cytolytic function;
- T-cell proliferation; and
- control of inflammatory mediators.

Drugs such as ciclosporin A and tacrolimus bind to cellular immunophilins and as a complex inhibit calcineurin (see Fig. 7.w1). This blockade dampens T-cell signalling mediated by NF-AT translocation and, in turn, decreases IL-2 and IFNγ production, impairing both T-cell activation and proliferation. The drug rapamycin (sirolimus) also binds an immunophilin; however, this interaction results in inhibition of the response to rather than the production of IL-2, again blocking both proliferation and activation in some lymphocyte subsets.

Interference with cellular proliferation is another mechanism of immune suppression. Drugs such as azathioprine or the more lymphocyte-specific inhibitor, mycophenolate mofetil, prevent B-cell and T-cell proliferation by affecting DNA synthesis.

Glucocorticosteroids and their functional analogues are potent anti-inflammatory drugs with effects on all branches of the immune response. In the light of their widespread use, we have included a more detailed discussion of this class of drugs.

Glucocorticoids are powerful immune modulators.
Among the pharmacological agents that dampen immune responses, the glucocorticoids have the broadest application. Glucocorticoids have pleiotropic effects that vary with both dose and duration of use; however, they are perhaps best known for their potent anti-inflammatory effect. They have been the front-line drugs for decades in the treatment of a variety of inflammatory and allergic conditions and continue to be a major component of immunosuppressive regimens after organ transplantation.

Patients can receive glucocorticoids:

- systemically, for example, during the early period immediately post-organ transplant (Chapter 21);
- locally, for example as an inhalant for treatment of asthma (Chapter 23);
- topically, for example as for treatment of poison ivy-induced contact hypersensitivity (Chapter 26).

Glucocorticoids are naturally occurring steroids produced by the adrenal cortex. In response to chronic stress or to inflammatory cytokines, a cascade of hormone signals originating in the hypothalamus drives adrenal production of the immunomodulatory steroid cortisol (Fig. 19.2 and see Fig. 12.21). Cortisol and its analogues are small steroid hormones that readily cross the cellular membrane and bind cytosolic glucocorticoid receptors. Activated glucocorticoid receptors enter the nucleus and can either directly bind DNA to affect gene transcription or regulate expression by disrupting other transcription factor complexes such as NF-κB and AP-1 (see Fig. 7.w1).

Functional effects of steroid treatment.
Glucocorticoids have significant effects on both the innate and adaptive branches of the immune response. There is profound suppression of

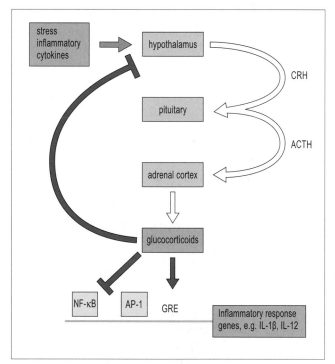

Fig. 19.2 The hypothalamus–pituitary–adrenal (HPA) axis Neuroendocrine signalling plays a key role in integrating feedback from the immune system to maintain homeostasis. Inflammatory cytokines trigger the hypothalamus to release corticotropin-releasing hormone (CRH). Increased CRH levels trigger pituitary production of adrenocorticotrophic hormone (ACTH), which in turn signals the adrenal glands to increase glucocorticoid production. Glucocorticoids bound to their receptor can interfere with NF-κB and AP-1 transcription factor complexes from binding to promoter regions. Additionally, they can interfere with transcription by directly binding to inhibitory glucocorticoid responsive elements (GRE). Under normal conditions, this signalling pathway serves as part of the negative feedback loop shutting down immune responses after infection is controlled.

inflammatory cytokine secretion (IL-1β, IL-6, IL-8, TNFα, IL-12) and chemokine expression, resulting in decreased recruitment of neutrophils and macrophages to sites of injury or infection. Glucocorticoids also interfere with prostaglandin synthesis, COX2 production and mast cell degranulation. Interestingly, while glucocorticoids enhance both phagocytosis of opsonized antigens and uptake via scavenger receptors, they reduce dendritic cell activation by impairing upregulation of MHC class II and co-stimulatory B7 molecules.

Within the adaptive branch of immunity, profound down-regulation of the inflammatory cytokines and the response of T cells to these cytokines preferentially shift the adaptive immune profile from TH1 towards a TH2-type (Chapter 12). In particular, glucocorticoids suppress both DC production of IL-12 and T-cell expression of the IL-12 receptor. In contrast, the effect of corticosteroids on B-cell responses is less profound, with humoral immune responses less impacted by corticosteroid treatment compared with cell-mediated responses.

Glucocorticoids are an invaluable tool, particularly for controlling inflammatory processes, and they are often used for only short periods because of the risk of potent side effects both infectious and non-infectious. In administering any of the immunosuppressant drugs, physicians must weigh the therapeutic benefits against the risks of broad immunosuppression.

Monoclonal antibody and fusion protein therapies. As a result of the non-specific immunosuppressive effects of steroids and other immunosuppressive drugs, an array of more targeted immunosuppressive therapies have been developed using antibodies or chimeric receptor constructs specifically to inhibit cytokines, cytokine receptors, lymphocyte surface molecules and cellular adhesion molecules (Table 19.1). Many of these medications are used to treat inflammatory and autoimmune diseases such as inflammatory bowel disease and rheumatological diseases and others are used in the context of solid organ and stem cell transplantation. This array of immunosuppressive medicines allows for more targeted suppression of specific areas of the immune system. Despite this improved specificity, these therapies still increase infection risk in ways that significantly impact clinical care.

TNF inhibitors were one of the first-developed classes of monoclonal antibody therapies. These drugs bind to both soluble and transmembrane forms of TNFα and are widely used in the treatment of inflammatory bowel disease and rheumatoid arthritis. Although widely successful at treating inflammatory diseases, TNF inhibitors carry a specific increased risk of tuberculosis and endemic fungal infection from *Histoplasma* and other endemic fungi.

Rituximab is an anti-CD20, B-cell-depleting agent commonly used in treatment of malignancies and autoimmune diseases. In some patients, B-cell function is slow to recover or never fully recovers. Some patients also suffer from neutropenia for a period of time after receiving this drug. Prolonged B-cell depletion can result in low IgG levels that place patients at risk for invasive infection with encapsulated bacteria such as *Streptococcus pneumoniae*. In many cases, these patients require administration of intravenous immunoglobulin (IVIG) to prevent infections.

In the past several years, a wide variety of other monoclonal antibody therapies have been developed, studied and deployed for use in a variety of settings (see Table 19.1). Drugs such as tocilizumab and anakinra target IL-6 and IL-1 signalling, respectively, and thereby decrease innate initiators of inflammation. The monoclonal antibodies ustekinumab and secukinumab inhibit IL-17-mediated neutrophilic inflammation; secukinumab targets IL-17A specifically and ustekinumab inhibits IL-12 and IL-23. The specific infection risks of these monoclonal antibodies can be somewhat predicted based on animal models and genetic immune deficiencies involving these cytokines and their signalling pathways. However, defining and quantifying

---

TABLE 19.1 Selected Monoclonal Antibodies and Fusion Proteins

Therapeutic Agent	Type of Agent	Target	Mechanism of Action	Major Infection Risk
Rituximab	Chimeric mAb	CD20	B-cell depletion	JC virus Encapsulated bacteria
Etanercept	Fusion protein	TNFα	Prevents cytokine receptor binding	Tuberculosis Histoplasmosis and other endemic fungi
Infliximab	Chimeric mAb			
Adalimumab	Human mAb			
Tocilizumab	Humanized mAb	IL-6 receptor	Prevents cytokine receptor binding	Bacterial lung and skin infections
Anakinra	Recombinant protein	IL-1α and IL-1β	Prevents cytokine receptor binding	Bronchopulmonary infections
Ustekinumab	Human mAb	p40 subunit of IL-17 and IL-23	Prevents cytokine receptor binding	Theoretical risk of bacterial and fungal infections
Secukinumab	Human mAb	IL-17A	Prevents cytokine receptor binding	Mucosal and cutaneous *Candida* infections
Natalizumab	Humanized mAb	α4-integrin	Prevents leukocyte trafficking	JC virus
Abatacept	Fusion protein	CD80/86	Inhibits co-stimulation	EBV-associated post-transplant lymphoproliferative disorder
Eculizumab	Humanized mAb	Complement 5 (C5)	Inhibits formation of complement membrane attack complex	Infection with *Neisseria meningitidis*

mAb, Monoclonal antibody.

specific infection risk is challenging given that patients can be on multiple immunosuppressive therapies at the same time. In addition, the comparison groups are often treated with combination immunosuppressive regimens that also increase infection risk.

OTHER CAUSES OF SECONDARY IMMUNODEFICIENCIES

There are several other clinical conditions that lead to immune suppression and increased susceptibility to infection. Many chemotherapy regimens, as well as irradiation treatment for cancer, target rapidly dividing cells and cause loss of bone marrow precursor cells. Similarly, cancer metastases to the bone and leukaemia involving bone marrow may decrease bone marrow output or lead to generation of immature or atypical leukocyte populations. Severe and prolonged neutropenia is the main immune impairment that results from cancer therapy regimens. Neutropenia in this setting places a patient at risk for a variety of invasive bacterial and fungal infections. In addition to neutropenia, mucosal breakdown from chemotherapy and breach of skin integrity resulting from central line placement further increase the risk of these infections.

Major surgery and/or trauma, as well as chronic stressors or debility and advanced age, all correlate with diminished immune function, in part caused by the upregulation of endogenous glucocorticoids. Some surgeries can also lead to immune dysfunction because of removal of immune tissue. For example, infants who undergo cardiac surgery often lose precious thymic tissue because of the organ's proximity to the heart. This can lead to T-cell deficiency, resulting from reduced thymic output. Lastly, viral infections can cause loss of immune function, or paradoxically, some cause immune activation or proliferation.

HIV causes AIDS. Infection with HIV is second only to malnutrition as a worldwide cause of immune deficiency and is a significant cause of morbidity and mortality across the globe. HIV is a retrovirus whose primary cellular targets upon infection are CD4 T cells, DCs and macrophages. Untreated, HIV leads to depletion of the immune system or acquired immunodeficiency syndrome (AIDS), leaving the host susceptible to fatal opportunistic infections. Disease caused by normally non-pathogenic infections, such as *Pneumocystis jiroveci* (pneumonia), cytomegalovirus (retinitis) and *Cryptococcus neoformans* (meningitis) occur, as do cancers driven by oncogenic viruses such as Kaposi's sarcoma (human herpes virus 8, HHV8), non-Hodgkin's lymphoma (Epstein–Barr virus, EBV) and cervical cancer (human papilloma virus, HPV).

Present primarily in blood, semen, vaginal secretions and breast milk of infected individuals, HIV is primarily transmitted via unprotected sex, contaminated needles/blood products or vertically from mother to child during the perinatal period. Globally, more than 37 million people are living with the virus, with over 1.5 million newly infected and an estimated 1 million deaths each year (WHO estimates, 2017). Roughly 35 million people have died from HIV since the descriptions of the first cases in 1981.

There are two main variants, HIV-1 and HIV-2:
- HIV-2 is endemic in West Africa and appears to be less pathogenic;
- HIV-1 has several subtypes (or clades), which are designated by the letters A through K, and the prevalence of the different clades varies by geographical region: over 90% of people infected with HIV-1 live in developing countries and spread is 80% by the sexual route.

HIV life cycle. HIV is a single-stranded RNA lentivirus. Each enveloped virion contains two copies of the 10-kilobase genome, each encoding nine genes flanked at each end by a long-terminal repeat (LTR) sequence. The LTR sequences are essential for integration of viral DNA into the host chromosome and also provide binding sites for initiating replication. The HIV genome contains *gag* (core proteins), *pol* (reverse transcriptase, protease and integrase enzymes) and *env* (envelope protein) genes as well as six regulatory and accessory proteins (Fig. 19.3).

HIV targets CD4$^+$ T cells and mononuclear phagocytes. HIV primarily targets CD4$^+$ T cells, CD4$^+$ macrophages and some DCs. *Env* encodes a 160 kDa precursor of the envelope glycoproteins and proteolytic cleavage generates gp120 and gp41. Infection of the target cells requires initial attachment of gp120 to the major receptor, CD4. Viral entry also requires additional binding through co-receptors, most commonly the chemokine receptors CCR5 and CXCR4. Once bound to the cells, interaction via gp41 mediates cell–virus fusion. Upon entry of the HIV capsid, reverse transcription of the RNA genome generates cDNA that subsequently integrates into the host DNA. These latter two steps occur primarily within activated cells.

Differences in the envelope glycoprotein sequence determine whether the virus can utilize the chemokine receptors CCR5 or CXCR4, or both, as co-receptor(s). HIV variants that utilize CCR5 or CXCR4 are referred to as R5 or X4 viruses, respectively. R5 viruses, therefore, can infect memory CD4$^+$ T cells and mononuclear phagocytes expressing CCR5. R5 tropism predominates early in HIV infection, while X4, R5 and R5/X4 dual tropic variants may be found in patients during later stages. Individuals homozygous for a 32 base pair deletion in the CCR5 allele (CCR5Δ32) are highly resistant to HIV infection by R5 viruses but remain susceptible to infection with X4 virus. Other receptors for HIV include DC-SIGN on DC and galactosyl ceramide (GalC), a major binding site for infection within the brain, gut and vagina.

Acute symptoms occur 2–4 weeks post-infection. Disease is generally the result of infection by a single virion. With infection via a mucosal surface (~80% of infections), the initial target cell is likely a tissue DC or macrophage that can then transport virus to the draining lymphoid tissue. Migration of virus to lymphoid tissue allows productive infection of an activated CD4$^+$ T cell or macrophage, inducing cytokine release and further recruitment of activated cells. Recent studies have shown the gut-associated lymphoid tissues (GALT), a site rich with memory CCR5$^+$ CD4$^+$ T cells, are an early locus of infection. HIV infection of GALT

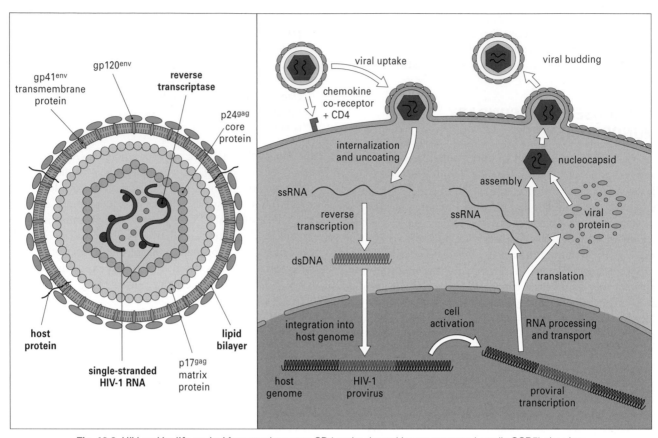

Fig. 19.3 HIV and its life cycle After attachment to CD4 and a chemokine co-receptor (usually CCR5), the virus membrane fuses with the cellular membrane to allow entry into the cell. Following uncoating, reverse transcription of viral RNA results in the production of double-stranded DNA (*dsDNA*). This is inserted into the host genome as the HIV provirus by a virally coded integrase enzyme, which is a target for new antiviral medications currently in development. Cell activation leads to transcription and the production of viral mRNAs. Structural proteins are produced and assembled. Free HIV viruses are produced by viral budding from the host cell, after which further internal assembly occurs with the cleavage of a large precursor core protein into the small core protein components by a virally coded protease enzyme, producing mature virus particles, which are released and can go on to infect additional cells bearing CD4 and the chemokine co-receptor.

CD4$^+$ T cells quickly leads to their depletion. Approximately 2–4 weeks post-infection, the patient experiences flu-like symptoms, with fever, swollen lymph nodes, malaise, occasionally rashes, headache and nausea. During acute viraemia, plasma virus levels can reach up to 10 million copies/mL, with wide dissemination of the virus throughout tissues, often also accompanied by acute depletion of CD4$^+$ T cells in the blood and, importantly, establishment of HIV reservoirs. It is estimated that more than half of all memory CD4 T cells are lost during this acute phase.

Viral latency is associated with chronic infection. Without anti-retroviral treatment, HIV levels peak 3–4 weeks post-infection, then gradually drop and plateau (Fig. 19.4). This reflects a combination of the decrease in readily available activated targets and, perhaps more importantly, control by the innate and adaptive immune responses. There is usually a moderate rebound in circulating CD4$^+$ T cell numbers at this point, although recent studies indicate the GALT CD4$^+$ T-cell populations do not recover. Simultaneously, the virus establishes stable viral reservoirs. This first consists of cells supporting low-level

viral replication in lymphoid and other tissues, likely with efficient cell-to-cell propagation of the virus. The second reservoir is within CD4$^+$ T cells in which the HIV genome is integrated as a provirus yet remains latent as a silent infection without viral protein transcription. Subsequent T-cell activation can then stimulate virus production.

The plasma viral load after acute infection has receded (viral set-point) can be an indicator of disease progression. The average period of stable infection is 10 years, with mean plasma viral load of ~30 000 copies/mL. Rapid progressors can experience increases in viraemia, CD4$^+$ T-cell depletion and onset of opportunistic disease within 6 months. Plasma viral RNA levels of >100 000 copies/mL 6 months after infection are associated with a 10-fold greater risk of progression to AIDS within 5 years compared with patients with HIV plasma load of <100 000 copies/mL. In contrast, long-term non-progressors (LTNPs) generally have a lower viral set-point and may remain asymptomatic for more than 25 years with stable CD4$^+$ T-cell numbers. During this chronic infection period, active immune responses keep viral levels in check. Most infected individuals are asymptomatic during this period but can still transmit infectious virus to others.

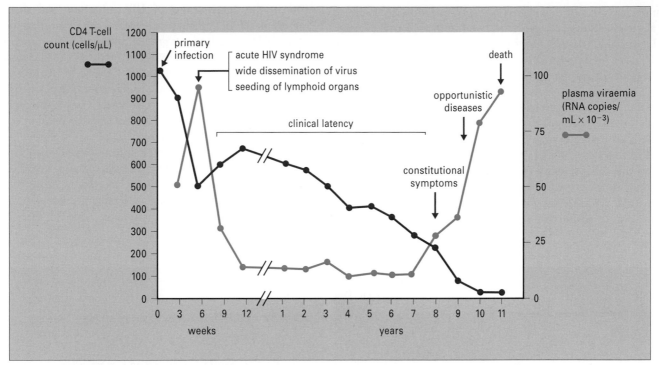

Fig. 19.4 Natural history of HIV A typical course of HIV infection. (Courtesy Dr AS Fauci. Modified with permission from Pantaleo G, Graziosi C. N Engl J Med 1993;328:327–335. Copyright 1993 Massachusetts Medical Society. All rights reserved.)

HIV infection induces strong immune responses. Both humoral and cellular immune responses develop after infection. Detectable HIV-specific antibodies are evident in the first few weeks of infection. Production of neutralizing antibodies (which prevent virus–cell fusion and correlate with protection) does not occur until at least 12 weeks after infection. Importantly, although antibodies are sufficient to drive evolution of viral epitopes, they are insufficient to prevent disease progression.

The drop in HIV viraemia to the set-point level coincides with the expansion of HIV-specific CD8 T cells. In $CD8^+$ T-cell-depleted animal models of infection, viral containment fails. Thus, as with many viruses, $CD8^+$ T-cell responses are important components in the control of infection. These responses are usually against peptides derived from multiple viral proteins and comprise a considerable portion (up to 25%) of total $CD8^+$ T cells; however, neither the breadth nor the magnitude of CTL responses correlates with control of viraemia. In contrast, the genetic background, specifically the HLA haplotype of the host, is important in determining viral control. Both the HLA-B*27 and HLA-B*57 class I alleles are associated with low viral set-point and long-term asymptomatic control of infection. These patients are often LTNP and may have stable infection for >10 years.

HIV can evade the immune response. HIV is a rapidly mutating virus. Both error-prone reverse transcription and high recombination frequencies during reverse transcription combine with an extremely high virus production rate to generate genetic diversity. Particularly during acute infection, immune clearance via antibody and CTL recognition favour survival of

virions with envelope or peptide sequence changes in regions targeted by host-protective epitopes. Additionally, the HIV protein Nef limits CTL detection of infected cells via selective downregulation of both HLA-A and HLA-B expression, reducing the surface display of viral epitopes. Viral escape, coupled with the existence of latent viral reservoirs undetectable by HIV-specific immune responses, prevents the immune system from eliminating HIV-infected cells. Exacerbating this issue, the immune responses become progressively weaker over time.

Immune dysfunction results from the direct effects of HIV and impairment of CD4 T cells. The chronic phase of HIV infection is marked by persistent generalized immune activation. Infected persons present with B-cell polyclonal activation and hypergammaglobulinaemia. Inflammatory cytokines such as IFNα, IFNγ, IL-18, IL-15 and TNFα are elevated during acute infection. Finally, increased translocation of bacteria through the gut barrier, due to extensive HIV infection within the GALT and lamina propria, increases circulating LPS levels, activating many immune effectors via Toll-like receptors. In patients with high viral load, HIV-specific CTL typically contain low levels of intracellular perforin (see Figs 8.9 and 8.11) and have a poor proliferative capacity. During this chronic phase, $CD8^+$ T cells often express PD-1, a receptor associated with programmed cell death. The points above are all consistent with persistent activation and eventual exhaustion of the supply of anti-HIV $CD8^+$ T cells that worsens over time.

Of equal, if not greater, impact on overall immune dysfunction from HIV infection, however, is the loss of the $CD4^+$ T cells. Although circulating $CD4^+$ T-cell counts often rebound (at least quantitatively if not qualitatively) to pre-infection levels after the acute phase, they do not recover within the mucosal associated lymphoid tissues. Furthermore, in untreated patients, CD4+ T-cell levels eventually decline although they may remain above critical levels for a period of 6 months to 10 years.

CD4+ T-cell loss is due to direct killing by HIV and activation-induced apoptosis. Additionally, infected CD4+ T cells present both gp120 and HIV peptide:HLA complexes on the cell surface, leaving them subject to anti-HIV antibodies and CTLs. Ongoing loss of CD4+ T-cell help ultimately contributes to the collapse of the CD8+ T-cell response. Progressive immunodeficiency is a hallmark of HIV and the eventual diminished CD4+ T-cell levels correlate tightly with the subsequent progression to advanced disease and death.

AIDS is the final stage of HIV infection and disease. Progression to AIDS includes a CD4+ T-cell count of <200/μL. As blood CD4+ T-cell counts gradually decline during the chronic phase, patients become susceptible to opportunistic infection and malignancies (Fig. 19.5). Below 500 CD4+ cells/μL, less severe conditions such as oral candidiasis, recurrent herpes virus outbreaks (e.g. shingles from varicella zoster virus and anogenital herpes from herpes simplex virus) and pneumococcal infections occur. CD4+ T-cell levels below 200/μL are associated with increased risk of life-threatening infections and malignancies including *Pneumocystis jiroveci* pneumonia and Kaposi's sarcoma, respectively. With CD4+ T-cell levels below 50/μL, patients become vulnerable to additional systemic infection with organisms such as *Mycobacterium avium* complex. The three main

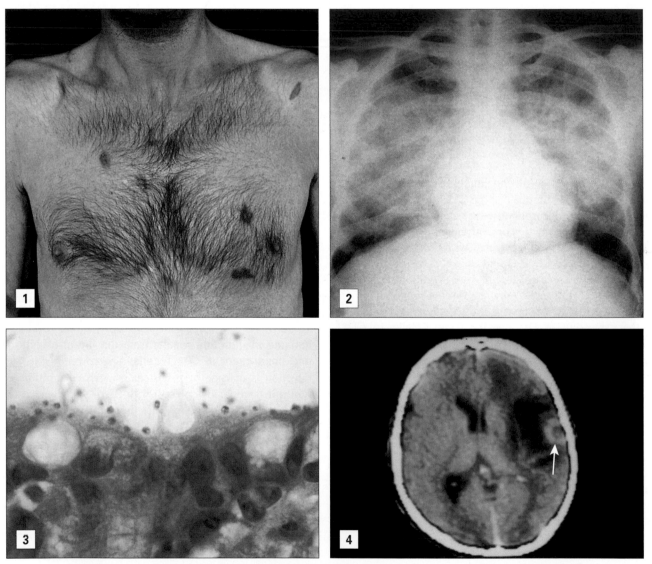

Fig. 19.5 Common features of late-stage HIV infection (**1**) Multiple Kaposi's sarcoma lesions on the chest and abdomen. (**2**) Chest radiograph of a patient with *Pneumocystis jiroveci* pneumonia, showing bilateral interstitial shadowing. (**3**) Small bowel biopsy from a patient with diarrhoea caused by cryptosporidia, showing intermediate forms of cryptosporidia (small pink dots) on the surface of the mucosa. (**4**) Computed tomography scan of the head of a patient with cerebral toxoplasmosis. The patient presented with a history of fits and weakness of the left arm and leg. Injection of contrast revealed a ring-enhancing lesion in the right hemisphere *(arrow)*, with surrounding oedema *(dark area)*.

organ systems affected are the respiratory system, gastrointestinal tract and central nervous system.

Pneumocystis jiroveci (previously *P. carinii*) is the most common opportunistic respiratory infection (see Fig. 19.5), but pulmonary bacterial infections, including *Mycobacterium tuberculosis,* also occur. Protozoa (cryptosporidia and microsporidia) are the most common pathogens isolated in patients with diarrhoea and weight loss (see Fig. 19.5). Enteric bacteria such as *Salmonella* and *Campylobacter* spp. may also afflict AIDS patients.

Neurological complications in AIDS are due to direct effects of HIV infection, opportunistic infections or lymphoma. AIDS-related dementia once affected between 10% and 40% of patients with other manifestations of AIDS, but with more effective antiviral treatment it has become less common. Neurological involvement can be due to a number of pathogens. *Cryptococcus neoformans* is a fungus and is the most common cause of AIDS-related meningitis. Toxoplasmosis, a protozoal infection, causes cysts in the brain and neurological deficit (see Fig. 19.5). Cytomegalovirus reactivation may cause inflammation of the retina, brain and spinal cord and its nerve roots, and a polyomavirus (JC virus), which infects oligodendrocytes in the brain, produces a rapidly fatal demyelinating disease—progressive multifocal leukoencephalopathy.

Kaposi's sarcoma (KS), caused by infection with human herpes virus 8 **(HHV8),** is the most common AIDS-associated malignancy (see Fig. 19.5). HHV8 infections, similar to CMV herpes virus infections, are often asymptomatic in individuals with competent T-cell immunity. With HIV co-infection, however, HHV8 titres increase and KS emerges with multifocal lesions (see Fig. 19.5) of mixed cellularity often resulting in widespread involvement of skin, mucous membranes, viscera (gut and lungs) and lymph nodes. Most of the opportunistic infections, as well as malignancies, are difficult to diagnose and treatment often suppresses rather than eradicates them. Relapses are common and continuous suppressive or maintenance treatment is necessary.

An effective vaccine remains an elusive goal. Currently, treatment for HIV focuses on antiviral drug cocktails that significantly reduce the patient's viral load. As a result of the rapid rate of mutation in the viral genome during replication, single drug therapy nearly always leads to rapid drug resistance. However, by providing the patient with a cocktail of antiviral drugs, each targeting a different aspect of the viral life cycle, it is possible to prolong the period of time before plasma viral load increases and T-cell counts drop. Anti-retroviral therapies, unfortunately, are not a cure, nor can they prevent transmission of the virus.

Despite increasing characterization of adaptive immune responses, the correlates of protection remain to be fully defined, and this has left the field with mostly empiric approaches. Ideally, investigators will develop a vaccine that provides sufficient protection to prevent viral transmission.

Encouraging early reports of persons repeatedly exposed to HIV who never became infected suggested that adaptive immune responses, particularly HIV-specific CD8$^+$ T-cell responses, might be responsible for apparent protection, but this remains somewhat controversial. Such a vaccine will almost certainly also require the induction of broadly neutralizing antibody responses, something that candidate vaccines have yet to achieve. To date, there have been clinical trials of numerous candidate HIV vaccines, but most would agree that an effective vaccine remains an elusive goal.

CRITICAL THINKING: SECONDARY IMMUNODEFICIENCY

See Critical thinking: Explanations, section 19

A 52-year-old record producer developed a severe cough with increasing shortness of breath. He also had a fever, chest pain and malaise. For the week before presentation he complained of pain on swallowing. His past medical history included gonorrhoeae and genital herpes within the previous 3 years. Over the previous 2 months, he had suffered from persistent diarrhoea and lost 9 kg in weight from a baseline of 68 kg. He lived with his girlfriend with whom he had been having unprotected intercourse for several years. There was no history of intravenous drug abuse.

On examination he was underweight and had enlarged lymph nodes in the neck, axillae and groin. Plaques of *Candida albicans* were visible in his throat. There were abnormal breath sounds in his lungs. The results of his blood tests are shown here.

Investigation	Result (normal range)
Haemoglobin (g/dL)	12.8 (13.5–18.0)
Platelet count ($\times 10^9$/L)	128 (150–400)
White cell count ($\times 10^9$/L)	6.2 (4.0–11.0)
Neutrophils ($\times 10^9$/L)	5.4 (2.0–7.5)
Eosinophils ($\times 10^9$/L)	0.24 (0.4–0.44)
Total lymphocytes ($\times 10^9$/L)	0.75 (1.6–3.5)
T lymphocytes	
CD4$^+$ ($\times 10^9$/L)	0.12 (0.7–1.1)
CD8$^+$ ($\times 10^9$/L)	0.42 (0.5–0.9)
B lymphocytes ($\times 10^9$/L)	0.11 (0.2–0.5)
ECG	Normal
Chest radiography	Bilateral diffuse interstitial shadowing
Bronchoscopy with bronchoalveolar lavage	Positive for *Pneumocystis jirovecii*

Because of his sexual history, the patient was counselled about having a human immunodeficiency virus (HIV) test and he consented. An ELISA was positive for anti-HIV antibodies and a polymerase chain reaction (PCR) demonstrated HIV-1 RNA in the plasma.

Examination of an induced sputum specimen revealed *P. jirovecii,* which together with the positive HIV ELISA is an AIDS-defining illness. Thus, a clear diagnosis of AIDS was made and the patient's *P. jirovecii* pneumonia was treated with oxygen by mask and parenteral co-trimoxazole. He was discharged from hospital taking oral co-trimoxazole and a set of anti-retroviral drugs.

1. Which diagnostic tests are available for HIV infection?
2. Which serological and cellular indices can be used to monitor the course of HIV infection?

FURTHER READING

Archin NM, Sung JM, Garrido C, et al. Eradicating HIV-1 infection: seeking to clear a persistent pathogen. Nat Rev Microbiol 2014;12:50–764.

Bourke C, Berkley J, Predergast A. Immune dysfunction as a cause and consequence of malnutrition. Trends Immunol 2016;37:386–398.

Buttgereit F. Molecular mechanisms of glucocorticoid action and selective glucocorticoid receptor agonists. Mol Cell Endocrinol 2007;275:71–78.

Caskey M, Klein M, Nussenzweig MD. Broadly neutralizing antibodies for HIV-1 prevention or immunotherapy. N Engl J Med 2016;375:2019–2021.

Cunningham-Rundles S, McNeeley DF, Moon A. Mechanisms of nutrient modulation of the immune response. J Allergy Clin Immunol 2005;115:1119–1128.

Fishman JA. Infection in organ transplantation. Am J Transplant 2017;17:856–879.

Hricik DE. Transplant Immunology and immunosuppression: core curriculum 2015. Am J Kidney Dis 2015;65:956–966.

Murdaca G, Spano F, Contatore M, et al. Infection risk associated with anti-TNFα agents: a review, 2015;14:571–582.

Paczesny S, Hanauer D, Sun Y, Reddy P. New perspectives on the biology of acute GVHD. Bone Marrow Transplant 2010; 45:1–11.

Stahn C, Löwenberg M, Hommes DW, et al. The immune system in children with malnutrition: a systematic review. PLoS One 2014 Aug 25;9(8)e105017.

Wintergerst E, Maggini S, Hornig D. Contribution of selected vitamins and trace elements to immune function. Ann Nutr Metab 2007;51:301–323.

Winthrop KL, Mariett X, Silva JT, et al. ESCMID Study Group for Infections in Compromised Hosts Consensus Document on the safety of targeted and biological therapies. an infectious diseases perspective. Clin Microbiol Infect 2018; 24:S21–S40.

Yarchoan R, Uldrick TS. HIV-associated cancers and related diseases. N Engl J Med 2018;378:1029–1041.

Autoimmunity and Autoimmune Disease

SUMMARY

- **Autoimmunity is associated with disease.** Autoimmune mechanisms underlie many diseases, some organ-specific, others systemic in distribution. Autoimmune disorders can overlap.
- **Genetic factors play a role in the development of autoimmune diseases.** Twin studies show that there is a heritable component to autoimmunity. The majority of diseases are polygenic but HLA genes are particularly important.
- **Self-reactive B and T cells persist even in healthy subjects,** but in disease are selected by autoantigen in the production of autoimmune responses.
- **Controls on the development of autoimmunity can be bypassed.** Microbial cross-reacting antigens and cytokine dysregulation can lead to autoimmunity.
- **In most diseases associated with autoimmunity, the autoimmune process produces the lesions.** This can be demonstrated in experimental

models and human autoantibodies can be directly pathogenic. Immune complexes are associated with systemic autoimmune disease. Autoantibody tests are valuable for diagnosis, identification of disease subgroups and, in some diseases, for monitoring and prognosis.
- **Treatment of autoimmune disease has a variety of aims.** Treatment of organ-specific diseases usually involves metabolic control. Treatment of systemic diseases includes the use of anti-inflammatory and immunosuppressive drugs. Biological therapies, using monoclonal antibodies against pro-inflammatory cytokines and individual cell markers, have revolutionized the treatment of autoimmune rheumatic diseases. B-cell-directed therapies have proved highly effective in many autoimmune diseases.

Like a highly trained army, the immune system has evolved to recognize and to destroy foreign invading forces. Sometimes immune recognition fails, resulting in 'friendly fire' against the body's own tissue. For example, 'friendly fire' directed against synovial tissue causes rheumatoid arthritis, whereas an attack on cells within the pancreas results in diabetes mellitus.

Non-specific inflammation (e.g. in response to infection) invariably leads to some degree of collateral damage, but because of efficient clearance of the inciting pathogen and negative feedback loops, this is usually self-limited. In contrast, once initiated, autoimmune reactions usually persist because the inciting self antigen cannot be cleared without complete destruction of the target tissue. Furthermore, the tissue destruction resulting from the autoimmune attack may expose previously hidden antigens, leading to further autoantibody production. This phenomenon is known as epitope spread.

AUTOIMMUNITY AND AUTOIMMUNE DISEASE

Because the repertoire of specificities expressed by the B cells and T cells is generated randomly, it includes many that are specific for self components. The body therefore requires self-tolerance mechanisms to distinguish between self and non-self determinants to avoid autoreactivity (see Chapter 11). However, such mechanisms may fail and a number of diseases have been

identified in which there is autoimmunity, with copious production of autoantibodies and autoreactive T cells. The targets of the autoimmune attacks vary widely.

Not every autoimmune event leads to clinically overt disease. For example, anti-nuclear antibodies may be observed in the healthy relatives of patients with systemic lupus erythematosus (SLE), as well as a small number of unrelated, healthy individuals.

Autoimmunity strictly refers to an inappropriate adaptive immune response, i.e. a loss of self tolerance. Although the terms 'autoinflammatory' and 'autoimmune' are often used interchangeably, they are not synonymous. Autoinflammatory diseases can occur without autoimmunity. For example, the periodic fever syndromes, which include familial Mediterranean fever and tumour necrosis factor receptor associated periodic syndrome (TRAPS), are caused by dysregulation of the innate immune system, without any adaptive immune response against self. Conversely, autoimmune diseases need not be inflammatory; examples include immune thrombocytopenia, haemolytic anaemia and myasthenia gravis.

Autoimmune conditions present a spectrum between organ-specific and systemic disease.

Hashimoto's thyroiditis is highly organ-specific. One of the earliest examples in which the production of autoantibodies was associated with disease in a given organ is **Hashimoto's**

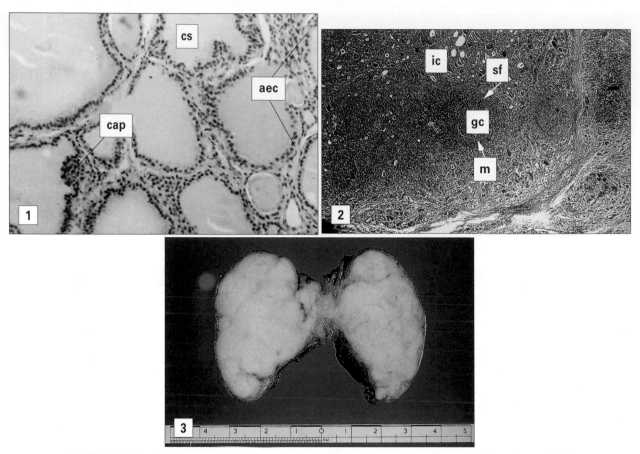

Fig. 20.1 Pathological changes in Hashimoto's thyroiditis In the normal thyroid gland (**1**), the acinar epithelial cells *(aec)* line the colloid space *(cs)* into which they secrete thyroglobulin, which is broken down on demand to provide thyroid hormones *(cap*, capillaries containing red blood cells). In the Hashimoto gland (**2**), the normal architecture is virtually destroyed and replaced by invading cells *(ic)*, which consist essentially of lymphocytes, macrophages and plasma cells. A secondary lymphoid follicle *(sf)* is present with a germinal centre *(gc)* and a mantle of small lymphocytes *(m)*. H&E stain. × 80. (**3**) In contrast to the red colour and soft texture of the normal thyroid, the pale and firm gross appearance of the Hashimoto gland reflects the loss of colloid and heavy infiltration with inflammatory cells. ((**2**) Reproduced from Woolf N. Pathology: Basic and Systemic. London: WB Saunders; 1998.)

thyroiditis. Thyroiditis is a condition that is most common in middle-aged women and often leads to the formation of a goitre or hypothyroidism. The gland is infiltrated with inflammatory lymphoid cells. These are predominantly mononuclear phagocytes, lymphocytes and plasma cells, and secondary lymphoid follicles are common (Fig. 20.1). The gland often also has regenerating thyroid follicles.

The serum of patients with Hashimoto's disease usually contains antibodies to thyroglobulin. These antibodies are demonstrable by agglutination and by precipitin reactions when present in high titre. Most patients also have antibodies directed against a cytoplasmic or microsomal antigen, also present on the apical surface of the follicular epithelial cells (see Fig. 20.1), and now known to be thyroid peroxidase, the enzyme that iodinates thyroglobulin. The antibodies associated with Hashimoto's thyroiditis react only with the thyroid: hence the resulting lesion is highly localized.

SLE is a systemic autoimmune disease. By contrast, the serum from patients with diseases such as SLE reacts with many,

if not all, of the tissues in the body. In SLE, one of the dominant antibodies is directed against the cell nucleus (Fig. 20.2).

Hashimoto's thyroiditis and SLE represent the extremes of the autoimmune spectrum (Fig. 20.3):

- The common target organs in **organ-specific disease** include the thyroid, adrenal, stomach, and pancreas.
- The non-organ-specific diseases, often termed **systemic autoimmune diseases**, which include rheumatological disorders, characteristically involve the skin, kidney, joints and muscle (Fig. 20.4).

The location of the antigen determines where a disease lies in the spectrum. The autoantigen in organ-specific autoimmune disease is expressed only in that tissue. In contrast, autoantigens in systemic autoimmune disease are present in multiple tissues. Examples include tRNA synthetases in myositis (which in spite of its name may also involve the skin, joints, lungs and heart), small nuclear ribonucleoproteins (snRNPs) in SLE and topoisomerases in systemic sclerosis. These small proteins play a vital role in the cellular

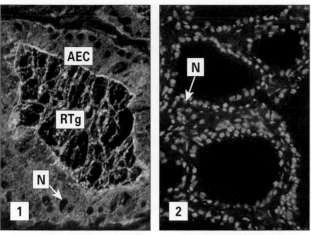

Fig. 20.2 Autoantibodies to thyroid Healthy, unfixed human thyroid sections were treated with patients' serum and then with fluoresceinated rabbit anti-human immunoglobulin. (**1**) Some residual thyroglobulin in the colloid *(RTg)* and the acinar epithelial cells *(AEC)* of the follicles, particularly the apical surface, are stained by antibodies from a patient with Hashimoto's disease, which react with the cells' cytoplasm but not the nuclei *(N)*. (**2**) In contrast, serum from a patient with systemic lupus erythematosus contains antibodies that react only with the nuclei of acinar epithelial cells and leave the cytoplasm unstained. (Courtesy Mr G Swana.)

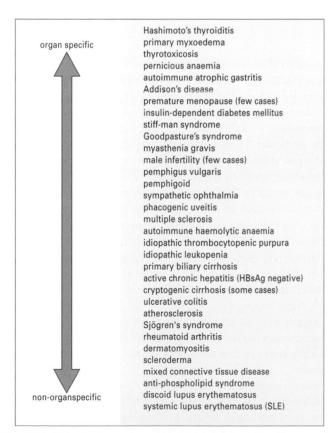

Fig. 20.3 The spectrum of autoimmune diseases Autoimmune diseases may be classified as organ specific or non-organ specific depending on whether the response is primarily against antigens localized to particular organs or against widespread antigens.

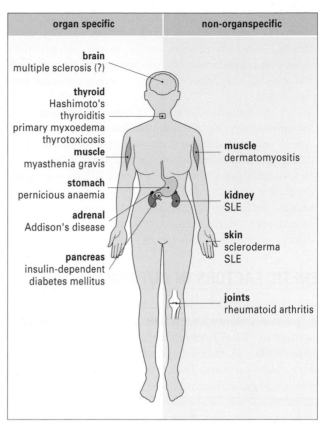

Fig. 20.4 Two types of autoimmune disease Although the non-organ-specific diseases characteristically produce symptoms in the skin, joints, kidney and muscle, individual organs are more markedly affected by particular diseases: for example, the kidney in systemic lupus erythematosus *(SLE)* and the joints in rheumatoid arthritis.

'machinery'. tRNA synthetases are involved in protein translation, snRNPs in mRNA splicing and topoisomerases in DNA replication.

An individual may have more than one autoimmune disease.
Autoimmune diseases 'hunt in packs': in patients with an autoimmune disease, the chance of developing an additional autoimmune disease is significantly elevated. This holds true for both organ-specific and systemic autoimmune disease.

- Thyroid antibodies occur with a high frequency in patients with pernicious anaemia who have gastric autoimmunity and these patients have a higher incidence of thyroid autoimmune disease than the normal population. Similarly, patients with thyroid autoimmunity have a high incidence of stomach autoantibodies and to a lesser extent the clinical disease itself (pernicious anaemia).
- Around 15% of patients with primary Sjögren's syndrome have concomitant autoimmune hypothyroidism and up to 40% have thyroid antibodies. Around 10% of SLE patients have thyroid antibodies in their serum.
- Thirty percent of patients with SLE and Sjögren's syndrome have a second, third or even fourth autoimmune disease.

The systemic autoimmune rheumatic diseases also show considerable overlap. This is typified by the so-called overlap syndromes in which patients exhibit mixed features of SLE, myositis and scleroderma. The mechanisms of immunopathological damage vary, depending on where the disease lies in the spectrum:

- Where the antigen is localized in a particular organ, type II hypersensitivity (e.g. autoimmune haemolytic anaemia) and type IV cell-mediated reactions, as in type I insulin-dependent diabetes, are most important (see Chapters 24–26).
- In systemic disorders such as SLE, type III immune complex deposition leads to inflammation through a variety of mechanisms, including complement activation and phagocyte recruitment. In rheumatoid arthritis, immune complexes directly stimulate production of cytokines such as TNFα.

GENETIC FACTORS IN AUTOIMMUNITY

There is an undoubted familial incidence of autoimmunity. For example, concordance for type I diabetes in identical twins may be as high as 50%. Concordance is largely genetic rather than environmental, as may be seen by comparison of identical and non-identical twins. Thus, if one of a pair of identical twins gets SLE, there is a 25% chance the other will develop it. In non-identical twins, the concordance rate is 2%–3%.

Within families, clustering of distinct autoimmune diseases has been reported. A large population-based survey found that families with a proband with rheumatoid arthritis were more likely to manifest other autoimmune disorders. This finding holds true for relatives of patients with other autoimmune diseases, such as multiple sclerosis (MS), which suggests the presence of shared pathogenic factors across the autoimmune diseases. However, the majority of individuals with autoimmune disease will not have an affected first-degree relative. Thus, whereas genetic factors are important in the pathogenesis of autoimmunity, they are usually not sufficient to cause disease without additional environmental influences.

Usually, several genes underlie susceptibility to autoimmunity. The vast majority of autoimmune diseases are not single-gene disorders but occur as a result of the complex interplay of multiple genetic and environmental factors. Evidence from genome-wide association studies (GWAS) has demonstrated that many genes contribute to disease susceptibility. Thus, the effect of variation in any one gene is, by itself, typically small.

There is emerging interest in how epigenetic modifications of DNA and associated histones may provide explanations of the molecular basis of complex polygenic disease traits such as autoimmunity. Epigenetic changes may occur as a result of environmental stimuli but may also be partly heritable.

Certain HLA haplotypes predispose to autoimmunity. Further evidence for the operation of genetic factors in autoimmune disease comes from their tendency to be associated with

TABLE 20.1 **HLA Associations in Autoimmune Disease**		
Disease	**HLA**	**Relative Risk**
Ankylosing spondylitis	B27	>150
Subacute thyroiditis	B35	14
Psoriasis vulgaris	Cw6	7
SLE	DR2/DR3	2–5
Hashimoto's thyroiditis	DR3	2–6
Graves' disease	DR3	4
Myasthenia gravis	DR3	2–5
Addison's disease	DR3	5–7
Rheumatoid arthritis	DR4	6–9
Juvenile arthritis	DR8	8
Coeliac disease	DQ2/DQ8	30
Multiple sclerosis	DQ6.02	12
Narcolepsy	DQ6.02	>40
Type I diabetes	DQ8	14

SLE, Systemic lupus erythematosus.
Relative risk is a measure of the increased chance of contracting the disease for individuals bearing the HLA antigen, relative to those lacking it. Virtually all autoimmune diseases studied have shown an association with some HLA specificity. The table gives some examples with indicative values. Actual values vary between studies as the relative risk depends on the population studied and the interaction of the specific HLA gene with environmental triggers and with other risk genes in each population.

particular HLA specificities (Table 20.1). For most autoimmune diseases, the major histocompatibility complex (MHC) region located on the short arm of chromosome 6 provides the strongest genetic component to disease susceptibility. It is important to appreciate that the increased risk associated with particular HLA haplotypes depends on the population under investigation and any other genetic and non-genetic risk factors that apply to them. Moreover, sets of MHC genes on one chromosome (haplotypes) are often in linkage disequilibrium. In this case, an MHC gene that is in linkage disequilibrium with a disease-susceptibility gene will also appear to give increased risk for the disease. For example, HLA-DR3 gives a relative risk (RR) for Addison's disease of RR ≈ 5; HLA-B8 is in linkage disequilibrium with HLA-DR3 and it also gives an increased risk for Addison's disease, albeit at a lower level, RR ≈ 2.

Recent high-density genome mapping in multiple autoimmune diseases has demonstrated complex, multi-loci effects that span the entire region, with both shared and unique loci across diseases.

Rarely, single HLA genes appear to determine disease susceptibility, e.g. HLA-B27 and ankylosing spondylitis. In others, such as rheumatoid arthritis, complex interactions between alleles at multiple genes within the HLA are involved. Rheumatoid arthritis shows no associations with the HLA-A and

HLA-B loci haplotypes but is associated with a nucleotide sequence known as the shared epitope (encoding amino acids 70–74 in the DRβ chain) that is common to DR1 and major subtypes of DR4; the MHC association with rheumatoid arthritis is restricted to patients who are positive for antibodies to citrullinated peptides. The nucleotide sequence of the shared epitope is also present in the dnaJ heat-shock proteins of various bacilli and EBV gp110 proteins, suggesting an interesting possibility for the induction of autoimmunity by a microbial cross-reacting epitope (see later). However, HLA-DR molecules bearing this sequence can bind to another bacterial heat-shock protein, dnaK, and to the human analogue hsp73, which targets selected proteins to lysosomes for antigen processing.

The haplotype B8-DR3 is common in both the organ-specific diseases and systemic autoimmune diseases such as SLE and myositis. Interestingly, for type I diabetes mellitus, DQ2/8 heterozygotes have a greatly increased risk of developing the disease.

Genes of the MHC, including HLA-A1, B8, DR2 and DR3, have been linked to SLE, although over a dozen other genes (including those regulating IFNα) have shown a stronger linkage.

The occurrence of different autoimmune conditions in one individual can be partly explained by the observation that specific MHC haplotypes confer susceptibility to more than one autoimmune disease (Fig 20.5). However, this is not the whole explanation, because other susceptibility genes and non-genetic factors may also contribute to different autoimmune conditions. It should also be noted that some MHC haplotypes are relatively protective (RR < 1). For example, in one study HLA-DQ0602 was associated with lower incidence of type I diabetes (RR = 0.02).

Genes outside the HLA region also confer susceptibility to autoimmunity.

Although HLA risk factors tend to dominate, autoimmune disorders are genetically complex and genome-wide searches for mapping the genetic intervals containing genes for predisposition to disease also reveal a plethora of non-HLA genes (Table 20.2) affecting:

- loss of tolerance;
- lymphocyte activation (receptor signalling pathways and co-stimulation);
- microbial recognition;
- cytokines and cytokine receptors;
- end-organ targeting.

One of the commonest genes outside the HLA region to be associated with autoimmune disease is the protein tyrosine phosphatase gene (PTPN22), which is expressed in lymphocytes. The minor allele of PTPN22 (Trp620) is associated with type I diabetes, rheumatoid arthritis, autoimmune thyroiditis and SLE. Crohn's disease, in contrast, is linked to the more common allele (Arg620). The minor allele results in gain of function causing inhibition of B-cell and T-cell activation and homozygous individuals have a profound defect in lymphocyte receptor signalling. The mechanisms by which this leads to autoimmunity are not clear, but possibilities include failure to delete autoreactive T cells in the thymus, impaired regulatory T-cell function and ineffective clearance of pathogens. It is interesting

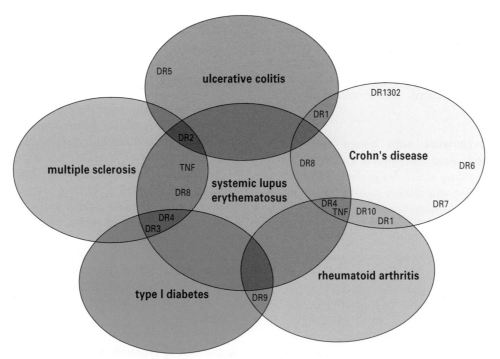

Fig. 20.5 HLA genes are associated with susceptibility to more than one condition Individual major histocompatibility complex haplotypes or gene loci (e.g. TNF) may be associated with different clinical conditions. (Based on Fernando MA et al. Defining the role of MHC in autoimmunity: a review and pooled analysis. PLoS Genet 2008;4(4):e1000024)

TABLE 20.2   Some Genetic Loci Associated With Autoimmune Disease

Chromosomal Location	Candidate Genes	Function of Protein Encoded by Gene	Diseases
1p13	PTPN22	T-cell and B-cell receptor signalling	RA, T1D, SLE, IBD, AT
	CD2/CD58	T-cell activation	RA, MS
1p31	IL-23R	Component of IL-23 receptor	IBD, psoriasis, AS
1q23	CRP	Innate immunity	SLE
	FCGR2A	Phagocytosis and immune complex clearance	SLE
	FCGR2B	B-cell regulation Phagocytosis of immune complexes	SLE
	FCGR3A	Expressed on natural killer cells Mediates antibody-dependent cellular cytotoxicity	SLE
	FCGR3B	Clearance of immune complexes	SLE, AAV
1q32	IL-10	Downregulates immune responses	IBD, T1D, SLE
1q41-42	PARP	Apoptosis	SLE
	TLR5	Innate immunity	SLE
2q33	CTLA-4	Transmits inhibitory signals to T cells	RA, TID
2q35-37	PDCD1	Transmembrane protein; activation leads to cytokine inhibition and control of cellular activation and antibody production	SLE
5q33	IL-12B	p40 subunit common to both IL-12 and IL-23	IBD, psoriasis
6p21	MHC region: multiple genes, e.g. TNFα, C2, C4	Multiple	Majority of autoimmune diseases
6q23	TNFAIP3	Induced by TNF and pattern recognition activation Inhibits NF-κB signalling	RA, SLE, psoriasis
10p15	IL2RA	IL 2 receptor α chain	MS, T1D, SLE, Graves' disease, AAV

AAV, ANCA-associated vasculitis; *AS*, ankylosing spondylitis; *AT*, autoimmune thyroiditis; *CRP*, C-reactive protein; *CTLA-4*, cytotoxic T-lymphocyte-associated protein 4; *FCGR*, Fc gamma receptor; *IBD*, inflammatory bowel disease; *IL*, interleukin; *MHC*, major histocompatibility complex; *MS*, multiple sclerosis; *PARP*, poly-ADP-ribose polymerase; *PDCD1*, programmed cell death 1; *PTPN22*, protein tyrosine phosphatase, non-receptor type 22; *RA*, rheumatoid arthritis; *SLE*, systemic lupus erythematosus; T1D, *type I diabetes mellitus*; *TLR5*, Toll-like receptor 5; *TNFα*, tumour necrosis factor α.

to note that two alleles with contrasting effects on lymphocyte receptor signalling are associated with distinct autoimmune diseases.

Autoimmunity is associated with genes that control lymphocyte activation. Autoimmunity is associated with a multitude of genes encoding molecules expressed by lymphocytes, which modulate co-stimulation signals. These include CD2/CD58 and TNFSF15. A notable example is a single nucleotide polymorphism (SNP) linked to CTLA-4, a molecule present on Tregs (see Chapter 12).

Mutations in the transcriptional autoimmune regulator (*AIRE*) gene are associated with the multi-organ disorder known as autoimmune polyglandular syndrome type 1, characterized by Addison's disease, hypoparathyroidism and type I diabetes mellitus. Deficiency in AIRE inhibits the establishment of self tolerance to a number of organ-specific antigens such as glutamic acid decarboxylase, GAD65, one of the key autoantigens in type 1 diabetes mellitus, by preventing its expression in the thymus. In SLE, variants in the promoter for BLK, which encodes kinases involved in signalling and regulation of the B-cell development (see Fig. 9.6), also associate with disease through alteration in survival and tolerance.

AUTOIMMUNITY AND AUTOIMMUNE DISEASE

Despite the complex selection mechanisms operating to establish self tolerance during lymphocyte development, the body contains large numbers of lymphocytes, which are potentially autoreactive.

Thus, many autoantigens, when injected with adjuvants, induce autoantibodies in normal animals, demonstrating the presence of autoreactive B cells, and it is possible to identify a small number of autoreactive B cells (e.g. anti-thyroglobulin) in the normal population.

Autoreactive T cells are also present in normal individuals, as shown by the fact that it is possible to produce autoimmune lines of T cells by stimulation of normal circulating T cells with the appropriate autoantigen (e.g. myelin basic protein (MBP)) and IL-2.

Autoantibody production alone does not equal autoimmune disease. Healthy individuals may have autoantibodies without clinical disease. Thus, healthy individuals have significant levels of anti-nuclear antibodies (ANAs) whose prevalence in the general population aged over 60 rises to 20%–30%. Transiently positive ANAs may occur following infection. In patients who eventually develop autoimmune disease, autoantibody production may predate clinical disease by years: in one study, autoantibodies preceded the onset of clinical manifestations of lupus by up to 9 years.

The autoantibodies typically appear in a stereotyped order, providing insight into the sequential pathogenic changes that occur as SLE develops. Antinuclear antibodies, antibodies to Ro and antibodies to β_2-glycoprotein 1 appear first; anti-dsDNA antibodies typically appear 1–2 years before symptom onset; antibodies to Sm and RNP appear in the months immediately preceding symptoms. Similarly, rheumatoid factors and anti-CCP antibodies have been identified in the serum of individuals years before they develop clinically overt rheumatoid arthritis.

Progression to autoimmune disease occurs in stages.

Autoimmune diseases thus seem to result from a multistep process. The first stage is predisposition of an individual to autoimmunity by his or her genes and other factors such as female hormones.

The second phase is initiated by an event, probably stochastic or perhaps caused by an environmental trigger such as infection or ultraviolet radiation, leading to loss of self tolerance and autoantibody production. A further step is required before progression to a third phase involving tissue damage by the autoimmune attack. This autoimmune attack leads to further release of self antigens, which are not removed in the normal efficient manner (see later), and propagation of the autoimmune response, resulting in the clinical manifestations of disease.

During the propagation phase, not only is there an autoimmune response to an increasing number of autoantigens (demonstrated by the sequential development of multiple autoantibodies in patients with SLE), but also to more epitopes within each antigen – a phenomenon termed **epitope spread**. Epitope spread can involve multiple epitopes on the same molecule (intramolecular spread) or epitopes on different molecules associated as part of a macromolecular complex (intermolecular spread). The latter provides a mechanism for how antibodies to non-protein self antigens such as DNA and phospholipid can occur.

Autoimmunity results from antigen-driven self-reactive lymphocytes.

The question remains whether autoreactive B cells are stimulated to proliferate and to produce autoantibodies by interaction with autoantigens or by some other means, such as non-specific polyclonal activation or interactions between idiotypes (clone-specific antigenic determinants on the V region of antibody) (Fig. 20.6).

Evidence that B cells are selected by antigen comes from the existence of high-affinity autoantibodies, which arise through somatic mutation, a process that requires both T cells and autoantigen. In addition, patients' serum usually contains autoantibodies directed to epitope clusters occurring on the same autoantigenic molecule. Apart from the presence of autoantigen itself, it is very difficult to envisage a mechanism that could account for the co-existence of antibody responses to

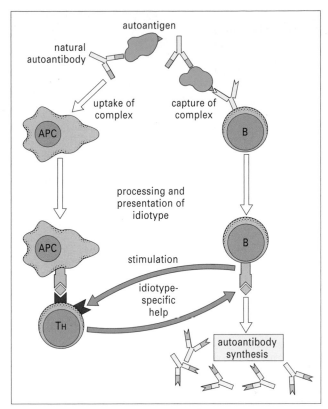

Fig. 20.6 Possible model of T-cell help via processing of intermolecular complexes in the induction of autoimmunity An immune complex consisting of autoantigen (e.g. DNA) and a naturally occurring (germline) autoantibody is taken up by an antigen-presenting cell *(APC)* and peptides derived by processing of the idiotypic segment of the antibody (Id) are presented to T$_H$ cells. B cells that express the pathogenic autoantibody can capture the complex and so can receive T-cell help via presentation of the processed Id to the T$_H$ cell. Similarly, an anti-DNA-specific B cell that had endocytosed a histone–DNA complex could be stimulated to autoantibody production by histone-specific T$_H$ cells.

different epitopes on the same molecule. A similar argument applies to the induction, in a single individual, of autoantibodies to organelles (e.g. nucleosomes and spliceosomes, which appear as blebs on the surface of apoptotic cells) or antigens linked within the same organ (e.g. thyroglobulin and thyroid peroxidase).

The most direct evidence for autoimmunity being antigen-driven comes from studies of the obese strain chicken, which spontaneously develops thyroid autoimmunity. If the thyroid gland (the source of antigen) is removed at birth, the chickens mature without developing thyroid autoantibodies (Fig. 20.7). Furthermore, once thyroid autoimmunity has developed, later removal of the thyroid leads to a gross decline of thyroid autoantibodies, usually to undetectable levels.

Comparable experiments have shown that in the non-obese diabetic (NOD) mouse, which models human autoimmune diabetes, chemical destruction of the β cells leads to decline in pancreatic autoantibodies.

The rate of clearance of any autoreactive B cells is also important. Elevated levels of B-cell activating factor (BAFF) in mouse models promote the survival of autoreactive B cells

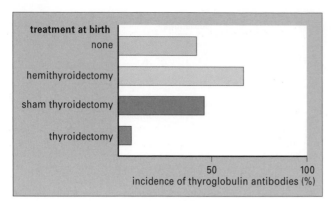

Fig. 20.7 Effect of neonatal thyroidectomy on Obese chickens Because removal of the thyroid at birth prevents the development of thyroid autoantibodies, it would appear that the autoimmune process is driven by the autoantigen in the thyroid gland. (Based on data from de Carvalho P et al. The role of self antigen in the development of autoimmunity in obese strain chickens with spontanoues allergic thyroiditis. J Exp Med 1982;155:1255.)

and elevated levels are also observed in the sera of patients with SLE.

In organ-specific disorders, there is ample evidence for T cells responding to antigens present in the organs under attack. But in non-organ-specific autoimmunity, identification of the antigens recognized by T cells is often inadequate. However, histone-specific T cells are generated in patients with SLE and histone could play a piggyback role in the formation of anti-DNA antibodies by substituting for natural antibody in the mechanism outlined in Figure 20.6.

Another possibility is that the T cells do not 'see' conventional peptide antigen (possibly true of anti-DNA responses) but instead recognize an antibody's idiotype. In this view, SLE, for example, might sometimes be initiated as an idiotypic disease, following the model shown in Figure 20.6. In this scheme, autoantibodies are produced normally at low levels by B cells using germline genes. If these then form complexes with the autoantigen, the complexes can be taken up by antigen-presenting cells (APCs) (including B cells) and components of the complex, including the antibody idiotype, may be presented to T cells. Idiotype-specific T cells would then provide help to the autoantibody-producing B cells.

Evidence for the induction of anti-DNA and glomerulonephritis by immunization of mice with the idiotype of germline 'natural' anti-DNA autoantibody supports this hypothesis.

INDUCTION OF AUTOIMMUNITY

Normally, naive autoreactive T cells recognizing cryptic self epitopes are not switched on because the antigen is presented on 'non-professional' APCs such as pancreatic β-islet cells or thyroid epithelial cells, which lack co-stimulator molecules, or because it is presented only at low concentrations on 'professional' APCs. However, the normal mechanisms that maintain self tolerance may be bypassed.

Molecular mimicry by cross-reactive microbial antigens can stimulate autoreactive lymphocytes. Infection with microbe-bearing antigens that cross-react with the cryptic self epitopes (i.e. have shared epitopes) will load the professional APCs with sufficient levels of processed peptides that can activate the naive autoreactive T cells. Once primed, these T cells are able to recognize and to react with the self epitope on the non-professional APCs because they:

- no longer require a co-stimulatory signal; and
- have a higher avidity for the target, because of upregulation of accessory adhesion molecules (Fig. 20.8).

Cross-reactive antigens that share B-cell epitopes with self molecules can also break tolerance, but by a different mechanism. Many autoreactive B cells cannot be activated because the CD4+ TH cells they need are unresponsive, either because:

- these TH cells are tolerized at lower concentrations of autoantigens than the B cells; or
- because they recognize only cryptic epitopes.

However, these 'helpless' B cells can be stimulated if the cross-reacting antigen bears a 'foreign' carrier epitope to which the T cells have not been tolerized (Fig. 20.9). The autoimmune process may persist after clearance of the foreign antigen if the activated B cells now focus the autoantigen on their surface receptors and present it to normally resting autoreactive T cells, which then proliferate and act as helpers for fresh B-cell stimulation.

Molecular mimicry operates in rheumatic fever. An example of a disease in which such molecular mimicry may operate is rheumatic fever, in which autoantibodies to heart valve antigens can be detected. These develop in a small proportion of individuals several weeks after a streptococcal infection of the throat. Because carbohydrate antigens on the streptococci cross-react

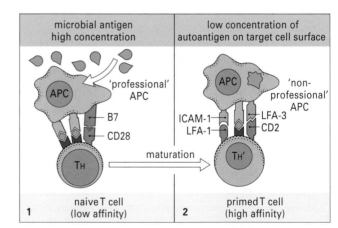

Fig. 20.8 Cross-reactive antigens induce autoimmune TH cells The inability of naive TH cells to recognize autoantigen on a tissue cell, whether because of low concentration or low affinity, can be circumvented by a cross-reacting microbial antigen at higher concentration or with higher innate affinity, together with a co-stimulator such as B7 on a 'professional' antigen-presenting cell (*APC*); this primes the TH cells (**1**). Due to increased expression of accessory molecules (e.g. LFA-1 and CD2), the primed TH cells now have high affinity and, because they do not require a co-stimulatory signal, they can interact with autoantigen on 'non-professional' APCs such as organ-specific epithelial cells to produce autoimmune disease (**2**).

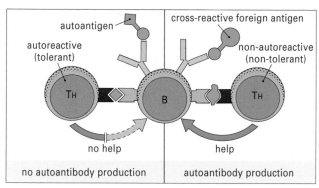

Fig. 20.9 Induction of autoantibodies by cross-reactive antigens The B cell recognizes an epitope present on autoantigen but coincidentally present also on a foreign antigen. Normally the B cell presents the autoantigen but receives no help from autoreactive TH cells, which are functionally deleted. If a cross-reacting foreign antigen is encountered, the B cell can present peptides of this molecule to non-autoreactive T cells and thus be driven to proliferate, differentiate and secrete autoantibodies.

with an antigen on heart valves, the infection may bypass T-cell self tolerance to heart valve antigens. Historically, many concepts about autoimmunity arose because the early immunologists often had a background in infectious diseases and brought with them ideas about cross-reactivity and molecular mimicry extrapolated from rheumatic fever. However, the evidence for molecular mimicry in most chronic autoimmune diseases is lacking or absent. A notable exception is post-infective polyneuropathy (Guillain–Barré syndrome) (see Fig. 24.11).

There is circumstantial evidence for molecular mimicry in antineutrophil cytoplasmic antibody (ANCA)-associated vasculitis (AAV). Antibodies to lysosomal membrane protein-2 (LAMP-2) are a subtype of ANCA found in most patients with pauci-immune focal necrotizing glomerulonephritis (FNGN). The autoantibodies to LAMP-2 commonly recognize an epitope with 100% homology to the bacterial adhesion FimH. Rats injected with FimH develop antibodies to LAMP-2 and pauci-immune FNGN. Furthermore, many humans with pauci-immune FNGN have evidence of recent infection with fimbriated organisms.

In some cases foreign antigen can directly stimulate autoreactive cells.

Another mechanism to bypass the tolerant autoreactive TH cell is where antigen or another stimulator directly triggers the autoreactive effector cells.

For example, lipopolysaccharide or Epstein–Barr virus causes direct B-cell stimulation and some of the clones of activated cells will produce autoantibodies, although in the absence of T-cell help these are normally of low titre and affinity. However, it is conceivable that an activated B cell might pick up and process its cognate autoantigen and present it to a naive autoreactive T cell.

Infection may trigger relapse in autoimmune disease.

Many autoimmune diseases have a relapsing–remitting phenotype, characterized by periods of disease activity punctuated by periods of quiescence. This relapsing–remitting phenotype suggests there are varying influences on the autoimmune process. Clinical observation suggests that infections appear to trigger

increased autoimmune disease activity, although precise mechanisms are unclear. In Wegener's granulomatosis, relapses are closely correlated with recent infection and chronic *Staphylococcus aureus* nasal carriage is linked with more frequent relapses of upper respiratory tract disease.

The 'waste disposal' hypothesis of SLE. Antibodies to nuclear components are the serological hallmark of SLE. The question arising from this observation is how nuclear components normally hidden are detected by the immune system as antigen. The answer appears to lie with apoptosis. There is strong evidence that SLE, and possibly other autoimmune diseases, are diseases of failure of clearance of apoptotic cells, i.e. due to decreased macrophage 'scavenger' function. When a cell undergoes apoptosis (programmed cell death), blebs of cellular material are formed on the cell surface. Antigens normally buried deep within the cell (and therefore not detected by the immune system) are exposed on the cell surface. In healthy individuals, these apoptotic cells are efficiently cleared. However, in SLE, apoptosis is defective; it has been demonstrated that scavenging of apoptotic debris in vitro by macrophages from lupus patients is less efficient than by macrophages from healthy controls. Thus, the antigens contained within the apoptotic blebs may trigger an autoimmune response in systemic autoimmune diseases such as SLE, Sjögren's syndrome and myositis (Fig. 20.10).

A defective complement pathway may also contribute to ineffective clearance of apoptotic cells as C1q binds to cell debris, allowing macrophages with C1q receptors to engulf the apoptotic cells. Complement deficiency in SLE is usually attributed to consumption as a secondary consequence of immune complex formation. However, it is clear that in a very small number of patients complement deficiency is

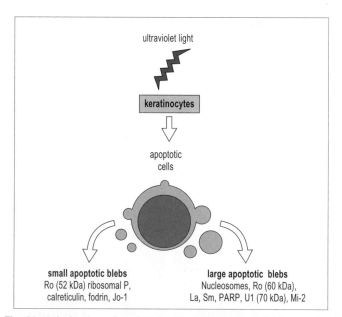

Fig. 20.10 Induction of surface blebs during apoptosis Apoptosis of keratinocytes exposed to ultraviolet light is illustrated. The different constituents of developing small and large surface blebs during apoptosis are shown. *PARP*, Poly-ADP-ribose polymerase. (Based on Rahman A, Isenberg DA. Systemic lupus erythematosus. N Engl J Med 2008;358:929–939.)

the cause rather than the effect of SLE. In patients with these rare genetic disorders of deficiency of complement components (including C1q, C2 and C4, as discussed previously), there is a hugely increased risk of developing a lupus-like disease. Reduced clearance of immune complexes by the spleen has been demonstrated in a patient with C2 deficiency and SLE. This problem was correctable with transfusions of fresh-frozen plasma containing C2. The C1q knock-out mouse also provides evidence for the role of complement in clearance of apoptotic cells. This mouse develops a lupus-like glomerulonephritis and renal biopsy reveals multiple apoptotic fragments.

Cytokine dysregulation, inappropriate MHC expression and failure of suppression may induce autoimmunity.

Dysregulation of the cytokine network can also lead to activation of autoreactive T cells and, as noted earlier, genes affecting cytokines and their receptors (e.g. IL-2RA) are implicated in autoimmune disease by genome-wide association studies.

Consider the introduction of a transgene for interferon-γ (IFNγ) into pancreatic β-islet cells. If the transgene for IFNγ is fully expressed in the cells, MHC class II genes are upregulated and autoimmune destruction of the islet cells results. This is not simply a result of a non-specific chaotic IFNγ-induced local inflammatory milieu because normal islets grafted at a separate site are rejected, implying clearly that T-cell autoreactivity to the pancreas has been established.

The surface expression of MHC class II in itself is not sufficient to activate the naive autoreactive T cells, but it may be necessary to allow a cell to act as a target for the primed autoreactive TH cells. It was therefore most exciting when cells taken from the glands of patients with Graves' disease were found to be actively synthesizing class II MHC molecules (Fig. 20.11) and therefore could be recognized by CD4+ T cells.

Thus, it is interesting that isolated cells from several animal strains that are susceptible to autoimmunity are also more readily induced by IFNγ to express MHC class II molecules than cells from non-susceptible strains.

The argument that imbalanced cytokine production may also contribute to autoimmunity receives further support from the unexpected finding that tumour necrosis factor (TNF; introduced by means of a TNF transgene) ameliorates the spontaneous SLE-like disease of F$_1$ (NZB × NZW) mice. Furthermore, serological (and less commonly clinical) features of SLE have developed in humans treated with TNF blockade.

Aside from the normal 'ignorance' of cryptic self epitopes, other factors that normally restrain potentially autoreactive cells may include:

- regulatory T cells;
- hormones (e.g. steroids);
- cytokines (e.g. transforming growth factor-β (TGFβ)); and
- products of macrophages.

Deficiencies in any of these factors may increase susceptibility to autoimmunity.

The feedback loop on TH cells and macrophages through the pituitary–adrenal axis is particularly interesting because defects at different stages in the loop appear in a variety of autoimmune disorders (Fig. 20.12).

For example, patients with rheumatoid arthritis have low circulating corticosteroid levels compared with controls. After surgery, although they produce copious amounts of IL-1 and IL-6, a defect in the hypothalamic paraventricular nucleus prevents the expected increase in adrenocorticotrophic hormone (ACTH) and adrenal steroid output.

There is currently intense interest focused on the role of Tregs. Patients with rheumatoid arthritis, for example, have a deficiency of Treg function (see later).

A subset of CD4 regulatory cells present in young healthy mice of the NOD strain, which spontaneously develop IDDM, can prevent the transfer of disease provoked by injection of

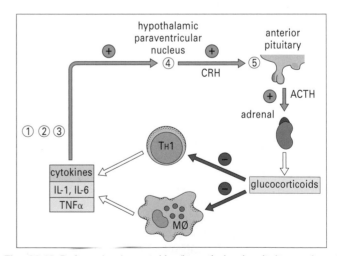

Fig. 20.12 Defects in the cytokine/hypothalamic–pituitary–adrenal feedback loop in autoimmunity Production of IL-1 is defective in the NOD mouse *(1)* and diabetes-prone BB rat *(2)*; the disease can be corrected by injection of the cytokine. The same is true for the production of TNFα by the NZB × W lupus mouse *(3)*. Patients with rheumatoid arthritis have a poor hypothalamic response to IL-1 and IL-6 *(4)*. The hypothalamic–pituitary axis is defective in the Obese strain chicken and in the Lewis rat, which is prone to the development of Freund adjuvant-mediated experimental autoimmune disease *(5)*. *ATCH*, Adrenocorticotrophic hormone; *CRH*, corticotrophin-releasing hormone; *MØ*, macrophage, *NOD*, non-obese diabetic.

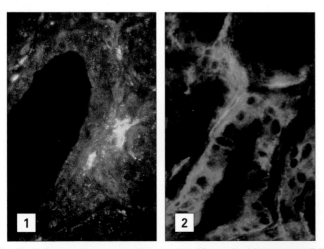

Fig. 20.11 Human thyroid sections stained for major histocompatibility complex (MHC) class II (1) Normal thyroid with unstained follicular cells and an isolated dendritic cell that is strongly positive for MHC class II. **(2)** Thyrotoxic (Graves' disease) thyroid with abundant MHC class II molecules in the cytoplasm, indicating that rapid synthesis of MHC class II molecules is occurring.

spleen cells from diabetic animals into NOD mice congenic for the severe combined immunodeficiency (SCID) trait; this regulatory subset is lost in older mice.

Pre-existing defects in the target organ may increase susceptibility to autoimmunity. Target cells are sensitive to upregulation of MHC class II molecules by IFNγ in animals susceptible to certain autoimmune diseases. Other evidence also favours the view that there may be a pre-existing defect in the target organ. For example:

- diabetes mellitus, in which one of the genetic risk factors is linked to a transcription factor controlling the rate of insulin production; and
- rheumatoid arthritis, in which the agalacto IgG glycoform is abnormally abundant.

The post-translational modification of arginine to citrulline, producing a new autoantigen in rheumatoid arthritis, represents yet another mechanism by which autoimmunity can be evoked.

AUTOIMMUNE PROCESSES AND PATHOLOGY

Autoimmune processes are often pathogenic. When autoantibodies are found in association with a particular disease, there are three possible inferences:

- the autoimmunity is responsible for producing the lesions of the disease;
- there is a disease process that, through the production of tissue damage, leads to the development of autoantibodies;
- there is a factor that produces both the lesions and the autoimmunity.

Autoantibodies secondary to a lesion (the second possibility) are sometimes found. For example, cardiac autoantibodies may develop after myocardial infarction.

However, sustained production of autoantibodies rarely follows the release of autoantigens by simple trauma. In most diseases associated with autoimmunity, the evidence supports the first possibility, that the autoimmune process produces the lesions.

Human autoantibodies can be directly pathogenic. There is much evidence to suggest that autoantibodies may be important in pathogenesis, as discussed later.

Autoantibodies can give rise to a wide spectrum of clinical thyroid dysfunction. Several diseases have been recognized in which autoantibodies to hormone receptors may actually mimic the function of the normal hormone and produce disease. Graves' disease (thyrotoxicosis) was the first disorder in which such **anti-receptor antibodies** were recognized.

The phenomenon of neonatal thyrotoxicosis provides us with a natural passive transfer study, because IgG antibodies from the thyrotoxic mother cross the placenta and react directly with the thyroid-stimulating hormone (TSH) receptor on the neonatal thyroid. Many babies born to thyrotoxic mothers and showing thyroid hyperactivity have been reported, but the problem spontaneously resolves as the antibodies derived from the mother are catabolized in the baby over several weeks.

Whereas autoantibodies to the TSH receptor may stimulate cell division and/or increase the production of thyroid hormones, others can bring about the opposite effect by inhibiting these functions, a phenomenon frequently observed in receptor responses to ligands that act as agonists or antagonists.

Different combinations of the various manifestations of thyroid autoimmune disease (chronic inflammatory cell destruction and stimulation or inhibition of growth and thyroid hormone synthesis) can give rise to a wide spectrum of clinical thyroid dysfunction (Table 20.3).

TABLE 20.3 The Spectrum of Autoimmune Thyroid Disease

Thyroid disease	Thyroid destruction	CELL DIVISION		THYROID HORMONE SYNTHESIS	
		Stimulation	Inhibition	Stimulation	Inhibition
Hashimoto's thyroiditis	■				
Hashimoto's persistent goitre	■	■			
Autoimmune colloid goitre		■			
Graves' disease		■		■	
Non-goitrous hyperthyroidism				■	
'Hashitoxicosis'	■			■	
Primary myxoedema	■		■		■

TSH, Thyroid-stimulating hormone.
Responses involving thyroglobulin and the thyroid peroxidase (microsomal) surface microvillous antigen lead to tissue destruction, whereas autoantibodies to TSH receptors can stimulate or block metabolic activity or thyroid cell division. Hashitoxicosis is an unconventional term that describes a gland showing Hashimoto's thyroiditis and Graves' disease simultaneously.

A variety of other diseases are associated with autoantibodies. Myasthenia gravis provides an example of a disease where some of the autoantibodies can act as a receptor antagonist, blocking the acetylcholine receptor on the post-synaptic membrane of the neuromuscular junction, thus causing muscle weakness and fatigability. A parallel with neonatal hyperthyroidism has been observed – **antibodies to acetylcholine receptors** from mothers who have myasthenia gravis cross the placenta into the fetus and may cause transient muscle weakness in the newborn baby.

A similar phenomenon, the neonatal lupus syndrome, is seen in 5% of women who have anti-Ro antibodies (found in both SLE and Sjögren's syndrome). These antibodies can cross the placenta into the fetal circulation, causing heart-block and/or transient lupus-like rash in the neonate, providing direct evidence of their pathogenicity.

Somewhat rarely, **autoantibodies to insulin receptors and to α-adrenergic receptors** can be found, the latter associated with bronchial asthma.

Neuromuscular defects can be elicited in mice injected with serum containing **antibodies to presynaptic calcium channels** from patients with the Lambert–Eaton syndrome, while **sodium channel autoantibodies** have been identified in Guillain–Barré syndrome.

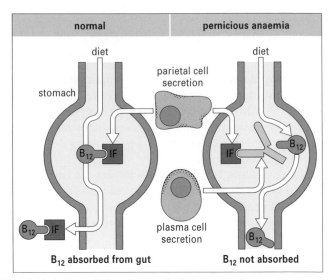

Fig. 20.13 Failure of vitamin B_{12} *(B_{12})* absorption in pernicious anaemia Normally, dietary vitamin B_{12} is absorbed by the small intestine complexed with intrinsic factor *(IF)*, which is synthesized by parietal cells in gastric mucosa. In pernicious anaemia, locally synthesized autoantibodies, specific for intrinsic factor, combine with intrinsic factor to inhibit its role as a carrier for vitamin B_{12}.

In pernicious anaemia an autoantibody interferes with the normal uptake of vitamin B_{12}. Vitamin B_{12} is not absorbed directly but must first associate with a protein called intrinsic factor; the vitamin–protein complex is then transported across the intestinal mucosa.

Early passive transfer studies demonstrated that serum from a patient with pernicious anaemia (PA), if fed to a healthy individual together with intrinsic factor–B_{12} complex, inhibited uptake of the vitamin.

Subsequently, the factor in the serum that blocked vitamin uptake was identified as **antibody against intrinsic factor**. It is now known that plasma cells in the gastric mucosa of patients with PA secrete this antibody into the lumen of the stomach (Fig. 20.13).

Antibodies to the glomerular capillary basement membrane cause Goodpasture's disease. Goodpasture's disease is characterized clinically by rapidly progressive glomerulonephritis and pulmonary haemorrhage. Patients with Goodpasture's disease have circulating **antibodies to the glomerular capillary basement membrane** (GBM), which bind to the kidney and lung (see Fig. 25.15). Evidence for the direct pathogenicity of these antibodies was demonstrated by the passive transfer of antibodies eluted from renal biopsy specimens into primates (whose renal antigens were similar to humans). The injected monkeys subsequently died from glomerulonephritis. Subsequent work has shown that these antibodies bind to the several non-collagenous-1 (NC-1) domains of type IV collagen in the GBM. Moreover, immunization of animals with NC-1 domains induces glomerulonephritis, providing a causal link between autoantigen and antibody.

Blood and vascular disorders caused by autoantibodies include AHA and ITP. Autoimmune haemolytic anaemia (AHA) and idiopathic thrombocytopenic purpura (ITP) result from the synthesis of **autoantibodies to red cells and platelets**, respectively.

The primary antiphospholipid syndrome characterized by recurrent thromboembolic phenomena and fetal loss is triggered by the reaction of autoantibodies with a complex of β₂-glycoprotein 1 and cardiolipin.

The β₂-glycoprotein is an abundant component of atherosclerotic plaques and autoimmunity may initiate or exacerbate the process of lipid deposition and plaque formation in this disease, the two lead candidate antigens being **heat-shock protein 60** (Fig. 20.14) and the low-density lipoprotein, **apoprotein B**.

Immune complexes appear to be pathogenic in systemic autoimmunity. In SLE, it can be shown that complement-fixing complexes of antibody with DNA and other nucleosome components such as histones are deposited in the kidney, skin, joints and choroid plexus of patients and must be presumed to produce type III hypersensitivity reactions as outlined in Chapter 25. A variety of different antibodies have been eluted from the kidney biopsies of patients with SLE. These include anti-dsDNA (nucleosomes), anti-Ro and anti-Sm/RNP. Whilst placing these antibodies at the scene of the crime, their mere presence does not prove they 'pulled the trigger'. However, experiments using murine monoclonal anti-dsDNA antibodies in a rat kidney perfusion system, and other evidence from the use of human hybridoma derived anti-dsDNA antibodies in SCID mice, provide compelling

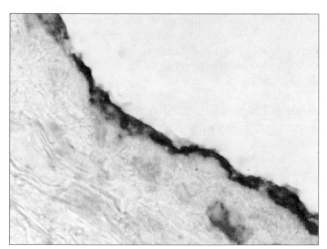

Fig. 20.14 Upregulation of heat-shock protein 60 (Hsp60) in endothelial cells at a site of haemodynamic stress Hsp60 expression *(red)* co-localized with intercellular adhesion molecule-1 (ICAM-1) expression *(black)* by endothelial cells and cells in the intima (macrophages) at the bifurcation of the carotid artery of a 5-month-old child. × 240. (Courtesy Professor G Wick.)

evidence that some anti-dsDNA antibodies are genuinely pathogenic.

It has been proposed that anti-dsDNA/nucleosome antibodies bind to the negatively charged surface of the renal glomerulus via a histone (positively charged) 'bridge'. The histone is part of the nucleosome complex. The formation of immune complexes at the glomerular surface membrane is thought to induce an inflammatory response, leading to the kidney damage frequently seen in patients with SLE, although the precise mechanisms have yet to be elucidated.

Autoantibodies to IgG provoke pathological damage in rheumatoid arthritis. The erosions of cartilage and bone in rheumatoid arthritis are mediated by macrophages and fibroblasts, which become stimulated by cytokines from activated T cells and immune complexes generated by a vigorous immunological reaction within the synovial tissue (Fig. 20.15).

The complexes can arise through the self-association of IgG rheumatoid factors specific for the Fcγ domains – a process facilitated by the striking deficiency of terminal galactose on the biantennary N-linked Fc oligosaccharides (Fig. 20.16). This agalacto glycoform of IgG in complexes can exacerbate inflammation through reaction with mannose-binding lectin and production of TNFα.

Evidence for directly pathogenic T cells in human autoimmune disease is hard to obtain. Adoptive transfer studies have shown that Th1 cells are responsible for directly initiating the lesions in experimental models of organ-specific autoimmunity.

In humans, evidence for a pivotal role of T cells in the development of autoimmune disease includes:

- the production of high-affinity, somatically mutated IgG autoantibodies characteristic of T-dependent responses;
- the isolation of thyroid-specific T-cell clones from the glands of patients with Graves' disease;

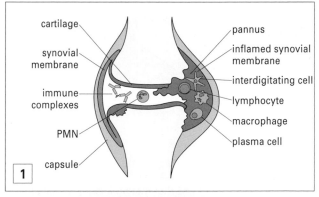

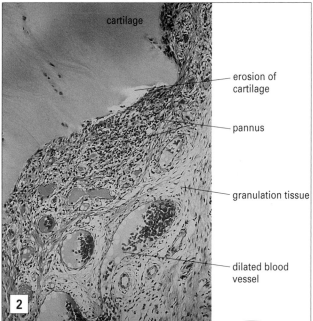

Fig. 20.15 Pathology of rheumatoid arthritis In the rheumatoid arthritis joint, an inflammatory infiltrate is found in the synovial membrane, which hypertrophies, forming a pannus (**1** and **2**). This covers and eventually erodes the synovial cartilage and bone. Immune complexes and neutrophils (polymorphonuclear leukocytes *(PMNs)*) are detectable in the joint space and in the extra-articular tissues where they may give rise to vasculitic lesions and subcutaneous nodules. (Histological section reproduced from Woolf N. Pathology: Basic and Systemic. London: WB Saunders; 1998.)

- the beneficial effect of ciclosporin in pre-diabetic individuals; and
- the close associations with certain HLA haplotypes.

However, it is difficult to identify a role for the T cell as a pathogenic agent as distinct from a Th function in the organ-specific disorders.

The central role of Th1 cells in some autoimmune diseases has been challenged. Many autoimmune diseases such as rheumatoid arthritis (RA) were thought to be primarily driven by Th1 cells. Initially, the proposal to use rituximab (a monoclonal antibody against the CD20 molecule which is expressed on B cells but not plasma cells) in rheumatoid arthritis was met with great scepticism. However, rituximab's success in the treatment of RA has emphasized that B cells play a key

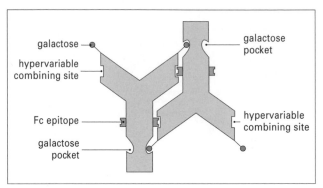

Fig. 20.16 Self-associated IgG rheumatoid factors forming immune complexes The binding between the Fab on one IgG rheumatoid factor and the Fc of another involves the hypervariable region of the combining site. As it has been established that the Fab oligosaccharides, which occur on approximately one in three different immunoglobulin molecules, are not defective with respect to glycosylation in rheumatoid arthritis, a Fab galactose residue could become inserted in the Fc pocket left vacant by a galactose-deficient Cγ2 oligosaccharide, increasing the strength of intermolecular binding. The stability and inflammatory potency of these complexes is increased by binding IgM rheumatoid factor and Clq.

role its pathogenesis and has led some to doubt that RA is TH1 driven. However, the precise mechanisms by which B-cell depletion has a therapeutic effect are unclear. B cells are more than simply precursors to antibody-producing plasma cells – they also act as APCs, interacting with T cells in several ways. Thus, rituximab's efficacy in RA cannot necessarily be used as proof that T cells are not important in its pathogenesis.

The role of TH17 cells. Recent interest has focused on the role of TH17 cells in autoimmunity. Their initial discovery came about when it was noted that deletion of key TH1 molecules such as IL-12 and IFNγR did not abrogate EAE and collagen-induced arthritis (CIA) in mice. In fact, these animals showed enhanced susceptibility, casting doubt on the role of TH1 cells as the fundamental players in autoimmunity. This led to the identification of a new cytokine IL-23: knockout of IL-23 is protective against experimentally induced autoimmunity and IL-23 was subsequently shown to induce IL-17 from activated T cells. Such IL-23-driven TH cells show a unique pattern of gene expression (which differs from that of IL-12-driven TH1 cells) and are now known to be TH17 cells. Whereas TGFβ, IL-1β and IL-6, but not IL-23, are the key cytokines for the induction of TH17 cells, IL-23 is important for their maintenance; IL-23-deficient mice show normal numbers of TH1 cells but a reduction in TH17 cells. Tregs also play an important role here; the balance of Tregs to TH17 cells appears to be involved in the loss of tolerance as Treg defects have been reported in patients with SLE.

In humans, high levels of IL-17 and its receptor are found in the synovial fluid and tissue of patients with RA. However, the number of TH17 cells is not elevated in the synovial fluid or peripheral blood mononuclear cells (PBMCs) with RA compared with healthy controls. Multiple SNPs in the IL-23 receptor

gene region, as well as other genes involved in the IL-23/TH17 pathway, are associated with inflammatory bowel disease. The results of trials of anti-IL-17 monoclonal antibodies in patients with RA and MS will help clarify the role of TH17 cells in these diseases.

The role of Tregs in autoimmune disease. Dysregulated function and numbers of Tregs have been reported in several autoimmune diseases, including type I diabetes, multiple sclerosis, rheumatoid arthritis and SLE. Mice with a mutation in the FOXp3 gene that leads to the absence of Tregs display a lupus-like disease and, interestingly, have antibodies seen in SLE (ANA, anti Sm and anti dsDNA). This suggests that absence or dysregulation of Tregs can result in B-cell dysfunction. Scalapino and colleagues demonstrated control by Tregs in lupus-prone B/W mice: restoring Treg populations reduced autoantibody production and hence delayed disease progression. In addition, they modulated APCs by expressing inhibitory CTLA-4, which interfered with co-stimulatory signals from CD80/CD86 essential for T-cell activation. Treatments for SLE, including methyl-prednisolone and the B-cell depleting agent rituximab (anti-CD20), increase Treg numbers and function transiently.

The role of regulatory B cells in autoimmune disease. The term 'regulatory' B cells was first coined in 2002 by Mizoguchi et al., who found that B cells secreting IL-10 had a suppressive role in colitis. Several mouse models of autoimmune disease have demonstrated a role for Bregs, including NOD mice in type I diabetes, multiple sclerosis, RA and SLE. An increase of regulatory B cells has been reported in the peripheral blood of patients with SLE; however, their function is thought to be impaired. In RA patients, there is a negative correlation between Bregs and disease severity, lending evidence to the hypothesis of a suppressive role.

AUTOANTIBODIES FOR DIAGNOSIS, PROGNOSIS AND MONITORING

Autoantibodies frequently provide valuable markers for diagnostic purposes. A particularly good example is the test for mitochondrial antibodies, used in diagnosing primary biliary cirrhosis (Fig. 20.17). Other examples include:

- Antibodies to cyclic citrullinated peptides (CCP) in the diagnosis of RA.
- The presence of anti-nuclear antibodies is one of the revised ACR criteria for SLE but is non-specific. In contrast, anti-dsDNA antibodies (also an ACR criterion) are highly specific for SLE, but only present in 60%–70% of SLE patients and in less than 0.5% of controls. Anti-Sm antibodies are highly lupus specific and found in 10% of Caucasian and 30% of Afro-Caribbean SLE patients; like dsDNA antibodies, they have a high specificity for SLE.
- Autoantibodies may have predictive value. For instance, individuals testing positively for antibodies to both insulin and glutamic acid decarboxylase have a high risk of developing type I diabetes mellitus.

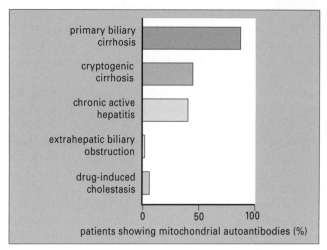

Fig. 20.17 Diagnostic value of anti-mitochondrial antibodies Mitochondrial antibody tests using indirect immunofluorescence, together with percutaneous liver biopsy, can be used to assist in the differential diagnosis of these diseases. Many patients with primary biliary cirrhosis, but less than half of patients with cryptogenic cirrhosis or chronic active hepatitis, have anti-mitochondrial antibodies. The antibodies are rare in the other diseases.

Prognosis and disease subtype:

- In rheumatoid arthritis, CCP antibodies are associated with a poor prognosis and predict erosive disease.
- Within the context of SLE, specific autoantibodies are associated with specific disease manifestations. For example, anti-La antibodies are associated with features of Sjögren's syndrome; anticardiolipin antibodies and anti-β_2-glycoprotein 1 antibodies with thrombosis and miscarriage; anti-dsDNA antibodies with glomerulonephritis; anti-RNP with pulmonary hypertension; and anti-Ro with photosensitivity and the neonatal lupus syndrome.

Disease monitoring:

- Anti-dsDNA antibodies can be used as a measure of disease activity in SLE. A rising titre of anti-dsDNA antibodies often heralds a disease flare, especially if accompanied by a falling C3 level, and should prompt the clinician to monitor the patient more frequently.
- Similarly, a rising ANCA titre may indicate impending relapse in AAV. However, the association between ANCA titre and disease activity in AAV is much less robust than that between anti-dsDNA antibody titre and lupus activity.

TREATMENT OF AUTOIMMUNE DISEASES

Many autoimmune diseases can be treated successfully. Often, in organ-specific autoimmune disorders, the symptoms can be corrected by metabolic control. For example:

- hypothyroidism by administration of thyroxine;
- type I diabetes mellitus by administration of insulin;
- in pernicious anaemia, metabolic correction is achieved by injection of vitamin B_{12};

- in myasthenia gravis by administration of cholinesterase inhibitors.

If the target organ is not completely destroyed, it may be possible to protect the surviving cells by transfection with *FasL* or *TGFβ* genes.

Where function is completely lost and cannot be substituted by hormones, as may occur in lupus nephritis or chronic rheumatoid arthritis, tissue grafts or mechanical substitutes may be appropriate. In the case of tissue grafts, protection from the immunological processes that necessitated the transplant may be required.

Conventional immunosuppressive therapy with anti-mitotic drugs at high doses can be used to damp down the immune response, but, because of the dangers involved, tends to be used only in organ or life-threatening disorders such as SLE, myositis and AAV. Advances in treatment have transformed the 5-year survival rate in severe systemic autoimmune diseases such as SLE and AAV from around 50% and less than 10%, respectively, in the mid-20th century to over 90% today. However, the cost of this success in controlling autoimmune disease activity includes the adverse effects of immunosuppressants, especially glucocorticoids. Most of the early mortality in SLE or AAV is now a result of infection secondary to immunosuppressive therapy rather than uncontrolled autoimmune disease. Drugs such as cyclophosphamide and azathioprine may cause bone marrow dysfunction. The challenge now is to minimize treatment toxicity. This is likely to be achieved through several means. First, the rational design of targeted therapies (in contrast to the 'shotgun' approach of non-specific cytotoxics such as cyclophosphamide) should reduce the toxicity of treatment regimes. Second, it should become possible to identify patients through means of biomarkers in whom immunosuppression can be safely reduced. Some such biomarkers have already been identified but require further validation before translation into clinical practice. For example, CD8$^+$ T-cell transcription signatures from blood samples taken at time of diagnosis in patients with AAV and SLE identify subgroups of patients with high and low risk of subsequent relapse.

Biologics: key players in the treatment of autoimmune disease. The most recent treatments for autoimmune disease are therapeutic antibodies (see Figs 10.18 and 10.19) that target individual elements of the immune system, including:

- TNFα and IL-6 in rheumatoid arthritis;
- B cells in several autoimmune diseases (RA, SLE, AAV);
- co-stimulatory interactions in rheumatoid arthritis;
- small molecules that inhibit intracellular signalling pathways such as inhibitors of the JAK-STAT pathway
- trans-endothelial migration in multiple sclerosis (Fig. 20.18).

The treatment of patients with rheumatoid arthritis has been revolutionized by the introduction of biological agents (biologics). Infliximab, a murine-human chimeric antibody against TNFα, not only markedly alleviates the symptoms of RA such as joint pain, stiffness and swelling, but also halts the progression of joint destruction (Fig. 20.19). A number of other anti-TNF agents have subsequently become available,

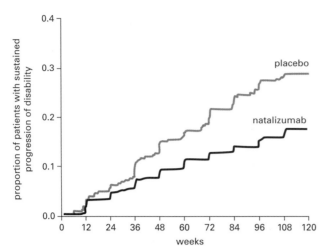

Fig. 20.18 Treatment of multiple sclerosis with antibody to α4β1-integrin A group of patients with relapsing–remitting multiple sclerosis were treated for 2 years with antibody to α4β1-integrin (natalizumab), which interferes with leukocyte migration. The rate of disease progression (disability score) was compared with a placebo-treated group. (Data from Polman et al. N Engl J Med 2006;354:899–910.)

including adalimumab (a fully humanized monoclonal antibody against TNF), etanercept (a soluble TNF receptor), certolizumab (a pegylated anti-TNF antibody) and golimumab (humanized monoclonal antibody against TNF). It is fascinating to record that the compromised regulatory T-cell function in the patients is reversed by such therapy (Fig. 20.w4). Similarly impressive results in RA are seen with B-cell depletion using rituximab, an anti-CD20 monoclonal antibody, and

tocilizumab, a monoclonal antibody against IL-6. Other biologics licensed for use in RA include abatacept, which inhibits the co-stimulatory interaction between T cells and APCs, and anakinra, an IL-1 blocker. More recently, inhibitors of the janus kinase (JAK)/signal transducers and activators of transcription (STAT) signal transduction pathway have been licensed in RA. Tofacitinib inhibits the JAK1 and JAK 3 pathways, whereas baricitinib inhibits JAK1 and 2. These drugs block the continuous activation of this pathway and thereby reducing aberrant cytokine signalling, MMP (matrix metalloproteinase) gene expression and apoptosis, resulting in an overall reduction in inflammation.

Biologic agents have also become key players in the treatment of psoriasis, psoriatic arthritis and axial spondyloarthropathies. Although there is as yet no discernible autoantibody in these conditions, regulation of the T-cell axis appears to ameliorate disease. The IL-12/23 axis has been targeted through ustekinumab, with positive effects on both joints and the skin. Similarly, secukinumab, a monoclonal antibody that binds to IL-17a, has shown efficacy in both psoriasis and AS by inhibiting the pathogenic effects of IL-17 produced by TH17 cells.

Rituximab has shown notable efficacy across the spectrum of autoimmune disease from ITP to multiple sclerosis. Randomized controlled trials show that it has equivalent efficacy to cyclophosphamide in AAV. It is particularly useful in patients with AAV who are refractory to cyclophosphamide treatment. Rituximab treatment results in reduction of the titre of the pathogenic anti-neutrophil cytoplasmic antibodies. Despite initial encouraging results from uncontrolled series, two randomized

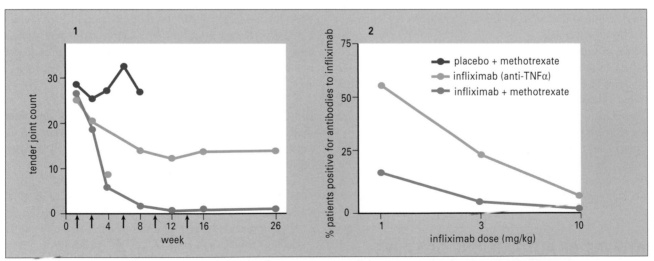

Fig. 20.19 Synergy of anti-TNFα and methotrexate in the treatment of rheumatoid arthritis (1) Infusions were given at times indicated by the arrows. Median joint scores were more effectively reduced by a combination of anti-TNFα with methotrexate, which **(2)** eliminated the anti-idiotypic response to infliximab (a humanized anti-TNFα monoclonal antibody). (Data reproduced from Maini RN, et al. Arthritis Rheum 1998;41:1552, with permission of the authors and publishers.)

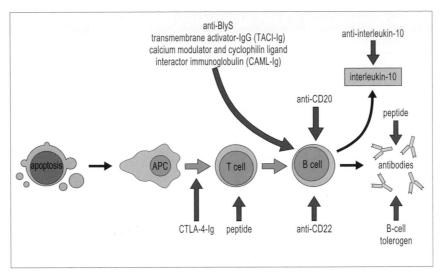

Fig. 20.20 Targeted therapeutic approaches in systemic lupus erythematosus This simplified diagram, which is based on our increased understanding of the immunologic events thought to occur in lupus, indicates the targets of current therapeutic interventions. *APC*, Antigen-presenting cell; *BlyS*, B-lymphocyte stimulator; *CAML*, calcium modulator and cyclophilin ligand; *CTLA-4-Ig*, cytotoxic T-lymphocyte-associated protein 4 IgG1; *TACI-Ig*, transmembrane activator and CAML interactor immunoglobulin. (Based on Rahman A, Isenberg DA. Systemic lupus erythematosus. N Engl J Med 2008;358:929–939.)

controlled trials did not demonstrate benefit from rituximab in SLE. The reasons for this have been widely debated in the literature and this may be accounted for by poor trial design. More recently, data from 270 SLE patients on biologics (261 on rituximab) between 2010 and 2015 showed a reduction in disease activity indices.

Belimumab, which targets the B-cell survival factor BAFF (also known as BLyS), has, in contrast to rituximab, demonstrated efficacy in SLE in two randomized trials. In the future, the combination of an anti-CD20 agent such as rituximab with anti-BLyS therapy using belimumab may produce longer-lasting disease remission.

Less well-established approaches to treatment may become practicable. As we understand more about the molecular mechanisms underlying autoimmunity, targeted therapy is becoming increasingly possible (Fig. 20.20):
- Several centres are trying out autologous stem cell transplantation after haematoimmunoablation with cytotoxic drugs for patients with severe SLE and vasculitis.
- Repeated injection of Cop 1 (a random copolymer of alanine, glutamic acid, lysine and tyrosine) reduces relapse rate in relapsing–remitting multiple sclerosis. Cop 1 was originally designed to simulate the postulated 'guilty' autoantigen, MBP, and induce experimental autoimmune

encephalitis; paradoxically it had the opposite effect. This suggests it is possible to achieve antigen-specific immune suppression.
- Eculizumab, a monoclonal antibody against complement component C5, has been used successfully in paroxysmal nocturnal haemoglobinuria. It may prove effective in SLE.
- Inhibiting key cytokines in the development of disease may still have a role. Initial studies of IFNα inhibition did not show a benefit, but drugs such as anifrolumab (blocks the type I interferon receptor) are still in development.
- Restoring the balance of regulatory cells may play a role as selectively increasing Breg or Tregs could be a strategy to enhance immune regulation.
- Regulation of the TH1 and TH17 pathways may prove pivotal in autoimmune disease.
- Depletion of long-lasting plasma cells through proteasome inhibitors, which enhance the accumulation of unfolded proteins and promote apoptotic cell death, such as bortezomib, has proved successful in some patients.

Targeting immune checkpoints is currently a strategy mainly used in cancer treatments, but may be applicable to certain immune-mediated disease.

The prospects for these new treatments either individually or in combination with therapeutic antibodies are very positive.

CRITICAL THINKING: AUTOIMMUNITY AND AUTOIMMUNE DISEASE

See Critical thinking: Explanations, section 20

Miss Jacob, a 30-year-old Caribbean woman, was seen in a rheumatology clinic with stiff painful joints in her hands, which were worse first thing in the morning. Other symptoms included fatigue, a low-grade fever, a weight loss of 2 kg and some mild chest pain. Miss Jacob had recently returned to the UK from a holiday in Jamaica and was also noted to be taking the combined oral contraceptive pill. Past medical history of note was a mild autoimmune haemolytic anaemia 2 years previously.

On examination, Miss Jacob had a non-specific maculopapular rash on her face and chest and patchy alopecia (hair loss) over her scalp. Her mouth was tender and examination revealed an ulcer on the soft palate. She had moderately swollen and tender proximal interphalangeal joints. Her other joints were unaffected, but she had generalized muscle aches. The results of investigations are shown in the table.

Investigation	Result
Radiograph of hands	Soft tissue swelling, but no bone erosions
Chest radiograph	A small pleural effusion at the right lung base
Full blood count	A mild normocytic, normochromic anaemia and mild lymphocytopenia
C-reactive protein levels	Normal
Erythrocyte sedimentation rate	Raised
Rheumatoid factor	Negative

Serum IgG levels	Raised
Anti-nuclear antibodies (ANA)	Positive by immunofluorescence
Anti-double-stranded DNA, anti-RNA and anti-histone	Positive by ELISA antibodies
Complement (C3 and C4) levels	Low
Skin biopsy from an area unaffected by the rash	Deposition of IgG and complement components at the junction between dermis and epidermis (lupus band test)

A diagnosis of SLE was made. Miss Jacob was treated with hydroxychloroquine, an anti-malarial drug, for the rash and the arthritis.

At a follow-up appointment, urinalysis showed protein and red cells. Serum creatinine was mildly elevated as was her blood pressure. A renal biopsy showed membranous lupus nephritis. She was prescribed oral corticosteroids, mycophenolate mofetil and an angiotensin-converting enzyme (ACE) inhibitor, which improved her renal function and blood pressure. Her physician also gave advice regarding birth control and pregnancy and regular check-ups were arranged.

1. What is the immunological mechanism leading to the glomerulonephritis?
2. Are immune complexes the main mediator of systemic damage?
3. What is the mechanism for the vasculitis seen in SLE?
4. Are anti-double-stranded DNA (anti-dsDNA) antibodies pathognomonic of SLE?

FURTHER READING

Arbuckle MR, McClain MT, Rubertone MV, et al. Development of autoantibodies before the clinical onset of systemic lupus erythematosus. N Engl J Med 2003;349:1526–1533.

Damsker JM, Hansen AM, Caspi RR. TH1 and TH17 cells: adversaries and collaborators. Ann N Y Acad Sci 2010;1183:211–221.

Hadaschik EN, Wei X, Leiss H, et al. Regulatory T cell-deficient scurfy mice develop systemic autoimmune features resembling lupus-like disease. Arthritis Res Ther 2015;17:35.

Hedrich CM. Epigenetics in SLE. Curr Rheumatol Rep 2017;19(9):58.

Isenberg DA, Manson JJ, Ehrenstein MR, et al. Anti-dsDNA antibodies – at journey's end? Rheumatology 2007;46:1052–1056.

Kain R, Exner M, Brandes R, et al. Molecular mimicry in pauci-immune focal necrotizing glomerulonephritis. Nat Med 2008;14:1088–1096.

Lyn-Cook BD, Xie C, Oates J, et al. Increased expression of Toll-like receptors (TLRs) 7 and 9 and other cytokines in systemic lupus erythematosus (SLE) patients: ethnic differences and potential new targets for therapeutic drugs. Mol Immunol 2014;61(1):38–43.

McKinney E, Lyons PA, Carr EJ, et al. A CD8[b] T cell transcription signature predicts prognosis in autoimmune disease. Nat Med 2010;16:586–591.

Mizoguchi A, Bhan AK. A case for regulatory B cells. J Immunol 2006;176(2):705–710.

Niewold TB, Hua J, Lehman TJ, et al. High serum IFN-alpha activity is a heritable risk factor for systemic lupus erythematosus. Genes Immun 2007;8:492–502.

Notley CA, Ehrenstein MR. The yin and yang of regulatory T cells and inflammation in RA. Nat Rev Rheumatol 2010;6:572.

Rioux JD, Goyette P, Vyse TJ, et al. International MHC and Autoimmunity Genetics Network: mapping of multiple susceptibility variants within the MHC region for 7 immune-mediated diseases. Proc Natl Acad Sci USA 2009;106:18680–18685.

Yamada H, Nakashima Y, Okazaki K, et al. TH1 but not TH17 cells predominate in the joints of patients with rheumatoid arthritis. Ann Rheum Dis 2008;67:1299–1304.

Transplantation and Rejection

SUMMARY

- **Transplantation is the only form of treatment** for most end-stage organ failure.
- **The barrier to transplantation** is the genetic disparity between donor and recipient.
- **The immune response in transplantation depends on a variety of factors.** Host versus graft responses cause transplant rejection. Histocompatibility antigens are the targets for rejection. The primary targets for rejection are major histocompatibility complex (MHC) molecules but minor histocompatibility antigens can be targets of rejection even when donor and recipient MHC are identical. Graft versus host reactions result when donor lymphocytes attack the graft recipient.
- **Rejection results from a variety of different immune effector mechanisms.** Hyperacute rejection is immediate and caused by antibody. Acute rejection occurs days to weeks after transplantation and is initiated by T cells. Chronic rejection is seen months or years after transplantation.
- **MHC matching is one of two major methods for preventing rejection of allografts.** The better the MHC matching of donor and recipient, the less the strength of the rejection response.

- **Successful organ transplantation depends on the use of immunosuppressive drugs.** 6-MP, azathioprine and MPA are anti-proliferative drugs. Ciclosporin, tacrolimus and sirolimus are inhibitors of T-cell activation. Corticosteroids are anti-inflammatory drugs used for transplant immunosuppression. Antibodies designed to deplete immune cells or to block key cellular interactions are now important tools in preventing graft failure.
- **The ultimate goal in transplantation is to induce donor-specific tolerance.** There is evidence of the induction of tolerance in humans and novel methods for inducing tolerance are being developed.
- **The strength of the rejection response depends on the nature of the transplant.** The relative immune privilege of some grafts (such as the cornea) is a result of both the nature of the tissue and the site of the transplant.
- **Shortage of donor organs and chronic rejection limit the success of transplantation.** Living donation is one way to overcome the shortage of donor organs, as is the increased use of marginal donors, who in previous years would not have been considered for organ donation. Alternative approaches are being investigated.

Transplantation is the only form of treatment for most end-stage organ failure and it is a central topic for immunologists for two reasons:

- transplantation is an important clinical procedure;
- transplantation has proved an important tool for understanding immunological mechanisms. For example, the major histocompatibility complex (MHC; see Chapter 6) was first described in the context of transplantation and transplantation models continue to be widely used as tools in basic and applied immunology.

As a clinical procedure, transplantation is used to replace tissues or organs that have failed. The first successful transplants were those of the cornea, first described in 1906.

World War II provided an important impetus, with the problems of skin grafting airmen who had extensive burns motivating a number of scientists, most notably Peter Medawar, to investigate the immunological basis of graft rejection.

The demonstration by the Medawar group that it was possible to manipulate a recipient animal so that it accepted grafts from an unrelated donor animal encouraged the subsequent clinical development of transplantation. The discovery (by Roy Calne and others) of immunosuppressive drugs and agents allowed surgeons to undertake a range of organ transplants. Initially, these had relatively poor outcomes and it has taken decades of clinical development and experimentation to achieve the high success rates that are now seen.

TRANSPLANTATION IN CLINICAL PRACTICE

Many solid organs are now routinely transplanted. In modern practice many transplants are performed routinely (Table 21.1). The most common transplants performed are the cornea, kidney, liver, heart, lungs and pancreas. Combined transplants (heart and lung or kidney and pancreas) are often clinically indicated and there is continued work on other organs (such as intestine). In recent years, there have been increased numbers of vascularized composite tissue allografts, in which grafts containing blood vessels, nerves, skin, bone or muscle are transplanted. These include face and limb transplants. However, while these attract considerable media attention and raise interesting ethical, immunological, surgical and psychological challenges, the numbers of such operations remains relatively low.

In general most transplants use organs from dead donors (**cadaveric transplants**), although there is an increasing number of living donors (usually related to the recipients) for kidney transplantation (see later). In some cases, organs come from patients who are receiving a transplant. For example, someone who receives a heart–lung transplant may be able to donate their healthy heart to another person.

TABLE 21.1 Transplant Activity

Kidney (cadaveric donor)	2379
Kidney (living donor)	1020
Kidney and pancreas	168
Kidney and pancreas islets	4
Pancreas	17
Pancreas islets	22
Heart	197
Heart and lung	12
Lung (single and double)	201
Liver	892
Domino liver	1
Liver lobe (cadaveric donor)	98
Liver lobe (living donor)	29
Intestinal (including with liver and pancreas)	26
Kidney and liver	22
Heart liver or liver and lung	2
Cornea	3999

The table shows the number of transplants carried out in the UK from March 2017 to March 2018. Similar proportions would be seen in other countries with advanced transplantation services. Data were obtained from NHSBT Organ Donation and Transplant Activity Report 2017/18 and NHSBT Annual Statistics 2018.

Stem cell transplants are used to treat inherited immune deficiencies and leukaemia.
Haematopoietic stem cell transplants are performed for two main reasons. One is to treat children who have inherited immune deficiencies. These children are susceptible to infection and will normally die young as a consequence. However, if they are given stem cells from a healthy donor, the infused stem cells can replace the defective bone marrow stem cells. The stem cells can then mature into fully effective immune cells, thus giving the child a functioning immune system.

The second major application is for patients with leukaemia. It is possible to eradicate the patient's leukaemic cells with chemotherapy and radiotherapy. However, this also results in destruction of the patient's stem cells in the bone marrow and circulation. The patient therefore becomes immunodeficient and will die of infection. Stem cell transplantation can 'rescue' the patient by providing a fresh source of stem cells. In some cases the stem cells are autologous: they are harvested before chemotherapy, stored and then infused back into patients after the therapy is over. In these settings there is no risk of graft versus host disease (GvHD; see later). However, there is a risk that leukaemic cells will be present in the stored stem cells and will then grow in the patient. In other cases the stem cells come from a well-matched donor. This removes the chance of carry-over of leukaemic cells but does run the risk of GvHD. In some forms of leukaemia it has been shown that there is a graft versus leukaemic effect, in which the allogeneic T cells mount a response against any leukaemic cells remaining in the patient and prevent them from growing.

These forms of stem cell are increasingly combined with gene therapy. So a child with immunodeficiency may be given autologous stem cells that have been genetically modified to replace the defective gene that is causing the immune deficiency. Immune cells (often T cells) will be genetically modified to express receptors so that they can recognize and kill neoplastic cells.

Clinical trials of stem cell therapy, using mesenchymal stem cells or embryonic stem cells, are now also underway for the repair of damaged organs.

GENETIC BARRIERS TO TRANSPLANTATION

The main immunological problem with transplantation is that the grafted organ or tissue is seen by the immune system as foreign and is recognized and attacked, leading to rejection of the organ.

Transplantation is normally performed between individuals of the same species who are not genetically identical and the antigenic differences are known as **allogeneic differences**, resulting in an **allospecific immune response** against the **allograft** (Fig. 21.1).

However, it is also possible in experimental circumstances (and possibly in the future in the clinical setting) to perform grafting between different species (**xenograft**).

Transplantation can also be performed within an individual (e.g. skin grafting), when it is known as an **autograft**.

Syngeneic grafts or **isografts** can be performed between genetically identical individuals. This can occur clinically for identical twins but is more commonly seen in experimental settings with inbred strains of animals.

In the case of autografts and isografts there should be no antigenic differences between donor and recipient and therefore no

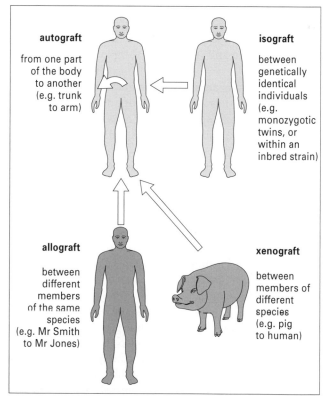

Fig. 21.1 Genetic barriers to transplantation The genetic relationship between the donor and recipient determines whether or not rejection will occur. Autografts or isografts are usually accepted, whereas allografts and xenografts are not.

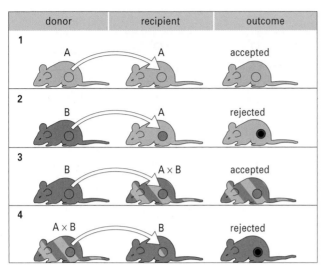

Fig. 21.2 Host versus graft reactions Grafts between genetically identical animals are accepted. Grafts between genetically non-identical animals are rejected with a speed that is dependent on where the genetic differences lie. For example, syngeneic animals (strain A) that are genetically identical accept grafts from each other (**1**). Animals that are genetically different (strain B transplanted into strain A) reject grafts from each other (**2**). The ability to accept a graft is dependent on the recipient sharing all the donor's antigens; this is illustrated by the difference between grafting from parental (strain B) to (A × B) F$_1$ animals (**3**) and vice versa (**4**). B into (A × B) F$_1$ are not rejected because all the donors do not express any antigens that are not in the recipient. The (A × B) F$_1$ into B are rejected as the donor expresses additional antigens (derived from the A strain parent) that are not present in the recipient.

immune response. This can be readily illustrated using transplantation of skin or organs between inbred strains of animals (Fig. 21.2).

GRAFT REJECTION

Host versus graft responses cause transplant rejection.
Immune recognition of the antigenic differences between the donor organ and the recipient will, unless treated, lead to an immune response in which the host immune system responds to, and attacks, the donor tissue. The nature of the host versus graft response is discussed in more detail later.

Similar to any other adaptive immune response, the immune response against a graft shows memory of previous encounters with an antigen. Therefore, once an animal has rejected a graft for the first time, if a second graft is performed from the same strain or donor then it is rejected more rapidly (**second set rejection**).

There is a high frequency of T cells recognizing the graft.
One of the main features of the immune response against a transplanted organ is that it is much more vigorous than the response against a pathogen, such as a virus. This is largely reflected by the frequency of T cells that recognize the graft as foreign and react against it.

Thus, in a naive or unimmunized individual fewer than 1/100 000 T cells respond upon exposure to a virus or a protein immunization. However, 1/100–1/1000 T cells respond to allogeneic antigen-presenting cells (APCs). This is reflected in the

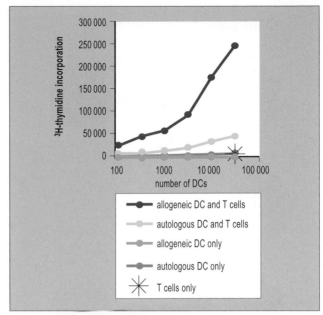

Fig. 21.3 Measuring the strength of the alloresponse The strength of the alloresponse can be measured in a mixed lymphocyte reaction. In this assay, T cells from an individual were mixed with varying numbers of dendritic cells (*DCs*) from either the same (autologous DC) or a different (allogeneic DC) donor. The DCs were irradiated to prevent their proliferation. As a control, cultures were included that contained just the dendritic cells or just the T cells. Five days later, T-cell proliferation was measured by incorporation of ^{3}H-thymidine, which is incorporated into the DNA of dividing cells. There is strong proliferation of T cells exposed to allogeneic dendritic cells, even though these T cells have not previously been exposed to the allogeneic cells, i.e. it represents a primary immune response.

strong T-cell response (proliferation) seen when naive T cells are stimulated with allogeneic dendritic cells (Fig. 21.3).

Histocompatibility antigens are the targets for rejection.
Early experiments showed that the bulk of the allospecific response is against molecules of the MHC. We now know that these molecules are MHC class I or class II molecules, which are responsible for presenting antigen (in the form of peptides) to either:
- CD8 T cells (MHC class I); or
- CD4 cells (MHC class II).

As discussed in Chapter 6, MHC molecules are highly polymorphic, and it is these polymorphic differences that are seen by alloreactive T cells. This is known as direct recognition, or the **direct response**.

What do allospecific T cells recognize?
In a primary alloresponse (see Fig. 21.3), most of the alloreactive CD4$^+$ or CD8$^+$ T cells directly recognize the donor MHC molecules. There are two models that explain the high frequency of allospecific T cells that directly recognize donor MHC: the high determinant density and the multiple determinant models.

However, there are other forms of alloresponse, including:
- those against **minor MHC antigens** (see later); or
- the **indirect response** in which the recipient CD4 T cells recognize donor MHC molecules that have been processed by recipient APCs and are presented as peptides in the context of recipient MHC class II molecules (Fig. 21.4).

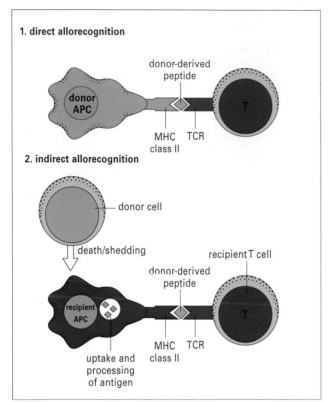

Fig. 21.4 Direct and indirect allorecognition (1) In direct allorecognition, the recipient CD4⁺ or CD8⁺ T cell *(red)* directly recognizes the donor antigen-presenting cells *(APC)* *(blue)*, with the T-cell receptor *(TCR)* binding donor major histocompatibility complex *(MHC)* molecules bearing donor peptide. **(2)** Indirect allorecognition is more similar to conventional T-cell recognition, in that the recipient CD4⁺ T cells recognize foreign (donor-derived) antigen that has been taken up and processed by recipient APCs. The TCR therefore recognizes recipient MHC-bearing donor peptide. CD8⁺ cells only see alloantigen by the direct pathway.

The indirect response is very similar to conventional T-cell recognition of normal antigens, such as those from a pathogen, which are processed by host APCs and presented in the context of host MHC molecules.

The indirect pathway of recognition is important during chronic rejection, when the number of donor-derived professional APCs is no longer high enough to stimulate a direct immune response. It is also important in the rejection of corneal grafts because the cornea lacks large numbers of APCs.

Minor antigens can be targets of rejection even when donor and recipient MHC are identical. Although the MHC is the major target of the alloimmune response, there are also minor histocompatibility antigens. These can serve as targets of rejection even when the MHC is identical between donor and recipient.

The nature of most minor histocompatibility antigens is unknown, although they are assumed to be peptides of normal polymorphic molecules, which bind to host MHC and to induce an immune response. In some cases they are expressed in a tissue-specific manner.

The best studied minor histocompatibility antigen system is the H–Y system. These are antigens encoded by the Y chromosome and are expressed only on male cells. Thus, after

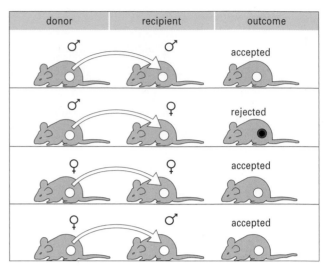

Fig. 21.5 H–Y minor histocompatibility antigens The H–Y antigens are minor histocompatibility antigens expressed on male animals only. Their existence can be demonstrated by skin grafting between animals of the same strain. As would be expected, grafts from female mice are always accepted, while those from male mice are accepted on male recipients, but not female recipients.

immunization, it is possible to demonstrate immune responses and rejection of male organs or skin after transplantation mediated by female animals (two X chromosomes) against male cells (X and Y chromosome). It is not possible to show responses against female antigens by male animals because the male animals have one X chromosome and are therefore tolerant to all antigens encoded on it (Fig. 21.5).

Graft versus host reactions result when donor lymphocytes attack the graft recipient. Although it is usual to think of the immune response recognizing and destroying the transplanted organ, the situation is different when competent immune cells are transplanted into a recipient. This can happen during haematological stem cell transplantation, when normal donor T cells may be infused into the recipient. In such circumstances the T cells can recognize the MHC molecules and/or minor histocompatibility antigens of the recipient as foreign and produce an immune response against the recipient. This is known as **graft versus host disease (GvHD)**.

GvHD can be lethal, causing damage in particular to the skin and gut. It can be demonstrated in animal models by transfer of bone marrow to irradiated recipient animals (Fig. 21.6). It can be avoided by:

- careful matching of the donor and recipient;
- removal of all T cells from the graft; and
- immunosuppression.

IMMUNE EFFECTOR MECHANISMS IN GRAFT REJECTION

Rejection of organs or tissues can occur at various times following transplant, each of which is associated with different immune effector mechanisms (Table 21.2). These are:

- hyperacute rejection, which occurs within minutes to hours and is principally mediated by antibody;

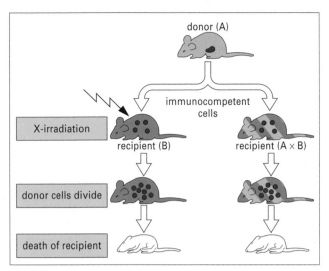

Fig. 21.6 Graft versus host disease Graft versus host disease is caused by immunocompetent cells reacting against their host animal. Immunocompetent cells from a donor of type A are injected into an immunosuppressed (X-irradiated) host of type B, or a normal (A × B) F₁ recipient. The immunosuppressed individual is unable to reject the cells and the F₁ animal is fully tolerant to parental type A cells. In both cases, the donor cells recognize the foreign tissue type B of the recipient. They divide and react against the recipient tissue cells and recruit large numbers of host cells to inflammatory sites. Very often the process leads to the death of the recipient.

TABLE 21.2		**Tempo of Rejection Reactions**
Type of Rejection	**Time Taken**	**Mechanisms of Rejection**
Hyperacute rejection	Minutes to hours	Preformed anti-donor antibodies
Acute rejection	Days to weeks	Activation of alloreactive T cells
Chronic rejection	Months to years	Slow cellular response, response of organ to injury, unknown causes

Rejection of organs or tissues can occur at various times, each of which is associated with different immune effector mechanisms, ranging from antibody-mediated to acute and chronic cellular responses.

- acute rejection, which usually occurs in days to weeks and is initiated by alloreactive T cells; and
- chronic rejection, which is seen months to years after transplantation.

Hyperacute rejection is immediate and mediated by antibody.
Hyperacute rejection is seen when the recipient has pre-existing antibodies that are reactive with the donor tissue. This may be because:

- the recipient has been sensitized to the donor MHC, for example by previous transplants, multiple blood transfusions or pregnancy; or
- the recipient may have natural pre-existing antibodies (e.g. as a result of ABO blood group incompatibility).

A special case is seen in xenotransplantation, where humans and Old World monkeys and apes all have pre-existing antibodies to the carbohydrate antigen α-galactosyl. This carbohydrate is expressed on cell surface proteins of all other mammals. Therefore, a xenotransplant of a cellular organ from a pig (or most other species) into a primate is at risk of hyperacute rejection.

Hyperacute rejection is seen within minutes of connecting the circulation into the transplanted organ. It is caused by the pre-existing antibodies binding to the endothelial cells lining the blood vessels and initiating immune effector functions.

Complement activation can lead to death of the endothelium or, when the damage is sublethal, activation of the endothelial cells. This not only causes an inflammatory response, increasing vascular leakage, but also can cause blood coagulation. The result is rapid destruction of the graft (Fig. 21.7).

Prevention of hyperacute rejection is achieved by carefully avoiding transplanting an organ into an individual with pre-existing antibodies to that tissue. This is done by:
- ABO matching individuals; and
- cross-matching the donor and recipient.

Cross-matching involves incubating donor leukocytes with recipient serum in the presence of complement; cell death indicates the presence of anti-donor antibody and is a contraindication to proceeding with transplantation. Such cross-matching is normally performed immediately before surgery. There is increasing success in transplanting across ABO-incompatible barriers, although this requires very careful preparation, to remove antibodies against the ABO blood group antigens from the recipient's blood; additional immunosuppressive measures may be included to limit antibody formation after transplantation.

Depleting circulating antibodies can also be used when patients have antibodies against HLA antigens. This is important for people who have already rejected an organ and may have developed antibodies against HLA antigens from that donor.

Acute rejection occurs days to weeks after transplantation.
Acute rejection is normally seen days to weeks after transplantation and is caused by activation of allospecific T cells capable of damaging the graft.

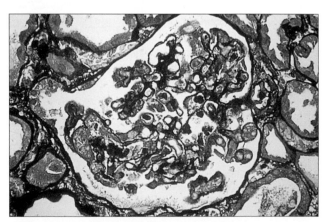

Fig. 21.7 Renal histology showing hyperacute graft rejection Hyperacute rejection is caused by pre-existing antibody at the time of transplantation. There is extensive necrosis of the glomerular capillary associated with massive interstitial haemorrhage. This extensive necrosis is preceded by an intense polymorphonuclear infiltration, which occurs within the first hour of the graft's revascularization. The changes shown here occurred 24–48 hours after this. H&E stain. × 200.

Donor dendritic cells (sometimes called passenger leukocytes) play an important role in triggering acute rejection. Dendritic cells that are present in the organ, following transplantation into the recipient, migrate to the lymph nodes draining the organ and stimulate a primary alloimmune response.

The importance of these dendritic cells can be shown by 'parking experiments' in which:

- a kidney is transplanted from one strain of rat to another under cover of immunosuppression (to prevent rejection) (Fig. 21.8);
- the kidney is kept in that animal long enough to ensure that all the resident dendritic cells have migrated out of the organ;
- the kidney is then transplanted into a third animal, of the same strain as the original recipient, where it shows prolonged graft survival.

However, if the third animal is injected with donor-derived dendritic cells, there is rapid graft rejection. These data highlight the contribution of donor dendritic cells in initiating the alloresponse.

Although the direct pathway is thought to predominate in acute rejection, the indirect alloresponse, although significantly weaker, can also cause acute rejection in some animal models.

Once activated, the T cells migrate to the organ and lead to tissue damage by standard immunological effector mechanisms (Fig. 21.9). These include:

- the generation of Tc cells; and
- the induction of delayed-type hypersensitivity reactions. The role of the T cells in graft rejection can be demonstrated by depletion studies in which antibodies against T-cell subsets

are administered in vivo. Both of the major T-cell subsets, CD4$^+$ and CD8$^+$, can cause graft rejection.

If the animal or patient has already been exposed to the alloantigens expressed by the graft, and as a consequence has been immunized, there will be alloreactive memory cells. This will lead to a much more rapid (accelerated) rejection of the graft (Fig. 21.10).

Chronic rejection is seen months or years after transplantation. In vascularized organs, chronic rejection presents as occlusion of blood vessels, which on histological analysis show a thickening of the intima, similar in some respects to the thickening seen as a result of atherosclerosis (Fig. 21.11). Smooth muscle cell proliferation is often seen, together with a macrophage infiltrate and some lymphocytes. This eventually leads to blockage of the blood vessels and subsequent ischaemia of the organ.

A number of mechanisms can lead to chronic rejection. They include:

- a low-grade T-cell response (mainly of the indirect allospecific pathway as a result of the loss of passenger leukocytes that activate T cells with direct pathway specificity);
- antibody can also be involved in chronic rejection, as indicated by the deposition of complement components (C4d) in tissues.

Non-immunological processes are also important, such as:

- the response of the graft to injury caused at the time of transplantation or by acute rejection episodes;
- recurrence of the original underlying disease; and
- drug-related toxicities (e.g. the immunosuppressive drug ciclosporin A is nephrotoxic and can damage the kidneys).

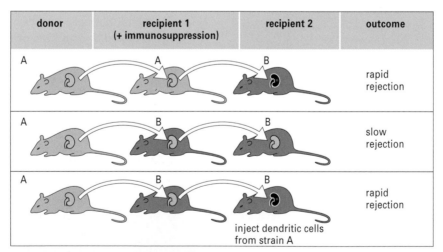

Fig. 21.8 Importance of passenger leukocytes in graft sensitization The role of passenger leukocytes (dendritic cells) can be shown by 'parking' experiments in which kidneys are grafted from a rat of strain A into a recipient of strain B. Immunosuppression is used to prevent the animal from rejecting the graft. After a period, the grafts are then re-transplanted into a fresh strain B rat. There is very slow rejection of the graft (when compared with the rapid rejection seen when the kidney is transferred first into a strain A rat), which is thought to be a result of the inability of the kidney from the strain A rat to immunize the strain B recipient because of the loss of dendritic cells during the period when the graft was 'parked' in the first strain B animal. The slow rejection probably occurs via the indirect pathway. The rejection occurs at the normal rapid tempo if strain A dendritic cells are injected into the recipient animal at the same time as the graft, suggesting that dendritic cells are capable of sensitizing the animal to the graft.

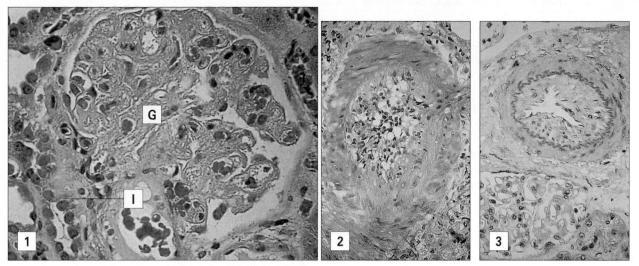

Fig. 21.9 Renal histology showing acute graft rejection (**1**) Small lymphocytes and other cells are accumulating in the interstitium of the graft. Such infiltration *(I)* is characteristic of acute rejection and occurs before the appearance of any clinical signs. H&E stain. (**2**) H&E stain of acutely rejecting kidney showing vascular obstruction. (**3**) van Gieson stain of acutely rejecting kidney showing the end stage of this process. *G*, Glomerulus.

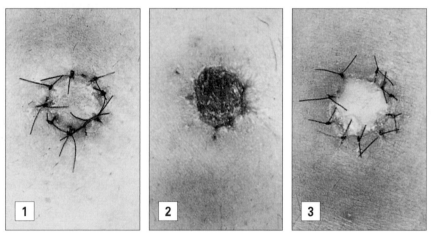

Fig. 21.10 Graft rejection displays immunological memory A human skin allograft at day 5 (**1**) is fully vascularized and the cells are dividing but by day 12 (**2**) is totally destroyed. A second graft (second-set graft) from the same donor shown here on day 7 (**3**) does not become vascularized and is destroyed rapidly. This indicates that sensitization to the first graft produces immunological memory.

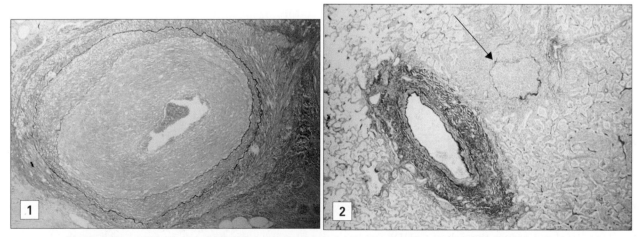

Fig. 21.11 Chronic rejection Grafts that survive acute rejection are still capable of undergoing chronic rejection. (**1**) Section taken from a patient with chronic rejection of their heart graft. The lumen of the blood vessel in the heart has been narrowed as a result of thickening of the wall of the vessel, limiting the blood supply to the heart. (**2**) Section taken from a patient with chronic rejection of the lung, showing obliterative bronchiolitis *(arrow)* blocking the airways. (Courtesy Professor Marlene Rose, Imperial College London, Harefield Hospital, and Dr Margaret Burke, Pathology Department, Royal Brompton Hospital and Harefield Hospital.)

In some cases, initiation of chronic rejection may be immunological in nature, but its progression is caused by non-immunological mechanisms.

Chronic rejection responds poorly to current immunosuppressive therapy. Therefore, although there has been considerable improvement in overall graft survival over the past decades, this improvement is mostly seen in the first year after transplantation – the subsequent survival of grafts has hardly altered over the past 20–30 years. This indicates the need to improve the treatment of chronic rejection.

PREVENTING REJECTION

The two major methods for preventing rejection of allografts are:
- to match the donor and recipient to minimize the antigenic differences; and
- to use immunosuppressive regimens that block the immune response against the organ.

However, in animal models (and hopefully in the clinic) there are techniques that can induce tolerance to an organ such that the immune system of the recipient learns to treat the donor organ as self and not to destroy it. The ability to induce donor-specific tolerance is the Holy Grail of transplantation immunology.

The better the HLA matching of donor and recipient, the less the strength of rejection. The major antigenic differences recognized by the alloimmune response are found on the MHC molecules (HLA in humans). These highly polymorphic molecules have a vital role in presenting antigens to T cells.

There are many different alleles of the MHC molecules and one way to reduce the strength of a rejection response is to match the donor and recipient so that they share as many alleles as possible. In general, matching is now performed using molecular techniques.

In humans, HLA matching is rarely perfect between unrelated donors because of the difficulty in matching all MHC class I and class II gene loci and the high level of polymorphism at each locus (there are 1000s of alleles for each HLA locus).

In cases where the transplant is between living related donors (such as brothers and sisters), there is a greater opportunity for a match because, in general, the HLA locus is inherited as a single set (or haplotype) from each parent.

Loci outside the MHC can also lead to rejection (the minor histocompatibility antigens). However, there is no attempt to match for these antigens because there is little possibility of getting a good match and the effect of matching any single minor antigen is too small to be significant.

It should be noted that even when siblings are perfectly matched at the MHC locus, they will not be matched (unless they are identical twins) for the minor histocompatibility antigens.

HLA matching is not always crucial. HLA matching is very important in bone marrow transplantation (where a large potential donor pool can reduce the risk of GvHD) and has a significant influence on the outcome in kidney transplantation. For other organs, the importance is less clear. For example:
- in corneal transplantation, there is no benefit of HLA matching;

- for those organs where transplantation is essential to maintain life (such as heart and liver), there is no possibility of waiting for a well-matched organ to become available.

Immunosuppressive drugs prevent graft rejection. The success of organ transplantation is entirely dependent on the use of immunosuppressive drugs that control the alloimmune response. Although rejection episodes still occur, they are usually kept in check by the drugs so that lasting damage is minimized.

Over recent decades, there has been a marked improvement in short-term success rates, such that over 90% of kidney transplants are functioning 1 year after transplantation. The major reason for these improved success rates is the advent of more powerful immunosuppressive agents.

Despite the continuing interest in strategies to promote specific immunological tolerance, clinical transplantation is likely to require non-specific immunosuppression for some years to come. The present challenge is to use the currently available agents intelligently to minimize side effects while preserving graft function.

The commonest cocktail of drugs used for kidney transplant patients involves four types of drug, each of which has a distinct mode of action:
- anti-proliferatives;
- inhibitors of T-cell activation;
- anti-inflammatory agents; and
- biologics, in particular antibodies.

There is ongoing research to optimize how best to use these agents so that they can be withdrawn or reduced. The drug therapy is often considered in three phases: induction therapy soon after transplantation, where relatively aggressive drug doses and combinations are given; maintenance therapy, where the doses and number of drugs are reduced to minimize side effects; and then therapy to treat rejection episodes when they happen. Active monitoring of critical markers of rejection results in drug regimens that are continually adapted in consideration of the risk to the patient of rejection and the side effects.

6-MP, azathioprine and MPA are anti-proliferative drugs. The first anti-proliferative drug to be used in patients was **6-mercaptopurine (6-MP)**. This was followed by **azathioprine**, which is converted in vivo to 6-MP. Azathioprine was given to all patients until a more potent alternative arrived on the scene, **mycophenolic acid (MPA)**.

These anti-proliferative drugs inhibit the synthesis of purines that are required for cell division:
- azathioprine is a purine antagonist and competes with inosine monophosphate;
- MPA inhibits the enzyme inosine monophosphate dehydrogenase, which is essential in the de novo synthesis of purines.

Purine synthesis is clearly needed in all cell types. Consequently, the risk of such agents is inhibition of other populations of rapidly dividing cell systems, such as the bone marrow. Indeed, close monitoring of white cell and platelet numbers is necessary in patients on anti-proliferative drugs.

T cells are particularly sensitive to anti-proliferative agents, partly because they are largely dependent on the de novo synthesis of purines, whereas other cell types have a more efficient salvage pathway. Consequently, at conventional doses there is selective inhibition of T-cell-dependent immunity.

Ciclosporin, tacrolimus and sirolimus are inhibitors of T-cell activation.

Drugs that inhibit T-cell activation are the mainstay of immunosuppressive regimens. The first such drug to be discovered was **ciclosporin**, a fungal metabolite (Fig. 21.w2). The introduction of ciclosporin revolutionized clinical transplantation because it led to a marked improvement in early success rates, which rose from approximately 70% to over 90%. Furthermore, the doses of other drugs that were required were substantially lower, so that drug side effects were less troublesome. This made transplantation a much more viable prospect for many patients.

The key effect of ciclosporin is to inhibit the production of the major growth factor for T cells, interleukin-2 (IL-2). The intracellular mechanism of action of ciclosporin involves binding to **cyclophilin** and the consequent inhibition of the calcium-dependent phosphatase **calcineurin**, which would otherwise activate the **NF-AT complex** and lead to IL-2 gene transcription (see Fig. 7.w1).

A few years after the introduction of ciclosporin, another fungal metabolite was discovered with a similar mode of action and greater molar potency, **tacrolimus (FK506)**. Tacrolimus binds to an intracellular protein, FK-binding protein 12 (FKBP12). The resulting complex inhibits calcineurin and the consequences of calcium-dependent signalling, in the same manner as ciclosporin.

Ciclosporin and tacrolimus have different toxicities, with ciclosporin being more nephrotoxic and tacrolimus being diabetogenic in some patients.

The third drug in the category of inhibitors of T-cell activation is **sirolimus (rapamycin)**.

Sirolimus is a fungal metabolite that was discovered on Easter Island (Rapa Nui) and its mechanism of action is quite distinct. Rather than inhibiting the production of IL-2, it blocks the response to IL-2 by interfering with some of the signals resulting from IL-2 binding to its receptor.

Sirolimus inhibits signalling through several growth factor receptors; consequently, it has quite widespread anti-proliferative effects and was written off as being too non-specific when first studied in vitro.

Sirolimus has attracted much attention recently, for two reasons:

- It appears to be a tolerance-permissive drug; i.e. if T cells are exposed to antigen in tolerance-promoting conditions, such as co-stimulatory blockade, sirolimus allows tolerance to occur, while the calcineurin inhibitors can inhibit the development of tolerance under similar circumstances.
- The broader anti-proliferative effects of sirolimus may be beneficial because they reduce the incidence of some malignancies.

Corticosteroids are anti-inflammatory drugs used for transplant immunosuppression.

Corticosteroids, given in combination with azathioprine, were the mainstay of immunosuppression for several decades.

Corticosteroids are pharmacological derivatives of the glucocorticoid family of steroid hormones and act through intracellular receptors that are almost ubiquitously expressed.

The anti-inflammatory effects of steroids are highly complex, reflecting the fact that as many as 1% of genes may be regulated by glucocorticoids. Some of their most important effects are:

- inhibition of pro-inflammatory cytokine secretion (IL-1, IL-3, IL-4, IL-5, IL-8 (CXCL8), TNFα);
- inhibition of nitric oxide synthase;
- inhibition of adhesion molecule expression, leading to reduced inflammatory cell migration;
- induction of endonucleases, leading to apoptosis in lymphocytes and eosinophils.

The problem of side effects is a major issue with the use of corticosteroids, particularly at high doses. Protracted corticosteroid use can result in central weight gain, fluid retention, diabetes mellitus, bone mineral loss and thinning of the skin. Therefore, most protocols seek to minimize steroid use, particularly after the initial post-transplant period. However, for corneal transplants, where topical (local) administration of the drug is possible (thus minimizing side effects), corticosteroids are the main form of immunosuppression used.

Biologic agents are increasingly being used to prevent graft rejection.

Biologic agents, in particular antibodies, have been widely used to prevent graft rejection. Indeed the first monoclonal antibody licensed for human use was to prevent acute rejection (anti-CD3 muromonab). The antibodies used to prevent rejection can be classified as those that deplete cells or molecules and those that block interactions (for example between a cytokine and its receptor). Most of the biologics used in transplantation are monoclonal antibodies, although polyclonal antibodies have been in use since the late 1960s. In addition, recombinant fusion proteins have been developed (see Figs 10.18 and 10.19). It must be noted that, while some biologic agents have been licensed for use in transplantation, many are licensed for other indications and are used by clinicians 'off label'.

Biologics can be used at different stages in management of the patient. In addition to the three phases of therapy described earlier (induction, maintenance and rejection therapy), antibodies are also used in the desensitization of patients prior to transplantation and in the treatment of primary disease in order to protect the organ from damage (Fig. 21.12).

Desensitization reduces the titre of antibodies that recognize the graft.

One strategy in patients with preformed antibodies to the donor graft is to reduce the antibody titre. This can be achieved using plasmapheresis, as described earlier. The infusion into the patient of a preparation of non-specific immunoglobulin (intravenous immunoglobulin or IVIG) can further reduce the titre, probably by shortening the half-life of the anti-graft antibody through competition for FcRn (see Fig. 10.14). Rituximab, which is a chimeric anti-CD20 antibody that depletes B cells, can also be used as part of the desensitization protocol.

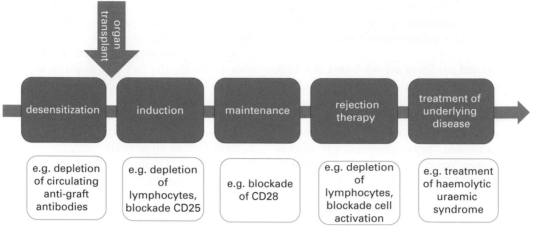

Fig. 21.12 Use of antibodies in transplantation. Antibodies (both monoclonal and polyclonal) have been used for five purposes in transplantation: desensitization of patients with pre-existing antibodies against the graft; induction therapy immediately after transplantation; longer-term maintenance therapy; the treatment of rejection episodes; and the prevention or treatment of underlying disease. Antibodies work either by depletion or by blocking molecular interactions.

Agents that deplete lymphocytes or block IL-2 signalling are used in induction. Anti-thymocyte globulin (ATG) is a preparation of polyclonal antibodies produced in horses or rabbits immunized with human thymocytes. It has been used for many years as part of induction therapy, particularly in patients who are at high risk of rejection. Its main action is to deplete T cells, although other lymphocytes can also be removed. While the antibody preparation is less well defined than a monoclonal antibody, ATG continues to be used because it is effective and the side effects are tolerable.

Alemtuzumab, perhaps better known as CAMPATH-1H, was the first therapeutic antibody to be humanized (see Chapter 10). It recognizes CD52 expressed mainly on lymphocytes and is a strong depleting antibody. It has been widely used off label for induction and can be used to treat rejection episodes. However, consideration has to be made of the side effects that occur mostly because of the induction of cytokine release.

The most widely used biologic induction agents are antibodies against IL-2 receptor (CD25), which is expressed on activated T cells. The two main antibodies in this category are daclizumab (a humanized antibody that has now been withdrawn from the market) and basiliximab (a chimeric antibody), neither of which depletes T cells but they block IL2 interaction with CD25. They have a relatively good safety profile.

Agents that block the interaction between CD28 and its ligands are used in maintenance. Belatacept and abatacept are fusion proteins between CTLA-4 and the Fc region of immunoglobulin (CTLA-4-Ig), which block the interaction between CD28 and its ligands CD80 and CD86. Blocking this interaction can induce anergy in alloreactive T cells (see Chapter 7). This

class of agents has been shown to be effective in replacing calcineurin inhibitors in maintenance therapy.

Biologic agents can also be used to treat rejection and underlying disease. The first monoclonal antibody licensed for clinical use, muromonab (anti-CD3), was designed to reverse acute rejection episodes. Its application was limited by side effects that were caused by cytokine release and it was withdrawn from the market, but several of the biologic agents developed for induction and maintenance are still in use to treat rejection, such as alemtuzumab and ATG.

While transplantation can replace a failed organ, it does not block any disease that damaged the organ in the first place. Therefore, if the patients have an ongoing primary disease that led to organ failure, it is likely that the transplanted organ will undergo damage. Biologics can be used to treat this ongoing disease, thus preserving graft function. Eculizumab, an inhibitor of complement C5, has been used to prevent or treat haemolytic-uraemic syndrome (HUS).

INDUCTION OF DONOR-SPECIFIC TOLERANCE

Although generalized immunosuppression has been highly successful in preventing graft rejection, it comes at a price. This includes:

- the non-specific toxicity of the drugs;
- the need to stay indefinitely on medication; and
- the consequences of generalized immunosuppression such as the increased incidence of cancer and infection.

It would therefore be desirable to induce tolerance to the graft whereby the immune system specifically becomes non-responsive to the donor antigens yet is still capable of responding normally to other antigens.

Tolerance to grafts was first demonstrated by Peter Medawar's group. They showed that if allogeneic cells were injected into a neonatal animal, when the animal became adult it would be tolerant to tissue from the donor and would accept grafts without the need for immunosuppression. There have since been numerous examples of inducing tolerance to grafts in animal models, but it has been difficult to translate this into the clinical setting.

One of the difficulties in the clinical setting is to demonstrate that tolerance really exists. It is relatively easy to demonstrate tolerance in an animal model by:

- performing a second graft (showing that the immune system will no longer respond to the antigen); while
- demonstrating that an irrelevant third-party graft is still rejected (demonstrating that graft survival is not a result of a generalized immunosuppression).

However, this is more difficult in humans.

There is evidence for the induction of tolerance in humans.
There are three sources of evidence for the induction of tolerance in humans.

First, there are patients who have received grafts but are no longer on immunosuppressive regimens because they cannot tolerate the drugs. They can show long-term graft survival. This is not formal evidence of tolerance, but it is highly suggestive that some people can have an operational tolerance whereby they fail to destroy their organ graft.

Second, it is possible to look at the frequency of alloreactive T cells in patients with grafts. In some groups, there is a reduced frequency of these cells, but the response to other antigens remains normal (Fig. 21.13). Again, this is not a formal proof of tolerance because it is not yet known how the in vitro assays

relate to the response in patients. However, it does indicate that it might be possible to develop tests that will allow us to monitor the development of tolerance in patients and hence know how to tailor treatment to the individual (e.g. removing them from immunosuppression when indicated).

Third, there are studies that demonstrate long-term graft survival (and hence apparent tolerance) in a limited number of patients who have received combined renal and haematopoietic stem cell transplants. These patients had a short course of immunosuppression, resulting in long-term graft survival with no rejection. While this combination of treatments is rare, the use of stem cells is a promising strategy to induce operational graft tolerance.

Novel methods for inducing tolerance are being developed.
There are various ways in which tolerance (or the appearance of tolerance) can occur. Most of these are discussed in more detail in Chapter 11. An understanding of the mechanisms by which tolerance is induced and maintained allows the development of novel methods for inducing tolerance.

Central tolerance results from deletion of T cells in the thymus and is the most important form of tolerance induction for preventing autoimmunity. It has been harnessed for the induction of tolerance in experimental systems by transplanting the thymus from the donor into the recipient. This approach may be particularly useful in the context of xenotransplantation, where there is an opportunity to manipulate the donor and/or recipient before grafting of the organ.

Alloreactive cells can be made anergic.
In peripheral organs, tolerance induction can result from deletion. However, it is also possible for alloreactive cells to be anergized. Anergy describes a

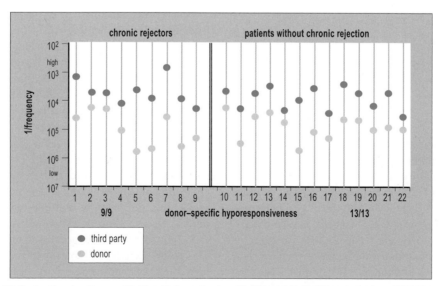

Fig. 21.13 Reduction in allospecific T cells in patients with kidney grafts The graph shows the frequency of T cells capable of producing IL-2 from patients with long-term kidney grafts that react with cells bearing the donor alloantigen or control (third-party) alloantigens. The data show two groups of patients – those with evidence of chronic rejection and those without. Both groups of patients show a reduced frequency of T cells capable of recognizing alloantigen from the donor of the organ when compared with the frequency against third-party alloantigen. This indicates that the patients show a degree of reduced reactivity to alloantigens.

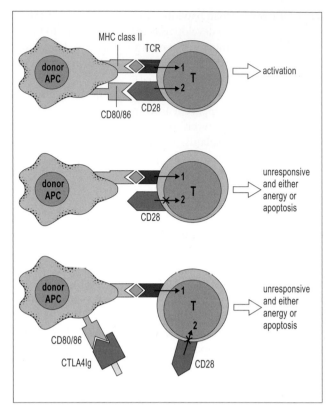

Fig. 21.14 Co-stimulation blockade For full T-cell activation to occur, the T cell needs to receive two signals: signal 1 through the TCR binding the appropriate peptide–MHC complex (which provides antigenic specificity) and signal 2 through co-stimulatory molecules (the most important of which for naive T cells is CD28 on the T-cell binding CD80 or CD86 on the APC). Interaction of a T cell with an APC that lacks CD80 or CD86, so that only signal 1 is received, fails to activate the T cell and can result in apoptosis or anergy of the lymphocyte. In experimental or clinical settings, it is possible to block the CD28 interaction with CD80/86 by addition of a soluble molecule, CTLA-4–Ig, which consists of the extracellular part of CTLA-4 (an alternative ligand for CD80/86) fused to the Fc of immunoglobulin. This molecule prevents the interaction of CD28 with CD80/86. It can also result in upregulation of immunoregulatory enzyme, indoleamine 2,3-dioxygenase (IDO). *APC*, Antigen-presenting cell; *MHC*, major histocompatibility complex; *TCR*, T-cell receptor.

state in which the cell is not deleted but has been rendered unresponsive to further stimulation by the same antigen.

Blockade of co-stimulatory molecules such as CD80 and CD86 with agents such as CTLA-4-Ig (a fusion protein between CTLA-4, a ligand for CD80 and CD86, and the Fc part of immunoglobulin, available as belatacept or abatacept) can be used to induce anergy in alloreactive cells (Fig. 21.14). However, it should be noted that the situation could be more complex than this. In many APCs, cross-linking of CD80 and CD86 with CTLA-4–Ig results in upregulation of an immunomodulatory enzyme indoleamine 2,3-dioxygenase (IDO). This enzyme catabolizes tryptophan and, as a result, prevents T-cell activation both as a result of:

- depriving T cells of this essential amino acid; and
- the products of tryptophan breakdown acting directly on the T cells.

The role of IDO in immune regulation was first recognized in the placenta, where it protects the fetus from immunological rejection – inhibition of IDO causes rejection of histoincompatible fetuses.

Another alternative is to induce a regulatory response to the alloantigen. The phenomenon of T-cell regulation has long been recognized (Fig. 21.15) and can be shown in experimental models by transferring T cells from a tolerant animal to a naive recipient and showing that this results in a transfer of the tolerance. Regulatory cells are discussed further in Chapter 12 and strategies that develop regulatory cells either in situ or ex vivo followed by administration to the recipient are being investigated.

Immune privilege can be a property of the tissue or site of transplant. Although a failure to reject a graft could be the result of tolerance (or immunosuppression), an alternative is that the graft is immune privileged and protected from the immune response against it (see Chapter 13):

- When corneal transplantation is performed in an animal model, the rejection response is weaker than for other forms of transplantation, indicating the immune privileged nature of the graft.
- Skin transplanted onto the anterior chamber (where the cornea is) shows a lower rate of rejection than skin transplanted into other sites.

It is important to note that immune privilege is not an absolute term. Corneal grafts are rejected, albeit less vigorously than other grafts. It is probably best to think of immune privilege as a spectrum ranging from grafts that show a high degree of privilege (cornea) to those where the immune response against them is very strong (skin), with other grafts somewhere in between.

Several mechanisms can be responsible for immune privilege. These include 'ignorance' – the immune system does not come in contact with the graft (see Fig. 13.8). The cornea is not vascularized and has poor lymphatic drainage. It also has a very low concentration of dendritic cells in the centre. These features reduce the ability of the graft to stimulate an immune response against it. If this ignorance is disrupted (e.g. by inducing vascularization in the graft bed), the cornea is more rapidly rejected.

In addition, the tissue itself can modify the immune response. In the anterior chamber of the eye, there is a cytokine environment (high in TGFβ and α-melanocyte-stimulating hormone) that deviates the immune response away from a tissue destructive to a non-inflammatory response.

Finally, the tissue being transplanted can itself be privileged. This is also seen in the cornea, which expresses high levels of Fas ligand that can induce apoptosis in invading T cells.

Limitations on transplantation. Two major issues limit success of transplantation:

- The first is the shortage of donor organs: this means that not everyone who would benefit from a transplant receives one and, given the high success rate of transplantation, an increasing number of patients would benefit.

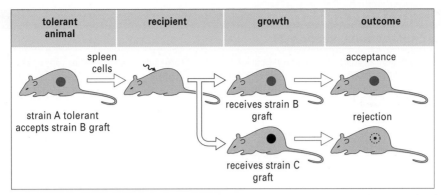

Fig. 21.15 Tolerance to grafts can be transferred by regulatory cells An animal of strain A that has been made tolerant to a graft B can contain regulatory cells. If these cells are removed from the animal and transferred to a lightly irradiated strain A recipient, and this animal is then given a skin graft from strain B, that graft might be accepted. In most cases, this tolerance is specific, therefore if a mouse treated this way received a graft of strain C, it would be rejected.

- The second is chronic rejection, which results in a continual loss of transplanted organs and necessitates patients remaining on immunosuppression, with the consequences of drug toxicity, systemic immunosuppression, increased incidence of malignancy and infection.

The second of these problems, chronic rejection, would be solved if we were able to induce tolerance to grafts in patients. To do this, it is necessary to develop assays that will allow us to determine when tolerance has been induced and to translate the therapies developed in animal models to the clinic.

These assays are still under development but may involve measuring the frequency of alloreactive and/or regulatory T cells in patients, as well as other immunological biomarkers. At present, it is not clear which tolerance induction procedure is most likely to work in clinical transplantation and further work is needed to address this issue.

Alternative approaches to overcoming the shortage of donor organs are being investigated. Although it is very important to increase the donor pool, the approaches discussed earlier will never provide all the organs needed. Alternatives include:
- the development of artificial mechanical organs;
- in the longer term, use of cloning and/or tissue engineering strategies to make artificial biological organs; and
- xenotransplantation (the use of animal organs).

Xenotransplantation may increase the supply of organs. The most favoured animal for developing xenotransplantation is the pig, for reasons that include the physiological and anatomical compatibility between pigs and humans and the ability to breed large numbers of animals rapidly.

There are several barriers to xenotransplantation, including public acceptability, safety and scientific issues.

The main safety concern is the risk of transmission of viruses from the pig to the human, although this is a diminishing concern. It should be noted that acellular xenografts have been performed for many years and are highly successful. For example, pig heart valves are used to replace diseased valves. These are not subject to immunological rejection, nor are they potential sources of viral infection. It is also possible to produce animals where the viruses are knocked out using gene-editing approaches.

The scientific issues revolve around preventing graft rejection. As indicated, a pig organ transplanted into a human would undergo hyperacute rejection as a result of preformed anti-α-galactosyl antibodies in the recipient's circulation. One solution has been to engineer pigs (by nuclear cloning from cell lines) that lack the galactosyl transferase enzyme responsible for creating α-galactosyl residues. Organs from these pigs show reasonably long-term survival in primates, with no evidence of hyperacute rejection.

Although offering scientific challenges, there are opportunities for using pig organs. The ability to engineer the pig genetically should make it easier to develop tolerance to the organ. This, as well as the ability to carry out transplants in a pre-planned manner, offers considerable advantages over conventional transplantation.

CRITICAL THINKING: TRANSPLANTATION

See Critical thinking: Explanations, section 21

A research team is experimenting with new approaches to inducing tolerance to cardiac (heart) grafts. They do this by carrying out heart transplants between two different strains of mice, BALB/c and C57/BL6 mice, which are totally MHC mismatched. In initial experiments using mice that they had not treated in any way, the grafts were performed heterotopically (which means that they did not replace the recipient's normal heart but were placed in the abdominal cavity of the animal) and graft survival was measured by palpitation (to see if the donor heart was still beating). In each group they used six recipients.

Group	Donor	Recipient	Median Graft Survival
1	BALB/c	C57/BL6	7 days
2	C57/BL6	C57/BL6	>100 days

1. Comment on these results

The research team had developed a new approach to blocking the expression of co-stimulatory molecules CD40 and CD80 by injecting gene therapy vectors that prevent the transcription of their genes. In a second experiment, recipient animals were lightly irradiated before transplantation and treated with either control vector, with the vector that blocks CD40 or CD80 or both. They obtained the following results.

Group	Donor	Recipient	Gene Therapy Vector	Median Graft Survival
3	BALB/c	C57/BL6	None	13 days
4	BALB/c	C57/BL6	Control	15 days
5	BALB/c	C57/BL6	Blocking CD40	32 days
6	BALB/c	C57/BL6	Blocking CD80	25 days
7	BALB/c	C57/BL6	Blocking CD40+CD80	>100 days

2. Comment on these results. Are the animals in group 7 tolerant to their grafts? Which further experiments might the research team do to test whether tolerance had been induced?

3. The researchers suspect that in group 5 they have induced regulatory T cells that are preventing the graft being rejected. How can they test this?

4. The researchers used groups of six animals in their experiments. Discuss why they might have chosen this number.

5. The researchers hope that their study might one day lead to treatments that could induce tolerance in clinical transplantation, reducing the need to use immunosuppressive drugs. What are the disadvantages to patients of being on immunosuppressive drugs to prevent graft rejection?

6. A kidney is available from a blood group A donor. There are two potential recipients: Jane has blood group O and Seema blood group AB. What should be considered when deciding which recipient should get the organ?

FURTHER READING

Alelign T, Ahmed MM, Bobosha K, Tadesse Y, Howe R, Petros B. Kidney transplantation: the challenge of human leukocyte antigen and its therapeutic strategies. J Immunol Res 2018;5986740.

Altaf SY, Apperley JF, Olavarria E. Matched unrelated donor transplants – state of the art in the 21st century. Semin Hematol 2016;53:221–229.

Boardman DA, Jacob J, Smyth LA, Lombardi G, Lechler RI. What is direct allorecognition? Curr Transplant Rep 2016;3:275–283.

Crepeau RL, Ford ML. Challenges and opportunities in targeting the CD28/CTLA-4 pathway in transplantation and autoimmunity. Expert Opin Biol Ther 2017;17:1001–1012.

Garcia de Mattos Barbosa M, Cascalho M, Platt JL. Accommodation in ABO-incompatible organ transplants. Xenotransplantation 2018;25:e12418.

George AJT, Larkin DFP. Corneal transplantation: the forgotten graft. Am J Transpl 2004;4:678–685.

Grgic I, Chandraker A. Significance of biologics in renal transplantation: past, present, and future. Cur Opin Org Transp 2018;23:51–62.

Mahdi BM. A glow of HLA typing in organ transplantation. Clin Transl Med 2013;2:6.

Meier RPH, Muller YD, Balaphas A, et al: Xenotransplantation: back to the future? Transpl Int 2018;31:465–477.

Moreau A, Varey E, Anegon I, Cuturi MC. Effector mechanisms of rejection. Cold Spring Harb Perspect Med 2013;3: a015461.

Rosen SJ, Harris PE, Hardy MA. State of the art: role of the dendritic cell in induction of allograft tolerance. Transplantation 2018;102:1603–1613.

Safinia N, Grageda N, Scottà C, et al. Cell therapy in organ transplantation: our experience on the clinical translation of regulatory T cells. Front Immunol 2018;26(9):354.

Schwarz C, Mahr B, Muckenhuber M, Wekerle T. Belatacept/CTLA4Ig: an update and critical appraisal of preclinical and clinical results. Expert Rev Clin Immunol 2018;14:583–592.

Zhao H, Alam A, Soo AP, George AJT, Ma D. Ischemia-reperfusion injury reduces long term renal graft survival: mechanism and beyond. EBioMedicine 2018;28:31–42.

22

Immunity to Cancers

SUMMARY

- **The immune system can survey the body for several types of developing tumours**.
- **Tumours elicit immunity against themselves**. Mice, rats, hamsters and frogs can be immunized against tumours. In most tumours in animals, tumour immunity elicited by immunization is specific (or strongest) to the individual tumour that was used to immunize.
- **Tumour antigens have been characterized by four means: immunization-challenge experiments, T-cell reactivity, antibody reactivity and, most recently, genomic analyses**. Immunization-challenge experiments have uncovered the immunogenicity of individual tumour-specific mutated antigens (neo-epitopes). Antigens identified by reactivity to T cells include individual tumour-specific mutated antigens,

cancer/testes antigens, differentiation antigens and viral tumour antigens. Antigens defined by antibody reactivity are mostly those that are expressed on tumour cells ectopically or at higher levels than on normal tissues. Genomically defined antigens, much like the antigens identified by immunization-challenge experiments, are overwhelmingly individual tumour-specific mutated antigens (neo-epitopes).

- **Vigorous anti-tumour immune responses are compromised by regulatory mechanisms**. Tumours elicit immunity in their primary host, but such immunity is actively downregulated. Anti-tumour T cells may be inhibited via CTLA-4 and PD-1. Tregs are also involved in the downregulation of tumour immunity. Blockade of CTLA-4 and PD-1 mediates enhanced immunological activity in patients with a variety of cancers.

Cancer has engaged the minds of immunologists since the beginning of immunology. Ehrlich, who opined on all things immunological, believed that the immune system could protect the host from cancer.

Burnet and Thomas refined that idea into the **immune surveillance hypothesis** of cancer. This idea derived considerable support from the clinical observation that transplant patients receiving immunosuppressive medication had a significantly higher incidence of a variety of cancers than comparable control populations. Yet, the hypothesis lived in limbo for several decades, failing to thrive and failing to die, until recently when work from several independent investigators (mainly in Denmark and the USA) demonstrated that mice with a compromised immune status were more prone to developing new cancers than immunocompetent mice.

The immune surveillance hypothesis is often regarded as the intellectual underpinning of cancer immunology. Although the hypothesis itself has contributed little to our attempts to treat cancer through immunological means, it has profound implications for understanding the functions of the immune system.

Non-specific stimulation of the immune system can have an anti-cancer effect. German physicians in the 19th century noted dramatic regressions of cancer in occasional patients who developed streptococcal infections. These anecdotes led to a systematic exploration of infections/fever as an immunotherapeutic modality by William Coley, a New York City surgeon.

The work of Coley and his predecessors, suggesting that non-specific stimulation of the immune system, such as by an infection, can have an anti-cancer effect, remains a key idea in cancer immunology. Indeed, the first approved immunotherapy for human cancer (intravesical instillation of BCG for non- or minimally invasive bladder cancer) is predicated upon enhancement of non-specific stimulation. It is only a small exaggeration to say that every idea in cancer immunity has been interpreted at some time or another, in terms of Coley's observations.

TUMOUR IMMUNITY IN THE PRIMARY HOST

Entirely unrelated to these lines of enquiry, the study of cancer immunity saw a revival at the hands of those who were transplanting chemically induced tumours into the many inbred mice that became available in the 1950s. These investigators showed highly successful immunization against the transplantable tumours and expressed great hopes about cancer vaccination. In hindsight, these successful immunizations were simply a result of allogeneic differences between tumours and the host strain of mouse, a theme that played a seminal role in definition of the major histocompatibility complex (MHC) but had no relevance for cancer immunity.

Nonetheless, amidst the barrage of experiments where MHC-mismatched tumours were transplanted into mice, the experiments of Ludwik Gross, and later those of Prehn and Main and of George and Eva Klein, showed that, even when MHC-matched tumours were used to immunize mice, protection against subsequent tumour growth could be achieved (Fig. 22.1). These studies led to two principles, which have informed much of cancer immunology since and are discussed later.

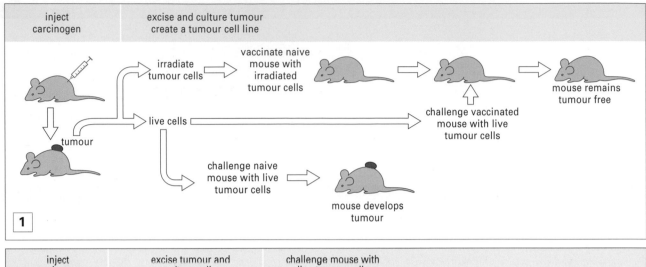

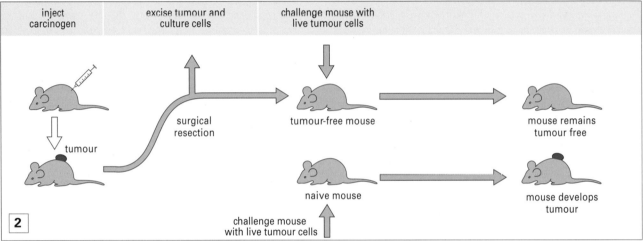

Fig. 22.1 Immunogenicity of chemically induced tumours (**1**) Mice immunized with tumour cells are protected against subsequent tumour growth. (**2**) The primary animal that develops the tumour is also immune to subsequent challenges with the same tumour.

Cancers elicit protective immunity in the primary and syngeneic host. Mice and rats of a given haplotype can be immunized with irradiated cancer cells that arose in animals of the same haplotype. When they are challenged with live cancer cells, they are able to resist the tumour challenge. The following observations and deductions have been derived from these results:

- The immunogenicity of tumours has provided the foundation stone for the idea of **tumour-specific antigens**. If immunization is possible, then antigens must exist.
- Tumour immunity depends on many factors. The degree of tumour immunity depends upon the type of cancer and the method of its induction or lack of induction. UV-induced cancers are highly immunogenic, methylcholanthrene-induced tumours less so and spontaneous tumours even less so. Nonetheless, immunogenicity of tumours has been demonstrated in all model systems tested.
- The primary animal develops immunity to subsequent tumour challenge. Furthermore, it is also immune to subsequent challenges with the same tumour (see Fig. 22.1).

- Protective immunity is only seen in prophylactic immunization and not therapeutic immunization: once a mouse has been implanted with a tumour, immunization with irradiated cancer cells (derived from the growing tumour) does nothing to mitigate tumour growth (Fig. 22.2). Exploration of differences between prophylaxis and therapy has led to fundamental insights into tumour immunity.

It is obviously not possible to test immunogenicity of tumours in humans by doing transplantation-challenge experiments. There is no other reliable method of determining immunogenicity of tumours. It is therefore impossible to comment on the immunogenicity of human tumours in vivo.

Specific immunity to induced and spontaneous tumours may develop. When mice are immunized against a given fibrosarcoma, they are rendered immune to it, but only to that individual fibrosarcoma or lines derived from it. If the mice are challenged with another fibrosarcoma, even one induced by the same carcinogen, tumour growth is unaffected by the prior immunization.

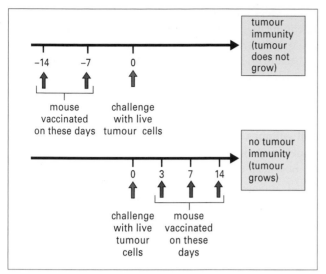

Fig. 22.2 Difference between prophylaxis against future tumours and therapy of pre-existing tumours Protective immunity is only seen in prophylactic immunization and not therapeutic immunization. Once a mouse has been implanted with a tumour, immunization with irradiated cancer cells (derived from the growing tumour) does nothing to mitigate tumour growth.

The most extensive interrogation of the individually distinct antigenicity of chemically induced tumours was carried out by Basombrio and Prehn. They induced fibrosarcomas in 25 syngeneic BALB/c mice using methylcholanthrene and tested the immunogenicity of each one against all other tumours in an immunization-challenge model. They concluded that, even though all tumours were induced at the same time, in the same strain of mice of the same age, by the same carcinogen and were histologically all fibrosarcomas, they were antigenically distinct. Independent tumours induced by the same carcinogen in the same mouse are also antigenically distinct.

Spontaneous tumours are also antigenically distinct. Cross-reactivity among tumours does occur occasionally. Typically, such cross-reactive immunity has been observed to be significantly weaker than the cell-line specific antigenicity. Efforts at characterization of such cross-reactive tumour-protective antigens have not made much headway, except in the case of virally induced tumours. In contrast, there has been considerable success in identification of individually distinct antigens.

In addition to these experimental studies, several clinical observations point to the existence of tumour-protective immunity in humans. These include the increased relative risk of cancers in patients who are immunosuppressed because they are kidney transplant recipients (Table 22.1) or for a variety of other reasons (Table 22.2). The association between immunosuppression/immunodeficiency and virus-induced tumours can be explained in two ways that are not mutually exclusive:

- The individual may be unable to control the viral infection effectively, or
- Immunosurveillance of primary tumours that arise may be impaired.

TABLE 22.1 Relative Risk of Tumours in Immunosuppressed Patients

Tumour Type	Approximate Relative Risk
Kaposi's sarcoma	50–100
Non-Hodgkin's lymphoma	25–45
Carcinoma of the liver	20–35
Carcinoma of the skin	20–50
Carcinoma of the cervix	2.5–10
Melanoma	2.5–10
Lung	1–2

In patients, immunosuppressed because of kidney transplantation, the relative risk of developing tumours in which viruses are known to play a role is greatly increased. This is the case for all those listed except cancer of the lung. The relative risks vary in different studies according to the duration of follow-up and the presence of co-factors such as sunlight for skin cancer.

TABLE 22.2 Tumour Viruses and Immunodeficiency

Cause of Immunodeficiency	Common Tumour Types	Viruses Involved
Inherited immunodeficiency	Lymphoma	EBV
Immunosuppression for organ transplants or because of AIDS	Lymphoma	EBV
	Cervical cancer	Papilloma viruses
	Skin cancer	Probably papilloma viruses
	Liver cancer	Hepatitis B and C viruses
	Kaposi's sarcoma	Human herpes virus 8
Malaria	Burkitt's lymphoma	EBV
Autoimmunity	Lymphoma	EBV

Skin cancer is the most common form of tumour in absolute numbers in organ transplant recipients. In other forms of immunodeficiency, tumours of the immune system dominate. Most normal adults carry both Epstein–Barr virus (EBV) and many papilloma viruses throughout life with no ill effects because they have antiviral immunity.

CHARACTERIZATION OF TUMOUR ANTIGENS

The broad approaches to the identification of tumour antigens are shown in Table 22.3 and discussed later. Not surprisingly, the approaches have yielded results that are not fully concordant. These differences have helped highlight a fascinating interplay between immunity and tolerance to tumours, discussed later.

Tumour-specific antigens recognized by T cells show a wide spectrum of specificity. Many studies have identified tumour-reactive T cells in blood or within a tumour and these findings have thus supported the idea of tumour antigens.

The work of Thierry Boon and his colleagues first made it technically possible to identify the CTL epitopes of cancer cells being recognized by the tumour-reactive T cells.

TABLE 22.3 Comprehensive List of Major Types of Tumour Antigen

Method of Identification	Category of Antigen	Examples of Individual Antigens
T-cell/antibody reactivity	Cancer/testes antigens	NY-ESO-1, MAGE
	Differentiation antigens (lineage specific)	Melan A, tyrosinase Gp100, PSA
	Antigens with broader expression	Human: CEA, MUC, HER2, G250 Murine: P1A, gp70
	Common tumour-specific antigens	Mutated p53, mutated Ras, BCR-ABL, papilloma virus
	Viral antigens	(see Table 22.4)
Tumour transplantation	Autologous tumour-derived heat-shock protein-peptide complexes (conceptually the same as the genomics/bio-informatics defined antigens below)	Autologous tumour-derived Gp96-peptide complexes, hsp90-peptide complexes, hsp70-peptide complexes
Genomics/bio-informatics-defined antigens	Unique tumour-specific antigens (mutations)	A very large and increasing number of mouse and human unique mutational antigens (neo-epitopes)

Although the idea of tumour-specific antigens in mouse models of cancer was based on tumour rejection in vivo and thus had connotations of tumour specificity, the tumour antigens defined by tumour-reactive T cells show a wider spectrum of specificity and their connection with tumour immunity in vivo is tenuous.

The T-cell-defined tumour antigens of murine tumours have been defined in a mastocytoma, two fibrosarcomas, a squamous cell carcinoma and a colon carcinoma because these tumour lines are in popular use. Similarly, much of the corresponding work in human tumours has been carried out in melanomas because melanoma cell lines are easier to establish in culture, rather than because of any unique immunogenicity of human melanomas.

The tumour antigens identified as T-cell epitopes fall into a number of categories, discussed later (see Table 22.3).

Cancer/testes antigens are expressed on cancer cells and in testes.
Cancer/testes (CT) antigens, as the name suggests, are expressed on cancer cells and in testes, but not in other normal adult tissues. MAGE, BAGE, GAGE and NY-ESO1 are examples of this class of antigen. Individual epitopes within CT antigens have been defined for CD8 and CD4 lymphocytes. Two large randomized clinical trials with the MAGE antigen (in melanoma and lung cancers) failed to show clinical benefit in immunized cancer patients.

Differentiation antigens are expressed on normal tissues and tumours.
Differentiation antigens, which are lineage specific but not tumour specific, are expressed on normal tissues (melanocytes) and tumours (melanomas). Examples of such antigens include MART-1/Melan-A, tyrosinase, gp100, Trp1 and Trp2. Individual epitopes within differentiation antigens have been defined for CD8 and CD4 lymphocytes. Most differentiation antigens have been identified in human melanomas but, in randomized clinical trials, immunization with such antigens has not conferred clinical benefit to cancer patients.

T-cell epitopes of viral antigens have been identified.
T-cell epitopes of viral antigens of virus-induced tumours have been identified, such as:
- the T antigen of SV40 and the polyoma viruses;
- the E6 and E7 antigens of the human papilloma viruses (HPV) that cause cervical cancer; and
- a number of antigens of Epstein–Barr virus (EBV) (Table. 22.4).

Some of these, such as the HPV antigens, have been approved (as Cervarix and Gardasil) for prophylactic vaccination (see Chapter 17) of boys and girls.

Tumour-specific antigens defined by antibodies are rarely tumour specific.
The search for antibodies that discriminate between cancer cells and normal cells has a long pedigree and has been carried out with the whole range of tools starting from antisera to panning antibody libraries. This search has been largely unsuccessful and rarely have tumour-specific antibodies been generated. Most anti-tumour antibodies, like anti-tumour T cells, recognize CT antigens, differentiation antigens and even more broadly distributed common antigens (see Table 22.3).

Antibodies to a B-cell surface antigen, CD20, epidermal growth factor receptor and HER2/Neu have now been approved for treatments, respectively, of B-cell lymphoma, colorectal cancers and breast cancers. Although these antibodies have shown some efficacy in the treatment of certain cancers at certain stages, they:
- do not recognize tumour-specific antigens;
- act on tumour cells as many pharmacological agents (such as various platinum derivatives and other small molecules) do. They are not understood to elicit an immune response per se.

TABLE 22.4 Microorganisms and Human Tumours

Tumour	Organism
Adult T-cell leukaemia	Human T-leukaemia virus-I (HTLV-I)
Burkitt's lymphoma and lymphoma in immunosuppression	EBV
Cervical cancer	Human papilloma viruses (HPV 16 and 18 and others)
Liver cancer	Hepatitis B and C
Nasopharyngeal cancer	EBV
Skin cancer	Probably human papilloma viruses
Stomach cancer	*H. pylori*

Epstein–Barr virus (EBV) causes Burkitt's lymphoma in endemic malaria areas of Africa and nasopharyngeal carcinoma in China, suggesting that co-factors, either genetic or environmental, are required for tumour development. *Helicobacter pylori* is the only bacterium so far known to be involved in the aetiology of human cancer.

Antibodies used in the diagnosis and treatment of cancer may not be tumour specific. As serum antibodies are technically easy to measure, they have always attracted the attention of diagnosticians (Table 22.w1). Thus, antibody to carcinoembryonic antigen (CEA) is often used as a marker for progression or status of certain carcinomas; however, CEA or other such antigens are not tumour-specific antigens and diagnostic markers need not necessarily have the specificity required of a tumour-specific antigen. Nevertheless, antibodies targeting normal cell proteins have been used therapeutically to treat a variety of cancers (Table 22.w2). These antibodies may be cytotoxic for a particular cell type (e.g. antibody to CD20 targeting B-cell lymphoma) or aimed at interfering with tumour growth (e.g. antibody to human epidermal growth factor receptor-2 (HER2) to treat breast cancer).

Mutated oncogenes could be a source of tumour-specific antigens. The discussion thus far has dealt with tumour antigens defined by experimental tools. Several additional antigens have been tested as tumour antigens because of their restricted or relatively restricted expression on cancer cells, with the reasonable assumption that they would elicit tumour-specific and perhaps tumour-protective immune responses. Antigenic epitopes generated by mutated oncogenes such as *ras* and *p53* as well as gene fusion-generated oncogenes such as *bcr-abl*, which are, by definition, tumour specific, come into this category. These antigens could, in principle, be broadly applicable tumour antigens, particularly in those instances where specific mutations are seen in different individuals.

The idea that proteins encoded by mutant oncogenes are recognized by the immune system has been explored to a degree in murine and human systems and immune reactivity to peptides derived from such mutated oncogenes has been detected. However, no evidence of their general tumour-protective immunogenicity has emerged.

It is conceivable that the immune response to these alterations is tolerized early in tumorigenesis and, indeed, such tolerization may be a pre-condition for tumorigenesis.

Tumour-specific antigens can be defined using genomics and bioinformatics. The advent of high-throughput genomics and associated bioinformatics capabilities has allowed an unprecedented opportunity to identify tumour-specific changes by comparing the DNA sequences of the normal tissue and the tumours. This technological revolution has led to identification of tumour-specific mutations in thousands of tumours over the last 10 years. This work has confirmed two fundamentals of cancer immunology, previously deduced from murine work: (a) that tumours do have specific changes with respect to the normal tissues of the hosts in which they arise; (b) aside from the oncogenic or driver mutations, tumours contain vast numbers of incidental or passenger mutations. While the driver mutations are common to many tumours, the passenger mutations are unique to each patient's tumour.

It seemed straightforward in the beginning to identify the tumour-specific mutations and then predict which mutations would lead to MHC (class I or II) binding of the resulting peptides. Such epitopes created as a result of mutations are known as neo-epitopes. Since publicly available algorithms such as NetMHC are increasingly effective at predicting the binding affinity of a given peptide to a given MHC allele (and such exercise successfully predicts epitopes of viral or model antigens), considerable efforts have gone into predicting MHC-binding epitopes of mouse and human cancers. These efforts already suggest that of all the potential neo-epitopes, only a very small proportion (*estimated* to be anywhere between 0.1% and 5%, without any actual data) can actually mediate a change in the course of tumour growth. Although these are early days, it is already clear that the method of neo-epitope protection that works so well for foreign antigens does not work well for cancer neo-epitopes.

Available algorithms, such as NetMHC, rely overwhelmingly on the binding affinity of the mutant peptides to the MHC molecule (high, intermediate, low, non-binding) in order to predict a set of potential neo-epitopes. Although a small number of cancer neo-epitopes that bind MHC class I molecules with high affinity have been reported to mediate tumour rejection, a larger number of successful anti-tumour neo-epitopes do not show any significant measurable affinity for MHC class I. It has been suggested that the degree of difference in binding affinities of a neo-epitope and an unmutated sequence to an MHC class I molecule (differential agretopic index) is a better predictor of true anti-tumour neo-epitopes than the neo-epitope–MHC I binding affinity alone. The rules for predicting true neo-epitopes are still under intense examination and are largely unclear. Elucidation of such rules is necessary for clinical exploitation of these exciting tumour-specific antigens.

Although the genomics revolution has propelled neo-epitopes into the forefront, they have actually been known for over 25 years. They were originally defined as CD8 T-cell epitopes (and in some instances CD4 T-cell epitopes) of a number of mouse and human tumours and were shown to mediate tumour rejection in mice. The autologous tumour-derived heat shock protein-peptide vaccines, which showed limited clinical activity in phase III clinical trials, were also premised on the idea of a neo-epitope chaperoned by heat shock proteins gp96, hsp90 and hsp70.

A number of early-stage clinical trials using neo-epitope-based vaccines have been completed or are now ongoing in patients with melanoma, epithelial ovarian cancer, renal cell carcinoma, pancreatic cancer, follicular lymphoma, lymphocytic leukaemia, glioblastoma, urothelial and breast cancers.

ANTI-TUMOUR IMMUNE RESPONSES

Successful tumour immunity is rare in patients who have cancer. Mechanisms of tumour immunity have been examined mostly in mouse models, partly because successful tumour immunity is rare in patients who have cancer. Moreover, as successful tumour immunity is rare in the tumour-bearing setting in mouse models, much of the work has been done in a prophylactic setting, which is not applicable to the human situation.

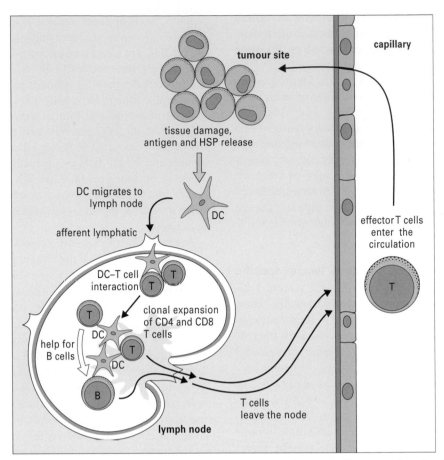

Fig. 22.3 A working diagram of the possible mechanism of tumour immunity The tumour inoculum (with its antigenic load) is taken up by antigen-presenting cells at the site of immunization and is cross-presented by them to the naive CD8 cells in the draining lymph nodes. *DC*, Dendritic cell.

Not surprisingly, the pathways to elicitation of immune response to tumours are straightforward (Fig. 22.3). The tumour inoculum (with its antigenic load) is taken up by the antigen-presenting cells (APCs) at the site of immunization and is cross-presented by them to the naive CD8 and CD4 cells in the draining lymph nodes. Both responses are necessary in the mouse models tested and both responses have been shown to be present in the cancer patients studied.

Generally speaking, antibodies have not been shown to be protective in the natural setting.

Natural killer (NK)-cell activity has been demonstrated most commonly, but its necessity has rarely been examined critically. In the few studies where it has been examined, NK cells play a crucial role in the immune response to cancers. The cytokines necessary for the effector functions of CD4, CD8 and NK cells, such as IL-2, IFNγ, IL-12 and others, are also necessary.

Despite an immune response, tumours continue to grow. Despite clear evidence of the existence of tumour-specific antigens and the immune response elicited by them, tumours continue to grow. In this regard, Ehrlich made a curious observation that remains at the centre of cancer immunity. He noted that animals with already growing tumours were strangely resistant to a second tumour challenge even as the first tumour kept growing (Fig. 22.4).

This phenomenon, termed **concomitant immunity** as early as 1908, remained unexamined until recently.

Concomitant immunity shows two aspects of tumour immunity

- First, a growing tumour elicits in the primary host a tumour-protective immune response.
- Second, although this response is sufficient to eliminate a nascent tumour, it fails to eliminate the tumour that elicited the response.

It was shown that concomitant immunity was tumour specific and operational only within a narrow window of 7–10 days after tumour implantation; if the second tumour was implanted beyond this time, it was not rejected. The lack of immunity beyond the narrow window was attributable to a new population of Tregs that appear at that time (Fig. 22.5). Similar to the phenomenon of concomitant immunity, it was also noted that mice in the process of rejecting a skin allograft were unable to reject concomitantly a growing tumour bearing the same allo-antigens as the allograft.

Immunization is effective prophylactically but rarely as therapy. The findings discussed earlier fit in well with the observations that, although naive mice can be immunized successfully using irradiated tumour cell vaccines in almost any

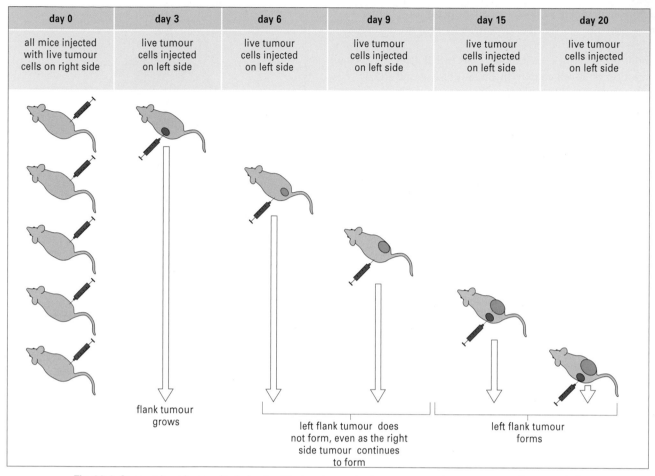

day 0	day 3	day 6	day 9	day 15	day 20
all mice injected with live tumour cells on right side	live tumour cells injected on left side	live tumour cells injected on left side	live tumour cells injected on left side	live tumour cells injected on left side	live tumour cells injected on left side

flank tumour grows

left flank tumour does not form, even as the right side tumour continues to form

left flank tumour forms

Fig. 22.4 Concomitant immunity Animals with already-growing tumours are resistant to a second tumour challenge even as the first tumour continues to grow.

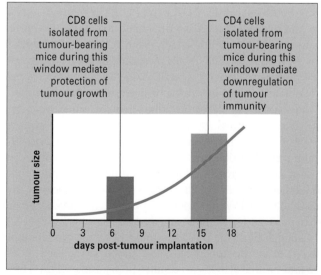

CD8 cells isolated from tumour-bearing mice during this window mediate protection of tumour growth

CD4 cells isolated from tumour-bearing mice during this window mediate downregulation of tumour immunity

tumour size

days post-tumour implantation

Fig. 22.5 Effector CD8 and regulatory CD4 cells in concomitant immunity Concomitant immunity is tumour specific and operational only within a narrow window of 7–10 days after tumour implantation. If the second tumour is implanted beyond this time, it is not rejected. The lack of immunity beyond the narrow window is attributable to a new population of regulatory T cells that appear at that time.

tumour model, the same irradiated cell vaccine is ineffective at treating established tumours. Prophylaxis is effective, even if begun as late as 3 days before tumour implantation, but therapy is ineffective even if begun as early as 2 days after tumour implantation (see Fig. 22.2).

It is easy, and incorrect, to infer from these observations that the tumour-bearing mice or cancer patients are generally immunosuppressed. Tumour-bearing mice generally mount a vigorous immune response to model antigens and even unrelated tumours, almost until the very end of their lives. Similarly, patients with cancer do not succumb to the opportunistic infections that are the hallmark of general immunosuppression.

The naive state and tumour-bearing state are essentially different. Collectively, the observations above have shaped the thinking that, immunologically, the tumour-bearing host is in a radically different state compared with the naive host.

What are the mechanisms behind this change of status? They are exactly the same as envisaged for the mechanisms for the initiation and maintenance of peripheral tolerance. None of the explanations is fully satisfactory by itself, but each may contribute to the final state of tolerance in some measure. Immune unresponsiveness per se is addressed in detail in Chapter 11. Aspects that are of specific relevance to tumour immunity include:

- inhibitory cytokines, including TGFβ and IL-10;
- inhibition of T-cell activity through CTLA-4 and PD-1;
- downregulation of the immune response through regulatory T cells;
- reversible or irreversible exhaustion of T cells;
- resistance to CD8 T-cell recognition by downregulation of MHC class I molecules; and
- generation of antigen-loss variants.

Downregulation of MHC I expression may result in resistance to recognition and lysis. A number of studies have shown:

- downregulation of expression of one or more MHC class I alleles;
- loss of β2-microglobulin; or
- loss or downregulation of any of the several components of the antigen-processing machinery.

Although these alterations are clearly likely to inhibit recognition of tumour cells by T cells, they are also more likely to make tumours more susceptible to NK cells.

On the whole, it is not clear what effect, if any, these alterations have on the net ability of a tumour to escape the immune response in vivo.

Generation of antigen-loss variants is another mechanism that no doubt plays a role in the immunological escape of tumour cells. However, because we do not yet have a significant knowledge of the identity of truly tumour-protective antigens, the role of antigen-loss variants cannot be critically examined.

T-cell activity is inhibited through CTLA-4 and PD-1. A likely explanation for unresponsiveness is the role of inhibition of T-cell activity through CTLA-4, which is an inhibitory molecule expressed by T cells upon activation (see Fig. 7.13).

CTLA-4 inhibits the T cell by raising the stimulatory threshold or by inhibiting the proliferative drive of T cells (Fig. 22.6). The biological role of CTLA-4 appears to lie in limiting the T-cell response to foreign antigens and to autoantigens. CTLA-4 is also expressed on other immune cells such as regulatory T cells and there is evidence that a substantial part of the anti-cancer activity of anti-CTLA-4 antibodies derives from their effect on inhibition of regulatory T cells, leading to a better T-cell immune response. Administering antibodies that inhibit CTLA-4:B7 interactions to mice bearing a broad array of tumours inhibited tumour growth, even when the antibody was administered after the tumours were visible and palpable (Fig. 22.w1). Such activity was seen only against the more immunogenic tumours and not against a poorly immunogenic melanoma (e.g. B16). In that instance, combination of anti-CTLA-4 antibody with a vaccine consisting of irradiated melanoma cells that were also transfected with the cytokine granulocyte–macrophage colony stimulating factor (GM-CSF) resulted in a stronger anti-tumour response than by anti-CTLA-4 antibody or the vaccine alone. Similar results have been observed in other tumour models. These results support the

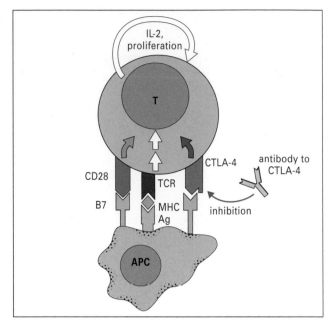

Fig. 22.6 Mechanism of action of anti-CTLA-4 antibody Normally, CTLA-4 delivers an inhibitory signal to the T cell by acting as an alternative receptor for the co-stimulatory signal delivered by B7 (CD80/86) binding to CD28. Antibody to CTLA-4 interferes with the inhibitory signalling and can thus increase T-cell activity. *APC*, Antigen-presenting cell; *MHC*, major histocompatibility complex; *TCR*, T-cell receptor.

notion derived from studies on concomitant immunity that progressive tumour growth results in the generation of inhibitory influences on the anti-tumour immune response. Antibodies to CTLA-4 have shown significant clinical benefit in a small proportion of melanoma patients and have been approved for human use (see later).

Programmed death-1 (PD-1) is also an inhibitory molecule transiently expressed by T cells upon their activation and by exhausted T cells at all times (see Chapter 7). Interaction of PD-1 with its ligands, PD-L1 and PD-L2, regulates the induction and maintenance of the peripheral tolerance and protects tissue from autoimmune attack. Such interaction inhibits the activity of effector CD8 T cells by suppression of cytokine production and cytotoxicity. The PD-1/PD-L1 interaction appears to facilitate tumour growth or progression in some tumours. A wide variety of cells, including a broad range of human tumour cells, express PD-L1, while PD-L2 is mostly expressed by APCs during inflammation. Administration of anti-PD-1 or anti-PD-L1 antibodies to tumour-bearing mice showed significant tumour growth inhibition in different tumour models. Antibodies to PD-1 or its ligands have shown significant clinical benefit in patients with a wide array of human cancers and have been approved for human use (see later).

Although blockade of CTLA-4 and PD-1 is often commonly referred to as checkpoint blockade, antibodies to each mediate their anti-tumour activities by distinct mechanisms. CTLA-4 blockade is considered to influence T-cell proliferation early in the immune response, largely in the lymph nodes, in addition to its anti-Treg activity. PD-1 blockade on the other hand acts on T cells at a later point in an immune response, i.e. in tumours and peripheral tissues.

Abrogation of CD25$^+$ Tregs leads to protective tumour immunity. The notion that progressive tumour growth results in the generation of inhibitory influences on the anti-tumour immune response is further supported by the recent work on the CD25$^+$ CD4$^+$ Treg cells (see Chapter 12). These cells have been shown to suppress CD8$^+$ T-cell responses in general, including autoimmune responses.

Recent studies have shown that abrogation of the CD25$^+$ subpopulation (through anti-CD25 antibodies or genetic manipulation) in tumour-bearing mice leads to a robust T-cell response and protective tumour immunity even in an aggressive tumour model such as the B16 melanoma. Conversely, re-addition of these cells can suppress the anti-tumour immune response.

Results consistent with these have been observed in patients with melanoma whose regulatory CD4$^+$ T cells specifically inhibit the CD8$^+$ activity against autologous melanoma cells, but not against other targets.

More recent studies have examined this paradigm through the prism of the CD25$^+$ T cells. In a study of patients with ovarian cancer, such cells were shown to be associated with a higher risk of death and reduced survival. Interestingly, the CD25$^+$ T cells were shown to migrate preferentially to the solid tumours and the ascites, but rarely to the draining lymph nodes.

Such results indicate that, despite the poor clinical outcomes in advanced cancer, the host mounts a vigorous anti-tumour immune response, which is compromised by regulatory mechanisms. Manipulation of such regulatory mechanisms for enhancing cancer immunity is bound to influence the fine balance between tolerance and autoimmunity. In certain contexts, that may be a reasonable price to pay.

Myeloid-derived suppressor cells inhibit the immune response to tumours. Myeloid-derived suppressor cells (MDSCs) are a heterogeneous population of immature myeloid cells with a mixture of granulocytic or monocytic morphology, which are defined by the expression of particular surface markers (these markers differ between humans and mice). Accumulating evidence has shown that factors associated with the tumour micro-environment, such as cytokines and pro-inflammatory signals, can induce, recruit and activate MDSCs in both murine and human cancers. MDSCs' immunosuppressive functions are mediated by a number of potential mechanisms of direct suppressive activity on the T-cell and NK-cell compartments. Further complicating a clear understanding of MDSCs' functions is the work demonstrating that the different MDSC subsets utilize different means of suppression. However, the main methods of MDSC-mediated immune suppression include expression of suppressive factors (e.g. arginase, inducible NOS, TGFβ, IL-10, COX2 and prostaglandin E$_2$), cysteine sequestration, reducing T-cell L-selectin expression and Treg induction. These mechanisms serve to reinforce a pro-tumour micro-environment through disruption of T-cell metabolism, activation, proliferation and, in turn, their tumour-cell killing capacity. Although MDSCs have a multitude of means for suppression, it is likely that, at any given time, one mechanism serves as the dominant force, which is dependent upon the immunological contexts, and can change as the tumour progresses and treatments are introduced. In addition to immunosuppressive functions, MDSCs can have a role in tumour progression and metastases through direct tumour-cell interactions.

Extracellular adenosine suppresses T-cell anti-tumour functions. Extracellular adenosine produced by Tregs in a paracrine manner can play a major role in immune suppression. Specifically, Tregs express the ecto-enzymes CD39 and CD73 on their cell surface, which are able to convert ATP to AMP and AMP to adenosine, respectively. This peri-cellular adenosine is able to bind to the adenosine A2A receptor on effector T cells and suppress their anti-tumour function by the activating cyclic AMP (cAMP)–PKA signalling cascade. However, the exact mechanism of how this results in T-cell dysfunction is yet to be elucidated. Extracellular ATP, which is essential as a substrate for CD39, is presumed to be derived from apoptosis of cells in the tumour micro-environment.

Antagonists of MDSCs and the adenosine pathway are under early phases of clinical testing.

IMMUNOTHERAPY FOR HUMAN CANCER

Animal models are limited in the translation of therapy. There exists a common wisdom but incorrect belief that treatment of cancers of mice is easy and has no bearing on treatment of human cancers. Mouse tumours are hard to cure – not a single publication reports curing a mouse with stage IV disseminated disease.

Most approaches study prophylactic vaccination in mice; a smaller number begin treatment on the day of tumour challenge and only a handful of studies begin treatment more than 10 days after tumour challenge. In most mouse tumour models, mice die within 4–6 weeks of tumour challenge and thus the window of treatment is extremely narrow.

Most approaches to immunotherapy of human cancer have either never been tested in appropriate mouse models or have failed to show anti-tumour activity when tested. It is important to bear this in mind while examining the three major categories of approaches to immunotherapy of human cancer, discussed later.

Antibodies have been used successfully. As antibodies are the oldest known immunological reagents, it is only to be expected that the first, and thus far among the most successful, approaches to human cancer immunotherapy have been made using these reagents.

In the 1980s, Ronald Levy and colleagues treated patients with B-cell lymphomas using individual patient's tumour-specific anti-idiotypic antibodies on the premise that the antibodies will recognize and help eliminate their targets (the surface immunoglobulin on the monoclonal lymphomas). The treatment was successful clinically, leading to significant objective tumour regressions, but was limited by the re-emergence of escape variants that did not express the idiotype. This approach has not been pursued further but remains a powerful reminder of what true tumour-specific antibodies can do to real-life tumours.

Selected antibodies are now approved for clinical use (see Table 22.w2) and include antibodies to:

- CD20 (rituximab) against B-cell lymphoma;
- HER2/Neu (trastuzumab, Herceptin) against breast cancer;
- epidermal growth factor receptor (cetuximab, Erbitux) against colon cancer.

It is ironic that the anti-tumour antibodies that may recognize truly or relatively tumour-specific molecules and that were the earliest hopes of much of the efforts in this area have yet to enter the phase of randomized clinical testing. Such antibodies are difficult to characterize and therefore have been slow in development.

Vaccination can be used to treat cancer. Although the term 'vaccination' is typically used to indicate prophylactic vaccination, cancer researchers use it to indicate the treatment of someone who already has cancer with agents that stimulate an anti-cancer immune response, with a view to causing regression of cancers, slowing down the growth of progressing cancers or preventing or delaying recurrence of cancer. Several vaccination approaches have been pursued in the past and yet others are being pursued now. The overwhelming majority of cancer vaccines tested in the past, including whole cancer cells, cancer lysates, purified autologous tumour-derived heat shock protein-peptide complexes or defined T-cell epitopes of differentiation antigens or cancer/testes antigens, have failed to show clinical benefits to immunized patients in randomized trials. Nonetheless, these failures have helped advance the research. Most importantly, they have clarified that, unlike for infectious agents, one-size-fits-all or shared antigen vaccines are unsuitable as cancer vaccines, simply because each cancer is antigenically distinct, as observed even in the very early studies by Gross, Prehn and Main and George and Eva Klein. Some of the previous approaches, such as vaccination with the autologous tumour-derived heat shock protein-peptide complexes, were based on the individuality of cancers and have now evolved into the currently ongoing studies using personalized neo-epitopes of individual cancers as cancer vaccines.

Idiotypes of B-cell lymphomas have been used as vaccines. Following the use of anti-idiotypic antibodies and the attendant limitations discussed earlier, the idiotypes of B lymphomas have been used as vaccines. In this approach, a patient's idiotype is determined by polymerase chain reactions from the tumour tissues and a synthetic idiotype, conjugated to a carrier such as keyhole limpet haemocyanin, is administered with GM-CSF. In a phase III trial of 117 patients who were in complete remission after chemotherapy, median time to relapse for 76 patients vaccinated using this approach was 44.2 months, compared with 30.6 months for the 41 who received placebo. This was the first and thus far the only vaccine that has shown significant clinical activity in B-cell lymphoma. For obvious reasons, this approach is limited to B-cell haematological malignancies.

Immunization with defined MHC I restricted epitopes does not lead to clinical benefit. The antigenic epitopes of differentiation antigens and cancer/testes antigens have been used extensively and several hundred melanoma patients have been treated with these. Although anti-peptide CD8 responses have been detected in most studies, these have not generally translated into clinical benefit even for those patients who have shown good CD8 responses. A recent randomized trial using a gp100 peptide showed no evidence of clinical benefit.

Efforts to vaccinate using altered peptide epitopes with higher affinity for the cognate T-cell receptors are particularly interesting. Immunization with such altered peptides is able to break tolerance against these self antigens where immunization with native peptides is not.

Immunotherapy with DCs presenting a prostate antigen shows clinical benefit. DCs can be isolated from a cancer patient, pulsed with antigenic peptides, whole proteins or tumour lysates and infused back into the patient. The most advanced clinical trials using this approach have been carried out in patients with prostate cancer, using the protein prostatic acid phosphatase because of the prostate-specific distribution of this protein and because of its low homology with non-prostate proteins. Patients' APCs are pulsed with a fusion protein consisting of prostatic acid phosphatase and GM-CSF and are re-infused into the patient. In a randomized phase III trial in 512 subjects, prostate cancer patients who received the acid phosphatase pulsed autologous APCs (Sipuleucel-T) showed a median survival of 25.8 months compared with 21.7 months for patients who received placebo. This trial formed the basis of the FDA approval of this treatment for patients with asymptomatic or minimally symptomatic prostate cancer but, in spite of an FDA approval, Sipuleucel-T has not received an enthusiastic reception in actual clinical practice.

Checkpoint blockade of CTLA-4, PD-1 or PD-L1/2 shows significant clinical benefit. Antibodies to CTLA-4 and PD-1 have shown dramatic success in cancer immunotherapy, even though only a minority of the patients treated with them benefit from the treatment. PD-1 blockade acts by removing the brake from the anti-tumour immune response by blocking the inhibitory PD-L1/2–PD-1 interaction. CTLA-4 blockade inhibits CTLA-4–B7 interaction and may act, additionally, through inhibition of Treg activity. James Allison and Tasuku Honjo were awarded the 2018 Nobel Prize in Physiology or Medicine for their discoveries using CTLA-4 and PD-1, respectively.

Antibodies to PD-1 (pembrolizumab and nivolumab) have been shown to mediate durable tumour shrinkage and to improve survival and progression-free survival significantly in several cancers. Such antibodies have been approved for treatment of advanced melanoma, non-small cell lung cancer, urothelial cancer, Hodgkin's lymphoma, head and neck squamous cell carcinoma and cancers that are microsatellite instability-high or mismatch-repair deficient. Additionally, the FDA has approved pembrolizumab for gastric and cervical cancer and nivolumab for advanced liver cancer and small cell lung cancer. Anti-PD-L1 antibody atezolizumab has also been approved for advanced non-small cell lung and urothelial carcinoma. Additional anti-PD-L1 antibodies avelumab and durvalumab have both been approved for urothelial carcinoma and avelumab has been approved for Merkel cell carcinoma. Clinical efficacy of anti-PD-L2 antibody is currently under evaluation.

Antibodies to CTLA-4 have been shown to mediate durable tumour shrinkage in a small proportion of melanoma patients and have been shown to prolong overall survival. Such antibodies have been approved for treatment of advanced melanoma. PD-1 blockade elicits higher response rates (tumour shrinkage) than CTLA-4 blockade. As may be expected from the fact that blockade of each antibody (to CTLA-4 and PD-1) works by a distinct immunological mechanism, combination of the two antibodies has proven to be more effective than either antibody alone in treatment of advanced melanoma.

In spite of the dramatic successes of antibodies to CTLA-4 and PD-1, most patients do not benefit from these treatments. There is an enormous amount of effort ongoing to determine biomarkers that predict response to each therapeutic modality, but so far no compelling biomarkers have emerged.

CTLA-4 and PD-1 have important functions in normal immune response and its regulation. There is no cancer specificity to these molecules. It may then be expected that their blockade will have significant adverse effects. Indeed, both treatments elicit serious immune-mediated adverse events, such as rashes, gastrointestinal disorders and endocrinopathies. Treatment-related adverse events occur more frequently with CTLA-4 than with PD-1 blockade, perhaps as a consequence of the differences in their mechanisms of action. Dual blockade, while more efficacious, elicits significantly more toxicity than either monotherapy.

Adoptive immunotherapy using T cells: the clinical benefits.

Adoptive immunotherapy using T cells has a successful pedigree in murine models of cancer (Fig. 22.7). Clinical experience with bone marrow transplant recipients also provides a strong rationale for the approach.

Patients undergoing high-dose chemotherapy lose their bone marrow and are re-constituted with allogeneic stem cells, which engraft in the recipient. However, the T cells from the donor may see the normal tissues of the host as foreign, thus causing graft versus host disease (GvHD).

Interestingly, patients who develop GvHD also have a lower cancer relapse. This is thought to be a result of a graft versus tumour (GVT), sometimes also called a graft versus leukaemia (GVL), effect. The clinical experience with GvHD and GVT has long remained a compelling piece of evidence for the premise that T cells can eliminate human cancers in vivo (Fig. 22.8).

A number of studies have isolated tumour-infiltrating T cells from cancer patients, expanded them in vitro and infused the expanded cells back into the patients. Such studies have shown remarkable shrinkage of tumours in significant proportions of patients in non-randomized clinical studies.

In a variation of this approach, cloned T cells with defined specificity have been expanded to very large numbers and infused into patients with melanoma, producing dramatic tumour shrinkage.

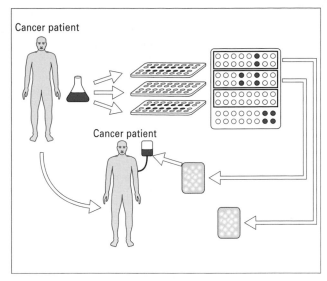

Fig. 22.7 Adoptive immunotherapy with T cells Lymphocytes removed from a patient with a tumour are expanded in vitro. Cells that recognize the tumour are selected and re-infused into the original patient. Adoptive therapy with allogeneic lymphocytes may also be carried out. (Redrawn from Dudley ME, Rosenberg SA. Adoptive-cell-transfer therapy for the treatment of patients with cancer. Nat Rev Cancer 2003;3:666–675. Copyright 2002, Nature Reviews Cancer, Macmillan Magazines Ltd.)

However, hurdles to expansion of T cells and their effector functions in vivo remain and there is considerable ongoing experimental effort to engineer T cells that will retain specificity and autonomy of growth and will be relatively refractory to downregulatory influences of the host.

T cells with chimeric antigen receptors are highly effective in therapy of several haematological malignancies.

Chimeric antigen receptor (CAR) T-cell therapy is a form of adoptive T-cell transfer that involves nultifaceted methods of T-cell engineering and ex vivo culture, typically using autologous T cells, prior to patient re-infusion (Fig. 22.9). Specifically, CAR T-cell methodologies entail the genetic engineering of T cells to express a CAR, most commonly implemented as a single-chain variable fragment (scFv) from an antibody as the extracellular antigen-binding domain coupled with the intracellular signalling domains of the TCRζ chain and additional co-stimulatory domains from other T-cell activating receptors (e.g. CD28, OX40 and CD137). Therefore, engagement of the CAR antigen-recognition ecto-domain results in potent intracellular signalling and T-cell activation. In turn, this approach is associated with a number of advantages and disadvantages compared with other forms of adoptive cell transfer, such as ex vivo tumour-infiltrating lymphocyte (TIL) expansion/reinfusion and engineered TCR T cells.

One key advantage is that CAR T cells do not require MHC expression and antigen presentation on target cells in order to achieve targeted killing, thus limiting a major mechanism of tumour cell escape: namely, MHC loss and/or decreased antigen presentation. However, CAR T cells require target antigens to be expressed on the surface of tumour cells. This profound

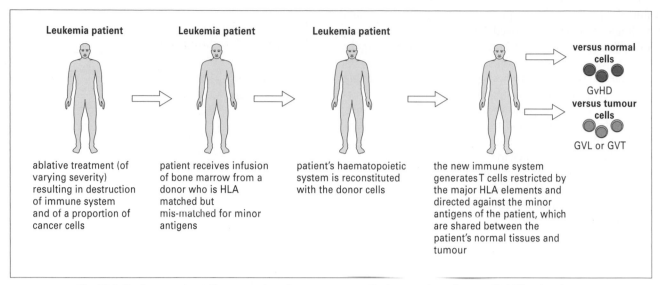

Leukemia patient **Leukemia patient** **Leukemia patient**

versus normal
cells

GvHD

versus tumour
cells

GVL or GVT

ablative treatment (of
varying severity)
resulting in destruction
of immune system
and of a proportion of
cancer cells

patient receives infusion
of bone marrow from a
donor who is HLA
matched but
mis-matched for minor
antigens

patient's haematopoietic
system is reconstituted
with the donor cells

the new immune system
generates T cells restricted by
the major HLA elements and
directed against the minor
antigens of the patient, which
are shared between the
patient's normal tissues and
tumour

Fig. 22.8 Graft versus host disease and graft versus tumour Graft versus host disease *(GvHD)* and graft versus leukaemia *(GVL)* effects. Both responses are restricted by the major histocompatibility complex (MHC) alleles and directed against the minor antigens. The minor antigens are the same between the patient's normal tissues and tumour; hence the GvHD (immune response against normal tissues) and GVL (immune response against leukaemia or other tumour) are generally inextricably linked. *GVT,* Graft versus tumour.

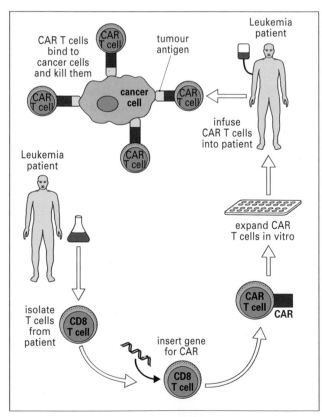

Fig. 22.9 CAR T-cell therapy CD8 T cells are isolated from a cancer patient's blood. A gene for a chimeric antigen receptor, which recognizes the patient's tumour, is introduced into the cells. The T cells expressing the new receptor are expanded in vitro and infused back into the patient, where they recognize and kill the cancer cells.

disadvantage of CAR T cells limits the number/type of antigenic targets to those found on the tumour's surface. In addition, the antigens would ideally be expressed only on tumour cells because on-target, off-tumour toxicities associated with the targeting of shared antigens have been severe.

With this in mind, initial successes in the CAR T therapy have been limited to haematological malignancies with well-defined and highly restricted surface antigens specific to particular cell types, such as CD19. CAR T-cell therapies against CD19 have produced robust clinical responses of up to 90% remission rates in a number of B-cell malignancies such as acute lymphoblastic leukaemia (ALL), diffuse large B-cell lymphoma (DLBCL), chronic lymphocytic leukaemia (CLL) and other B-cell non-Hodgkin's lymphomas. This has resulted in the FDA approval of tisagenlecleucel (KYMRIAH, Novartis) for B-ALL in August 2017 and DLBCL in May 2018 as well as ciloleucel (YESCARTA, Kite Pharmaceuticals) for DLBCL in October 2017. However, this treatment results in a near complete ablation of the B-cell compartment because of its ubiquitous CD19 expression and necessitates infusion of immunoglobulins to mitigate associated morbidities. Other targets, such as B-cell maturation antigen (BCMA) and CD22, for targeting multiple myeloma and ALL, respectively, are being investigated in ongoing clinical trials given their restricted B-cell lineage expression. Other trials targeting tumour-associated antigens (for example, ERBB2/HER2) have had limited success partly because of severe on-target, off-tumour related toxicities and the inherent T-cell suppressive qualities of the tumour micro-environment in solid tumours.

Further limiting the success of CAR T therapies against both solid and haematological malignancies have been incidences of the severe and sometimes fatal inflammatory condition known as cytokine release syndrome (CRS). CRS is the result of exceedingly high levels of circulating cytokines and chemokines that are released from over-activated CAR T cells and other endogenous immune cell populations, which can cause neurological, haematological and other organ-specific dysfunctions. Even in the face of these challenges and shortcomings, CAR T-cell therapies are a very promising and active field of study, as highlighted by the fact that, worldwide, there are more than 250 clinical trials as of the beginning of 2018. Looking to the future, advances in T-cell engineering, tumour immunology, T-cell biology and other related fields will continue to increase our understanding of the complex interactions between cancer and the immune system, leading to changes in CAR T-cell approaches that will almost certainly result in increased efficacy of these therapies. Ideas that are already in the process of pre-clinical and clinical implementation include combinatorial approaches with other immunomodulatory agents (e.g. immune checkpoint blockade, cytokines), further genetic alterations to T cells to decrease expression of inhibitory checkpoint molecules, allogeneic universal CAR T cells for off-the-shelf delivery and many other novel approaches.

CRITICAL THINKING: IMMUNITY TO CANCERS

See Critical thinking: Explanations, section 22

The head of a cancer institute has decided that the institute should focus more heavily on pancreatic cancer. She recruits a cancer immunologist to develop a new immunotherapy for pancreatic cancer. The immunologist has previously developed CAR T-cell therapies for B-cell malignancies and decides to take a similar approach here.

1. What kind of tumour antigens are suitable targets for CAR T-cell therapy?

The immunologist thinks that a protein called mesothelin might be a suitable target, because it is highly expressed in pancreatic cancers. He develops a CAR that recognizes mesothelin and expresses it in T cells. He begins by testing the safety of his CAR T cells in 10 healthy volunteers.

2. Three of the volunteers experience fever, muscle and joint pain and low blood pressure. What could be the reason for this?

3. The immunologist notices that these three volunteers have unusually high serum IL-6. What does this suggest about the way that this side effect could be treated?

4. Two of the 10 volunteers experience pleuritis (inflammation of the lining of the lungs). What could be the reason for this?

5. The immunologist feels that the CAR T-cell therapy is not yet safe enough to move forward to trials in patients. What adjustments could be made to improve the safety of the therapy?

FURTHER READING

Callahan MK, Postow MA, Wolchok JD. Targeting T cell co-receptors for cancer therapy. Immunity 2016;44:1069–1078.

Klein G. The strange road to the tumor-specific transplantation antigens (TSTAs). Cancer Immun 2001;1:6.

Marvel D, Gabrilovich DI. Myeloid-derived suppressor cells in the tumor microenvironment: expect the unexpected. J Clin Invest 2015;125(9):3356–3364.

Maus MV, Fraietta JA, Levine BL, et al. Adoptive immunotherapy for cancer or viruses. Annu Rev Immunol 2014;32:189–225.

Nishikawa H, Sakaguchi S. Regulatory T cells in cancer immunotherapy. Curr Opin Immunol 2014;27:1–7.

North RJ. Down-regulation of the antitumor immune response. Adv Cancer Res 1985;45:1–43.

Rosenberg SA, Restifo NP. Adoptive cell transfer as personalized immunotherapy for human cancer. Science 2015;348(6230):62–68.

Sitkovsky MV, Hatfield S, et al. Hostile, hypoxia-A2-adenosinergic tumor biology as the next barrier to overcome for tumor immunologists. Cancer Immunol Res 2014;2:598–605.

Srivastava PK. Neoepitopes of cancers: looking back, looking ahead. Cancer Immunol Res 2015;3:969–977.

Wei SC, Duffy CR, Allison JP. Fundamental mechanisms of immune checkpoint blockade therapy. Cancer Discov 2018;8(9):1069–1086.

23

Immediate Hypersensitivity (Type I)

SUMMARY

- **The classification of hypersensitivity reactions is based on the system proposed by Gell and Coombs**. However, type I hypersensitivity is now seen as part of type 2 immunity.
- **Historical observations have shaped our understanding of immediate hypersensitivity**. The severity of symptoms depends on IgE antibodies, the quantity of allergen, the route of administration and a variety of factors that can enhance the response, including viral infections and environmental pollutants.
- **Most allergens are proteins**, but worms and ticks can induce IgE to oligosaccharide epitopes.
- **In genetically predisposed individuals, IgE production occurs to many different allergen sources.**
- **Allergens are the antigens that give rise to immediate hypersensitivity** and contribute to asthma rhinitis or food allergy.
- **Mast cells and basophils contain histamine**. IgE antibodies bind to a specific receptor, FcεRI, on mast cells and basophils. This Fc receptor has a very

high affinity and, when bound, IgE is cross-linked by specific allergen and mediators, including histamine, leukotrienes and cytokines, are released.
- **Multiple genes have been associated with asthma in different populations**. Multiple genetic loci influence the production of IgE, the inflammatory response to allergen exposure, and the response to treatment. Polymorphisms have been identified in the genes, in promoter regions and in the receptors for IgE, cytokines, leukotrienes and the β_2-receptors.
- **Skin tests and IgE assays are used for diagnosis and as a guide to the treatment**.
- **Several different pathways contribute to the chronic symptoms of allergy**.
- **Immunotherapy can be used for allergic rhinitis, asthma and anaphylactic sensitivity to venoms**. In addition, many different monoclonal antibodies are now being used to help treat allergic disease.

CLASSIFICATION OF HYPERSENSITIVITY REACTIONS

The adaptive immune response provides specific protection against infection with bacteria, viruses, parasites and fungi. Some immune responses, however, give rise to an excessive or inappropriate reaction, which is usually referred to as **hypersensitivity**.

The term 'hypersensitivity' evolved in the early years of the 20th century from the observations of Richet and Portier, who described the catastrophic result of exposing a presensitized animal to systemic antigen. The resulting outcome, termed **anaphylaxis**, became the prototype of immediate hypersensitivity responses.

In 1963, Coombs and Gell proposed a classification scheme in which allergic hypersensitivity of the type described by Portier and Richet was termed 'type I' and broadened the definition of hypersensitivity to include:

- **Immediate (type I) hypersensitivity responses** are characterized by the production of IgE antibodies against foreign proteins that are commonly present in the environment (e.g. pollens, animal dander or house dust mites) and can be identified by wheal and flare responses to skin tests, which develop within 15 minutes.

- **Antibody-mediated (type II) hypersensitivity reactions** occur when IgG or IgM antibodies are produced against surface antigens on cells of the body. These antibodies can trigger reactions either by activating complement (e.g. autoimmune haemolytic anaemia) or by facilitating the binding of natural killer cells (see Chapter 24).

- **Immune complex diseases (type III hypersensitivity)** involve the formation of immune complexes in the circulation that are not adequately cleared by macrophages or other cells of the mononuclear phagocyte system. The formation of immune complexes requires significant quantities of antibody and antigen (typically microgram quantities of each). The classic diseases of this group are systemic lupus erythematosus (SLE), chronic glomerulonephritis and serum sickness (see Chapter 25).

- **Cell-mediated reactions (type IV hypersensitivity)** are those in which specific T cells are the primary effector cells (see Chapter 26). Examples of T cells causing unwanted responses are:
  - contact sensitivity (e.g. to nickel or plants such as poison ivy);
  - delayed hypersensitivity responses of leprosy or tuberculosis;

type I	type II	type III	type IV
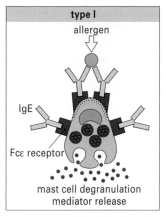	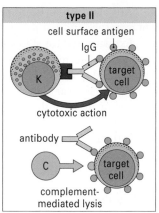	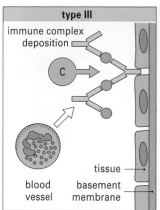	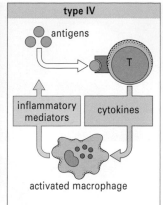

Fig. 23.1 The Coombs and Gell classification of hypersensitivity reactions In type I hypersensitivity, mast cells bind IgE via their Fc receptors. On encountering allergen the IgE becomes cross-linked, inducing degranulation and release of mediators that produce allergic reactions. In type II, antibody is directed against antigen on an individual's own cells (target cell) or foreign antigen, such as transfused red blood cells. This may lead to cytotoxic action by K cells or complement-mediated lysis. In type III, immune complexes are deposited in the tissue. Complement is activated and polymorphs are attracted to the site of deposition, causing local tissue damage and inflammation. In type IV, antigen-sensitized T cells release cytokines following a secondary contact with the same antigen. Cytokines induce inflammatory reactions and activate and attract macrophages, which release inflammatory mediators.

- exaggerated response to viral infections such as measles;
- persistent symptoms of allergic disease.

The original Coombs and Gell classification is shown in Figure 23.1.

In the past several years it has become apparent that the Coombs and Gell classification artificially divided mechanistically related antibody reactions (such as types I, II and III), which contribute to the pathophysiology of many common immune-mediated diseases, while including the T-cell-mediated reactions of delayed-type hypersensitivity (DTH) in a common classification (termed type IV).

There are important common features of types I, II and III hypersensitivity in that many or most of the functions of antibodies are dependent on specific Fc receptors (see Chapter 10). This is particularly true for the function of IgE where the two receptors FcεR1 or FcεR2 are specific for IgE and completely different in function.

HISTORICAL PERSPECTIVE ON IMMEDIATE HYPERSENSITIVITY

The first allergic disease to be defined was seasonal hay fever caused by pollen grains (which have a defined season of weeks or months) entering the nose (rhinitis) and eyes (conjunctivitis). In severe cases, patients might also get seasonal asthma and seasonal dermatitis. In 1873, Charles Blackley demonstrated that pollen grains placed into the nose could induce symptoms of rhinitis. He also demonstrated that pollen extract could produce a wheal and flare skin response in patients with hay fever.

The **wheal and flare skin response** (see Fig. 23.13) is an extremely sensitive method of detecting specific IgE antibodies. The timing and form of the skin response is similar to the response to histamine. However, pseudopods (lateral extensions of the wheal), severe reactions and delayed or late reactions only occur with allergen in the skin of allergic patients. Furthermore,

the immediate skin response can be effectively blocked with antihistamines.

In 1903, Portier and Richet discovered that immunization of guinea pigs with a toxin from the jellyfish *Physalia* could sensitize them so that a subsequent injection of the same protein would cause rapid onset of breathing difficulty, influx of fluid into the lungs and death. They coined the term **anaphylaxis** (from the Greek *ana*, non, and *phylaxos*, protection) and speculated about the relationship to other hypersensitivity diseases. They noted that:

- human anaphylaxis had no familial characteristics (unlike most of the other allergic diseases); and
- natural exposure to inhaled allergens did not cause anaphylaxis or urticaria.

Subsequently, it became clear that injection of any protein into an individual with immediate hypersensitivity to that protein could induce anaphylaxis (Fig. 23.2). Thus, anaphylaxis occurs when a patient with immediate hypersensitivity is exposed to a relevant allergen in such a way that the antigen enters the circulation rapidly.

Anaphylaxis may also occur as a result of eating an allergen such as peanut or shellfish or after the rupture of hydatid cysts with the rapid release of parasite antigens.

The term **allergen** was first used by von Pirquet in 1906 to cover all foreign substances that could produce an immune response. Subsequently, the word 'allergen' came to be used selectively for the proteins that cause 'supersensitivity'. Thus, an allergen is an antigen that gives rise to immediate hypersensitivity.

CHARACTERISTICS OF TYPE I REACTIONS

Most allergens are proteins. Substances that can give rise to wheal and flare responses in the skin and to the symptoms of allergic disease are derived from many different sources. When purified, they are almost all found to be proteins and their sizes

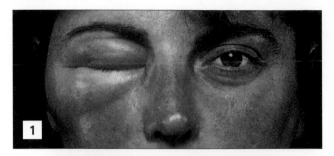

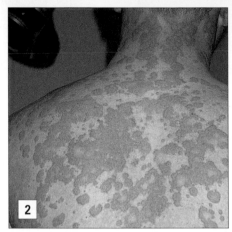

Fig. 23.2 Anaphylaxis and urticaria (1) The anaphylactic response to bee venom in a patient who has IgE antibodies to the venom protein phospholipase A. The immediate reaction occurred within 20 minutes and was caused by the release of histamine and other mediators from mast cells. This patient had been stung on the face, but the reaction can become generalized, leading to a fall in blood pressure, generalized urticaria and/or bronchospasm (i.e. anaphylaxis). **(2)** Diffuse urticaria on a patient with severe chronic urticaria. The lesions have a raised edge and come up within minutes or hours. The lesions almost always resolve within 12 hours, leaving no trace on the skin.

range from 10 to 40 kDa. These proteins are all freely soluble in aqueous solution but have many different biological functions, including digestive enzymes, carrier proteins, calycins and pollen recognition proteins.

Any allergen can be described or classified by its source, route of exposure and nature of the specific protein (Table 23.1).

Extracts used for skin testing or in vitro measurement of IgE antibodies are made from the whole material, which contains multiple different proteins, any of which can be an allergen. Indeed, it is clear that individual patients can react selectively to one or more of the different proteins that are present in an extract.

Estimates of exposure can be made either by visual identification of particles (e.g. pollen grains or fungal spores) or by immunoassay of the major allergens (e.g. Fel d1 or Der p1).

IgE is distinct from the other dimeric immunoglobulins. In 1921, Küstner, who was allergic to fish, injected his own serum into the skin of Prausnitz, who was allergic to grass pollen but not fish, and demonstrated that it was possible to transfer immediate hypersensitivity passively (the Prausnitz–Küstner or P–K test). Prausnitz also noticed that an immediate wheal and flare occurred at the site of passive sensitization when he ate fish. This showed that some protein or part of fish proteins sufficient to trigger mast cells can be absorbed into the circulation.

Over the next 30 years, it was established that P–K activity was a general property of the serum of patients with immediate hypersensitivity and that it was allergen specific (i.e. it behaved like an antibody).

In 1967, Ishizaka and his colleagues purified the P–K activity from a patient with ragweed hay fever and proved that this was a novel isotype of immunoglobulin – IgE. However, it was obvious that the concentration of this immunoglobulin isotype in serum was very low i.e. ≤ 1 μg/mL.

IgE is distinct from the other dimeric immunoglobulins because it has:
- an extra constant region domain;
- a different structure to the hinge region; and
- the primary binding sites for both FcεR1 and FcεR2 are on the C3 domain of IgE. This domain has an unusual form of internal flexibility, such that on binding with IgE it rearranges and becomes thermodynamically more stable. In turn,

TABLE 23.1	**Properties of Allergens**					
			ALLERGEN		
Source	**Airborne Particles**	**Dimension of Airborne Particle (μm)**	**Name**	**MW (kDa)**	**Function/Homologies**
Dust mite: *Dermatophagoides pteronyssinus*	Faeces	10–40	Der p1 Der p2	25 13	Cysteine protease (epididymal protein)
Cats: *Felis domesticus*	Dander particles	2–15	Fel d1	36	Uteroglobin
German cockroach: *Blattella germanica*	Frass, saliva and other debris	≥5	Bla g2 Bla g4 Bla g5	36 21 23	Aspartic protease Calycin Glutathione-*S*-transferase
Rat: *Rattus norvegicus*	Urine on bedding?	2–20	Rat n1	19	Pheromone-binding protein
Grass	Pollen	30	Lol p1	29	Not known
Fungi: *Alternaria alternata,* *Aspergillus fumigatus*	Spores Spores	14 × 10 2	Alt a1 Asp f1	28 18	Not known Mitogillin

The terminology of specific allergens is based on the first three letters of the genus (i.e. Der), followed by the first letter of the species (i.e. Der p) and the order in which the allergen was purified and defined, i.e. Der_p1 or Fel_d_1 or Bet_v_1. The size of the particles is important, because it affects how much becomes airborne and where it is deposited in the respiratory tract.

this results in a very low off rate and very high affinity (see Fig. 10.19).

The primary cells that bear FcεRI are **mast cells** and **basophils**, which are the only cells in humans that contain significant amounts of histamine.

Low-affinity receptors for IgE (FcεRII or CD23) are also present on B cells and may play a role in antigen presentation.

In addition, in atopic dermatitis, dendritic cells in skin can express a high-affinity receptor for IgE, but this receptor lacks the β chain of FcεRI.

The properties of IgE can be separated into three areas:
- the characteristics of the molecule, including its half-life and binding to IgE receptors;
- the control of IgE and IgG antibody production by T cells; and
- the consequences of allergen cross-linking IgE on the surface of mast cells or basophils.

The half-life of IgE is short compared with that of other immunoglobulins. The concentration of IgE in the serum of normal individuals is very low compared with all the other immunoglobulin isotypes. Values range from <10 to 10 000 IU/mL and the international unit (IU) is equivalent to 2.4 ng. Most sera contain <400 IU/mL (i.e. <1 μg/mL). The reasons serum IgE is so low include:
- Serum IgE has a much shorter half-life than other isotypes (~2 days compared with 21–23 days for IgG).
- IgE is produced in small quantities and is only produced in response to a select group of antigens (allergens and parasites).
- IgE antibodies are sequestered on the high-affinity receptor on mast cells and basophils.

The half-life of IgE in the serum has been measured both by injecting radiolabelled IgE and by infusing plasma from allergic patients into normal and immune-deficient patients.

The half-life of IgE in serum is less than 2 days; by contrast, IgE bound to mast cells in the skin has a half-life of approximately 10 days.

The low quantities of IgE in the serum must reflect a more rapid breakdown of IgE, as well as removal from the circulation by binding onto mast cells.

The most important site of breakdown of IgE is thought to be within **endosomes** where the low pH facilitates breakdown of free immunoglobulin by cathepsin.

Serum is constantly being taken up by endocytosis. Many macromolecules, including IgE, degrade in the endosome. One major exception is IgG, which is protected by binding to the neonatal Fc gamma receptor, FcγRn (Fig. 23.3).

IgG4 is transferred across the placenta, but IgE is not. In cord blood, the concentration of IgE is very low, generally <1 IU/mL (i.e. <2 ng/mL). Thus, there appears to be almost no transfer across the placenta.

By contrast, IgG, including IgG4 antibodies to allergens such as those from dust mite or cat, is very efficiently transferred across the placenta. This process also involves endocytosis and receptor-mediated transport.

Passive transfer of IgE to the fetus may be blocked because IgE is broken down in the endosomes or because an Fc receptor that is essential for transport is absent on the cells that comprise the placental tissues. In prenatal transfer, IgG is protected in endosomes by binding to FcγRn.

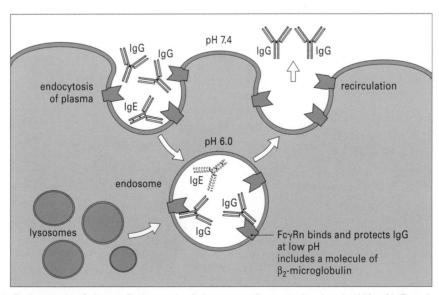

Fig. 23.3 Endocytosis of plasma Endocytosis of plasma contributes to the short half-life of IgE as plasma proteins are taken up and the pH falls because of lysosomes combining with the endosome. At low pH, IgG, including IgG4 molecules, bind to the neonatal Fc γ receptor (FcγRn). By contrast, IgE molecules do not bind to FcγRn and are therefore not protected and are digested by cathepsin. As the endosomes recirculate, the pH rises to 7.4 and the undamaged IgG molecules are released into the circulation. The FcγRn includes a molecule of β2-microglobulin. In keeping with this model, the half-life of IgG is shorter than normal in mice that have had the gene for β2-microglobulin knocked out.

T cells control the response to inhalant allergens.

IgE production is dependent on TH2 cells. Experiments in animals have established that the production of IgE is dependent on T cells. It is also clear that T cells can suppress IgE production.

T cells that suppress TH2 responses that include IgE production:

- act predominantly by producing interferon-γ (IFNγ); and
- are produced when the animal (e.g. mouse, rat or rabbit) is primed in the presence of Freund complete adjuvant.

This adjuvant, which includes bacterial cell walls and probably bacterial DNA, is a very potent activator of macrophages.

With the discovery of TH1 and TH2 cells, it became clear that IgE production is dependent on TH2 cells and that any priming that generates a TH1 response will inhibit IgE production.

The primary cytokines relevant to a TH2 response are:

- IL-4 and IL-13;
- IL-5; and
- IL-10 (Fig. 23.4).

It is clear from experiments in mice and humans that the expression of the gene for IgE is dependent on IL-4. Thus, if immature human B cells are cultured with anti-CD40 and IL-4, they will produce IgE antibodies.

Cytokines regulate the production of IgE. In humans, IgE antibodies are the dominant feature of the response to a select group of antigens and most other immune responses do not include IgE.

The classical allergens are inhaled in very small quantities (5–20 ng/day) either perennially indoors or over a period of weeks or months outdoors. Immunization of mice with repeated low-dose antigen is a very effective method of inducing IgE responses.

By contrast, the routine immunization of children with diphtheria and tetanus toxoid does not induce persistent production of IgE antibodies. This is clear because we do not routinely take precautions against anaphylaxis when administering a booster injection of tetanus.

Because T cells differentiate, TH1 cells express the functional IL-12 receptor with the IL-12 β2 chain. By contrast, TH2 cells express only part of the IL-12 receptor and this part is non-functional.

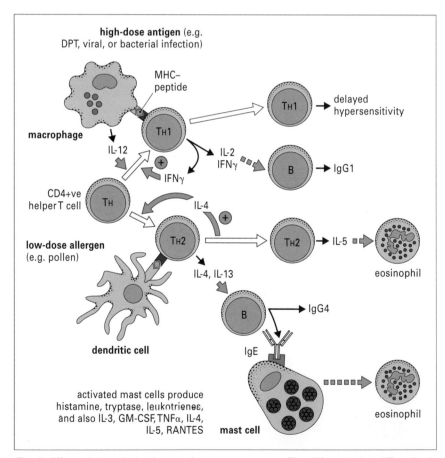

Fig. 23.4 T-cell differentiation during human immune responses The differentiation of TH cells depends on the antigen source, the quantity of allergen and the cytokines produced. Bacterial antigens or a high dose of antigen will induce IL-12 from macrophages. In addition, the developing TH1 cells produce IFNγ, which further enhances the production of TH1 cells. Low-dose antigen without adjuvant will induce TH2 cells, which produce both IL-4 and IL-5. IL-4 plays a role in enhancing the growth of TH2 cells and the expression of the gene for IgE. In turn, IgE binds to the high-affinity receptor for IgE (FcεRI) on mast cells. IL-5 plays a critical role in the production of eosinophils.

IL-4 is important in the differentiation of TH2 cells and is also a growth factor for these cells. Because it is produced by TH2 cells, it is at least in part acting on the cell that produced it (i.e. in an autocrine fashion). The interaction of IL-4 with T cells can be blocked either with:

- an antibody to IL-4;
- a soluble form of the IL-4 receptor (IL-4R); or
- a monoclonal antibody specific for the common chain of teh IL-4 receptor and the IL-13 receptor.

The release of soluble IL-4R from T cells may be a natural mechanism for controlling T-cell differentiation. However, recent evidence suggests that in vivo responses are controlled by T cells producing either IL-10 or transforming growth factor-β (TGFβ).

Group 2 innate lymphoid cells (ILC2) is an innate lymphoid subset present in tissues where the host interacts with the environment to direct immune responses against pathogens, especially helminths. ILC2 produce a cytokine profile that is very similar to CD4$^+$ TH2 cells, such as IL-4, IL-5, IL-9 and IL-13; however, the amount of these cytokines is much greater than is produced by TH2 cells. ILC2 have many features of lymphocytes but lack rearranged antigen receptors, and, instead of responding to specific antigens, these cells are activated by soluble mediators that include IL-33, IL-25 and thymic stromal lymphopoietin (TSLP). IL-33, IL-25 and TSLP are all expressed by epithelial cells in response to proteases. Proteases are important constituents of many allergens, such as *Alternaria* and dust mites. ILC2 indirectly activated by allergens infiltrate the lung and are a major innate source of IL-13. There is very strong evidence suggesting ILC2 may be critical in the genesis and propagation of allergic responses.

Both IgE and IgG4 are dependent on IL-4. The genes for immunoglobulin heavy chains are in sequence on chromosome 14. The gene for ε occurs directly after the gene for γ4. Although IgG4 and IgE may be expressed sequentially, there is now good evidence that direct switch from IgM is more important (Fig. 23.5).

The mechanisms by which IgG4 is controlled separately from IgE are not well understood, but this may include a role for IL-10. Thus, immunotherapy for patients with anaphylactic sensitivity to honeybee venom will induce IL-10 production by T cells, decreased IgE and increased IgG4 antibodies to venom antigens.

Recently, it has been shown that children raised in a house with a cat can produce an IgG response, including IgG4 antibody, without becoming allergic. A modified TH2 response (increased IgG4 and decreased IgE) therefore represents an important mechanism of tolerance to allergens (Fig. 23.6). IgG4 antibody responses without IgE antibody are a feature of immunity/tolerance to insect venom, rat urinary allergens and food antigens as well as cat allergens.

CHARACTERISTICS OF ALLERGENS

Allergens have similar physical properties. In mice, a wide range of proteins can be used to induce an IgE antibody response. The primary factors that influence the response are:

- the strain of mouse;
- the dose; and
- adjuvants used.

Thus, repeated low-dose immunization with alum or pertussis (but not complete Freund adjuvant) will produce IgE responses. However, the dose necessary to induce an optimal response varies greatly from one strain to another.

The allergens that have been defined have similar physical properties (i.e. freely soluble in aqueous solution with a molecular weight of 10–40 kDa) but are diverse biologically. Cloning has revealed sequence homology between allergens and proteins, including calycins, pheromone-binding proteins, enzymes and pollen recognition proteins. Although many of the allergens have homology with known enzymes, this is not surprising because enzymic activity is an important property of proteins in general. Some important allergens, for example Der p2 from mites, Fel d1 from cats and Amb a5 from

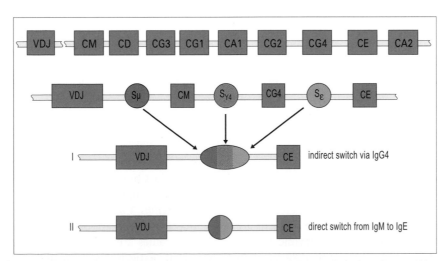

Fig. 23.5 Two models of rearrangement allow expression of the IgE gene Switch regions and heavy chain genes for immunoglobulin are arranged sequentially on chromosome 14. Both Cγ4 and Cε expression are dependent on IL-4 produced by T cells. The switch region of IgE often includes elements from Sγ4 indicating that the switching can occur sequentially. However, IgG4 responses can occur without IgE antibody responses.

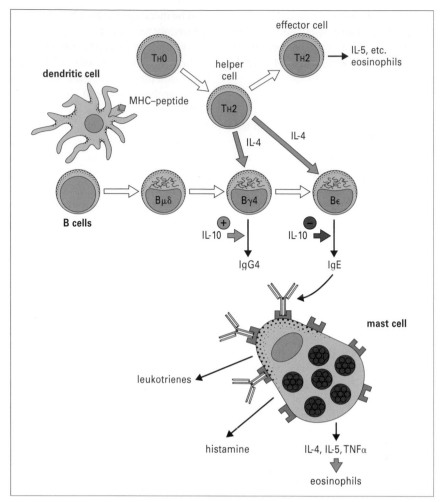

Fig. 23.6 Modified TH2 response The TH2 response includes T-effector cells as well as help for IgE and IgG4 antibody production. In turn, IgE plays a major role in triggering mast cells. However, increasing evidence shows that higher doses of allergen (e.g. bee venom, cat dander or rat urine) can induce a modified or tolerant TH2 response. This response includes IgG4 antibodies, but not IgE. The cytokine IL-10 may well play a role in enhancing IgG4 antibody while suppressing production of IgE. *MHC*, Major histocompatibility complex.

ragweed pollen, have neither enzymic activity nor homology with known enzymes. Thus, enzymic activity is not essential for immunogenicity.

Nevertheless, the group I allergens of dust mites are cysteine proteases and in several model situations it has been shown that this enzymic activity influences the immunogenicity of the protein. Thus, cleavage of CD23 or CD25 on lymphocytes by Der p1 can enhance immune responses. Alternatively, it has been shown that Der p1 can disrupt epithelial junctions and alter the entry of proteins through the epithelial layer. The interest in this property is increased because many different mite allergens are inhaled together in the faecal particles so the enzymic activity of one protein (i.e. Der p1) could facilitate either the physical entry or the immune response to other mite proteins.

The primary characterization of allergens relates to their route of exposure. The routes of exposure include:

- inhaled allergens, primarily to the nasal passages;
- oral exposure to foods;
- exposure of the skin to:
  - foods such as peanut
  - tick bites
  - parasites going through the skin, such as schistosomules
  - venom from wasps, bees or fire ants
  - scabies burrows in the skin;
- antigens from fungi growing in the lungs or the skin, e.g. *Aspergillus, Candida*;
- injected or oral antibiotics.

The routes are important because they define the ways in which the antigens are presented to the immune system. Antigen presentation may well be the site at which genetic influences play the biggest role; the properties of the different groups of allergen need to be considered separately.

The inhalant allergens cause hay fever, chronic rhinitis and asthma. The inhalant allergens are the primary causal agents in hay fever, chronic rhinitis and asthma among school-aged children and young adults and they play an important role in atopic dermatitis.

Allergens can only become airborne in sufficient quantity to cause an immune response or symptoms when they are carried on particles. Pollen grains, mite faecal particles, particles of fungal hyphae or spores and animal skin flakes (or dander) are the best-defined forms in which allergens are inhaled (Fig. 23.7).

In each case it is possible to define the approximate particle size and the quantity of protein on the particle as well as the speed with which the proteins in the particle dissolve in aqueous solution (see Fig. 23.3).

Thus, for grass pollen, mite faecal pellets and cat dander:
- the relevant allergens are present in high concentrations within the particles (up to 10 mg/cm^3);

- the particles are large (i.e. 3–30 μm diameter); and
- the allergens elute rapidly in aqueous solution.

The allergens within these particles will be delivered to the nasal epithelium and the local lymph nodes because a large proportion of particles of this size will impact on the mucous membrane during passage of inhaled air through the nose.

Small quantities of inhalant allergen cause immediate hypersensitivity. Estimates of the quantity of mite or pollen-derived proteins inhaled vary from 5 to 50 ng/day. Thus, exposure to some allergens may be as little as 1 μg/year. This is important because it probably explains:
- why the immune response is consistently of this one kind (i.e. immediate hypersensitivity); and
- why no respiratory diseases, other than asthma, have been associated with these allergens.

The quantities inhaled also seriously restrict the models about how allergens contribute to asthma. Inhaling a small number (i.e. 10–100) of large particles (10–30 μm in diameter) per day could produce local areas of inflammation but would not be expected to give rise to alveolitis, acute bronchospasm or progressive lung fibrosis.

Only a small number of food proteins are common causes of allergic responses. Although many food proteins can occasionally give rise to IgE responses, only a small number are common causes of food allergy. These include egg, milk, wheat, soy, tree nuts, peanut, fish and shellfish. In contrast to inhaled allergens, these proteins are often eaten in very large quantities (i.e. ≈ 10–100 g/day). In general, only a small fraction of these food proteins is absorbed. However, small peptides can be freely absorbed and may be recognized by T cells and even by IgE antibodies in a minority of individuals. Nevertheless, the bulk of the allergic and anaphylactic responses to foods are thought to be related to food proteins that have not been digested, either triggering mast cells in the intestine or entering the circulation.

Evidence from Dr Sampson and his colleagues has shown that some children produce IgE antibodies against linear epitopes on food allergens, indicating that cooking, which does not affect linear epitopes (e.g. Ara h), might not always destroy allergenicity.

Desensitization can be used to control type I hypersensitivity. Given the importance of T cells to the control of IgE antibody production and their potential role in the recruitment of inflammatory cells, it is logical to try treatments that directly desensitize T cells. The approaches used include treatments with modified allergens, including:
- allergen molecules modified in vitro by formaldehyde or glutaraldehyde (allergoids);
- site-directed mutagenesis;
- allergens combined with two to four molecules of CpG;
- peptides of 12–35 amino acids.

Therapeutic trials have been carried out with peptides from ragweed pollen antigens and the cat allergen Fel d1. The results show that peptide recognition is restricted by the HLA-DR type

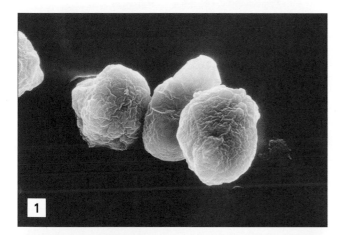

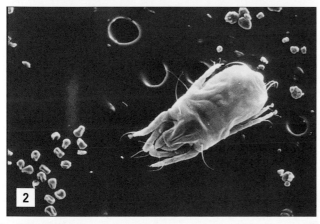

Fig. 23.7 Particles carrying airborne allergens—mite faecal pellets and pollen grains The dust mite is the most important source of allergen in house dust, largely as faecal particles (**1**). A mite is shown in (**2**) with pollen grains lower left and faecal particles upper right. The mite is approximately 300 μm in length (i.e. just visible but not small enough to become airborne). Mite faecal particles are approximately 10–40 μm in diameter and become airborne during domestic disturbance. Pollen grains are similar in size to mite faecal particles (i.e. approximately 30 μm in diameter). The important allergic sources of pollen (i.e. grass, ragweed and trees) are wind pollinated and the grains are designed to travel in the air for long distances.

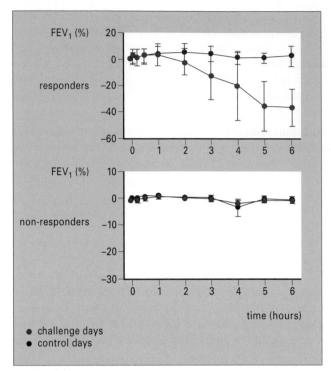

Fig. 23.8 Late asthmatic response to peptides from cat allergen Late asthmatic reactions induced in cat allergic patients by the intradermal injection of peptides derived from the cat allergen Fel d1. The nine responders show a mean fall in forced expiratory volume in 1 second (*FEV₁*) of approximately 30%. The response to the peptides is major histocompatibility complex (MHC)-restricted and correlated with the ability of the patients' T cells to respond to these peptides in vitro. On challenge days *(red filled circles)* injection of peptides was associated with a fall in FEV_1, which did not occur on the control days *(black filled circles)*. Data are shown for 9 responders *(upper graph)* and 31 non-responders *(lower graph)*. (Courtesy Dr Mark Larché from J Exp Med 1999;189:1885.)

of the patient, which means that a wide range of peptides is necessary for treatment. In addition, there is clear evidence that peptides can produce a significant response in the lungs (Fig. 23.8), indicating that T cells in the lung can contribute to an asthmatic response.

MEDIATORS RELEASED BY MAST CELLS AND BASOPHILS

The only human cell types that contain histamine are mast cells and basophils. In addition, these are the only cells that express the high-affinity receptor for IgE (FcεRI) under resting conditions.

The primary and most rapid consequence of allergen exposure in an allergic individual is cross-linking of IgE receptors on mast cells and basophils:

- Basophils are circulating polymorphonuclear leukocytes that are not present in normal tissue but can be recruited to a local site by cytokines released from either T cells or mast cells.

- Mast cells cannot be identified in the circulation but are present in connective tissue (including skin) and at mucosal surfaces throughout the body.

Mast cells in different tissues are morphologically and cytogenetically distinct.

Cells that contain histamine and their structure may be very different in other species. For example:
- in rabbits, the histamine content of the peripheral blood is almost all in platelets;
- in mice, there are few if any circulating basophils; and
- in rats, the degranulation of mast cells appears to be one granule at a time.

In contrast, in human mast cells and basophils the granules fuse with the exterior membrane and release their contents as a solution. The membrane of the granule then becomes part of the plasma membrane (Fig. 23.9).

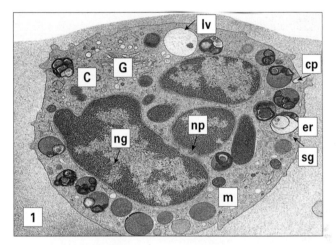

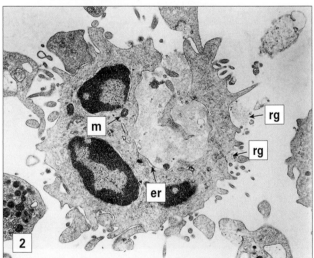

Fig. 23.9 Human basophils Basophils are circulating mononuclear cells that have multi-lobed nuclei and distinctive granules that stain with metachromatic stains (**1**). Basophils can be recruited into local tissues such as the skin, nose, lungs or gut by allergic and other immune responses. (**2**) A basophil degranulating 4 minutes after adding allergen. The degranulation that releases histamine occurs by fusion of the granule membrane with the external membrane of the cell. *C*, Centriole; *cp*, coated pit; *er*, endoplasmic reticulum; *G*, Golgi apparatus; *lv*, lucent vesicle; *m*, mitochondria; *ng*, nuclear granule; *np*, nuclear pore; *rg*, residual material from granules; *sg*, small granules. (Courtesy of Robin Hastie.)

Mast cells in different tissues have distinct granule proteases.

Mast cells were originally identified by Ehrlich, who named them based on the distinctive, tightly packed granules (*mast* means well fed, or fattening, in German.) Mast cells in different tissues can be distinguished by staining for proteases and the content of these enzymes may be relevant to their role in allergic diseases. The granule proteases of mast cells have been cloned and sequenced and are distinct for two types of mast cell (Table 23.2):

- mucosal mast cells are characterized by the presence of tryptase without chymase (MCT);
- by contrast, connective tissue mast cells contain both chymase and tryptase (MCTC).

These enzymes may play a direct role in the lung inflammation of asthma, either by breaking down mediators or, in the case of tryptase, by acting as a fibroblast growth factor. Basophils contain very little of either of these proteases.

Staining of basophils in tissue sections requires special fixation and staining. Without this staining, the granules in basophils cannot be identified and the cells appear as neutrophils (i.e. polymorphonuclear cells without eosinophilic or basophilic granules).

Cross-linking of FcεRI receptors results in degranulation.

The process of degranulation in human mast cells and basophils involves fusing of the membrane of the granules containing histamine with the plasma membrane (Fig. 23.10). The granule

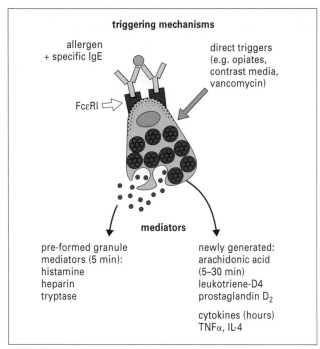

Fig. 23.10 Mast cell mediator release Mast cells release mediators after cross-linking of the IgE receptors on their surface. Preformed mediators are released rapidly and arachidonic acid metabolites such as leukotriene-D4 and prostaglandin D_2 are released more slowly. Mast cells can also be triggered by opiates, contrast media, vancomycin and the complement components C3a and C5a. The mediators, which are released by basophils, include histamine, TNFα, and IL-4. Histamine released by mast cells can be measured in serum following anaphylaxis or extensive urticaria, but it has a half-life of minutes. By contrast, tryptase can be measured in serum for many hours after an anaphylactic reaction.

TABLE 23.2 Differences Between Mast Cell Populations		
	MMC	**CTMC**
Location in vivo	Gut and lung	Ubiquitous
Life span	<40 days (?)	>40 days (?)
T-cell dependent	+	–
Number of Fcε R₁ receptors	25×10^5	3×10^4
Histamine content	+	+ +
Cytoplasmic IgE	+	–
Major AA metabolite LTC4 : PGD₂ ratio	25:1	1:40
DSGG/theophylline inhibits histamine release	–	+
Major proteoglycan	Chondroitin sulfate	Heparin

Mast cells are divided into two groups, mucosal (MMC) and connective tissue (CTMC), which have differences in morphology and pharmacology. MMC are strongly associated with parasitic disease. Both forms of mast cells are T-cell dependent but the CTMC are thought to have a longer life in the tissue, which may be 40 days or longer. The effects of cromolyn sodium or theophylline are more striking on CTMC. Mast cells contain several different enzymes that are not significant in basophils. These include tryptase and chymase, which may represent a large proportion of the mast cell protein. Tryptase is an important marker of anaphylaxis because it can be measured in the circulation for 6–24 hours after the allergic reaction.
AA, amino acid; *LTC4*, leukotriene-D4; *DSSG*, disodium cromoglycate; *PGD₂*, prostaglandin D₂.

contents rapidly dissolve and are secreted, leaving behind a viable degranulated or partially degranulated cell. Pairs of specific IgE molecules can be cross-linked by a relevant allergen with at least two epitopes or by anti-IgE experimentally.

When two IgE receptors (FcεRI) are cross-linked, signal transduction through the γ chains of the receptor leads to influx of calcium, which initiates both degranulation and the synthesis of newly formed mediators (see Fig. 23.10).

Other mechanisms can be involved. Experimentally, degranulation can be triggered through FcεRI by using anti-IgE. Lectins such as phytohaemagglutinin (PHA) or concanavalin A (Con A) and the bacterial peptide formyl-met-leu-phe (FMLP) can also trigger receptor-mediated degranulation.

Drugs such as codeine or morphine, the antibiotic vancomycin and contrast media used for imaging the kidneys also degranulate mast cells. Acute reactions to these agents, which are not thought to involve IgE antibodies, are referred to as **anaphylactoid**.

In allergic individuals mast cells can be recruited to the skin and nose.

Although mast cells are present in normal non-inflamed tissue, their numbers are increased in response to inflammation. It is assumed that this accumulation is T-cell dependent because in rats infected with *Nippostrongylus brasiliensis* accumulation of mast cells in the gut is dependent on T cells and can be suppressed by corticosteroids.

In guinea pigs, the immune response to tick bites includes a large local accumulation of basophils. Indeed, the tick is thought to be killed by basophils that it ingests.

In allergic individuals, mast cell recruitment has been demonstrated both:

- in the skin in response to repeated allergen exposure; and
- in the nose during the pollen season.

In both situations basophils are also recruited. In the nose, the recruitment of cells represents a shift so that mast cells move from the subepithelium into the epithelium and basophils appear in the nasal mucus. This process, which brings histamine-containing cells closer to the site of entry of allergen, is one of the ways in which allergic individuals become more sensitive. It is likely but less well established that equivalent processes occur in the human lung and gut.

GENETIC ASSOCIATIONS WITH ASTHMA

Hay fever, asthma and atopic dermatitis are common in allergic families. Children with one allergic parent have a 30% chance of developing allergic disease; those who have two allergic parents have a chance as high as 50%.

Systematic studies of allergic diseases are complicated because the phenotypes for diseases, such as hay fever and asthma, are not well defined and depend on the approach used to make the diagnosis. Although on average, total IgE values increase progressively from normal, in hay fever, asthma and atopic dermatitis, the individual values vary widely (Fig. 23.11).

Asthma defined by a patient questionnaire is less specific than asthma defined by testing of specific or non-specific

bronchial hyper-reactivity. Furthermore, studies on asthma are complicated because several aspects are under genetic control, including:

- IgE antibody responses;
- the inflammatory response to allergens;
- repair mechanisms; and
- bronchial reactivity.

Indeed, it is important not to confuse simple genetic diseases like cystic fibrosis or haemophilia with complex traits such as asthma or type II diabetes mellitus.

It is therefore not surprising that multiple genes (currently at least 50) have been associated with asthma in different populations.

A further major problem in interpreting genetic analyses of allergic disease comes from the progressive increase in the incidence of asthma between 1960 and 2000. Clearly this increase cannot be attributed to genetic change and implies that some of the genes identified would influence asthma only in the presence of other changes either in the environment or in lifestyle. This is referred to as a gene–environment interaction.

The genetics of asthma has been studied both by genomic screening and by using candidate genes. Genomic screening identifies regions of the genome that link to asthma so that this region can be examined to identify specific genes.

If a candidate gene is identified, it is possible to examine the gene for polymorphisms that link to asthma. However, a brief consideration of the possible targets (Table 23.3) makes it clear how complex the analysis of asthma is likely to be and indeed is proving to be. Typical examples include polymorphisms of the promoter region for IL-4 and polymorphisms of the gene for IL-5.

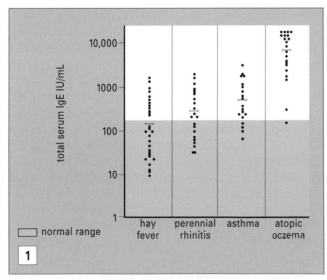

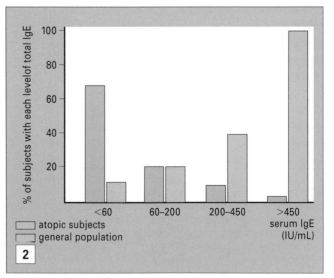

Fig. 23.11 **IgE levels and atopic disease** (**1**) The serum concentration of IgE, which is around 100 IU/mL (= 240 ng/mL), comprises less than 0.002% of the total immunoglobulin. Levels in atopic patients tend to be raised, especially in atopic eczema. (**2**) The higher the level of IgE, the smaller the percentage of the population included, but the greater the likelihood of atopic disease. Where the level is greater than 450 IU/mL the majority of subjects are atopic.

TABLE 23.3 Genetic Influences Over Asthma and Allergic Diseases

Allergen Specific IgE	HLA Related
IgE	Total production FcεRI, FcεRn
Cytokines	IL-4 promoter and receptor IL-5, IL-10, or IFNr TGFβ promoter IL-13 and receptor
Leukotriene pathway	Five lipoxygenase activating protein (FLAP) Lipoxygenase LTC4 synthase Leukotriene receptors: LTRI, LTRII
β₂-adrenergic receptor	Polymorphisms
Chemokines	CCR3 receptor

Allergic diseases run in families, but the inheritance is not simple. Population-based studies have established that the inheritance of allergic diseases is influenced by multiple genes. Some of these, such as HLA-linked control of the response to pollen antigens or genes controlling total IgE, are related to the immune response. However, many others are related to the mechanisms of inflammation (e.g. IL-4 and IL-5 gene polymorphisms) or to the response to treatment (e.g. leukotriene receptor genes or polymorphisms of the β₂-adrenergic receptor).

A further series of polymorphisms have been identified that influence the response of asthma to treatment. These include:
*   variants of the β₂-adrenergic receptor α chain; and
*   genetic differences that influence the therapeutic response to leukotriene antagonists.

As genetic screening becomes easier, pharmacogenetics might become an important method for identifying the best drugs for individual patients.

SKIN TESTS FOR DIAGNOSIS AND TO GUIDE TREATMENT

The primary method for diagnosing immediate hypersensitivity is skin testing. The characteristic response is a **wheal and flare** (Figs 23.12 and 23.13).
*   The wheal is caused by extravasation of serum from capillaries in the skin, which occurs as a direct effect of histamine and is accompanied by pruritus (also a direct effect of histamine).
*   The larger erythematous flare is mediated by an axon reflex.

This skin response takes 5–15 minutes to develop and may persist for 30 minutes or more. Techniques for skin testing include:
*   a prick test, in which a 25-gauge needle or a lancet is used to introduce ~0.2 µL of extract into the dermis;
*   an intradermal injection of 0.02–0.03 mL.

All allergen injections have the potential to cause anaphylaxis and for safety reasons the intradermal test, which introduces approximately 100 times more extract, should always be preceded by a prick test.

Skin tests are evaluated by the size of the wheal compared with a positive (histamine) and negative (saline) control. In general, a 3 × 3 mm wheal in children and a 4 × 4 mm wheal in adults can be considered a positive response to a prick test.

A positive skin test indicates that the patient has specific IgE antibodies on the mast cells in their skin. In turn, this implies

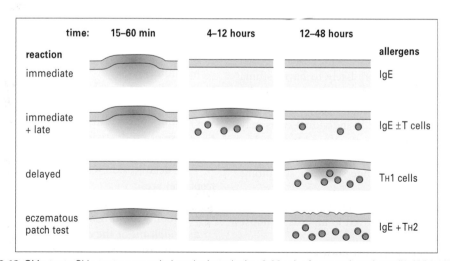

Fig. 23.12 Skin tests Skin tests are carried out by introducing 0.02 mL of extract intradermally. With allergens such as pollen, cat or dust mite, the positive reaction is an immediate (i.e. within 20 min) wheal, which in some cases is followed by an indurated response occurring late (i.e. at 4–12 hours). Non-allergic individuals make no discernible reaction to testing with these allergens. A delayed skin response is the commonest form of positive response to tuberculin, tetanus and mumps or to fungi such as *Trichophyton* and *Candida* spp. The skin typically shows no reaction up to 12 hours and then gradually develops an erythematous, indurated, delayed hypersensitivity response, which is maximal at 24–48 hours. Patch tests are performed by applying a gauze pad with allergen to a patch of skin that has been mildly abraded. This procedure may give an immediate wheal response, followed at 24–48 hours by an indurated, erythematous response, which has many of the features of eczema. The patch test is not a diagnostic test but has provided extensive information about the role of allergens in atopic dermatitis.

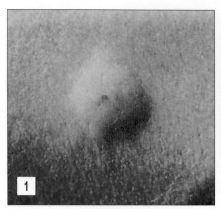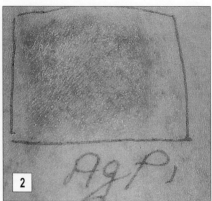

Fig. 23.13 Skin test reactions (**1**) A type I hypersensitivity reaction produces a raised wheal 5–7 mm in diameter and with a well-defined edge after about 15 minutes. (**2**) An erythematous and eczematous skin response 48 hours after the application of 5 μg of the mite allergen Der p1 to the skin of a patient with atopic dermatitis who had 56 IU/mL of IgE antibody to the dust mite *Dermatophagoides pteronyssinus*. Biopsy of the patch site demonstrated spongiosis and an infiltrate of eosinophils, basophils and lymphocytes. (Based on Mitchell et al. Basophils in allergen-induced patch test sites in atopic dermatitis. Lancet 1982;8264:127–130.)

that bronchial or nasal challenge would also be positive if sufficient antigen were administered.

In most cases (i.e. ≈80%) where the skin prick test is positive, IgE antibody will be detectable in the serum. However, blood tests for IgE antibody are generally less sensitive than intradermal skin tests.

Positive skin tests are common. Epidemiologically, sensitization to a relevant inhalant allergen is a risk factor for allergic disease. An individual with a positive skin test to grass pollen is therefore up to 10 times more likely to have hay fever during the grass pollen season (odds ratio ≥10) than a skin test-negative individual. Equally, an individual with a positive skin test to dust mite or cat allergen is more likely to have asthma (odds ratios 2.0 to >6.0). It is assumed that allergen exposure contributes to the risk, but the relationship is not simple.

Positive skin tests are common and in individual cases may not be relevant, because the patient is not exposed to the allergen. For example:

- Grass pollen is not relevant to understanding symptoms occurring during autumn.
- Equally, skin tests to cat dander or cockroach allergens may not be relevant if the patient has moved to an area or house where those allergens are not present.

There is epidemiological evidence that positive skin tests or serum IgE antibodies specific for major indoor allergens and seasonal exposures are a significant risk factor for asthma. In addition, up to one-third of skin test-positive individuals do not experience symptoms when they are exposed to the relevant allergen.

After a strongly positive skin test, the skin response may return at 6–12 hours as an indurated late response, which involves both the prolonged effects of mediators and a cellular influx.

Late skin reactions probably include several different events.
Late reactions can occur following an immediate response to an allergen, in either the skin or the lungs.

A late skin response is only common following a large immediate response (i.e. wheal size 10 × 10 mm). The late response, which is diffuse, erythematous and indurated, generally starts 2–3 hours after the wheal and may last for up to 24 hours. The late reaction is considered to be a model of the events that lead to persistent inflammation in the nose, lungs or skin.

Late reactions probably include several different events:

- the direct effects of prostaglandins, leukotrienes and cytokines released by mast cells following the initial release of histamine;
- infiltration of lymphocytes, eosinophils, basophils and neutrophils into the local site mediated by chemokines and other cytokines released from mast cells;
- release of products from the infiltrating cells.

In general, these events occur in parallel over a period of hours.

True delayed skin test responses (i.e. without an immediate response) are:

- characteristic of the response to tuberculin; and
- common with fungal antigens, particularly to the yeast *Candida albicans* or the dermatophyte fungus *Trichophyton* spp.

By contrast, true delayed responses are rare after skin testing with pollen, animal dander or dust mites.

Pathways that contribute to the chronicity of allergic diseases.
The release of histamine within 15 minutes after allergen exposure can only explain a proportion of allergic disease. The chronic inflammation in the lungs of patients with asthma and in the skin of patients with atopic dermatitis cannot be explained by histamine because:

- the time course is too long;

- there is a cellular infiltrate in these tissues; and
- there are major differences in disease between patients who have apparently similar titre and specificity of IgE in their serum.

Several different pathways contribute to chronic symptoms and can alter the severity or chronicity of allergic disease.

- Local recruitment of mast cells and basophils, combined with increased 'releasability' of these cells, allows an increased response to the same allergen challenge. This mechanism plays a major role in the increased symptoms in the nose during the pollen season.
- Release of leukotrienes, chemokines and cytokines from mast cells or basophils can have direct effects on blood vessels and smooth muscles. In addition IL-5, tumour necrosis factor (TNFα) and chemokines are thought to contribute to the recruitment of inflammatory cells.
- T cells can be recruited to local tissues and can release a wide range of cytokines, which have direct inflammatory effects.

Atopic Dermatitis and the Atopy Patch Test

Patients with atopic dermatitis (AD) have the highest levels of both specific IgE and total IgE. Thus, IgE antibodies of ≥100 IU/mL (class 6), specific for dust mite, cockroach, pollens or fungi, are common. Equally, total IgE levels in patients with severe AD are usually ≥2000 IU/mL. However, there are still major disagreements about the importance of allergen exposure to the symptoms of this disease. This is because:

- the time course of the disease is chronic;
- injection of allergen into the skin causes a wheal and flare response and does not consistently cause eczema;
- the disease is multifactorial, including a role for food allergy, skin infection, genetic variations in skin barrier function (based on filaggrin) and inhalant allergens.

The atopy patch test provides an important model of the ways in which allergen applied to the skin can induce eczema.

Epidermal spongiosis and a dermal infiltrate are features of a positive patch test. The infiltration of cells into the skin that occurs in the 24 hours after an allergen is applied can be studied in several ways:

- by local intradermal injections;
- by applying a patch of allergen on gauze that stays on the skin for 2 days; or
- by fixing a chamber containing allergen over a denuded area of skin.

The skin chamber allows repeated sampling, whereas the other two techniques require biopsy of the skin.

In the **patch test**, 10 μg allergen is applied on a gauze pad 2.5 cm^2 and the biopsy is carried out at 24 or 48 hours. A positive patch response induces:

- macroscopic eczema;
- spongiosis of the epidermis (a hallmark of eczema); and
- an infiltrate of cells into the dermis (see Fig. 23.14).

The cellular infiltrate includes eosinophils, basophils and lymphocytes.

With persistent allergen at a site (i.e. 6 days), the eosinophils degranulate locally. This is in keeping with the evidence that the skin of patients with eczema contains large quantities of the eosinophil granule major basic protein (MBP), even though very few whole eosinophils are visible (Fig. 23.14).

Biopsy of patch tests also yields T cells that are specific for the allergen used, which in most cases has been dust mite, thus establishing that antigen-specific T cells are present in the skin after antigen challenge.

Answering whether allergen-specific T cells are present at local sites is important because T cells could play a role both as effector cells and in the recruitment of other cells.

Establishing whether T cells play an effector role is also relevant to the nose in rhinitis, the lungs in asthma, the conjunctiva in hay fever and the skin in atopic dermatitis.

Biopsy of patch test sites has also established that the Langerhans cells in the skin of patients with eczema express FcεRI. It is assumed that these cells use IgE antibodies to help capture allergens and to increase the efficiency of antigen presentation.

Therefore, in any analysis of the factors influencing the severity of allergic disease (e.g. response to pharmacological treatment or response to immunotherapy), it is necessary to consider the relevance of both mast cells and effector T cells.

ALLERGENS CONTRIBUTE TO ASTHMA

The causal role of bee venom in anaphylaxis or grass pollen in seasonal hay fever is obvious because:

- these diseases occur in individuals who have positive skin tests; and
- the symptoms are directly related to increased exposure.

By contrast, the role of inhaled allergens in chronic asthma is less obvious because exposure is perennial, the patients are often not aware of the relationship and only a proportion of skin test-positive individuals develop asthma.

The evidence that allergens derived from dust mites, cats, dogs, the German cockroach or the fungus *Alternaria* spp. contribute to asthma comes from several different lines of evidence:

- The epidemiological evidence that positive skin tests or serum IgE antibodies are a major risk factor for asthma.
- Bronchial challenge with nebulized extracts can produce both rapid bronchospasm within 20 minutes and a late reaction in 4–8 hours, which is characterized by renewed mediator production and a cellular infiltrate.
- Reduced exposure to allergens can lead to decreased symptoms and decreased non-specific bronchial reactivity: this avoidance can be achieved either by moving patients to an allergen-free unit or by controlling exposure in the home.

Bronchi in the lungs of patients with asthma are characterized by increased mast cells, TH2 cells, eosinophils and products of eosinophils. In addition, there is increased mucus production secondary to goblet cell hyperplasia, epithelial desquamation and collagen deposition below the basement membrane. These changes are a reflection of chronic inflammation and it is generally considered that eosinophils play a major role in these events (Fig. 23.15). This view is supported

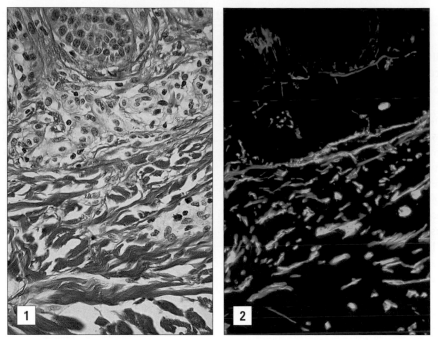

Fig. 23.14 Eosinophil major basic protein in the skin of atopic dermatitis Skin biopsy from a patient with severe atopic dermatitis. The haematoxylin and eosin (H&E) stain (**1**) shows an inflammatory infiltrate, but very few intact eosinophils are present. The same section stained with antibodies to eosinophil major basic protein (MBP) (**2**) shows extensive deposition of MBP in the dermis, demonstrating that eosinophils had degranulated in the skin. (Courtesy Dr K Lieferman.)

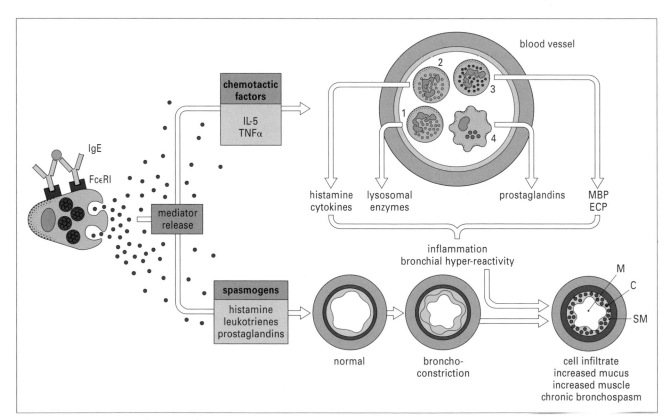

Fig. 23.15 Inflammatory response in asthmatic bronchi Mast cells release factors that can induce immediate bronchospasm (e.g. histamine and LTD4), but also release chemotactic factors such as LTB4, IL-5 and TNFα. The agents can induce oedema, increased mucus and smooth muscle constriction, resulting in an immediate decrease in airway conductance and a fall in FEV_1. By contrast, chemotactic factors recruit cells out of the circulation, including eosinophils, neutrophils, lymphocytes and macrophages. These cells can chronically modify the lung with goblet cell hyperplasia, collagen deposition below the basement membrane and possibly smooth muscle hyperplasia. In addition, these cells and their products produce non-specific bronchial hyper-reactivity. Thus, chronic bronchospasm includes elements of hyper-secretion, inflammatory infiltrate, thickening of the walls of the small bronchi and bronchial smooth muscle spasm. Evidence of this inflammatory response can be obtained from increased exhaled nitric oxide; increased eosinophils or eosinophil cationic protein *(ECP)* in induced sputum; and experimentally from biopsies of the lung. *1*, Neutrophils; *2*, basophils; *3*, eosinophils; *4*, monocytes; *C*, cells; *M*, mucus; *MBP*, major basic protein; *SM*, smooth muscle.

by the finding that treatment with monoclonal antibodies to both IL-5 and the IL-5 receptor decreases eosinophils and provides benefit to asthma over and above the effects of inhaled steroids.

BAL analysis after allergen challenge demonstrates mast cell and eosinophil products.
Analysis of bronchoalveolar lavage (BAL) after an allergen challenge demonstrates the presence of products derived from mast cells and eosinophils. Furthermore, MBP is present in biopsies of the lungs and can produce epithelial change typical of asthma in vitro (Fig. 23.16).

The subepithelial collagen deposition present in many patients with asthma is probably a reflection of fibroblast responses to local inflammation.

Although it has been suggested that these changes, which are referred to as remodelling, can lead to progressive decreases in lung function, the evidence for this view is not clear. In particular, progressive loss of lung function is unusual in asthma and there are no studies showing a correlation between the extent of collagen deposition and changes in lung function. Nonetheless, inhaled corticosteroids, which can block many different aspects of inflammation, are an effective long-term treatment that can control asthma. The effects of corticosteroids include:
* blocking the delayed response in the lungs;
* inhibiting influx of eosinophils, basophils and lymphocytes;
* reducing eosinophil production in the bone marrow;
* inhibiting transcription of genes for IL-5, TNFα and some chemokines;
* reducing T-cell activity.

Locally active corticosteroids are widely used in seasonal rhinitis, perennial rhinitis, asthma and atopic dermatitis. In addition, courses of systemic corticosteroids are used for the treatment of exacerbations of asthma.

Bronchial hyper-reactivity is a major feature of asthma.
Non-specific bronchial hyper-reactivity (BHR) is present in patients with asthma and is a major feature of the disease. Thus, airway obstruction, induced by cold air or exercise, and nocturnal asthma all correlate with non-specific bronchial reactivity. BHR can be demonstrated by challenging the lungs with histamine, methacholine or cold air.

The mechanism by which exercise or cold air induces a bronchial response is thought to be evaporation of water with associated cooling of the epithelium. However, it is unclear whether this process triggers nerve endings directly or by causing local mediator release.

Evidence of inflammation of the lungs of patients with asthma is indirect.
Bronchoscopy is not necessary in patients with asthma except as a research procedure. Therefore the only evidence for inflammation of the lungs that can be obtained routinely is indirect:
* Peripheral blood or nasal smear eosinophils are increased in most patients presenting with an acute episode of asthma (Fig. 23.17).
* Nasal secretions may contain increased eosinophil cationic protein (ECP) and IL-8 (CXCL8).

Additional evidence about inflammation in the lungs can be obtained either from exhaled air or from condensates of exhaled air. Exhaled nitric oxide (eNO) gas is increased in patients with asthma and this decreases after systemic or local corticosteroid treatment.

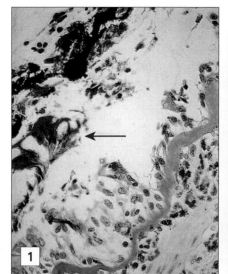
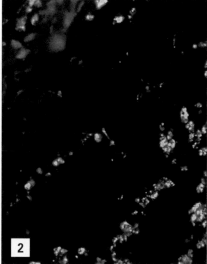

Fig. 23.16 Localization of MBP in the lung of a severe asthmatic (**1**) Respiratory epithelium showing striking submucosal eosinophil infiltration and a cluster of desquamated epithelial cells in the bronchial lumen *(arrow)* next to a 'stringy' deposit of soot. H&E stain. (**2**) The same section stained for major basic protein (MBP) showing immunofluorescent localization in infiltrating eosinophils. MBP deposits are also seen on desquamated epithelial cells on the luminal surface. (**3**) A control section stained with normal rabbit serum does not stain eosinophils or bronchial tissue but does show some non-specific staining of the sooty deposit. (Courtesy Dr G Gleich, reprinted from The late phase of the immunoglobulin E-mediated reaction: a link between anaphylaxis and common allergic disease? J. Allergy Clin Immunol 1982;70:160–169, with permission from American Academy of Allergy Asthma and Immunology.)

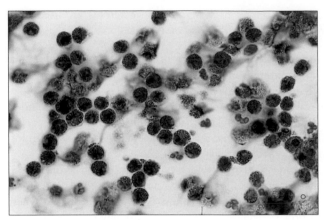

Fig. 23.17 Nasal eosinophils Nasal smear from an 8-year-old boy presenting with acute asthma. Most of the cells are eosinophils. He was known to be allergic to dust mites and had recently had a rhinovirus infection as judged by polymerase chain reaction for the virus in nasal secretions.

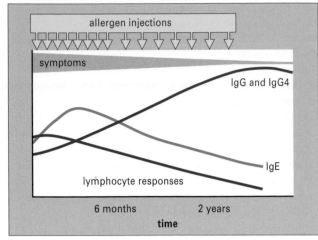

Fig. 23.18 Effects of immunotherapy on allergic rhinitis During desensitization or immunotherapy, the allergic patient receives regular subcutaneous injections of the relevant allergen. The immunological changes that occur include an initial increase in IgE antibodies followed by a gradual decline, which in pollen-allergic patients is largely caused by a blunting of the seasonal increase. Antibodies of the IgG, and specifically IgG4 isotype, increase progressively and may reach concentrations of 10 times those present before treatment. Symptoms decline, starting as early as 3 months, but generally not maximally until 2 years. Changes in T cells are less well defined but include decreased in vitro response to allergens and increased production of IL-10.

The increased eNO in asthma may reflect upregulation of the enzyme inducible nitric oxide synthase (iNOS) expressed in activated macrophages (see Fig. 5.18). In many studies, exhaled NO appears to be closely related to allergic inflammation. In adults, further information about the inflammation in the respiratory tract can be obtained from computed tomography (CT) of the nasal sinuses. Extensive opacification of the sinuses is present in approximately one-third of patients presenting with acute asthma. This reflects both:

- chronic sinusitis, which is a major feature of late-onset asthma; and
- sinus inflammation secondary to acute rhinovirus infection.

It is not clear whether the changes in the sinuses are a reflection of similar effects occurring in the lungs, a source of mediators or T cells that contribute to lung inflammation.

TREATMENTS FOR TYPE I HYPERSENSITIVITY

Immunotherapy is an effective treatment for hay fever and anaphylactic sensitivity to venom. Immunotherapy (or desensitization) with allergen extracts was introduced in 1911 by Noon and Freeman. At that time they were trying to establish immunity against pollen toxin.

Immunotherapy requires regular injections of allergen over a period of months. It is an established treatment for:

- seasonal hay fever; and
- anaphylactic sensitivity to bees, wasps, hornets and fire ants.

In addition, immunotherapy is an effective treatment for selected cases of other allergic diseases, including asthma.

The dose is increased progressively, starting with 1–10 ng and increasing up to approximately 10 µg allergen per dose.

The response to treatment includes:

- an increase in serum IgG antibodies;
- a striking decrease in the response of peripheral blood T cells to antigen in vitro; and
- a marked decrease in late reactions in the skin.

Over a longer period of time there is a progressive decrease in IgE antibodies in the serum (Fig. 23.18).

The change in antibodies, lymphocyte responses and symptoms could all be secondary to changes in T cells. Given the known mechanisms of allergic inflammation, a response of T cells to allergen injections could influence symptoms in several ways:

- decreased local recruitment of mast cells and basophils;
- decreased recruitment of eosinophils to the nose or lungs;
- increased IgG, including IgG4 antibodies, with progressive decreases in IgE: the IgG antibodies may act as blocking antibodies by binding allergen before it cross-links IgE on mast cells. Antigen-specific IgG may also bind to the inhibitory FcγRIIB on mast cells to prevent their degranulation.

Some studies of cytokine RNA have suggested that immunotherapy produces a shift in T cells from a TH2 profile (i.e. IL-4 and IL-5) towards a profile that is more typical of TH1 (i.e. IFNγ). Although this could explain decreased help for IgE and decreased eosinophil recruitment, it would not explain the production of IgG4. The expression of the gene for IgG4 is dependent on IL-4 and may also require the cytokine IL-10 (see Table 9.2). The response to immunotherapy is therefore better seen as a modification of the TH2 response.

Modified forms of allergen-specific immunotherapy.

Allergen peptides can stimulate T cells. Peptides from the primary sequence of an allergen, usually approximately 20 amino acids in length, stimulate T cells in vitro and in vivo.

In theory, peptides provide a mechanism for stimulating or desensitizing T cells without the risk of anaphylaxis, which is always present with traditional allergens.

Whether incomplete stimulation of T cells by peptides can lead to tolerance or a change in the cytokine profile is not clear. Problems with peptide immunotherapy include:

- significant reactions in the lung with a fall in FEV_1; and
- the fact that multiple peptides are necessary to allow presentation of antigen in patients with different HLA types.

Modified recombinant allergens have decreased binding to IgE. Genetically modified recombinant allergens that have decreased binding to IgE can be produced. Their advantage is that the primary sequence with the T-cell epitopes is preserved. Even if the molecule is extensively modified, any full-length protein has the potential to induce anaphylaxis in allergic individuals. Thus, the use of genetically modified molecules would always require precautions similar to those for traditional immunotherapy. A potential but unlikely problem is that patients would develop IgE antibodies against new epitopes.

Adjuvants can shift the immune response away from a simple TH2 response. Adjuvants attached to allergen molecules have been designed to shift the immune response from TH2 towards TH1. Possible co-molecules that act like an adjuvant include:

- the cytokine IL-12; or
- immunostimulatory sequences (ISSs). ISSs are DNA sequences such as cytosine phosphoguanidine (CpG) that are common in bacterial DNA and have a profound effect on the mammalian immune system.

In mice, combining an antigen with two or three molecules of CpG can induce a TH1 response or downregulate IgE responses.

Combining CpG with allergen not only influences the response but also reduces the reactivity of the allergen with IgE.

Thus, immunization with allergen and CpG may produce a greater immune response with less potential for an acute allergic reaction.

Although preliminary trials with CpG were encouraging, large trials were not. It is important to remember that CpG acts through TLR9, which is on the nuclear membrane. An alternative approach is to use flagellin attached to allergen because it binds to TLR5, which is on the cell surface.

DNA vaccines are being designed to change the immune response. The concept of immunizing with the gene for an antigen is well established (i.e. DNA vaccines). Experiments with DNA vaccines have been very successful in mice, both in inducing a TH1 response initially and in controlling an existing IgE antibody response. However, the consequences of expressing an allergen within the tissue of an allergic individual are not known. Equally, it is not clear whether inducing a TH1 response to a high-dose allergen such as cat dander, which is present in almost all houses, would give rise to other forms of inflammatory disease.

Other forms of immune-based non-specific therapy.

Humanized monoclonal anti-IgE. Humanized monoclonal anti-IgE treatment can reduce sensitivity and significantly decrease the number of acute episodes of asthma per year.

Antibodies directed against the binding site for FcεRI on IgE bind to IgE in the circulation, but not when it is attached to mast cells or basophils. An antibody of this kind can therefore remove IgE from the circulation but will not induce anaphylaxis. A mouse monoclonal antibody to IgE has been progressively humanized so that the molecule can be safely injected into patients and will bind IgE with high affinity.

Treatment of chronic urticaria with anti-IgE has also been established. Although the treatment is approved without IgE assays, it is more consistently effective in patients with higher levels of IgE. Treatment with anti-IgE antibodies has reduced exacerbations of asthma and the symptoms of hay fever. In addition, continued treatment that controls free IgE below 10 ng/mL leads to a progressive decrease in the number of IgE receptors on mast cells. Thus, the treatment may achieve a secondary effect, further decreasing the sensitivity of histamine-containing cells to allergen. Although there have been small studies on the role of anti-IgE in treating food allergy, atopic dermatitis, urticaria and drug allergy, this treatment remains to be established.

Monoclonal antibodies against IL-4Rα. IL-4Rα is a subunit common to both the IL-4 and IL-13. Inhibiting signalling through the IL-4Rα subunit thus blocks the activity of both IL-4 and IL-13, critical cytokines in allergic inflammatory responses. Monoclonal antibodies to IL-4Rα have been used to investigate the effect of blocking IL-4 and IL-13 signalling on asthma pathogenesis. Treatment with dupilumab, a fully human monoclonal antibody to IL-4Rα, reduced asthma exacerbations when long-acting β-agonists and inhaled glucocorticoids were withdrawn in patients with persistent, moderate-to-severe asthma and increased blood eosinophilia. In addition, the antibody improved lung function and blunted TH2-associated inflammatory markers. It also increased lung function and decreased severe exacerbations in patients with uncontrolled persistent asthma, irrespective of baseline blood eosinophil number. These results suggest that the combination of blocking IL-4 and IL-13 signalling through the IL-4Rα may be a robust strategy to inhibit TH2 inflammatory responses.

Humanized monoclonal anti-IL-5 and anti-IL-5 receptor antibodies. A recent Cochrane Database Systematic Review examined 13 studies that enrolled 6000 patients that included randomized trials comparing IL-5 neutralizing antibodies (mepolizumab and reslizumab) and an anti-IL-5 receptor antibody (benralizumab) versus placebo in adults and children with eosinophilic asthma refractory to existing treatments. In this review, all three of the anti-IL-5 treatments reduced rates of clinically significant asthma exacerbation by approximately 50% in participants with severe eosinophilic asthma on standard of care with poorly controlled disease who had experienced two or more exacerbations in the preceding year or an increased requirement for medication. This report supported the concept that IL-5 was a critical mediator in asthma characterized by eosinophilia.

Some new treatment approaches may not be practical. The primary treatment of allergic disease is based on:

- allergen avoidance;
- pharmacological management, including disodium cromoglycate, theophyline, leukotriene antagonists and local corticosteroids; and
- immunotherapy.

The treatment approaches using peptides, modified allergens or allergens linked to TLR ligands such as CpG or flagellin have the disadvantage that each allergen would have to go through clinical trials.

Although specific antagonists to other cytokines appear to be an attractive target for treatment, it is increasingly unlikely that they will be clinically successful in competition with anti-IgE, inhaled corticosteroids and leukotriene antagonists.

CRITICAL THINKING: SEVERE ANAPHYLACTIC SHOCK

See Critical thinking: Explanations, section 23

62-year-old Mrs Young was stung by a bee from a hive in her back garden. Harvesting the honey had left her with several stings during the course of the summer. Several minutes after the recent sting, she complained of an itching sensation in her hands, feet and groin accompanied by cramping abdominal pain. Shortly afterwards she felt faint and acutely short of breath. Moments later she collapsed and lost consciousness. Her husband, a doctor, noticed that her breathing was rapid and wheezy and that she had swollen eyelids and lips. She was pale and had patchy erythema across her neck and arms.

On examination, her apex beat could be felt, but her radial pulse was weak. Her husband immediately administered 0.5 mL of 1/1000 epinephrine (adrenaline) intramuscularly and 10 mg of chlorpheniramine (also known as chlorphenamine) (an H_1-receptor antihistamine) intravenously with 100 mg of hydrocortisone. She regained consciousness and her respiratory rate dropped. By the following day she had recovered completely. Results of investigations at this time are shown in the table.

Investigation	Result (Normal Range)
Haemoglobin (g/dL)	14.2 (11.5–16.0)
White cell count ($\times 10^9$/L)	7.5 (4.0–11.0)
Neutrophils ($\times 10^9$/L)	4.4 (2.0–7.5)
Eosinophils ($\times 10^9$/L)	0.40 (0.04–0.44)
Total lymphocytes ($\times 10^9$/L)	2.4 (1.6–3.5)
Platelet count ($\times 10^9$/L)	296 (150–400)
Serum immunoglobulins	
IgG (g/L)	10.2 (5.4–16.1)
IgM (g/L)	0.9 (0.5–1.9)
IgA (g/L)	2.1 (0.8–2.8)
IgE (IU/mL)	320 (3–150)
Antigen-specific IgE	
Bee venom	22.4 IU/mL
Wasp venom	<0.35 IU/mL
Skin prick tests	grade (0–5)
Bee venom (10 μg/mL)	0+

Mrs Young had no previous history of adverse reactions to bee venom, foods or antibiotics. In addition, there was no history of asthma, allergic rhinitis, food allergy or atopic dermatitis. A diagnosis of anaphylactic shock caused by bee venom sensitivity was made based on the history and investigations and a decision was taken to commence desensitization therapy. Her bee venom-specific IgE was elevated at 22.4 IU/mL (normal <0.35 IU/mL). Her skin test was negative to bee venom because she had experienced an anaphylactic reaction the day prior to skin testing and at that time the mast cells did not contain the mediators needed to elicit a positive skin test, even to antigen to which she had high levels of antigen-specific IgE. Skin testing 6 weeks later would have revealed a positive skin test when her mast cells had replenished their mediators and thus could have elicited a positive skin test when challenged by honeybee venom to which she made antigen-specific IgE.

Mrs Young was made aware of the possible risk of the procedure and consented to it. She was injected subcutaneously with gradually increasing doses of bee venom, the procedures being performed in the allergy clinic with access to resuscitation apparatus. No further allergic reactions occurred and she was maintained on a dose of bee venom at 1-month intervals for the next 2 years. She was stung by a bee the following summer and had no adverse reaction.

1. Which mechanisms are involved in anaphylaxis?
2. What are the clinical features and management of acute anaphylaxis?
3. How can such sensitivity be detected and what can be done to desensitize patients?

FURTHER READING

Akdis CA, Blaser K. IL-10-induced anergy in peripheral T cell and reactivation by microenvironmental cytokines: two key steps in specific immunotherapy. FASEB J 1999;13: 603–609.

Ali FR, Kay AB, Larche M. Airway hyperresponsiveness and bronchial mucosal inflammation in T cell peptide-induced asthmatic reactions in atopic subjects. Thorax 2007;62:750–757.

Commins SP, Satinover SM, Hosen J, et al. Delayed anaphylaxis, angioedema, or urticaria after consumption of red meat in patients with IgE antibodies specific for galactose-alpha-1,3-galactose. J Allergy Clin Immunol 2009;123:426–433.

Coyle AJ, Wagner K, Bertrand C, et al. Central role of immunoglobulin (Ig) E in the induction of lung eosinophil infiltration and T helper 2 cell cytokine production: inhibition by a non-anaphylactogenic anti-IgE antibody. J Exp Med 1996;183:1303–1310.

Ege MJ, Mayer M, Normand AC, et al. Exposure to environmental microorganisms and childhood asthma. N Engl J Med 2011;364:701–709.

Endo Y, Nakayama T. Pathogenic TH2 cells in airway inflammation. Oncotarget 2015;6:32303–32304.

Farne HA, Wilson A, Powell C, et al. Anti-IL5 therapies for asthma. Cochrane Database Syst Rev. 2017;9;CD010834.

Platts-Mills TAE, Vervloet D, Thomas WR, et al. Indoor allergens and asthma: report of the Third International Workshop. J Allergy Clin Immunol 1997;100:S2–S24.

Platts-Mills TAE, Vaughan JW, Squillace S, et al. Sensitisation, asthma and a modified T_H2 response in children exposed to cat allergen. Lancet 2001;357:752–756.

Rabe KE, Nair P, Brusselle G, et al. Efficacy and safety of dupilumab in glucocorticoid-dependent severe asthma. N Engl J Med 2018;378:2475–2485.

Stier MT and Peebles RS Jr. Innate lymphoid cells and allergic disease. Ann Allergy Asthma Immunol 2017;119:480–488.

Wan H, Winton HL, Soeller C, et al. Der p1 facilitates transepithelial allergen delivery by disruption of tight junctions. J Clin Invest 1999;104:123–133.

24

Hypersensitivity (Type II)

SUMMARY

- **Type II hypersensitivity is mediated by antibodies binding to specific cells.** Type II hypersensitivity reactions are caused by IgG, IgA, or IgM antibodies against cell surface and extracellular matrix antigens. IgG antibodies damage cells and tissues by activating complement and by binding and activating effector cells carrying Fcγ receptors.
- **Red blood cells (blood groups) must be cross-matched for transfusion.** Transfusion reactions to erythrocytes are produced by antibodies to blood group antigens, which may occur naturally or may have been induced by previous contact with incompatible tissue or blood after transplantation, transfusion or during pregnancy.
- **Type II hypersensitivity reactions may target tissues.** Damage to tissues may be produced by autoantibodies to extracellular matrix, cell surface molecules or intracellular proteins. Examples of diseases caused by these mechanisms are myasthenia gravis, pemphigus, Guillain–Barré syndrome and Goodpasture's syndrome.
- **Haemolytic disease of the newborn** occurs when maternal antibodies to fetal blood group antigens cross the placenta and destroy the fetal erythrocytes. Autoantibodies in the mother can also cross the placenta to produce symptoms in the unborn child, e.g. in myasthenia gravis.
- **Autoantibodies against intracellular components may be pathogenic.** Antibodies to intracellular components may be diagnostically useful and in conditions such as narcolepsy they may be pathogenic although the mechanisms are less well-defined.

MECHANISMS OF TISSUE DAMAGE

Type II hypersensitivity reactions are mediated by IgG and IgM antibodies binding to specific cells or components of the extracellular matrix. The damage caused is therefore restricted to the specific cells or tissues bearing those antigens. Type II reactions differ from type III reactions, which involve antibodies directed against soluble antigens in the serum, leading to the formation of circulating antigen–antibody complexes (see Chapter 25). Type-II and type-III reactions are often caused by autoantibodies directed against tissue-specific autoantigens (type II) or widely distributed autoantigens (type III). In practice however, there is much overlap between type-II and type-III reactions and both types of reaction can occur in a single disease. Moreover, autoantibodies to widely expressed antigens can produce symptoms that are confined to specific tissues. For example, Ro60 is a ribonucleoprotein that affects intracellular distribution of RNA; autoantibodies to Ro60 are characteristic of Sjögren's syndrome, which primarily affects salivary glands. One can therefore consider type-II and type-III reactions as related mechanisms that produce immunopathology.

Effector cells engage their targets using Fc and C3 receptors.

In type II hypersensitivity, antibodies directed against cell surface or tissue antigens interact with the **Fc receptors (FcR)** on a variety of effector cells and can activate complement to bring about damage to the target cells (Fig. 24.1).

Once the antibody has attached itself to the surface of the cell or tissue, it can bind and activate complement component C1, with the following consequences:
- Complement fragments (C3a and C5a) generated by activation of complement attract macrophages and polymorphs to the site and also stimulate mast cells and basophils to produce chemokines that attract and activate other effector cells.
- The classical complement pathway and activation loop lead to the deposition of C3b, C3bi and C3d on the target cell membrane.
- The classical complement pathway and lytic pathway result in the production of the C5b–9 membrane attack complex (MAC) and insertion of the complex into the target cell membrane.

Effector cells – in this case macrophages, neutrophils, eosinophils and natural killer (NK) cells – bind to either:
- the complexed antibody via their Fc receptors; or
- the membrane-bound C3b, C3bi and C3d, via their C3 receptors (CR1, CR3, CR4).

The mechanisms by which these antibodies trigger cytotoxic reactions in vivo have been investigated in FcR-deficient mice. Anti-red blood cell antibodies trigger erythrophagocytosis of IgG-opsonized red blood cells in an FcR-dependent manner. Fc receptor γ chain-deficient mice were protected from the pathogenic effect of these antibodies, whereas complement-deficient mice were indistinguishable from wild-type animals in their ability to clear the targeted red cells.

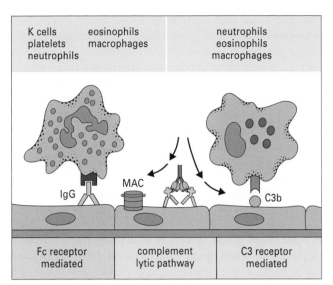

K cells	eosinophils	neutrophils
platelets	macrophages	eosinophils
neutrophils		macrophages

| Fc receptor mediated | complement lytic pathway | C3 receptor mediated |

Fig. 24.1 Antibody-dependent cytotoxicity Effector cells – natural killer cells, platelets, neutrophils, eosinophils and cells of the mononuclear phagocyte series – all have receptors for Fc, which they use to engage antibody bound to target tissues. Activation of complement C3 can generate complement-mediated lytic damage to target cells directly and also allows phagocytic cells to bind to their targets via C3b, C3bi or C3d, which also activate the cells. *MAC*, Membrane attack complex.

Cells damage targets by releasing their normal immune effector molecules. The mechanisms by which neutrophils and macrophages damage target cells in type II hypersensitivity reactions reflect their normal methods of dealing with infectious pathogens (Fig. 24.2).

Normally, pathogens would be internalized and then subjected to a barrage of microbicidal systems including reactive oxygen and nitrogen metabolites, hypohalites, enzymes, altered pH and other agents that interfere with metabolism (see Chapters 5 and 15).

If the target is too large to be phagocytosed, the granule and lysosome contents are released in apposition to the sensitized target in a process referred to as **exocytosis**. Cross-linking of the Fc and C3 receptors during this process causes activation of the phagocyte with production of reactive oxygen intermediates and activation of phospholipase A2 with consequent release of arachidonic acid from membrane phospholipids, the precursor of prostaglandins and leukotrienes. For example, leukotriene-B4 (LTB4) is a powerful chemoattractant for neutrophils; it also induces production of reactive oxygen intermediates and lysosomal enzyme release.

In some situations, such as the eosinophil reaction against schistosomes (see Chapter 16), exocytosis of granule contents is normal and beneficial. However, when the target is host tissue that has been sensitized by antibody, the result is damaging (Fig. 24.3).

Antibodies may also mediate hypersensitivity by NK cells. In this case, however, the nature of the target and whether it can inhibit the NK cells' cytotoxic actions are as important as the presence of the sensitizing antibody.

The resistance of a target cell to damage varies. Susceptibility depends on:

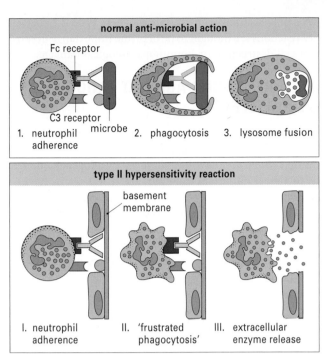

Fig. 24.2 Damage mechanisms Neutrophil-mediated damage is a reflection of normal ant-ibacterial action. *(1)* Neutrophils engage microbes that have bound anti-body and/or complement, via their Fc and C3 receptors. *(2)* The microbe is then phagocytosed and destroyed as lysosomes fuse to form the phagolysosome *(3)*. In type II hypersensitivity reactions, individual host cells coated with antibody may be similarly phagocytosed, but where the target is large, for example a basement membrane *(I)*, the neutrophils are frustrated in their attempt at phagocytosis *(II)*. They exocytose their lysosomal contents, causing damage to cells in the vicinity *(III)*.

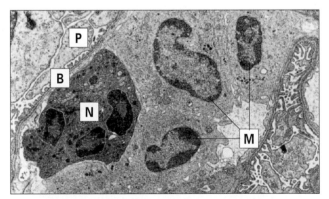

Fig. 24.3 Phagocytes attacking a basement membrane This electron micrograph shows a neutrophil *(N)* and three monocytes *(M)* binding to the capillary basement membrane *(B)* in the kidney of a rabbit containing anti-basement membrane antibody. × 3500. *P*, Podocyte. (Courtesy Professor GA Andres.)

- the amount of antigen expressed on the target cell's surface; and
- the inherent ability of different target cells to sustain damage.

For example, an erythrocyte may be lysed by a single active C5 convertase site, whereas it takes many such sites to destroy most nucleated cells – their ion-pumping capacity and ability to maintain membrane integrity with anti-complementary defences, such as decay-accelerating factor (CD55) and membrane cofactor protein (CD59), is so much greater.

We now examine some instances where type II hypersensitivity reactions are thought to be of prime importance in causing target cell destruction or immunopathological damage.

TYPE II REACTIONS AGAINST BLOOD CELLS AND PLATELETS

Some of the most clear-cut examples of type II reactions are seen in the responses to erythrocytes. These reactions may be autoimmune or they may have been induced by allogeneic (non-self) cells or tissue. Important examples are:

- incompatible blood transfusions, where the recipient becomes sensitized to antigens on the surface of the donor's erythrocytes;
- haemolytic disease of the newborn, where a pregnant woman has become sensitized to the fetal erythrocytes;
- autoimmune haemolytic anaemias, where the patient becomes sensitized to his or her own erythrocytes.

Reactions to platelets can cause thrombocytopenia and reactions to neutrophils and lymphocytes have been associated with systemic lupus erythematosus (SLE).

Transfusion reactions occur when a recipient has antibodies against donor erythrocytes. More than 20 blood group systems, generating over 200 genetic variants of erythrocyte antigens, have been identified in humans.

A blood group system consists of a gene locus that specifies an antigen on the surface of blood cells (usually, but not always, erythrocytes).

Within each system there may be two or more phenotypes. In the ABO system, for example, there are four phenotypes (A, B, AB and O) and therefore four possible blood groups.

An individual with a particular blood group can recognize erythrocytes carrying allogeneic blood group antigens and will produce antibodies against them. However, for some blood group antigens such antibodies can also be produced naturally (i.e. without previous sensitization by foreign erythrocytes).

Some blood group systems (e.g. ABO and Rhesus) are characterized by antigens that are relatively strong immunogens; such antigens are more likely to induce antibodies.

When planning a blood transfusion, it is important to ensure that donor and recipient blood types are compatible with respect to these major blood groups; otherwise, transfusion reactions will occur. Some major human blood groups are listed in Table 24.1.

The ABO blood group system is of primary importance. The epitopes of the **ABO blood group system** occur on many cell types in addition to erythrocytes and are located on the carbohydrate units of glycoproteins. The structure of these carbohydrates, and of those determining the related Lewis blood group system, is determined by genes coding for enzymes that transfer terminal sugars to a carbohydrate backbone (Fig. 24.4).

Most individuals develop antibodies to allogeneic specificities of the ABO system without previous sensitization by foreign erythrocytes. This sensitization occurs through contact

TABLE 24.1 Five Major Blood Group Systems Involved in Transfusion Reactions

System	Gene Loci	Antigens	Phenotype Frequency (%)	
ABO	1	A, B or O	A	42
			B	8
			AB	3
			O	47
Rhesus	2 closely linked loci: major antigen = RhD	C or c D or d E or e	RhD+	85
			RhD−	15
Kell	1	K or k	K	9
			k	91
Duffy	1	Fy^a, Fy^b or Fy	Fy^a Fy^b	46
			Fy^a	20
			Fy^b	34
			Fy	0.1
MN	1	M or N	MM	28
			MN	50
			NN	22

Not all blood groups are equally antigenic in transfusion reactions: thus, RhD evokes a stronger reaction in an incompatible recipient than the other Rhesus antigens; and Fy^a is stronger than Fy^b. Frequencies stated are for Caucasian populations—other races have different gene frequencies.

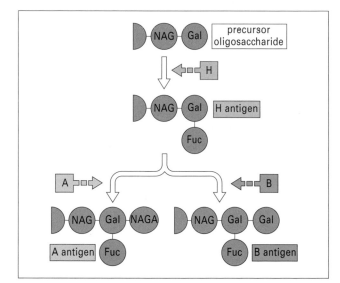

blood group (phenotype)	genotypes	antigens	antibodies to ABO in serum
A	AA, AO	A	anti-B
B	BB, BO	B	anti-A
AB	AB	A and B	none
O	OO	H	anti-A and anti-B

Fig. 24.4 ABO blood group antigens The diagram shows how the ABO blood groups are synthesized. The enzyme produced by the H gene attaches a fucose residue *(Fuc)* to the terminal galactose *(Gal)* of the precursor oligosaccharide. Individuals possessing the A gene now attach N-acetylgalactosamine *(NAGA)* to this galactose residue, whereas those with the B gene attach another galactose, producing A and B antigens, respectively. People with both genes make some of each. The table indicates the genotypes and antigens of the ABO system. Most people naturally make antibodies to the antigens they lack. *NAG, N-acetylglucosamine.*

with identical epitopes, coincidentally expressed on a wide variety of microorganisms.

Antibodies to ABO antigens are therefore extremely common, making it particularly important to match donor blood to the recipient for this system. However, all people are tolerant to the O antigen; therefore O individuals are **universal donors** with respect to the ABO system.

The Rhesus system is a major cause of haemolytic disease of the newborn.

The Rhesus system is also of great importance because it is potentially a major cause of **haemolytic disease of the newborn (HDNB)**.

Rhesus antigens are associated with membrane proteins of 30 kDa, which are expressed at moderate levels on the erythrocyte surface. The antigens are encoded by two closely linked loci, RhD and RhCcEe, with 92% homology.

RhD is the most important clinically because of its high immunogenicity, but in RhD⁻ individuals the RhD locus is missing completely. The RhCcEe locus encodes a molecule that expresses the RhC/c and RhE/e epitopes.

Cross-matching ensures that a recipient does not have antibodies against donor erythrocytes.

The aim of cross-matching is to ensure that the blood of a recipient does not contain antibodies that will be able to react with and destroy transfused (donor) erythrocytes. For example:

- Antibodies to ABO system antigens cause incompatible cells to agglutinate in a clearly visible reaction.
- Minor blood group systems cause weaker reactions that may only be detectable by an indirect Coombs, test (see Fig. 24.8).

With whole blood, it is also necessary to check that the donor's serum does not contain antibodies against the recipient's erythrocytes. However, transfusion of whole blood is unusual – most blood donations are separated into cellular and serum fractions to be used individually.

Transfusion reactions involve extensive destruction of donor blood cells.

Transfusion of erythrocytes into a recipient who has antibodies to those cells produces an immediate reaction. The symptoms include:

- fever;
- hypotension;
- nausea and vomiting; and
- pain in the back and chest.

The severity of the reaction depends on the class and the amounts of antibodies involved:

Antibodies to ABO system antigens are usually IgM and cause agglutination, complement activation and intravascular haemolysis. (IgM is not transported across the placenta; therefore, ABO incompatibility between mother and fetus is not usually problematical – see later, HDNB.) Other blood groups induce IgG antibodies, which cause less agglutination than IgM. The IgG-sensitized cells are usually taken up by phagocytes in the liver and spleen, although severe reactions may cause erythrocyte destruction by complement activation. This can cause circulatory shock and the released contents of the erythrocytes can produce acute tubular necrosis of the kidneys. These transfusion reactions are often seen in previously unsensitized individuals and develop over days or weeks as antibodies to the foreign cells are produced. This can result in anaemia or jaundice.

Transfusion reactions to other components of blood may also occur, but their consequences are not usually as severe as reactions to erythrocytes.

Hyperacute graft rejection is related to the transfusion reaction.

Hyperacute graft rejection occurs when a graft recipient has preformed antibodies against the graft tissue. It is only seen in tissue that is revascularized directly after transplantation: the most severe reactions in this type of rejection are the result of the ABO group antigens expressed on kidney cells. The damage is produced by antibody and complement activation in the blood vessels, with consequent recruitment and activation of neutrophils and platelets.

Donors and recipients are now always cross-matched for ABO antigens and this reaction has become extremely rare. Antibodies to other graft antigens (e.g. major histocompatibility complex (MHC) molecules) induced by previous grafting can also produce this type of reaction.

HDNB is due to maternal IgG reacting against the child's erythrocytes in utero.

HDNB occurs when the mother has been sensitized to antigens on the infant's erythrocytes and makes IgG antibodies to these antigens. These antibodies cross the placenta and react with the fetal erythrocytes, causing their destruction (Figs. 24.5 and 24.6).

A risk of HDNB arises when a Rh⁺-sensitized Rh⁻ mother carries a second Rh⁺ infant. Sensitization of the Rh⁻ mother to the Rh⁺ erythrocytes usually occurs during the birth of the first Rh⁺ infant, when some fetal erythrocytes leak back across the placenta into the maternal circulation and are recognized by the maternal immune system. The first incompatible child is therefore usually unaffected, whereas subsequent children have an increasing risk of being affected because the mother is re-sensitized with each successive pregnancy.

Reactions to other blood groups may also cause HDNB, the second most common being the Kell-system K antigen. Reactions resulting from anti-K are much less common than reactions to RhD because of the relatively low frequency (9%) and weaker antigenicity of the K antigen.

The risk of HDNB as a result of Rhesus incompatibility is known to be reduced if the father is of a different ABO group from the mother. This observation led to the idea that these Rh⁻ mothers were destroying Rh⁺ cells more rapidly because they were also ABO incompatible. Consequently, fetal Rh⁺ erythrocytes would not be available to sensitize the maternal immune system to RhD antigen.

This notion led to the development of **Rhesus prophylaxis**: preformed anti-RhD antibodies are given to Rh⁻ mothers immediately after delivery of Rh⁺ infants, with the aim of destroying fetal Rh⁺ erythrocytes before they can cause Rh⁻ sensitization. This practice has successfully reduced the

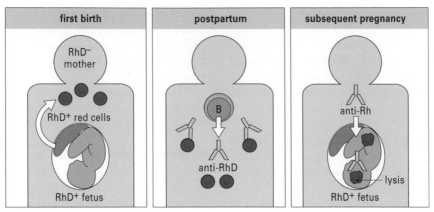

Fig. 24.5 Haemolytic disease of the newborn Erythrocytes from a RhD⁺ fetus leak into the maternal circulation, usually during birth. This stimulates the production of anti-Rh antibody of the IgG class postpartum. During subsequent pregnancies, IgG antibodies are transferred across the placenta into the fetal circulation (IgM cannot cross the placenta). If the fetus is again incompatible, the antibodies cause erythrocyte destruction.

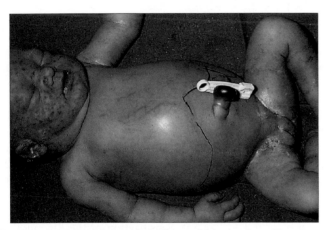

Fig. 24.6 A child with haemolytic disease of the newborn There is considerable enlargement of the liver and spleen associated with erythrocyte destruction caused by maternal anti-erythrocyte antibody in the fetal circulation. The child had elevated bilirubin (breakdown product of haemoglobin). The facial petechial haemorrhaging was caused by impaired platelet function. The most commonly involved antigen is RhD. (Courtesy Dr K Sloper.)

incidence of HDNB caused by Rhesus incompatibility (Fig. 24.7). Although the number of cases of HDNB has fallen dramatically and progressively, the proportion of cases caused by other blood groups, including Kell and the ABO system, has increased.

Autoimmune haemolytic anaemias arise spontaneously or may be induced by drugs.
Reactions to **blood group antigens** also occur spontaneously in the autoimmune haemolytic anaemias, in which patients produce antibodies to their own erythrocytes.

Autoimmune haemolytic anaemia is suspected if a patient gives a positive result on a **direct antiglobulin test** (Fig. 24.8), which identifies antibodies present on the patient's erythrocytes. These are usually antibodies directed towards erythrocyte antigens or immune complexes adsorbed onto the erythrocyte surface.

The direct antiglobulin test is also used to detect antibodies on red cells in mismatched transfusions and in HDNB.

Autoimmune haemolytic anaemias can be divided into three types, depending upon whether they are caused by:

- warm-reactive autoantibodies, which react with the antigen at 37°C;
- cold-reactive autoantibodies, which can only react with antigen below 37°C;
- antibodies provoked by allergic reactions to drugs.

Warm-reactive autoantibodies cause accelerated clearance of erythrocytes. Warm-reactive autoantibodies are frequently found against Rhesus system antigens, including determinants of the RhC and RhE loci as well as RhD. They differ from the antibodies responsible for transfusion reactions in that they appear to react with different epitopes.

Warm-reactive autoantibodies to other blood group antigens exist, but are relatively rare.

Most of these haemolytic anaemias are of unknown cause, but some are associated with other autoimmune diseases, including SLE and rheumatoid arthritis.

The anaemia appears to be a result of accelerated clearance of IgG-sensitized erythrocytes by spleen macrophages or IgM-sensitized erythrocytes by Kupffer cells, rather than complement-mediated lysis.

Cold-reactive autoantibodies cause erythrocyte lysis by complement fixation. Cold-reactive autoantibodies are often present in higher titres than the warm-reactive autoantibodies. The antibodies are primarily IgM and fix complement strongly. In most cases, they are specific for the Ii blood group system. The I and i epitopes are expressed on the precursor polysaccharides that produce the ABO system epitopes and are the result of incomplete glycosylation of the core polysaccharide.

The reaction of the antibody with the erythrocytes takes place in the peripheral circulation (particularly in winter), where the temperature in the capillary loops of exposed skin may fall

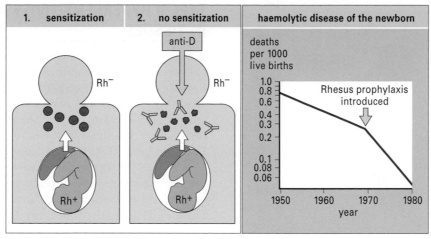

Fig. 24.7 Rhesus prophylaxis (1) Without prophylaxis, Rh⁺ erythrocytes leak into the circulation of a Rh⁻ mother and sensitize her to the Rh antigen(s). (**2**) If anti-Rh antibody (anti-D) is injected immediately postpartum, it eliminates the Rh⁺ erythrocytes and prevents sensitization. The incidence of deaths as a result of HDNB fell during the period 1950–1966 with improved patient care. The decline in the disease was accelerated by the advent of Rhesus prophylaxis in 1969.

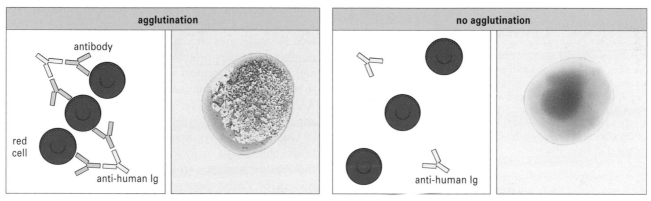

Fig. 24.8 Direct antiglobulin test This test, also called a Coombs' test, is used to detect antibody on a patient's erythrocytes. If antibody is present, the erythrocytes can be agglutinated by anti-human immunoglobulin. If no antibody is present on the red cells, they are not agglutinated by anti-human immunoglobulin.

below 30°C. In severe cases, peripheral necrosis may occur because of aggregation and microthrombosis in small vessels caused by complement-mediated destruction in the periphery.

The severity of the anaemia is therefore directly related to the complement-fixing ability of the patient's serum. (Fc-mediated removal of sensitized cells in the spleen and liver is not involved because these organs are too warm for the antibodies to bind.)

Most cold-reactive autoimmune haemolytic anaemias occur in older people. Their cause is unknown, but it is notable that the autoantibodies produced are usually of very limited clonality.

However, some cases may follow infection with *Mycoplasma pneumoniae* and these are acute-onset diseases of short duration with polyclonal autoantibodies. Such cases are thought to be caused by cross-reacting antigens on the bacteria and the erythrocytes, producing a bypass of normal tolerance mechanisms (see Chapter 11).

Drug-induced reactions to blood components occur in three different ways.

Drugs (or their metabolites) can provoke hypersensitivity reactions against blood cells, including erythrocytes and platelets. This can occur in three different ways (Fig. 24.9).

- **The drug binds to the blood cells and antibodies are produced against the drug.** In this case it is necessary for both the drug and the antibody to be present to produce the reaction. This phenomenon was first recorded by Ackroyd, who noted thrombocytopenic purpura (destruction of platelets leading to purpuric rash) following administration of the drug Sedormid. Haemolytic anaemias have been reported following the administration of a wide variety of drugs, including penicillin, quinine and sulfonamides. All of these conditions are rare.

- **Drug–antibody immune complexes are adsorbed onto the erythrocyte cell membrane.** When drug–antibody immune complexes are adsorbed on to the erythrocyte cell membrane, damage occurs by complement-mediated lysis.

- **The drug induces an allergic reaction.** The drug induces an allergic reaction and autoantibodies are directed against the erythrocyte antigens themselves, as occurs in 0.3% of patients

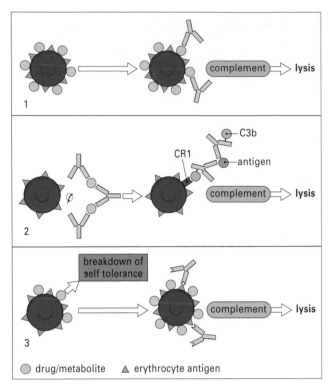

Fig. 24.9 Drug-induced reactions to blood cells Three ways that drug treatment can cause damage are illustrated. (**1**) The drug adsorbs to cell membranes. Antibodies to the drug bind to the cell and complement-mediated lysis occurs. (**2**) Immune complexes of drugs and antibody become adsorbed to the red cell via the C3b receptor CR1. Damage occurs by complement-mediated lysis. (**3**) Drugs, presumably adsorbed onto cell membranes, induce a breakdown of self tolerance, possibly by stimulating TH cells. This leads to the formation of antibodies to other blood group antigens on the cell surface. Note that in examples (**1**) and (**2**) the drug must be present for cell damage to occur, whereas in (**3**) the cells are destroyed whether they carry adsorbed drug or not.

given α-methyldopa. The antibodies produced are similar to those in patients with warm-reactive antibody. However, the condition remits shortly after the cessation of drug treatment.

Autoantibodies to platelets may cause thrombocytopenia. Autoantibodies to platelets are seen in up to 70% of cases of **idiopathic thrombocytopenic purpura** (ITP), a disorder in which there is accelerated removal of platelets from the circulation, mediated primarily by splenic macrophages. The mechanism of removal is via the immune adherence receptors on these cells.

ITP most often develops after bacterial or viral infections but may also be associated with autoimmune diseases, including SLE. In SLE, antibodies to cardiolipin, which is present on platelets, can sometimes be detected. Autoantibodies to cardiolipin and other phospholipids can dysregulate one aspect of blood clotting (**lupus anticoagulant**) and can be associated, in some cases, with venous thrombosis and recurrent abortions. Thrombocytopenia may also be induced by drugs by similar mechanisms to those outlined in Figure 24.9.

TYPE II HYPERSENSITIVITY REACTIONS IN TISSUES

A number of autoimmune conditions occur in which antibodies to tissue antigens cause immunopathological damage by activation of type II hypersensitivity mechanisms. The antigens are mostly extracellular and may be expressed on structural proteins or on the surface of cells. The resulting diseases discussed here include Goodpasture's syndrome, pemphigus, Guillain–Barré syndrome (GBS) and myasthenia gravis.

It is often possible to demonstrate autoantibodies to particular cytoplasmic proteins, including transcription factors, but it has been debated whether such antibodies could actually reach the intracellular antigens to cause damage. More recently, several conditions have been associated with autoantibodies to these intracellular antigens, although the pathogenic mechanisms have not been defined.

Antibodies against basement membranes produce nephritis in Goodpasture's syndrome. A number of patients with nephritis are found to have **antibodies to collagen type IV**, which is a major component of basement membranes. Collagen type IV undergoes alternate RNA splicing, which produces a number of variant proteins (**Goodpasture's antigen**), but the anti-glomerular basement membrane (GBM) antibodies appear to bind just those forms that retain the characteristic N-terminus. Anti-GBM is usually IgG and, in at least 50% of patients, it appears to fix complement.

Goodpasture's syndrome usually results in severe necrosis of the glomerulus, with fibrin deposition. The association of this type of nephritis with lung haemorrhage was originally noticed by Ernest Goodpasture and the syndrome was then named after him. Although the lung symptoms do not occur in all patients, the association of lung and kidney damage is caused by cross-reactive autoantigens in the basement membranes of the two tissues. In some cases, the condition is apparently triggered by exposure to organic solvents, lung infection or tobacco smoke, suggesting that modified antigen or antigen processing can induce autoimmune disease in susceptible individuals.

Pemphigus is caused by autoantibodies to an intercellular adhesion molecule. Pemphigus vulgaris is a serious blistering disease of the skin and mucous membranes. Patients have **autoantibodies against desmoglein-1 and desmoglein-3**, components of desmosomes, which form junctions between epidermal cells (Fig. 24.10). The antibodies disrupt cellular adhesion, leading to breakdown of the epidermis with separation of the superficial layers to form blisters.

Clinical disease profiles can be related to the specificity of the antibodies. For example:
- patients with only anti-desmoglein-3 tend to show mucosal disease;
- those with anti-desmoglein-1 and anti-desmoglein-3 have skin and mucosal involvement.

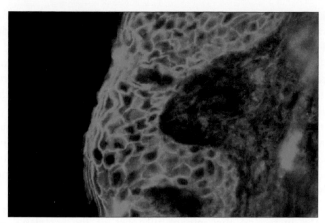

Fig. 24.10 Autoantibodies in pemphigus The antibodies in pemphigus bind to components of the desmosome involved in cell adhesion. Desmoglein-1 and desmoglein-3 are most commonly involved, but other molecules, including the plakins and desmocollin, may also act as auto-antigens. Immunofluorescence of human skin stained with anti-IgA. (Courtesy Dr R Mirakian and Mr P Collins.)

The disease profile is also partly dependent on the isotype of the antibodies produced; some patients show strong deposition of IgA (see Fig. 24.10) and others have particularly high titres of IgG4. Recently, antibodies to mitochondrial components have also been implicated in the pathology, by inducing apoptosis in keratinocytes.

Pemphigus is strongly linked to a rare haplotype of HLA-DR4 (DRB1*0402) and this molecule has been shown to present a peptide of desmoglein-3, which other DR4 subtypes cannot. This is therefore a clear example of an autoimmune disease producing pathology by type II mechanisms.

Autoantibodies to peripheral nerves are present in Guillain–Barré syndrome.

Guillain–Barré syndrome (GBS) is a group of autoimmune diseases characterized by inflammation, loss of myelin and loss of function in peripheral nerves. Many of the subgroups have autoantibodies against gangliosides, which are present in neurons. GBS is often preceded by a bacterial or viral infection, typically *Campylobacter jejuni* in 35% of cases, Epstein–Barr virus, cytomegalovirus or upper respiratory tract viruses. This link to infection indicates that autoimmunity may have been triggered by cross-reactive antigens in the pathogen, i.e. molecular mimicry. The target cells and the symptoms depend on the specificity of the autoantibodies. For example, in acute motor axonal neuropathy (AMAN) there are antibodies to GM1 associated with weakness in isolated muscles, but without sensory loss. In contrast, in Miller Fisher syndrome there are antibodies to GQ1b and GT1a, associated with ataxia and weakness in the eye muscles (Fig. 24.11). Variants of the triggering organism can lead to different autoantibodies and the different pathologies. For example, one variant of *C. jejuni* induces GD1-specific autoantibodies and AMAN, whereas another variant

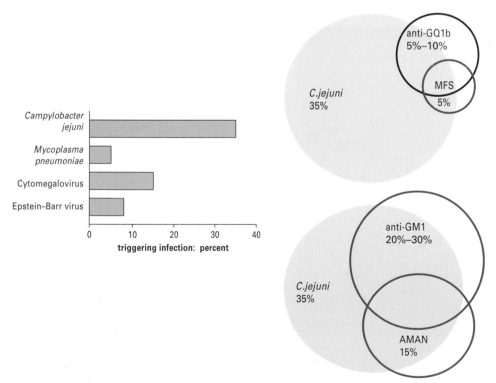

Fig. 24.11 Infection, autoantibodies and clinical subtypes in Guillain–Barré syndrome The bar chart shows the incidence of different infections preceding Guillain–Barré syndrome. The Venn diagrams show the overlap of clinical syndromes and different types of anti-ganglioside antibodies in patients with preceding *Campylobacter jejuni* infection. *MFS*, Miller Fisher syndrome – ataxia and eye muscle weakness, but no weakness in limbs. *AMAN*, Acute motor axonal neuropathy – isolated muscle weakness not affecting cranial nerves and usually with no sensory loss. Symptoms relate to the specificity of the autoantibodies and the neurons targeted.

with a single amino acid difference induces GQ1b-specific autoantibodies and Miller Fisher syndrome.

Different subgroups of disease are more common in some areas of the world and there are associations with MHC haplotypes and variants of CD1, which presents glycolipids.

In myasthenia gravis autoantibodies to acetylcholine receptors cause muscle weakness. Myasthenia gravis, a condition in which there is extreme muscular weakness, is associated with **antibodies to the acetylcholine receptors** on the surface of muscle membranes. The acetylcholine receptors are located at the motor endplate where the neuron contacts the muscle. Transmission of impulses from the nerve to the muscle takes place by the release of acetylcholine from the nerve terminal and its diffusion across the gap to the muscle fibre.

It was noticed that immunization of experimental animals with purified acetylcholine receptors produced a condition of muscular weakness that closely resembled human myasthenia. This suggested a role for antibodies to the acetylcholine receptor in the human disease.

Analysis of the lesion in myasthenic muscles indicated that the disease was not caused by an inability to synthesize acetylcholine, nor was there any problem in secreting it in response to a nerve impulse – the released acetylcholine was less effective at triggering depolarization of the muscle (Fig. 24.12).

Examination of neuromuscular endplates by immunochemical techniques has demonstrated IgG and the complement proteins C3 and C9 on the postsynaptic folds of the muscle (Fig. 24.13).

Further evidence for a pathogenetic role for IgG in this disease was the discovery of transient muscle weakness in babies born to mothers with myasthenia gravis. This is significant because it is known that IgG crosses the placenta, entering the circulation of the fetus.

IgG and complement are thought to act in two ways:
- by increasing the rate of turnover of the acetylcholine receptors; and
- by partial blocking of acetylcholine binding.

Cellular infiltration of myasthenic endplates is rarely seen; therefore, it is assumed that damage does not involve effector cells.

Lambert–Eaton syndrome is a condition with similar symptoms to myasthenia gravis, where the muscular weakness is caused by defective release of acetylcholine from the neuron. In this case, the autoantibodies are directed against components of voltage-gated calcium channels or the synaptic vesicle

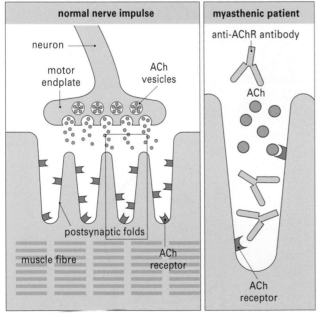

Fig. 24.12 Myasthenia gravis Normally a nerve impulse passing down a neuron arrives at a motor endplate and causes the release of acetylcholine *(ACh)*. This diffuses across the neuromuscular junction, binds ACh receptors *(AChR)* on the muscle and causes ion channels in the muscle membrane to open, which in turn triggers muscular contraction. In myasthenia gravis, antibodies to the receptor block binding of the ACh transmitter. The effect of the released vesicle is therefore reduced and the muscle can become very weak. Antibody-blocking receptors are only one of the factors operating in the disease.

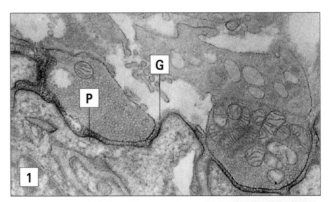
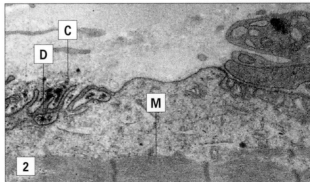

Fig. 24.13 Motor endplate in myasthenia gravis (1) Electron micrograph showing IgG deposits *(G)* in discrete patches on the postsynaptic membrane *(P)*. × 13 000. **(2)** Electron micrograph illustrating C9 *(C)* shows the postsynaptic region denuded of its nerve terminal. It consists of debris and degenerating folds *(D)*. There is a strong reaction for C9 on this debris. × 9000. *M*, Muscle fibre. (Courtesy Dr AG Engel.)

protein synaptotagmin. The different forms of Lambert–Eaton syndrome are thought to relate to the target antigen and the class and titre of antibodies involved.

AUTOANTIBODIES AND AUTOIMMUNE DISEASE

Although many autoantibodies react with tissue antigens, their significance in causing tissue damage and pathology in vivo is not always clear. For example, although autoantibodies to pancreatic islet cells can be detected in vitro using sera from some diabetic patients (Fig. 24.14), most of the immunopathological damage in autoimmune diabetes is thought to be caused by autoreactive T cells.

Until recently it was thought that autoantibodies against intracellular antigens would not usually cause immunopathology because they could not reach their antigen within a living cell. However, it now appears that antibodies such as anti-ribonucleoprotein (anti-RNP) and anti-DNA can reach the cell nucleus and modulate cell function or induce apoptosis.

Although the relative importance of antibody in causing cell damage is still debated, autoantibodies against internal antigens of cells often make excellent disease markers because they are frequently detectable before immunopathological damage occurs.

Finally, there is a group of conditions where autoantibodies actually stimulate the target cells. For example, in some forms of autoimmune thyroid disease, antibodies to the thyroid-stimulating hormone (TSH) receptor mimic TSH, thereby stimulating thyroid function (see Chapter 20).

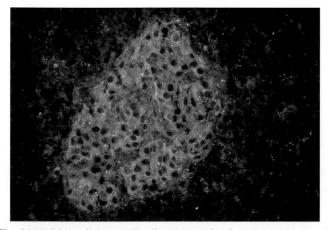

Fig. 24.14 Islet cell autoantibodies Autoantibodies to the pancreas in diabetes mellitus may be demonstrated by immunofluorescence. The antibodies are diagnostically useful and may contribute to the pathology. (Courtesy Dr B Dean.)

CRITICAL THINKING: BLOOD GROUPS AND HAEMOLYTIC DISEASE OF THE NEWBORN

See Critical thinking: Explanations, section 24

Mrs Chareston has the blood group O, Rhesus negative, and her husband Mr Chareston is A, Rhesus positive. They have had four children, two of whom have been affected by haemolytic disease of the newborn (HDNB), as follows:

- first child born 1968 – unaffected;
- second child born 1974 – mildly affected;
- third child born 1976 – seriously affected, required intrauterine blood transfusion;
- fourth child born 1980 – unaffected.

In both affected cases (second and third), the cause of the haemolytic disease was identified as antibodies to Rhesus D binding to the child's red cells. After the second, third and fourth deliveries, Mrs Chareston was given antibodies to the Rhesus D blood group (Rhesus prophylaxis was introduced in the UK in 1972).

1. From this information, what can you deduce about the blood group of the first child?
2. Why does HDNB usually become more serious with successive pregnancies?
3. What is the reason for giving anti-Rhesus D antibodies to the mother?
4. Why are the antibodies given postpartum and not earlier?
5. Give an explanation of why the Rhesus prophylaxis after the second delivery failed to prevent HDNB in the third child.
6. What explanation can be given to account for the fact that the fourth child is unaffected?

When the blood groups of the children are examined it is found that they are:
- first child – O, Rh⁺
- second child – B, Rh⁺
- third child – A, Rh⁺
- fourth child – A, Rh⁻

7. As Mrs Chareston has antibodies to blood group A, why was the fourth child not affected by HDNB caused by these antibodies?
8. One of these children was definitely not fathered by Mr Chareston. Which child?

FURTHER READING

Black M, Mignogna MD, Scully C. Pemphigus vulgaris. Oral Dis 2005;11:119–130.

Dean FG, Wilson GR, Li M, Edgtton KL, et al. Experimental autoimmune Goodpasture's disease: a pathogenetic role for both effector cells and antibody injury. Kidney Int 2005;67:566–575.

Diamond B, Honig G, Mader S, Brimberg L, Volpe BT. Brain-reactive antibodies and disease. Ann Rev Immunol 2013;31:345–385.

Engelfriet CP, Reesink HW, Judd WJ, et al. Current status of immunoprophylaxis with anti-D immunoglobulin. Vox Sang 2003;85:328–337.

Payne AS, Hanakawa Y, Amagai M, Stanley JR. Desmosomes and disease: pemphigus and bullous impetigo. Curr Opin Cell Biol 2004;16:536–543.

Salama AD, Pusey D. Goodpasture syndrome and other antiglomerular basement membrane diseases. In: Gilbert SJ, Weiner DE, eds, National Kidney Foundation Primer on Kidney Disease, 6th edn. 2014.

Vincent A. Antibody-mediated disorders of neuro-muscular transmission. Clin Neurophysiol Suppl 2004;57:147–158.

25

Hypersensitivity (Type III)

SUMMARY

- **Immune complexes are formed when antibodies meet antigens**. They are removed by the mononuclear phagocyte system following complement activation. Persistence of antigen from chronic infection or in autoimmune disease can lead to immune complex disease.
- **Immune complexes can trigger a variety of inflammatory processes.** Fc–FcR interactions are the key mediators of inflammation. Most importantly, Fc regions within immune deposits within tissues engage Fc receptors on activated neutrophils, lymphocytes and platelets to induce inflammation. During chronic inflammation, B cells and macrophages are the predominant infiltrating cell type and activation of endogenous cells within the organ contributes to fibrosis and disease progression.
- **Experimental models demonstrate the main immune complex diseases.** Serum sickness can be induced with large injections of foreign antigen. Autoimmunity causes immune complex disease in the NZB/NZW mouse. Injection of antigen into the skin of pre-sensitized animals produces the Arthus reaction.

- **Immune complexes are normally removed by the mononuclear phagocyte system.** Complement helps to disrupt antigen–antibody bonds and keeps immune complexes soluble. Primate erythrocytes bear a receptor for C3b and are important for transporting complement-containing immune complexes to the spleen for removal. Complement deficiencies lead to the formation of large, relatively insoluble complexes, which deposit in tissues.
- **The size of immune complexes affects their deposition.** Deposition of circulating, soluble immune complexes is limited by physical factors, such as the size and charge of the complexes. Small, positively charged complexes have the greatest propensity for deposition within vessels. Large immune complexes are rapidly removed in the liver and spleen.
- **Immune complex deposition in the tissues results in tissue damage.** Immune complexes can form both in the circulation, leading to systemic disease, and at local sites such as the lung. Charged cationic antigens have tissue-binding properties, particularly for the glomerulus, and help to localize complexes to the kidney. Factors that tend to increase blood vessel permeability enhance the deposition of immune complexes in tissues.

IMMUNE COMPLEX DISEASES

Immune complexes are formed when antibody meets antigen and generally they are removed effectively by the liver and spleen via processes involving complement, mononuclear phagocytes and erythrocytes.

Immune complexes may persist and eventually deposit in a range of tissues and organs. The complement and effector cell-mediated damage that follows is known as a type III hypersensitivity reaction or immune complex disease.

The sites of immune complex deposition are partly determined by the localization of the antigen in the tissues and partly by how circulating complexes become deposited.

Immune complex formation can result from (Table 25.1):
- persistent infection;
- inhalation of antigenic material;
- autoimmune disease;
- cryoglobulins.

Type II and type III hypersensitivity reactions are similar in concept and action and are not mutually exclusive. Both types of reactions may be seen in autoimmune rheumatic disorders, such as systemic lupus erythematosus (SLE), where autoimmune haemolytic anaemia and immune thrombocytopenic purpura may occur.

Persistent infection with a weak antibody response can lead to immune complex disease. The combined effects of a low-grade persistent infection and a weak antibody response lead to chronic immune complex formation and eventual deposition of complexes in the tissues (Fig. 25.1). Diseases with this aetiology include:
- leprosy;
- malaria;
- dengue haemorrhagic fever;
- viral hepatitis; and
- staphylococcal infective endocarditis.

Immune complexes can be formed with inhaled antigens. Immune complexes may be formed at body surfaces following exposure to extrinsic antigens.

Such reactions are seen in the lungs following repeated inhalation of antigenic materials from moulds, plants or animals. This is exemplified in:
- farmer's lung, where there are circulating antibodies to actinomycete fungi (found in mouldy hay); and
- pigeon fancier's lung, where there are circulating antibodies to pigeon antigens.

Both diseases are forms of **extrinsic allergic alveolitis** and occur only after repeated exposure to the antigen. Note that

TABLE 25.1 Three Categories of Immune Complex Disease

Cause	Antigen	Site of Complex Deposition
Persistent infection	Microbial antigen	Infected organ(s), kidney
Autoimmunity	Self antigen	Kidney, joint, arteries, skin
Inhaled antigen	Mould, plant or animal antigen	Lung

This table indicates the source of the antigen and the organs most frequently affected.

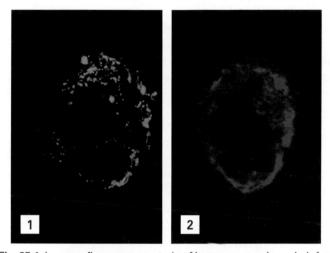

Fig. 25.1 Immunofluorescence study of immune complexes in infectious disease These serial sections of the renal artery of a patient with chronic hepatitis B infection are stained with fluoresceinated anti-hepatitis B antigen (**1**) and rhodaminated anti-IgM (**2**). The presence of both antigen and antibody in the intima and media of the arterial wall indicates the deposition of complexes at this site. IgG and C3 deposits are also detectable with the same distribution. (Courtesy Dr A Nowoslawski.)

the antibodies induced by these antigens are primarily IgG, rather than the IgE seen in type I hypersensitivity reactions. When antigens again enter the body by inhalation, local immune complexes are formed in the alveoli, leading to inflammation and fibrosis (Fig. 25.2).

Precipitating antibodies to actinomycete antigens are found in the sera of 90% of patients with farmer's lung. However, they are also found in some people with no disease and are absent from some patients; therefore, it seems that other factors are also involved in the disease process, including type IV hypersensitivity reactions.

Immune complex disease occurs in autoimmune rheumatic disorders. Immune complex disease is common in autoimmune disease, where the continued production of autoantibody to a self antigen leads to prolonged immune complex formation. As the number of complexes in the blood increases, the systems responsible for the removal of complexes (mononuclear phagocyte, erythrocyte and complement) become overloaded and complexes are deposited in the tissues (see Fig. 25.1). Systemic lupus erythematosus (SLE) is the classic disease characterized by immune complex deposition and others include Henoch–Schönlein purpura and primary Sjögren's syndrome.

Cryoglobulins precipitate at low temperature. Cryoglobulins are immunoglobulins that precipitate reversibly at low temperature. They can be divided into three classes:
- type I consists of a single monoclonal immunoglobulin and is typically found in association with lymphoproliferative diseases;
- type II is monoclonal IgM with rheumatoid factor activity, i.e. it binds to IgG;
- type III consists of polyclonal IgM rheumatoid factors.

Types II and III, also referred to as mixed cryoglobulins, are found in association with infectious, immunological and neoplastic diseases. Mixed cryoglobulinaemic vasculitis is a

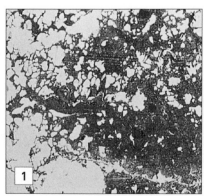
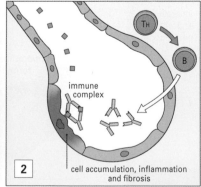
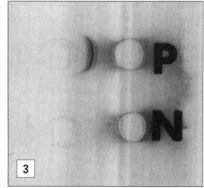

immune complex

cell accumulation, inflammation and fibrosis

Fig. 25.2 Extrinsic allergic alveolitis The histological appearance of the lung in extrinsic allergic alveolitis (**1**) shows consolidated areas as a result of cell accumulation. When fungal antigen is inhaled into the lung of a sensitized individual, immune complexes are formed in the alveoli (**2**). Complement fixation leads to cell accumulation, inflammation and fibrosis. Precipitin antibody *(P)* present in the serum of a patient with pigeon fancier's lung (**3**) is directed against the fungal antigen *Micropolyspora faeni*. Normal serum *(N)* lacks antibodies to this fungus.

major extra-hepatic manifestation of chronic hepatitis C virus infection. Clinical features include arthralgia, cutaneous purpuric vasculitis, glomerulonephritis and peripheral neuropathy. Hepatitis C virus-associated mixed cryoglobulinaemia is characterized by a clonal expansion of B cells secreting IgM-RF, which may be found in the liver, bone marrow and in the peripheral blood mononuclear cells of hepatitis C virus-infected patients.

IMMUNE COMPLEXES AND INFLAMMATION

Immune complexes are capable of triggering a wide variety of inflammatory processes:

* They interact directly with basophils and platelets (via Fc receptors) to induce the release of vasoactive amines (Fig. 25.3).
* Macrophages are stimulated to release cytokines, particularly tumour necrosis factor-α (TNFα) and interleukin-1 (IL-1), which have important roles in inflammation.

* They interact with the complement system to generate **C3a** and **C5a**, which stimulate the release of vasoactive amines (including histamine and 5-hydroxytryptamine) and chemotactic factors from mast cells and basophils; C5a is also chemotactic for basophils, eosinophils and neutrophils.

Studies with knockout mice indicate that complement has a less pro-inflammatory role than previously thought, whereas cells bearing Fc receptors for IgG and IgE appear to be critical for developing inflammation, with complement having a protective effect.

The vasoactive amines released by platelets, basophils and mast cells cause endothelial cell retraction and thus increase vascular permeability, allowing the deposition of immune complexes on the blood vessel wall (Fig. 25.4). The deposited complexes continue to generate C3a and C5a.

Platelets also aggregate on the exposed collagen of the vessel basement membrane to form microthrombi.

The aggregated platelets continue to produce vasoactive amines and to stimulate the production of C3a and C5a. Platelets are also a rich source of growth factors: they may be involved in the cellular proliferation seen in immune complex diseases such as **glomerulonephritis**.

Neutrophils are chemotactically attracted to the site by C5a. They attempt to engulf the deposited immune complexes but are unable to do so because the complexes are bound to the vessel wall. Therefore, they exocytose their lysosomal enzymes onto the site of deposition (see Fig. 25.4). If simply released into the

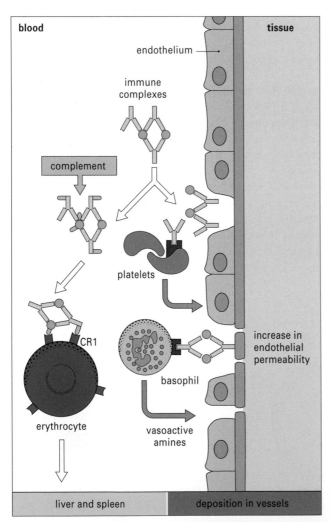

Fig. 25.3 Immune complexes trigger increased vascular permeability Immune complexes normally bind complement and are removed to the liver and spleen after binding to CR1 on erythrocytes. In inflammation, immune complexes act on basophils and platelets (in humans) to produce vasoactive amine release. The amines released (e.g. histamine, 5-hydroxytryptamine) cause endothelial cell retraction and thus increase vascular permeability.

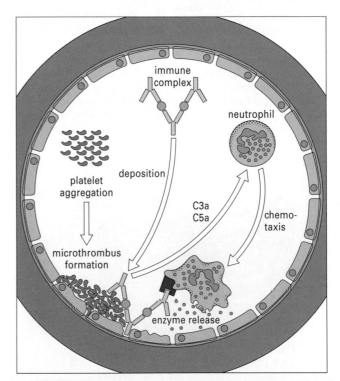

Fig. 25.4 Deposition of immune complexes in blood vessel walls Increased vascular permeability allows immune complexes to be deposited in the blood vessel wall. This induces platelet aggregation and complement activation. The aggregated platelets form microthrombi on the exposed collagen of the basement membrane of the endothelium. Neutrophils are attracted to the site by complement products but cannot ingest the complexes; therefore, they exocytose their lysosomal enzymes, causing further damage to the vessel wall.

blood or tissue fluids, these lysosomal enzymes are unlikely to cause much inflammation, because they are rapidly neutralized by serum enzyme inhibitors. But if the phagocyte applies itself closely to the tissue-trapped complexes through Fc binding, then serum inhibitors are excluded and the enzymes may damage the underlying tissue.

Complement is an important mediator of immune complex disease. In many diseases, complement activation is triggered inappropriately and drives a vicious cycle, causing:

- further tissue damage;
- increased inflammation; and
- perpetuation of the disease.

This scenario is particularly evident in autoimmune diseases where immune complexes deposit in tissues and activate complement, causing damage and destruction of host cells. Examples include:

- the kidney in various autoimmune glomerular diseases; and
- the skin in autoimmune diseases where cutaneous vasculitis is a feature such as SLE, Sjögren's syndrome and Henoch–Schönlein purpura.

Staining of these tissues for complement deposits reveals the full extent of involvement. The tissues are often packed with C3 fragments and other complement proteins. Complement activation is also evident in the blood in these diseases; complement activity and the plasma concentrations of the major components C3 and C4 are reduced due to consumption in the tissues and levels of complement activation fragments are increased.

In SLE, autoantibodies are generated against cell contents including DNA, cytoplasmic proteins and small nuclear ribonucleoproteins. The source of these autoantigens is apoptosis and failure to clear apoptotic bodies effectively has been demonstrated in SLE, resulting in the accumulation of apoptotic cell remnants. Immune complexes form when autoantibodies bind post-apoptotic debris, which deposit in capillary beds in sites such as skin, kidney, joint and brain where they activate complement causing further tissue damage. Here complement is playing two roles:

- The important immune complex solubilizing role will prevent immune complex deposition until the capacity of the system is exceeded.
- Beyond this threshold, complexes deposit and activate complement in the tissues, causing pathology.

Patients with active SLE often have markedly decreased plasma levels of complement activity and the components C3 and C4 as a result of the massive and widespread activation of the system. Genetic complement deficiencies are associated with the development of SLE.

Autoantibodies to complement components can modulate complement activity. Autoantibodies that directly target the complement components and complexes may also develop. For example, autoantibodies against C1q are commonly found in SLE, correlating particularly with renal involvement.

Antibodies against the alternative pathway C3 convertase bind and stabilize the complex, markedly increasing its functional half-life and thus consuming C3. These autoantibodies

were first identified in patients with **membranoproliferative glomerulonephritis (MPGN)** and were therefore termed **C3 nephritic factors (C3NeF)**, but they may also be found in SLE.

IMMUNE COMPLEXES CLEARANCE BY THE MONONUCLEAR PHAGOCYTE SYSTEM

Immune complexes are opsonized with C3b following complement activation and removed by the mononuclear phagocyte system, particularly in the liver and spleen. Removal is mediated by the complement C3b receptor, CR1.

In primates, the bulk of CR1 in blood is found on erythrocytes. (Non-primates do not have erythrocyte CR1 and must therefore rely on platelet CR1.) There are about 700 receptors per erythrocyte and their effectiveness is enhanced by the grouping of receptors in patches, allowing high-avidity binding to the large complexes.

CR1 readily binds immune complexes that have fixed complement, as has been shown by experiments with animals lacking complement (Fig. 25.5).

In normal primates, the erythrocytes provide a buffer mechanism, binding complexes that have fixed complement and effectively removing them from the plasma. In small blood vessels, streamline flow allows the erythrocytes to travel in the centre of the vessel surrounded by the flowing plasma. Thus it is only the plasma that makes contact with the vessel wall. Only

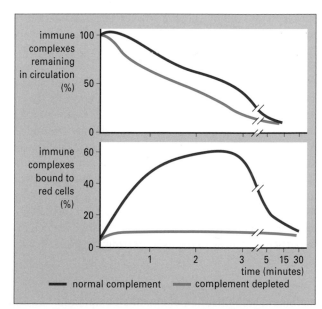

Fig. 25.5 Effects of complement depletion on handling of immune complexes A bolus of immune complexes was infused into the circulation of a primate. In animals with a normal complement system, the complexes were bound quickly by the CR1 on erythrocytes. In animals whose complement had been depleted by treatment with cobra venom factor, the erythrocytes hardly bound immune complexes at all. Paradoxically, this results in slightly faster removal of complexes in the depleted animals, with the complexes being deposited in the tissues rather than being removed by the spleen. (Based on data from Waxman FJ, et al. Complement depletion accelerates the clearance of immune complexes from the circulation of primates. J Clin Invest 1984;74:1329–1340.)

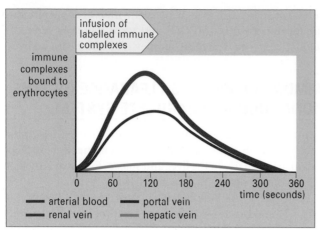

Fig. 25.6 Clearance of immune complexes in the liver ^{125}I-BSA/anti-BSA complexes were infused into a primate over a period of 120 seconds. Blood was sampled from renal, portal and hepatic veins and the level of immune complexes bound to the erythrocytes was measured by radioactive counting. The levels of complexes in the renal and portal veins were similar to that in arterial blood. However, complexes were virtually absent from hepatic venous blood throughout, indicating that complexes bound to erythrocytes are removed during a single transit through the liver. (Based on data from Cornacoff JB, et al. Primate erythrocyte-immune complex-clearing mechanism. J Clin Invest 1983;71:236–247.)

in the sinusoids of the liver and spleen, or at sites of turbulence, do the erythrocytes make contact with the lining of the vessels.

The complexes are transported to the liver and spleen, where they are removed by fixed tissue macrophages (Fig. 25.6). Most of the CR1 is also removed in the process; therefore, in situations of continuous immune complex formation the number of active receptors falls rapidly, impairing the efficiency of immune complex handling.

In patients with SLE, for example, the number of receptors may well be halved. With fewer complement receptors, the complexes are cleared rapidly to the liver, but these complexes, which arrive directly rather than on red cells, are later released into the circulation again and may then deposit in the tissues elsewhere and lead to inflammation.

Complexes can also be released from erythrocytes in the circulation by the enzymatic action of factor I. This action leaves a small fragment (C3dg) attached to the CR1 on the cell membrane. These soluble complexes are then removed by phagocytic cells, particularly those in the liver, bearing receptors for IgG Fc (Fig. 25.7).

Complement solubilization of immune complexes.

Since Heidelberger's work on the precipitin curve in the 1930s, it has been known that complement delays precipitation of immune complexes, although this information was forgotten for a long time.

The ability to keep immune complexes soluble is a function of the classical complement pathway. The complement components reduce the number of antigen epitopes that the antibodies can bind (i.e. they reduce the antigen valency) by intercalating into the lattice of the complex, resulting in smaller, soluble

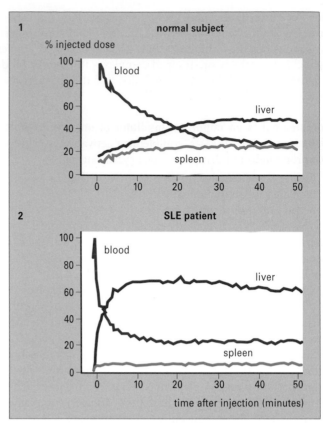

Fig. 25.7 Immune complex clearance (**1**) Immune complex clearance in a healthy normal subject. (**2**) Immune complex clearance in a patient with systemic lupus erythematosus *(SLE)*. Radiolabelled soluble complexes were injected intravenously and immune complex localization monitored by dynamic imaging. In the normal subject, complexes remained longer in the blood through binding to CR1 on red cells, followed by clearance to the liver and the spleen, where immune complexes take part in immunoregulation. In the hypocomplementaemic patient with SLE, there was little binding to red cells, but there was rapid clearance to organs such as the liver, with little localizing to the spleen, leading to impaired immunoregulation, which may be a factor in the persistence of autoimmunity.

complexes. In primates, these complement-bearing complexes are readily bound by the C3b receptor (CR1) on erythrocytes.

Complement can rapidly resolubilize precipitated complexes through the alternative pathway. The solubilization appears to occur by the insertion of complement C3b and C3d fragments into the complexes.

It may be that complexes are continually being deposited in normal individuals but are removed by solubilization. If this is the case, then the process will be inadequate in hypocomplementaemic patients and lead to prolonged complex deposition.

Solubilization defects have indeed been observed in sera from patients with systemic immune complex disease, but it is not known whether the defect is primary or secondary.

Complement deficiency impairs clearance of complexes.

In patients with low levels of classical pathway components, there is poor binding of immune complexes to erythrocytes. The complement deficiency may result from:
- depletion, caused by immune complex disease; or
- a hereditary disorder, as is the case in C2 deficiency.

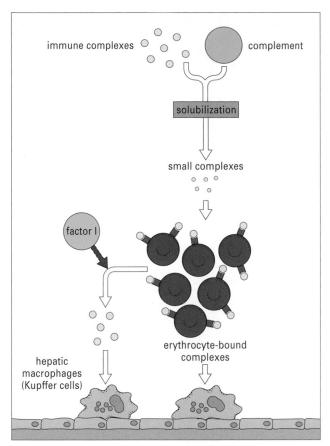

Fig. 25.8 Immune complex transport and removal In primates, complexes solubilized by complement are bound by CR1 on erythrocytes and transported to the liver where they are removed by hepatic macrophages. Complexes released from erythrocytes by factor I are taken up by cells (including macrophages) bearing receptors for Fc and complement.

This might be expected to result in persistent immune complexes in the circulation, but in fact the reverse occurs, with the complexes disappearing rapidly from the circulation. These non-erythrocyte-bound complexes are taken up rapidly by the liver (but not the spleen) and are then released to be deposited in tissues such as skin, kidney and muscle, where they might set up inflammatory reactions (Fig. 25.8).

Infusion of fresh plasma, containing complement, restores the clearance patterns to normal, illustrating the importance of complement in the clearance of immune complexes.

Failure to localize in the spleen not only results in immune complex disease but also may have important implications for the development of appropriate immune responses. This is because the spleen plays a vital role in antigen processing and the induction of immune responses (see Chapter 2).

The size of immune complexes affects their deposition. In general, larger immune complexes are rapidly removed by the liver within a few minutes, whereas smaller complexes circulate for longer periods (Fig. 25.9). This is because larger complexes are:

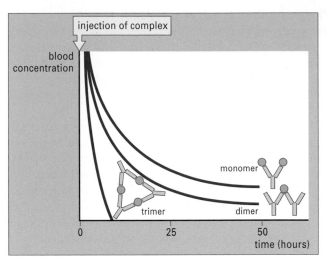

Fig. 25.9 Complex clearance by mononuclear phagocytes Large immune complexes are cleared most quickly because they present an IgG–Fc lattice to mononuclear phagocytes with Fc receptors, permitting higher avidity binding to these cells. They also fix complement better than small complexes.

- more effective at binding to Fc receptors and at fixing complement, so binding better to erythrocytes;
- released more slowly from the erythrocytes by the action of factor I.

Anything that affects the size of complexes is therefore likely to influence clearance.

It has been suggested that a genetic defect that favours the production of low-affinity antibody could lead to the formation of smaller complexes and hence to immune complex disease.

Antibodies to self antigens may have low affinity and recognize only a few epitopes. This results in small complexes and long clearance times because the formation of large, cross-linked lattices is restricted.

Affinity maturation is dependent on efficient somatic mutation and selection of B cells within germinal centres following binding of antigen. This process is far more effective when B cells are stimulated by antigen or immune complexes coated with complement. Patients with complement deficiencies are particularly prone to develop immune complex disease and recent evidence indicates that this is also brought about through poor targeting of antigen complexes to germinal centres, thus preventing affinity maturation.

Immunoglobulin classes affect the rate of immune complex clearance. Striking differences have been observed in the clearance of complexes with different immunoglobulin classes:

- IgG complexes are bound by erythrocytes and are gradually removed from the circulation;
- IgA complexes bind poorly to erythrocytes but disappear rapidly from the circulation, with increased deposition in the kidney, lung and brain.

Phagocyte defects allow complexes to persist. Opsonized immune complexes are normally removed by the mononuclear phagocyte system, mainly in the liver and spleen. However, when large amounts of complex are present, the mononuclear phagocyte system may become overloaded, leading to a rise in the level of circulating complex and increased deposition in the glomerulus and elsewhere.

Defective mononuclear phagocytes have been observed in human immune complex disease, but this might be the result of overload rather than a primary defect. In SLE, defects in macrophage clearance of apoptotic debris increase the exposure of intracellular constituents to the immune system. Immune complexes formed between autoantibodies and nucleic acids from apoptotic material can activate plasmacytoid dendritic cells, which then produce large quantities of pro-inflammatory type I interferons – a hallmark cytokine in SLE.

Dendritic cells can also capture immune complexes containing DNA fragments via FcγRIII receptors and TLR 9, generating TNFα production in the presence of granulocyte-macrophage colony-stimulating factor (GM-CSF). Dendritic cells can also be activated by immune complexes containing RNA fragments, which activate intracellular TLR7.

Carbohydrate on antibodies affects complex clearance.

Carbohydrate groups on immunoglobulin molecules have been shown to be important for the efficient removal of immune complexes by phagocytic cells.

Abnormalities of these carbohydrates occur in immune complex diseases such as rheumatoid arthritis, thus aggravating the disease process. Oligosaccharides associated with the Fc region of IgG lack the normal terminating galactose residue, which enhances rheumatoid factor binding. In addition, mannan-binding protein has been shown to bind agalactosyl IgG and, subsequently, activate complement.

IMMUNE COMPLEX DEPOSITION IN TISSUES

Immune complexes may persist in the circulation for prolonged periods of time. However, simple persistence is not usually harmful in itself; the problems start only when complexes are deposited in the tissues.

Two questions are relevant to tissue deposition:
- Why are complexes deposited?
- Why do complexes show affinity for particular tissues in different diseases?

The most important trigger for immune complex deposition is probably an increase in vascular permeability. Animal experiments have shown that inert substances such as colloidal carbon will be deposited in vessel walls after the administration of vasoactive substances, such as histamine or serotonin. Circulating immune complexes are deposited in a similar way after the infusion of agents that cause the liberation of mast cell vasoactive amines (including histamine). Pre-treatment with antihistamines blocks this effect.

In studies of experimental immune complex disease in rabbits, long-term administration of vasoactive amine antagonists,

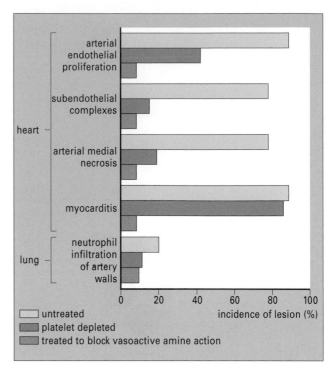

Fig. 25.10 Effect of a vasoactive amine antagonist on immune complex disease Serum sickness was induced in rabbits with a single injection of bovine serum albumin. The animals were either untreated, platelet depleted or treated with drugs to block vasoactive amine action. The incidence of serum sickness lesions in the heart and lung was scored. Drug treatment considerably reduced the signs of disease by lowering vascular permeability and thus minimizing immune complex deposition.

such as chlorpheniramine and methysergide, has been shown to reduce immune complex deposition considerably (Fig. 25.10). More importantly, young NZB/NZW mice, which normally develop proteinuria by 9 months old, have less renal pathology when treated with methysergide. Methysergide blocks the formation of the vasoactive amine 5-hydroxytryptamine (5-HT) and thus blocks a variety of inflammatory events (e.g. deposition of complexes, neutrophil infiltration of capillary walls and endothelial proliferation), all of which produce the glomerular pathology.

Increases in vascular permeability can be initiated by a range of mechanisms, which vary in importance, depending on the diseases and species concerned. This variability makes interpretation of some of the animal models difficult. In general, however, complement, mast cells, basophils and platelets must all be considered potential producers of vasoactive amines.

Immune complex deposition is most likely where there is high blood pressure and turbulence. Many macromolecules deposit in the glomerular capillaries, where the blood pressure is approximately four times that of most other capillaries (Fig. 25.11).

If the glomerular blood pressure of a rabbit is reduced by partially constricting the renal artery or by ligating the ureter, deposition is also reduced. If the glomerular blood pressure is increased by experimentally induced hypertension, immune complex deposition is enhanced as shown by the development

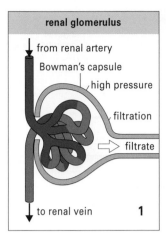
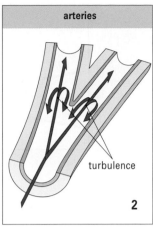

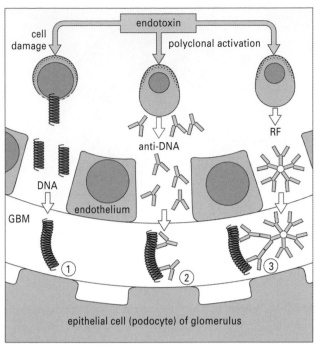

Fig. 25.11 Haemodynamic factors affecting complex deposition. Factors that affect complex deposition include filtration and high blood pressure, both of which occur in the formation of ultrafiltrate in the renal glomerulus (**1**). Turbulence at curves or bifurcations of arteries (**2**) also favour deposition of immune complexes.

Fig. 25.12 Tissue binding of antigen with local immune complex formation Endotoxin injected into mice increases vascular permeability and induces cell damage and release of DNA. The DNA can then become deposited *(1)* on the collagen of the glomerular basement membrane *(GBM)* in the kidney. Endotoxin can also induce a polyclonal stimulation of B cells, some of which produce autoantibodies such as anti-DNA and anti-IgG – the latter are known as rheumatoid factors *(RF)*. Anti-DNA antibody can then bind to the deposited DNA, forming a local immune complex *(2)*. RFs have a low affinity for monomeric IgG but bind with high avidity to the assembled DNA–anti-DNA complex *(3)*. Thus, further immune complex formation occurs in situ.

of serum sickness. Elsewhere, the most severe lesions also occur at sites of turbulence:

- at turns or bifurcations of arteries, where there are erratic shear forces and the platelets are not segregated from the vessel wall by laminar flow;
- in vascular filters such as the choroid plexus and the ciliary body of the eye.

Affinity of antigens for specific tissues can direct complexes to particular sites. Local high blood pressure explains the tendency for deposits to form in certain organs but does not explain why complexes are deposited on specific organs in certain diseases. In SLE, the kidney is a particular target, whereas in rheumatoid arthritis, although circulating complexes are present, the kidney is usually spared and the joints are the principal target.

It is possible that the antigen in the complex provides the organ specificity and a convincing model has been established to support this hypothesis. In the model, mice are given endotoxin causing cell damage and release of DNA, which then binds to healthy glomerular basement membrane. Anti-DNA is then produced by polyclonal activation of B cells and is bound by the fixed DNA, leading to local immune complex formation (Fig. 25.12). The production of rheumatoid factor (IgM anti-IgG) allows further immune complex formation to occur in situ.

It is possible that in other diseases antigens will be identified with affinity for particular organs.

The charge of the antigen and antibody may be important in some systems. For example, positively charged antigens and antibodies are more likely to be deposited in the negatively charged glomerular basement membrane.

The degree of glycosylation also affects the fate of complexes containing glycoprotein antigens because certain clearance mechanisms are activated by recognition of sugar molecules (e.g. mannan-binding protein).

In certain diseases, the antibodies and antigens are both produced within the target organ. The extreme of this is reached in

rheumatoid arthritis, where IgG anti-IgG rheumatoid factor is produced by plasma cells within the synovium; these antibodies then combine with each other (self association), setting up an inflammatory reaction.

The site of immune complex deposition depends partly on the size of the complex. The fact that the site of immune complex deposition depends partly on the size of the complex is exemplified in the kidney:

- Small immune complexes can pass through the glomerular basement membrane and end up on the epithelial side of the membrane.
- Large complexes are unable to cross the membrane and generally accumulate between the endothelium and the basement membrane or the mesangium (Fig. 25.13).

The size of immune complexes depends on the valency of the antigen and on the titre and affinity of the antibody.

The class of immunoglobulin in an immune complex can influence deposition. There are marked age- and sex-related variations in the class and subclass of anti-DNA antibodies seen in SLE. Similarly, as NZB/NZW mice grow older there is a class switch from predominantly IgM to IgG2a. This occurs earlier in females than in males and coincides with the onset of renal

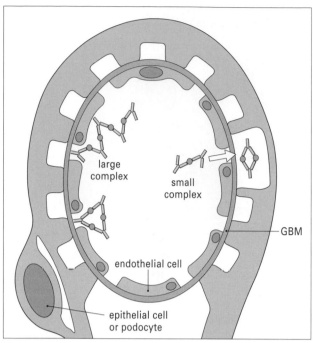

Fig. 25.13 Immune complex deposition in the kidney The site of complex deposition in the kidney is dependent on the size of the complexes in the circulation. Large complexes become deposited on the glomerular basement membrane *(GBM)*, whereas small complexes pass through the basement membrane and are seen on the epithelial side of the glomerulus.

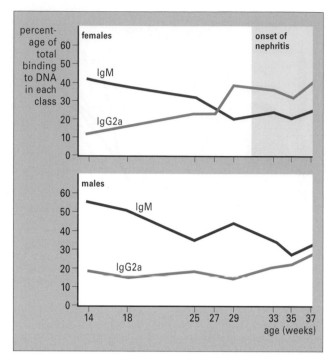

Fig. 25.14 Antibody classes in immune complex disease Immune complex disease is automatic in the NZB/NZW mouse and follows a class switch during early development from IgM to IgG2a. The graphs show the proportions of anti-DNA antibodies of the IgM and IgG2a isotypes in females and males. Both the class switch and fatal renal disease occur earlier in the female mice of this strain.

disease, indicating the importance of antibody class in the tissue deposition of complexes (Fig. 25.14).

DIAGNOSIS OF IMMUNE COMPLEX DISEASE

The ideal place to look for immune complexes is in the affected organ (see Fig 25.2 and Fig 25.15).

Tissue samples may be examined by immunofluorescence for the presence of immunoglobulin and complement. The composition, pattern and particular area of tissue affected all provide useful information on the severity and prognosis of the disease. For example:

- Patients with the continuous, granular, subepithelial deposits of IgG found in membranous glomerulonephritis have a poor prognosis with prolonged heavy proteinuria.
- In contrast, those whose complexes are localized in the mesangium have a good prognosis and respond to immunosuppressive therapies.

Not all tissue-bound complexes give rise to an inflammatory response; for example, in SLE, complexes are frequently found in skin biopsies from normal-looking skin and from inflamed skin.

Assays for immune complexes in serum are more readily performed than in situ immunofluorescence, although the results have to be interpreted carefully (Method Box 25.1 and Fig. 25.w5).

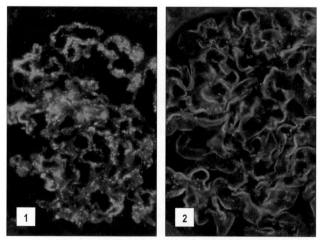

Fig. 25.15 Immunofluorescence study of immune complexes in autoimmune disease These renal sections compare the effect of systemic lupus erythematosus (type III hypersensitivity) (**1**) with Goodpasture's syndrome (type II hypersensitivity) (**2**). In each case, the antibody is detected with fluorescent anti-IgG. Complexes, formed in the blood and deposited in the kidney, form characteristic 'lumpy bumpy' deposits (**1**). The anti-basement membrane antibody in Goodpasture's syndrome forms an even layer on the glomerular basement membrane (**2**). (Courtesy Dr S Thiru.)

CRITICAL THINKING: TYPE III SERUM SICKNESS AFTER FACTOR IX ADMINISTRATION

See Critical thinking: Explanations, section 25

An 8-year-old boy with factor IX deficiency has had repeated episodes of bleeding into his joints and skin, despite administration of factor IX. Ten days after receiving a dose, he developed fever, swelling of multiple joints and a skin rash. On physical examination, his temperature was 39°C, he had a diffuse maculopapular skin rash involving his torso and extremities and both elbows and knees were red, warm and appeared inflamed. His mother thought the appearance and distribution were very different from the typical appearance after either minor trauma or bleeding into his joints, which he had sustained on multiple previous occasions. His paediatrician ordered tests (results shown here) and prescribed a short course of corticosteroids.

Variable	Result (normal range)
C3 (mg/dL)	38 (85–155)
C4 (mg/dL)	4 (12–45)
Anti-nuclear antibody	Negative
Haemoglobin (g/dL)	11.2
White cell count (cells/mm^3)	11 000
Eosinophils (%)	1

1. Which immunological mechanisms are involved in this inflammatory reaction after the boy received the factor IX?
2. Why were corticosteroids prescribed?
3. What is the likelihood that this type of reaction will develop again?
4. Which measures would you take to prevent this reaction from occurring again?

The boy responds to treatment and his symptoms resolve, but 1 year later his mother notices that his face is swollen in the morning and his feet are swollen at the end of the day. Otherwise he feels well.

On physical examination, his blood pressure is elevated at 140/90 mmHg and his ankles are very oedematous. His joints do not appear inflamed and the skin does not show evidence of recent bleeding or inflammation. Results of tests are shown here.

Variable	Result (normal range)
C3 (mg/dL)	142 (85–155)
C4 (mg/dL)	44 (12–45)
Anti-nuclear antibody	Negative
Haemoglobin (g/dL)	11.6
White cell count (cells/mm^3)	8600
Eosinophils (%)	< 1
Albumin (g/dL)	2.5 (3.5–5.5)
Urine protein (g/24 h)	8 (<0.2)

5. Which immunological mechanisms are involved in this inflammatory reaction after the boy received the factor IX? How do they differ from the previous episode?
6. What is the likelihood that this type of reaction will develop again?
7. Which measures would you take to prevent this reaction from occurring again?

FURTHER READING

Bruhns P, Samuelsson A, Pollard JW, Ravetch JV. Colony-stimulating factor-1-dependent macrophages are responsible for IVIG protection in antibody-induced autoimmune disease. Immunity 2003;18:573–581.

Davies KA, Hird V, Stewart S, et al. A study of in vivo immune complex formation and clearing in man. J Immunol 1990;144:4613–4620.

El-Ters M, Muthyala U, Philipneri MD, Hussein FA, Lentine KL. Immune complex deposits in pauci-immune glomerulonephritis; a case report and brief review of recent literature. Arch Med Sci 2015;6:633–637.

Johnston A, Auda GR, Kerr MA, et al. Dissociation of primary antigen–antibody bonds is essential for complement mediated solubilization of immune complexes. Mol Immunol 1992;29:659–665.

McKenzie SE, Taylor SM, Malladi P, et al. The role of the human Fc receptor Fc gamma RIIA in the immune clearance of platelets: a transgenic mouse model. J Immunol 1999;162:4311–4318.

Moll T, Nitschke L, Carroll M, et al. A critical role for Fc gamma RIIB in the induction of rheumatoid factors. J Immunol 2004;173: 4724–4728.

Park SY, Ueda S, Ohno H, et al. Resistance of Fc receptor-deficient mice to fatal glomerulonephritis. J Clin Invest 1998;102:1229–1238.

Ravetch JV. A full complement of receptors in immune complex diseases. J Clin Invest 2002;110:1759–1761.

Rosen A, Casciola-Rosen L. Autoantigens as partners in initiation and propagation of autoimmune rheumatic diseases. Ann Rev Immunol 2016;34:395–420.

Toong C, Adelstein S, Phan TG. Clearing the complexity: immune complexes and their treatment in lupus nephritis. Int J Nephrol Renovasc Dis 2011;4:17–28.

26

Hypersensitivity (Type IV)

SUMMARY

- **Delayed-type hypersensitivity (DTH) reflects the presence of antigen-specific T-cell-mediated inflammation.**
- **There are four subgroups of type IV hypersensitivity reaction**: these groups reflect the unique cytokine production by T cells and the participation of different inflammation-causing effector cells.
- **Type IVa hypersensitivity is induced by TH1-cell responses and leads to macrophage activation.** Persistence of antigen leads to chronic T-cell activation, differentiation of macrophages into epithelioid cells and their fusion to form giant cells. This macrophage effector cell reaction results in tissue pathology.
- **Type IVb is characterized by TH2 activation, leading to eosinophil-driven inflammation**. These include many drug reactions, chronic asthma and infections by nematodes.

- **Type IVc involves T cells as stimulatory and effector cells.** Sensitization occurs when skin dendritic cells (DCs) internalize and process epicutaneously applied hapten and migrate to the draining lymph nodes where they activate antigen-specific T cells, leading to recruitment of antigen-specific and non-specific T cells.
- **Type IVd hypersensitivity is defined by sterile neutrophilic effector cell inflammation in response to CD4$^+$ and CD8$^+$ T-cell stimulation.** These include acute generalized exanthematous pustulosis (AGEP), Behçet's disease and pustular psoriasis.
- **In general, type IV reactions often occur in connection with shared stimulatory pathways between subgroups and simultaneously with multiple types of effector cells.**

DELAYED-TYPE HYPERSENSITIVITY REACTIONS

Delayed-type hypersensitivity (DTH) is a T-cell-mediated inflammatory response in which the stimulation of antigen-specific T cells leads to effector cell activation and localized inflammation and oedema within tissues. This T-cell response is essential for the control of intracellular and other pathogens. If the response is excessive, however, it can damage host tissues.

The T-cell response may be directed against exogenous agents, such as microbial antigens and sensitizing chemicals, or against self antigens. Typically, T cells are sensitized to the foreign antigen during infection with the pathogen or by absorption of a contact-sensitizing agent across the skin.

Sensitizing agents behave as haptens. In type IV reactions, haptens include:

- low molecular weight chemicals (<1 kDa) that are not immunogenic by themselves;
- lipophilic molecules that can penetrate through the epidermis and dermis, or by oral or IV route, where they bind covalently to cysteine or lysine residues in self proteins to form new antigenic determinants.
- metal ions, which chelate with self peptides in the groove of major histocompatibility complex (MHC) class II molecules.

Some contact allergens are modified by detoxifying enzymes encountered in the skin to form highly reactive metabolites that bind to self proteins. Potent haptens, such as dinitrochlorobenzene (DNCB), sensitize nearly all individuals and are used in animal models of allergic contact dermatitis. Some drugs are pro-haptens, which require metabolism to become haptens such as sulfamethoxazole. Other chemicals appear to act outside the hapten pathway to cause sensitization. In these cases, the drug can bind directly to the T-cell receptor while being stabilized by an MHC/peptide interaction (known as pharmacological interaction with immune receptors, p-i concept) to cause T-cell activation.

Subsequent exposure of the sensitized individual to the exogenous antigen, either injected intradermally or applied to the epidermis, results in the recruitment of antigen-specific T cells to the site and the development of a local inflammatory response. If the foreign antigen persists in the tissues, chronic activation of T cells can lead to activation of other cell types, including macrophages, eosinophils, cytotoxic T cells and neutrophils. If the antigen is an organ-specific self antigen, autoreactive T cells may produce localized cellular inflammation and autoimmune disease, such as type I diabetes mellitus.

According to the Gell and Coombs classification, type IV or DTH reactions take more than 12 hours to develop and involve cell-mediated immune reactions rather than antibody responses to antigens. Some other hypersensitivity reactions may straddle this definition because they have:

- a rapid antibody-mediated phase;
- a later cell-mediated phase.

For example, the late-phase IgE-mediated reaction may peak 12–24 hours after contact with allergen and TH2 cells and eosinophils contribute to the inflammation as well as IgE (see Chapter 23).

Type IV hypersensitivity can be transferred from one animal to another by T cells, particularly CD4⁺ TH1 cells in mice, rather than by serum. Therefore, DTH can develop in antibody-deficient humans but is lost as CD4⁺ T cells fall in HIV infection and AIDS.

Type IV hypersensitivity reflects the presence of antigen-specific CD4⁺ T cells and is associated with protective immunity against intracellular and other pathogens. However, there is not a complete correlation between type IV hypersensitivity and protective immunity and progressive infections may develop despite the presence of strong DTH reactivity.

There are four subgroups of type IV hypersensitivity reaction. The Gell and Coombs classification originated before any significant T-cell subclassification and defined type IV reactions largely based on the T-helper type 1 (TH1) response seen in tuberculin reactions. Over recent years, subgrouping of type IV reactions has occurred to describe more accurately the T-cell-mediated immune mechanisms that underlie the specific hypersensitivity disease. Four subgroups of type IV hypersensitivity reaction are recognized (Fig. 26.1):

- **Type IVa**, in which TH1 cells secrete large amounts of interferon-γ (IFNγ) and lead to macrophage activation. This includes tuberculin and granulomatous reactions.
- **Type IVb** reactions develop after T-helper type 2 (TH2) cell activation of eosinophils via cytokines IL-4 and IL-5. Examples include chronic asthma, chronic allergic rhinitis, DRESS syndrome (drug reaction with eosinophilia and systemic symptoms) and schistosomiasis.
- **Type IVc** reactions involve CD8⁺ T cells acting as effector cells themselves to produce cytokines and drive cytotoxic activity. In vivo correlates include contact dermatitis and some bullous skin diseases.
- **Type IVd** reactions involve T-cell activation of neutrophils, causing sterile neutrophilic inflammations of the skin.

This subgrouping reflects the unique cytokine production by T cells and reflects the participation of the different effector cells, which underlie the cause of inflammation and tissue damage.

TYPE IVa REACTIONS REQUIRE MACROPHAGES AS EFFECTOR CELLS

Type IVa reactions are characterized by classic TH1-type immune reactions. TH1-type T cells activate macrophages by secreting IFNγ and other pro-inflammatory cytokines (tumour necrosis factor alpha (TNFα), IL-12). These T cells are able to drive the production of complement-fixing antibodies critical to types II and III reactions. In addition, TH1 cells can act as co-stimulators for a CD8⁺ T-cell response (type IVc, discussed later in this chapter). In vivo examples include monocyte activation seen in the skin test to tuberculin or granuloma formation seen in sarcoidosis or Crohn's disease.

In many type IVa reactions, the degree of the response is usually assessed in animals by measuring thickening of the skin. This local response is accompanied by evidence of T-cell activation systemically, such as antigen-specific T-cell proliferation and cytokine synthesis, such as IFNγ. While our understanding of the immunopathogenesis of many type IVa diseases such as sarcoidosis or Crohn's disease has advanced in recent years, much of our knowledge of type IVa hypersensitivity is based on tuberculin and granulomatous reactions.

Tuberculin-type hypersensitivity is a form of type IVa reaction. Tuberculin-type hypersensitivity was originally described by Koch. He observed that if patients with tuberculosis were injected subcutaneously with a tuberculin culture filtrate (antigens derived from the causative agent, *Mycobacterium tuberculosis*), they reacted with fever and generalized sickness. An area of hardening and swelling developed at the site of injection.

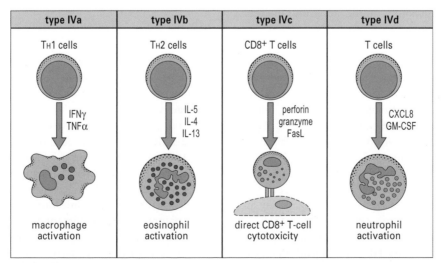

Fig. 26.1 Delayed hypersensitivity reactions The characteristics of type IV reactions comparing T-cell activation of subgroup specific effector cells.

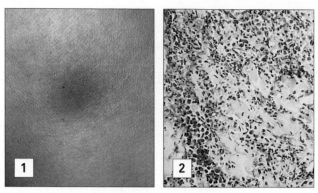

Fig. 26.2 Clinical and histological appearances of tuberculin-type sensitivity The response to an injection of leprosy bacillus into a sensitized individual is known as the Fernandez reaction. The reaction is characterized by an area of firm red swelling of the skin and is maximal 48–72 hours after challenge (**1**). Histologically (**2**), there is a dense dermal infiltrate of leukocytes. H&E stain. × 80.

Soluble antigens from other organisms, including *Mycobacterium leprae* and *Leishmania tropica*, induce similar tuberculin-type hypersensitivity reactions in sensitized people. The skin reaction is frequently used to test for T-cell-mediated responses to the organisms following previous exposure (Fig. 26.2). This form of hypersensitivity may also be induced by T-cell responses to non-microbial antigens, such as beryllium and zirconium.

The tuberculin skin test reaction involves monocytes and lymphocytes. The tuberculin skin test is an example of the recall response to soluble antigen previously encountered during infection. Dendritic cells (DCs) that take up *M. tuberculosis* in the lung undergo maturation and migrate to the draining mediastinal lymph nodes where they activate CD4+ and CD8+ T cells.

Following intradermal tuberculin challenge in a previously infected individual, mycobacteria-specific memory T cells are recruited and activated by dermal DCs to secrete IFNγ, which activates macrophages to produce TNFα and IL-1. These pro-inflammatory cytokines and chemokines from T cells and macrophages act on endothelial cells in dermal blood vessels to induce the sequential expression of the adhesion molecules E-selectin, intercellular adhesion molecule 1 (ICAM-1) and vascular cell adhesion molecule-1 (VCAM-1). These molecules bind receptors on leukocytes and recruit them to the site of the reaction.

The initial influx at 4 hours is of neutrophils, but this is replaced at 12 hours by monocytes and T cells. The infiltrate, which extends outwards and disrupts the collagen bundles of the dermis, increases to a peak at 48 hours. CD4+ T cells outnumber CD8+ cells by about 2:1. A few CD4+ cells infiltrate the epidermis between 24 and 48 hours.

Monocytes constitute 80%–90% of the total cellular infiltrate. Both infiltrating lymphocytes and macrophages express MHC class II molecules and this increases the efficiency of activated macrophages as antigen-presenting cells (APCs). CD1+ DCs also are present at 24–48 hours. Overlying keratinocytes express HLA-DR molecules 48–96 hours after the appearance of the lymphocytic infiltrate. These events are summarized in Figure 26.3.

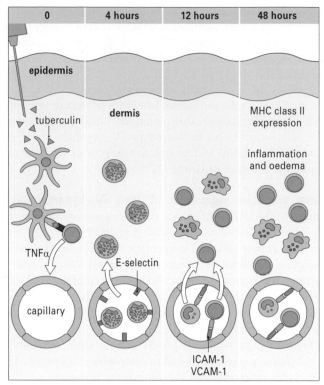

Fig. 26.3 Tuberculin-type hypersensitivity This diagram illustrates cellular movements following intradermal injection of tuberculin. Within 1–2 hours there is expression of E-selectin on capillary endothelium leading to a brief influx of neutrophil leukocytes. By 12 hours, intercellular adhesion molecule 1 (*ICAM-1*) and vascular cell adhesion molecule-1 (*VCAM-1*) on endothelium bind the integrins leukocyte functional antigen-1 and very late antigen-4 on monocytes and lymphocytes, leading to accumulation of both cell types in the dermis. This peaks at 48 hours and is followed by expression of the major histocompatibility complex (*MHC*) class II molecules on keratinocytes. There is no oedema of the epidermis. *TNFα*, tumor necrosis factor alpha.

The circulation of immune cells to and from the regional lymph nodes is thought to be similar to that for contact hypersensitivity. The tuberculin lesion normally resolves within 5–7 days, but if there is persistence of antigen in the tissues, it may develop into a granulomatous reaction.

Tuberculin-like DTH reactions are used practically in two ways. First, reaction to soluble antigens from a pathogen demonstrates past infection with that pathogen. Thus, tuberculin reactivity confirms past or latent infection with *M. tuberculosis*, but not necessarily active disease. However, subjects with latent tuberculosis infection have an increased lifelong risk of 7%–10% for the reactivation of active tuberculosis.

Second, DTH responses to frequently encountered microbes are a general measure of cell-mediated immunity. This can be tested with intradermal injection of single antigens from common pathogens or vaccine antigens, such as *Candida albicans* or tetanus toxoid. Loss of recall responses to specific antigens occurs in a wide range of diseases and infections, including HIV infection, which impair T-cell function, and during therapy with corticosteroids or immunosuppressive agents.

Granulomatous hypersensitivity is a special type of delayed hypersensitivity. Granulomatous hypersensitivity is clinically the most important form of type IV hypersensitivity, because it is responsible for the immunopathology in many diseases that involve T-cell-mediated immunity. It usually results from the persistence within macrophages of:

- intracellular microorganisms, which are able to resist macrophage killing; or
- other particles that the cell is unable to destroy.

This leads to chronic stimulation of T cells and the release of cytokines. The process results in the formation of epithelioid cell granulomas with a central collection of epithelioid cells and macrophages surrounded by lymphocytes.

The histological appearance of the granuloma reaction is quite different from that of the tuberculin-type reaction, although both types of reaction are caused by T cells sensitized to similar microbial antigens: for example, those of *M. tuberculosis* and *M. leprae*.

Granulomas occur with chronic infections associated with predominantly TH1-like T-cell responses, such as tuberculosis, leprosy and leishmaniasis, and with TH2-like T cells, as in schistosomiasis (see type IVb reactions).

Immune-mediated granuloma formation also occurs in the absence of infection, as in the sensitivity reactions to zirconium and beryllium, and in sarcoidosis and Crohn's disease where the antigens are unknown.

Foreign body granuloma formation occurs in response to talc, silica and a variety of other particulate agents, when macrophages are unable to digest the inorganic matter. These non-immunological granulomas may be distinguished by the absence of lymphocytes in the lesion.

Epithelioid cells and giant cells are typical of granulomatous hypersensitivity. Epithelioid cells are large and flattened with increased endoplasmic reticulum (Fig. 26.4). They:

- are derived from activated macrophages under the chronic stimulation of cytokines;
- continue to secrete TNFα and thus potentiate continuing inflammation.

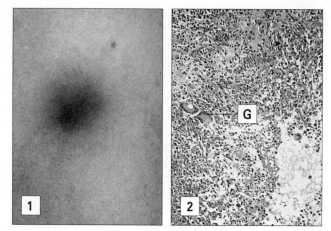

Fig. 26.5 Clinical and histological appearances of the Mitsuda reaction in leprosy At 28 days: (**1**) The resultant skin swelling (which may be ulcerated) is much harder and better defined than at 48 hours. (**2**) Histology shows a typical epithelioid cell granuloma (H&E stain. × 60). Giant cells *(G)* are visible in the centre of the lesion, which is surrounded by a cuff of lymphocytes. This response is more akin to the pathological granulomatous processes in delayed hypersensitivity diseases than the self-resolving tuberculin-type reaction. The reaction is caused by the continued presence of mycobacterial antigen.

Giant cells are formed when epithelioid cells fuse to form multinucleate giant cells (Fig. 26.5), sometimes referred to as Langhans giant cells (not to be confused with the Langerhans cell discussed earlier). Giant cells have several nuclei at the periphery of the cell. There is little endoplasmic reticulum and the mitochondria and lysosomes appear to be undergoing degeneration. The giant cell may therefore be a terminal differentiation stage of the monocyte/macrophage line.

A granuloma contains epithelioid cells, macrophages and lymphocytes. An immunological granuloma typically has a core of epithelioid cells and macrophages, sometimes with giant cells. In some diseases, such as tuberculosis, this central area

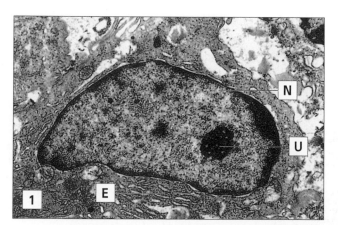

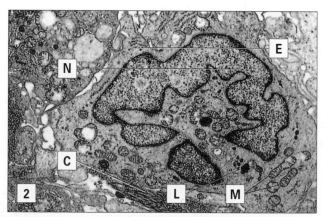

Fig. 26.4 Electron micrograph of an epithelioid cell The epithelioid cell is the characteristic cell of granulomatous hypersensitivity. Compare the extent of the endoplasmic reticulum *(E)* in the epithelioid cell (**1**, × 4800) with that of a tissue macrophage (**2**, × 4800). *C,* Collagen; *L,* lysosome; *M,* mitochondria; *N,* nucleus; *U,* nucleolus. (Courtesy MJ Spencer.)

may have a zone of necrosis, with complete destruction of all cellular architecture. The macrophage/epithelioid core is surrounded by a cuff of lymphocytes and there may also be considerable fibrosis (deposition of collagen fibres) caused by proliferation of fibroblasts and increased collagen synthesis. An example of a granulomatous reaction is the delayed Mitsuda reaction to dead *M. leprae* (see Fig. 26.5).

T cells bearing αβ TCRs are essential. Experiments with gene knockout mice have confirmed that T cells bearing αβ T-cell receptors (TCRs) rather than γδ TCRs are essential for initiating delayed hypersensitivity reactions in response to infection with intracellular bacteria.

Sensitized αβ T cells, stimulated with the appropriate antigen and APCs, undergo lymphoblastoid transformation before cell division (Fig. 26.6). This forms the basis of the lymphocyte stimulation test as a measure of T-cell function. Lymphocyte stimulation is accompanied by DNA synthesis and can be measured by assaying the uptake of radiolabelled thymidine, a nucleoside required for DNA synthesis. Lymphocytes from a patient are stimulated in culture with the suspect antigen to determine whether it induces proliferation. It is important to stress that this is a test for T-cell memory only and does not necessarily imply the presence of protective immunity.

Following activation by APCs, T cells release a number of pro-inflammatory cytokines, which attract and activate macrophages. These include IFNγ, lymphotoxin-α, IL-3 and granulocyte–macrophage colony stimulating factor (GM-CSF). The presence of memory T cells can be detected by antigen-specific IFNγ release assays. This TH1-like pattern of cytokines is enhanced by activation of the naive T cells in the presence of IL-12, which is released by DCs on exposure to bacterial products. IL-12 suppresses the cytokine response of TH2 cells.

IFNγ is required for granuloma formation in humans. The role of individual cytokines can be analysed in gene knockout mice deficient for a single cytokine. For example, IFNγ gene knockout mice are unable to activate macrophages and control infection with *M. tuberculosis* (Fig. 26.7). The absolute requirement of IFNγ for granuloma formation in humans is illustrated by the syndrome of Mendelian susceptibility to mycobacterial disease. Subjects deficient in the IFNγ receptor have markedly increased susceptibility to environmental mycobacteria and the vaccine strain BCG and fail to develop granulomas.

TNFα and lymphotoxin-α are essential for granuloma formation during mycobacterial infections. TNFα and the related cytokine lymphotoxin-α are both essential for the formation of granulomas during mycobacterial infections (Fig. 26.8) and act in part through the regulation of chemokine production. Both macrophage- and T-cell-derived TNFα contribute to this process, but within granulomas activated macrophages become the major source of TNFα, driving the differentiation of macrophages into epithelioid cells and the fusion of epithelioid cells to form giant cells (see Fig. 26.8 and Fig. 26.9). The maintenance of granulomas is also dependent on TNFα. Consequently, inhibition of TNFα activity suppresses the granulomatous inflammation in Crohn's disease and sarcoidosis.

Granulomatous reactions occur in many chronic diseases. There are many chronic human diseases that manifest type IVa hypersensitivity. Most are because of infectious agents, such as mycobacteria, although in other granulomatous diseases such as Crohn's disease, no infectious agent has been established. A common feature of these infections is that the pathogen causes a persistent, chronic, antigenic stimulus. Activation of macrophages by lymphocytes limits the infection, but continuing stimulation leads to tissue damage through the release of macrophage products, including reactive oxygen intermediates and hydrolases.

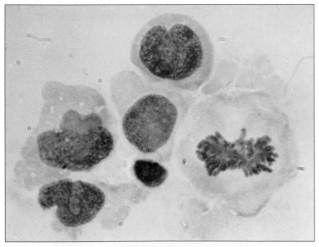

Fig. 26.6 Transformed lymphocytes Following stimulation with appropriate antigen, T cells undergo lymphoblastoid transformation before cell division. Blast cells with expanded nuclei and cytoplasm (as well as one lymphocyte in the metaphase of cell division) are shown. The resulting cell division can be measured by the uptake of tritiated thymidine.

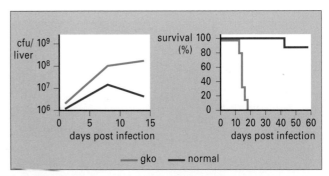

Fig. 26.7 The importance of IFNγ in the activation of macrophages Mice deficient in IFNγ (gene knockout *(gko)* mice), infected with a sublethal dose of *Mycobacterium tuberculosis*, are unable to activate macrophages in response to infection with an intracellular bacterium. Macrophages initially accumulate at the site of infection, but do not form typical granulomas. Uncontrolled infection (graph, *left*) causes widespread tissue necrosis and death (graph, *right*). *cfu*, Colony forming units of infectious agent in the liver.

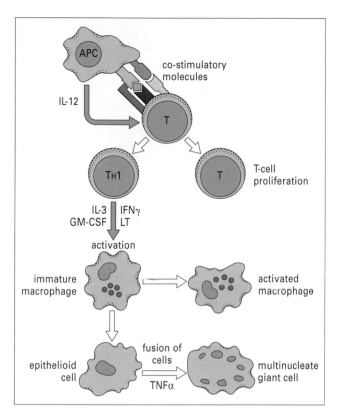

Fig. 26.8 Macrophage differentiation Bacterial products stimulate macrophages to secrete IL-12. Activation of T cells in the presence of IL-12 leads to the release of interferon-γ *(IFNγ)* and other cytokines, lymphotoxin *(LT)*, IL-3 and granulocyte -macrophage colony stimulating factor *(GM-CSF)*. These cytokines activate macrophages to kill intracellular parasites. Failure to eradicate the antigenic stimulus causes persistent cytokine release and promotes differentiation of macrophages into epithelioid cells, which secrete large amounts of tumour necrosis factor-α *(TNFα)*. Some fuse to form multinucleate giant cells. *APC*, Antigen-presenting cell.

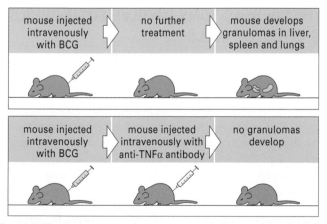

Fig. 26.9 The importance of tumour necrosis factor alpha *(TNFα)* in the formation of granulomas TNFα is essential for the development of epithelioid cell granulomas. If bacille Calmette-Guerin *(BCG)*-injected mice are injected with anti-TNFα antibodies, they do not develop granulomas.

Although delayed hypersensitivity is a measure of T-cell activation, the infection is not always controlled, with the result that protective immunity and delayed hypersensitivity do not necessarily coincide. Therefore, some subjects showing

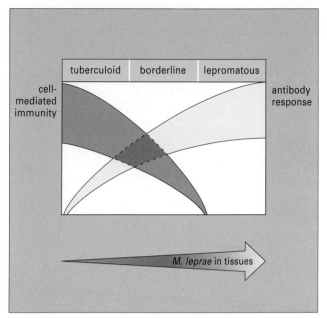

Fig. 26.10 The immunological spectrum of leprosy The clinical spectrum of leprosy ranges from tuberculoid disease with few lesions and bacteria to lepromatous leprosy, with multiple lesions and uncontrolled bacterial proliferation. This range reflects host immunity as measured by specific cellular and antibody responses to *Mycobacterium leprae* and the tissue expression of cytokines.

delayed hypersensitivity may not be protected against disease in the future.

The immune response in leprosy varies greatly between individuals. Leprosy is a chronic granulomatous disease of skin and nerves caused by infection with *M. leprae*. It is divided clinically into three main types – tuberculoid, borderline and lepromatous:

* In tuberculoid leprosy, the skin may have a few well-defined hypopigmented patches, which show an intense lymphocytic and epithelioid cell infiltrate and no microorganisms.
* By contrast, the polar reaction of lepromatous leprosy shows multiple confluent skin lesions characterized by numerous bacilli, 'foamy' macrophages and a paucity of lymphocytes.
* Borderline leprosy has characteristics of both tuberculoid and lepromatous leprosy (Fig. 26.10).

In leprosy, protective immunity is usually associated with cell-mediated immunity, but this declines across the leprosy spectrum towards the lepromatous pole with an increase in mycobacteria and a rise in non-protective anti-*M. leprae* antibodies.

The borderline leprosy reaction is a dramatic example of delayed hypersensitivity. Borderline reactions occur either spontaneously or after drug treatment. In these reactions, hypopigmented skin lesions containing *M. leprae* become swollen and inflamed (Fig. 26.11) because the patient is now able to mount a T-cell response to the mycobacteria, resulting in a delayed-type hypersensitivity reaction. The histological appearance shows a more tuberculoid pattern with an infiltrate of IFNγ-secreting lymphocytes. The process may occur in

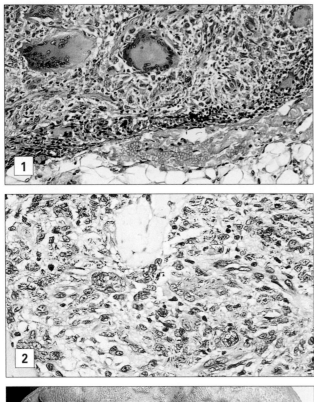

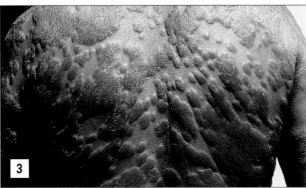

Fig. 26.11 Leprosy (1) A borderline leprosy reaction. This small nerve is almost completely replaced by the granulomatous infiltrate. (2) Lepromatous leprosy. Large numbers of bacilli are present. (3) Borderline lepromatous leprosy. There are gross infiltrated erythematous plaques with well-defined borders. ((2) Courtesy Dr Phillip McKee. (3) Courtesy Dr S Lucas.)

peripheral nerves, where Schwann cells contain *M. leprae*; this is the most important cause of nerve destruction in this disease. The lesion in borderline leprosy is typical of granulomatous hypersensitivity (see Fig. 26.11). In patients with a tuberculoid-type reaction, T-cell sensitization may be assessed in vitro by lymphocyte proliferation or the release of IFNγ following stimulation with *M. leprae* antigens.

Granulomatous reactions are necessary to control tuberculosis. In tuberculosis, the granuloma provides the microenvironment in which lymphocytes stimulate macrophages to kill the intracellular *M. tuberculosis*. The formation and maintenance of granulomas are essential to control the infection.

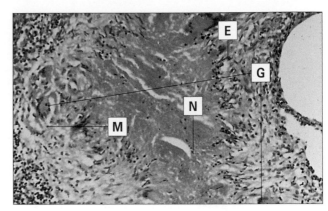

Fig. 26.12 Histological appearance of a tuberculous section of lung This micrograph shows an epithelioid cell granuloma *(E)* with giant cells *(G)*. Mononuclear cell infiltration can be seen *(M)*. There is also marked caseation and necrosis *(N)* within the granuloma. H&E stain. × 75.

In most (>90%) subjects with latent tuberculosis infection, the mycobacteria remain dormant within small granulomas in the lung. There is, however, a balance between the effects of activated macrophages:

- controlling the bacterial growth; and
- causing tissue damage in infected organs. In those who progress to clinical tuberculosis, granulomatous reactions erode airways, leading to cavitation in the lung and spread of bacteria. The reactions are frequently accompanied by extensive fibrosis and the lesions are visible in the chest radiographs of affected patients (Fig. 26.w1).

The histological appearance of the lesion is typical of a granulomatous reaction, with central caseous (cheesy) necrosis (Fig. 26.12). This is surrounded by an area of epithelioid cells with a few giant cells. Mononuclear cell infiltration occurs around the edge.

TYPE IVb REACTIONS INVOLVE EOSINOPHILS AS EFFECTOR CELLS

While type IVa reactions are driven by TH1 cells and macrophages, type IVb reactions are driven by T helper 2 (TH2) cells, which secrete IL-4, IL-13 and IL-5 cytokines to promote B-cell production of IgE and IgG4, with mast cell and eosinophil infiltration. IL-5 enhances chemotaxis and adhesion of eosinophils as well as promoting eosinophil activation, degranulation and cytotoxicity. This eosinophilic inflammation is seen in many drug-induced hypersensitivity reactions, including DRESS, asthma and infections with nematodes.

TH2-mediated inflammation of the airways is seen in asthma. Asthma is characterized by two phases: acute and chronic. The acute phase occurs rapidly after allergen exposure, usually within 1 hour. This reaction is the result of degranulation of mast cells by the binding of allergen to IgE (pre-bound to FcεR1 receptors on the mast cell surface) and the release of histamine, prostaglandins and other preformed or rapidly synthesized mediators that cause a rapid increase in vascular permeability and the contraction of smooth muscle (see Chapter 23).

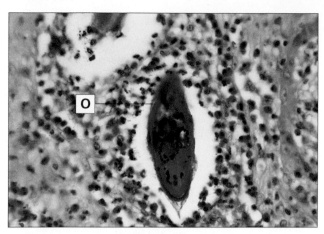

Fig. 26.13 Histological appearance of the liver in schistosomiasis The epithelioid cell granuloma surrounds the schistosome ovum *(O)* and eosinophils are prominent. H&E stain. × 300. (Courtesy Dr Phillip McKee.)

The chronic phase is a type IVb reaction that occurs within 6–12 hours of the initial allergen exposure. After the acute phase, there is an influx of inflammatory cells, including eosinophils and TH cells from the blood. Activated TH2 cells secrete cytokines that enhance eosinophil activation and degranulation, which causes further inflammation and recruitment of additional inflammatory cells. The result is chronic inflammation of the airways. Similar to the acute phase, there is a second phase of smooth muscle contraction, oedema and the development of airway hyper-reactivity to non-specific bronchoconstriction stimuli such as histamine and methacholine.

Granulomas surround the parasite ova in schistosomiasis.

In schistosomiasis, which is caused by parasitic trematode worms (schistosomes), the host becomes sensitized to the eggs of the worms, leading to a typical granulomatous reaction in the parasitized tissue mediated essentially by TH2 cells (Fig. 26.13; see also Chapter 16). In this case, the cytokines IL-5 and IL-13 are responsible for the recruitment of eosinophils and the formation of the granulomas around the ova. When the eggs have been deposited in the liver, the subsequent IL-13-dependent fibrosis causes hepatic scarring and portal hypertension.

TYPE IVc REACTIONS INVOLVE CD8⁺ T CELLS AS EFFECTOR CELLS

Type IVc reactions are responses in which CD8⁺ T cells function as the effector cells. In these reactions, T cells migrate to tissues and cause direct damage through perforin, granzyme B and Fas-ligand-dependent mechanisms. This process often occurs in conjunction with other type IV reactions including monocyte, eosinophil and neutrophil recruitment. In vivo correlates in which activated cytotoxic T cells participate in type IVc reactions include bullous skin diseases such as SJS (Stevens–Johnson syndrome) and TEN (toxic epidermal necrosis), as well as contact dermatitis. TH1 cells can activate CD8⁺ cells as seen in contact dermatitis, which is characterized by increased IFNγ (type IVa) and cytotoxic T-cell activation (type IVc)

Contact hypersensitivity requires sensitization by haptens.

Contact hypersensitivity is characterized by an eczematous skin reaction at the site of contact with an allergen (Fig. 26.14). Sensitizing agents for humans include metal ions, such as nickel and chromium, many industrial chemicals, including those in rubber and leather, and natural products present in dyes, drugs, fragrances and plants, such as pentadecacatechol, the sensitizing chemical in poison ivy. This is distinct from the non-immune-mediated inflammatory response to irritants.

A contact hypersensitivity reaction has two stages – sensitization and elicitation.

Antigen-presenting cells (APC) in the skin include Langerhans cells (LCs), located in the suprabasal epidermis and dermal dendritic cells (dDCs). Contact hypersensitivity is primarily an epidermal reaction and epidermal LCs were considered to be the APC responsible for initiating contact sensitivity (Fig. 26.15). More recent studies have established that dDCs are essential for stimulating hapten-specific T cells. LCs are specialized DCs that extend dendritic processes throughout the epidermis, allowing them to sample environmental antigens. LCs express MHC class II, CD1 and the C-type lectin, langerin (CD207), which is responsible for the development of Birbeck granules, the cell membrane-derived organelle characteristic of LCs (see Fig. 26.15). The majority of dermal DCs are Langerin⁻, but there is a small population of Langerin⁺ dDCs, which are distinct from LCs but also migrate rapidly to draining lymph nodes on exposure to sensitizers and activate hapten-specific CD8⁺ T cells. Both LCs and dDCs take up hapten-modified proteins by micropinocytosis, but they also absorb lipid-soluble haptens, which modify cytoplasmic proteins. Under the influence of IL-1 and TNFα secreted by keratinocytes and other cells, these DCs undergo maturation and increase expression of MHC and co-stimulatory molecules. Both LCs and dDCs are inactivated by ultraviolet B, which can therefore prevent or alleviate the effects of contact hypersensitivity.

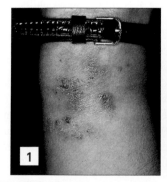
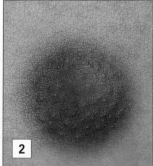

Fig. 26.14 Clinical and patch test appearances of contact hypersensitivity (**1**) The eczematous area at the wrist is due to sensitivity to nickel in the watch-strap buckle. (**2**) The suspected allergy may be confirmed by applying potential allergens, in the relevant concentrations and vehicles, to the patient's upper back (patch testing). A positive reaction causes a localized area of eczema at the site of the offending allergen 2–4 days after application.

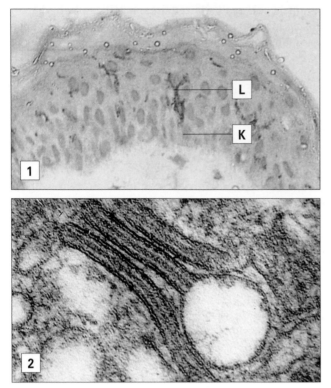

Fig. 26.15 Langerhans cells (1) These dendritic cells constitute 3% of all cells in the epidermis. They express a variety of surface markers, including Langerin and CD1. Here they have been identified in normal skin using an anti-CD1 monoclonal antibody (counterstained with Mayer's hemalum). × 312. **(2)** Electron micrograph of a Langerhans cell showing the characteristic Birbeck granule. This organelle is a plate-like structure derived from cell membranes, often with a bleb-like extension at one end. × 132 000. *L*, Langerhans cell; *K*, keratinocyte.

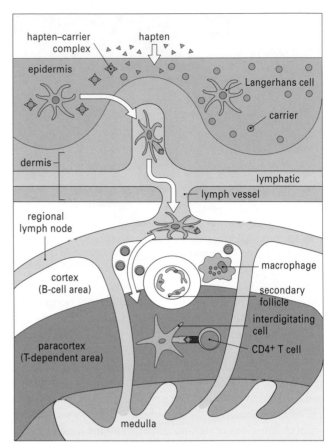

Fig. 26.16 Sensitization phase of contact hypersensitivity The hapten forms a hapten–carrier complex in the epidermis or within cytoplasm. Langerhans cells and dermal dendritic cells internalize the antigen, undergo maturation and migrate via afferent lymphatics to the paracortical area of the regional lymph node where peptide–MHC molecule complexes on the surface of the Langerhans cell can also be directly haptenated. As interdigitating cells, they present antigen to CD4⁺ and CD8⁺ T cells.

Keratinocytes produce cytokines important to the contact hypersensitivity response.

Keratinocytes provide the structural integrity of the epidermis and have a central role in epidermal immunology. Keratinocytes can be activated by a number of stimuli, including sensitizing agents and irritants. They may express MHC class II molecules and intercellular adhesion molecule-1 (ICAM-1) in the cell membrane.

Activated keratinocytes produce a wide range of cytokines, including:

- TNFα, IL-1 and GM-CSF, which activate LCs and dDCs;
- IL-3 which activates LCs and co-stimulates T-cell proliferative responses, recruits mast cells and induces secretion of immunosuppressive cytokines, such as IL-10 and transforming growth factor-β (TGFβ). These dampen the immune response and may induce clonal anergy or immunological unresponsiveness in TH1 cells.

Sensitization stimulates a population of memory T cells.

Sensitization takes 10–14 days in humans. Hapten-bearing LCs and dDCs bearing modified proteins migrate as veiled cells through the afferent lymphatics to the paracortical areas of regional lymph nodes, where they activate CD4⁺ and CD8⁺ T cells. MHC class I-restricted CD8⁺ T cells are important in contact hypersensitivity responses in humans and mice and are the major effector cells for many allergens. For example, lipid-soluble urushiol from poison ivy enters the cytoplasm of APCs and haptenated cytoplasmic proteins are processed through the MHC class I pathway, leading to the activation of allergen-specific CD8⁺ T cells. Hapten-specific CD4⁺ T cells are also activated by hapten–peptide conjugates in association with MHC class II molecules and become effector/memory CD4⁺ T cells, which contribute to the skin inflammation, or regulatory CD4⁺ T cells (Fig. 26.16). Activated T cells change the pattern of adhesion molecules on their surface by downregulating CD62L and the chemokine receptor, CCR7.

The expression of leukocyte functional antigen-1 (LFA-1), very late antigen-4 (VLA-4) and the chemokine receptors CXCR3 and CCR5 is increased. As a result, the activated/memory T cells remain within the circulation, rather than trafficking through lymphoid tissue, and are able to bind to adhesion molecules on the endothelium of inflamed tissues.

Elicitation involves recruitment of CD4+ and CD8+ lymphocytes and monocytes. The application of a contact allergen leads to:

- rapid expression of pro-inflammatory cytokines; and
- recruitment of effector T cells and monocytes to the site (Fig. 26.17).

There is induction of mRNA for TNFα, IL-1β and GM-CSF in Langerhans cells within 30 minutes of exposure to allergen and increased transcription of mRNA for IL-1α, macrophage inflammatory protein-2 (CXCL2) and interferon-induced protein-10 (CXCL10) by keratinocytes.

TNFα and IL-1 are potent inducers of endothelial cell adhesion molecules, including:

- E-selectin and vascular cell adhesion molecule-1 (VCAM-1) within 2 hours; and
- ICAM-1 within 8 hours (Fig. 26.18).

VCAM-1 and ICAM-1 are the receptors for VLA-4 and LFA-1, respectively, on the surface of effector/memory T cells and contribute to their recruitment across the endothelium.

These locally released cytokines and chemokines also produce a gradient signal for the movement of mononuclear cells towards the dermo-epidermal junction and epidermis.

The earliest histological change, seen after 4–8 hours, is the appearance of mononuclear cells around blood vessels. Macrophages and lymphocytes invade the dermis and epidermis, peaking at 48–72 hours (Fig. 26.19). The recruitment of memory T cells is antigen non-specific, with less than 1% of infiltrating lymphocytes bearing hapten-specific αβ T-cell receptors. However, the hapten-specific T cells are stimulated by dermal DCs expressing hapten–peptide complexes to expand and to increase the expression of adhesion molecules. This leads to the retention of hapten-specific T cells at the inflamed site. Infiltrating lymphocytes include CD4+ TH1 cells secreting IFNγ and up to 50% CD8+ T cells. CD8+ T cells are essential for inducing experimental allergic sensitivity through their direct cytolytic effect on keratinocytes and the release of IFNγ.

Effector αβ T cells are essential for experimental contact sensitivity in mice, but NKT cells and γδ T cells also contribute to

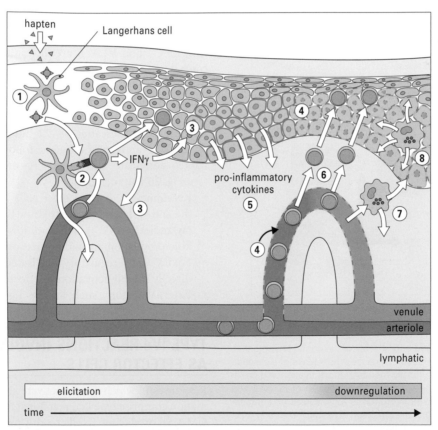

Fig. 26.17 Elicitation phase of contact hypersensitivity Langerhans cells carrying the hapten–carrier complex *(1)* move from the epidermis to the dermis, where they present the hapten–carrier complex to memory CD4+ and CD8+ T cells *(2)*. Activated CD4+ and CD8+ T cells release IFNγ, which induces expression of ICAM-1 *(3)* and, later, MHC class II molecules *(4)* on the surface of keratinocytes and on endothelial cells of dermal capillaries and activates keratinocytes, which release pro-inflammatory cytokines such as IL-1, IL-6 and GM-CSF *(5)*. Hapten-specific CD8+ T cells induce apoptosis of keratinocytes expressing haptenated self-peptides *(6)*. Non-antigen-specific T cells are attracted to the site by cytokines *(7)* and may bind to keratinocytes via ICAM-1 and MHC class II molecules. Activated macrophages are also attracted to the skin, but this occurs later. Thereafter the reaction starts to downregulate. This suppression is driven by eicosanoids such as prostaglandin E₂ (PGE₂), produced by activated keratinocytes and macrophages, and the inhibitory cytokines, IL-10 and TGFβ *(8)*.

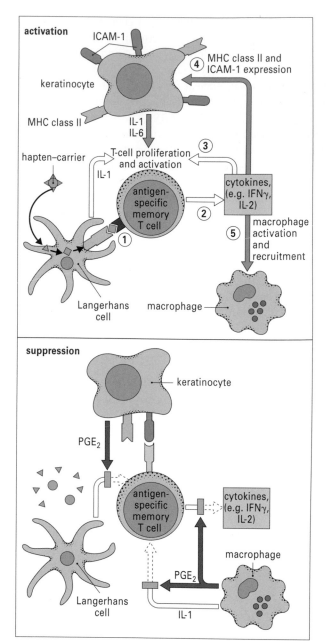

Fig. 26.18 Cytokines, prostaglandins and cellular interactions in contact hypersensitivity Cytokines and prostaglandins are central to the complex interactions between Langerhans cells, CD8⁺ and CD4⁺ T cells, keratinocytes, macrophages and endothelial cells in contact hypersensitivity. The act of antigen presentation *(1)* causes the release of a cascade of cytokines *(2)*. This cascade initially results in the activation and proliferation of CD4⁺ T cells *(3)*, the induction of expression of ICAM-1 and major histocompatibility complex *(MHC)* class II molecules on keratinocytes and endothelial cells *(4)* and the attraction of further T cells and macrophages to the skin *(3, 5)*. Subsequently, influx of FoxP3⁺ CD25⁺ CD4⁺ regulatory T cells inhibits T-cell activation and function by direct CTLA-4-mediated effects and secretion of IL-10 and TGFβ. IL-10 is also released by keratinocytes and mast cells, while keratinocytes and macrophages produce PGE₂, which inhibits IL-1 and IL-2 production. The combined effects of enzymatic and cellular degradation of the hapten–carrier complex, regulatory CD4⁺ T cells and suppressive cytokines and PGE₂ released by skin cells lead to downregulation of the reaction.

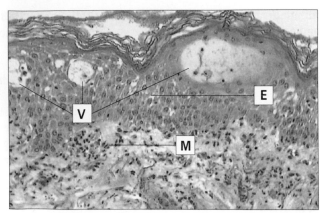

Fig. 26.19 Histological appearance of the lesion in contact hypersensitivity Mononuclear cells *(M)* infiltrate both dermis and epidermis. The epidermis is pushed outwards and micro-vesicles *(V)* form within it because of oedema *(E)*. H&E stain. × 130.

the induction and elicitation of this response. Interestingly, hapten-specific IgM antibodies from B-1 cells are also important during the elicitation phase in mice by activating complement and recruiting T cells to the challenge site. Experiments in gene-targeted mice show that selectins, ICAM-1, and the integrins, LFA-1 and VLA-4, are all required for the elicitation of contact and delayed hypersensitivity.

Suppression of the inflammatory reaction is mediated by multiple mechanisms. The reaction to cutaneous application of sensitizer wanes after 48–72 hours. This is because of the removal of antigenic stimulus following degradation of the hapten–conjugate and a variety of inhibitory mechanisms (see Fig. 26.18), including:

- Keratinocytes, dermal mast cells and macrophages secrete the anti-inflammatory cytokines IL-10 and TGFβ and prostaglandin E₂ (PGE₂), which inhibit T-cell proliferation, cytokine production and inflammation.
- FoxP3⁺ CD4⁺ regulatory T cells and IL-10 secreting TH1 cells directly inhibit activation of effector T cells.
- External factors, such as UV light, may also inhibit the expression of contact sensitivity.

TYPE IVd REACTIONS INVOLVE NEUTROPHILS AS EFFECTOR CELLS

Responses in which T cells activate sterile neutrophilic inflammation comprise type IVd reactions. Antigen activated, CXCL8/GM-CSF producing T cells recruit neutrophils via CXCL8 and promote survival through GM-CSF, resulting in a neutrophil-rich sterile inflammation. This is seen in acute generalized exanthematous pustulosis (AGEP), Behçet's disease and pustular psoriasis. Recent research has improved our understanding of the pathophysiology of type IVd reactions, showing that a deficiency in the IL-36 receptor antagonist (IL-36Ra) in some AGEP patients leads to, in addition to CXCL8 production, increased expression of various pro-inflammatory cytokines and chemokines such as IL-1, IL-6 and IL-17.

AGEP Is characterized by T-cell involvement.

AGEP is a type IVd reaction in which drugs, acute infections with enteroviruses or mercury act as hapten sources to drive a T-cell response. The disease is characterized by extensive formation of non-follicular sterile pustules, fever and increased numbers of blood neutrophils. In the acute phase of the pathogenesis of AGEP, there is activation of drug-specific T cells with subsequent migration of CD4$^+$ and CD8$^+$ cells to the skin. Similar to a type IVc reaction, the initial influx of CD8$^+$ cytotoxic T cells results in inflammation and tissue destruction, suggesting that granulysin may also play a role in the pathogenesis of AGEP. Next, infiltrating CD4$^+$ cells release high levels of CXCL8 and IL-17, which results in the recruitment of neutrophils, and GM-CSF, which prevents apoptosis of neutrophils. The influx of neutrophils results in conversion of vesicles into pustules. The disease process is exacerbated by T-cell release of IFNγ, which stimulates keratinocytes to secrete additional CXCL8, leading to further neutrophil recruitment.

CRITICAL THINKING: A HYPERSENSITIVITY TYPE IV REACTION

See Critical thinking: Explanations, section 26

An 8-year-old boy with recent weight loss and mild fever is found to have an enlarged lymph node on the right side of the neck. He has no cough and his chest radiograph is normal. Surgical biopsy of the lymph node reveals a granulomatous infiltrate with no evident acid-fast bacilli. The result of microbiological culture for *Mycobacterium tuberculosis* is awaited. Intradermal skin testing with tuberculin causes swelling and erythema of 20 mm in diameter after 48 hours.

1. Which cell types make up the granulomas in the lymph node and which cytokines are involved in their formation?
2. What is the pathology at the site of the skin testing and how does it differ from that in the lymph node?
3. What type of lymphocyte is responsible for the skin test reactivity?
4. What other conditions cause granulomas in lymph nodes and how are they diagnosed?
5. When the family members are tested, the boy's 5-year-old brother is found to have a positive tuberculin reaction (18 mm at 48 hours), but he is well with a normal chest radiograph. What does this result indicate about his immune responses and what is its significance?

FURTHER READING

Cavani A, De Luca A. Allergic contact dermatitis: novel mechanisms and therapeutic perspectives. Curr Drug Metabol 2010;11:228–233.

Cooper AM. Cell-mediated immune responses in tuberculosis. Ann Rev Immunol 2009;27:393–422.

Balakirski G, Merk H. Cutaneous allergic drug reactions: update on pathophysiology, diagnostic procedures and differential diagnosis. Cutan Ocul Toxicol 2017;36(4):307–316.

Hagge DA, Saunders BM, Ebenezer GJ, et al. Lymphotoxin-alpha and TNF have essential but independent roles in the evolution of the granulomatous response in experimental leprosy. Am J Pathol 2009;174:1379–1389.

Igyarto BZ, Kaplan DH. The evolving function of Langerhans cells in adaptive skin immunity. Immunol Cell Biol 2010;88:361–365.

Kaplan DH. In vivo function of Langerhans cells and dermal dendritic cells. Trends Immunol 2010;27:446–451.

Martin SF. Contact dermatitis: from pathomechanisms to immunotoxicology. Exp Dermatol 2012;21:382–389.

Martin SF, Esser PR, Schmucker S, et al. T cell recognition of chemicals, protein allergens and drugs: towards the development of in vitro assays. Cell Mol Life Sci 2010;67:4171–4184.

Pavlos R, Mallal S, Ostrov D, et al. T cell-mediated hypersensitivity reactions to drugs. Annu Rev Med 2015;66:439–454.

Pichler WJ. Delayed drug hypersensitivity reactions. Ann Intern Med 2003;139:683–693.

Salgame P. Host innate and Th1 responses and the bacterial factors that contain *Mycobacterium tuberculosis* infection. Curr Opin Immunol 2005;17:374–380.

Samitas K, Delimpoura V, Zervas E, et al. Anti-IgE treatment, airway inflammation and remodelling in severe allergic asthma: current knowledge and future perspectives. Eur Respir Rev 2015;24 (138):594–601.

Saunders BM, Britton WJ. Life and death in the granuloma: immunopathology of tuberculosis. Immunol Cell Biol 2007;85:103–111.

Szatkowski J, Schwartz RA. Acute generalised exanthematous pustulosis (AGEP): a review and update. J Am Acad Dermatol 2015;73:843–848.

Vocanson M, Hennino A, Rozieres A, et al. Effector and regulatory mechanisms in allergic contact dermatitis. Allergy 2009;64:1699–1714.

White KD, Chung W, Hung S, Mallal S, Phillips E. Evolving models of the immunopathogenesis of the T-cell mediated drug allergy: the role of the host, pathogens, and drug response. J Allergy Clin Immunol 2015;136(2):219–234.

Wynn TA, Thompson RW, Cheever AW, Mentink-Kane MM. Immunopathogenesis of schistosomiasis. Immunol Rev 2004;201:156–167.

CRITICAL THINKING: EXPLANATIONS

1. SPECIFICITY AND MEMORY IN VACCINATION

1.1 The immunological memory induced by vaccination does not depend just on the antibodies. Memory is due to long-lived memory lymphocytes, which persist in the lymphoid tissues for many years. They will be reactivated if the individual encounters the toxin or the vaccine on a later occasion.

1.2 The tetanus toxoid is a stable molecule – it does not change or mutate, with the result that antibodies and lymphocytes recognizing it continue to be effective. By contrast, influenza A mutates every year. Last year's antibodies are marginally effective or ineffective against this year's virus. Researchers must identify newly emerging virus strains and prepare vaccine from those strains they think will produce new epidemics. Often they get it right, but not always.

1.3 Recommendations are based on practicality. It is impossible to prepare sufficient vaccine each year to immunize everyone against influenza. There is not enough time to do it and not enough laboratory resources available. The highest-risk groups are therefore targeted – health workers because they are likely to be in contact with the disease and old people because the disease can lead to serious complications.

Discussion point: If we could immunize every person in the world against influenza A in 1 year, do you think that this would lead to total eradication of the disease?

2. DEVELOPMENT OF THE IMMUNE SYSTEM

2.1 The total numbers of blood lymphocytes are drastically reduced, with T cells being virtually absent and B cells significantly reduced – B cells require T cells to complete their own development. The lymph nodes are much reduced in size and this particularly affects the paracortex (T-cell areas). Compare this with DiGeorge's syndrome. The animals have a reduced ability to fight infections, but this is selective, affecting particularly some viruses and parasites – possibly because good NK-cell activity and macrophage-mediated antibacterial defences are still in evidence.

2.2 Adult thymectomy has very little effect on the individual's ability to fight infection. By adulthood, there is a large pool of peripheral T cells that may, to some extent, self-renew. The thymus progressively involutes and becomes less important as a site of T-cell development in the adult.

2.3 Because the lymphocyte precursors fail to make productive rearrangements of their antigen receptor genes, they die by apoptosis during development. This leads to a profound immune deficiency of all lymphocytes, which is analogous to severe combined immunodeficiency (SCID) in humans.

2.4 Interleukin-7 is required for lymphocyte development in primary lymphoid organs. There is a profound reduction in thymocytes and peripheral lymphocytes and a total absence of $\gamma\delta$ T cells.

2.5 The $\alpha_4\beta_7$-integrin is required for binding of cells to adhesion molecules on the high endothelial venule (HEV) of gut-associated lymphoid tissue (GALT). This knockout therefore results in drastically reduced lymphocyte numbers in these tissues.

3. THE ROLE OF ADHESION MOLECULES IN T-CELL MIGRATION

3.1 IL-1 induces the expression of a number of adhesion molecules, including ICAM-1 and VCAM-1, both of which can potentially mediate leukocyte migration by their interaction with the integrins LFA-1 and VLA-4, respectively.

3.2 Because it takes several hours to increase migration and ICAM-1 and VCAM-1 appear to be involved in the process, it can be inferred that their expression is increased as a result of protein synthesis (which takes several hours) rather than by a relatively rapid release from intracellular stores.

3.3 Antibodies to ICAM-1/LFA-1 reduce migration of cells across unstimulated endothelium. Therefore, this pair of adhesion molecules is required for migration across resting endothelium.

3.4 Antibodies to both ICAM-1/LFA-1 and VCAM-1/VLA-4 reduce migration across IL-1-activated cells; therefore both pairs of adhesion molecules control this event. In practice, it is known that ICAM-1 is present on unstimulated brain endothelium and is increased by IL-1, whereas VCAM-1 is virtually absent from unstimulated brain endothelium but may be synthesized following stimulation with inflammatory cytokines.

4. COMPLEMENT DEFICIENCY

4.1 Deficiencies of components of the classical or alternative pathways, particularly of C3, produce a reduced ability to opsonize bacteria, resulting in impaired phagocytosis by macrophages and neutrophils. Patients suffer from repeated bacterial infections from Gram-positive bacteria (e.g. staphylococci, streptococci). These children are unable to clear bacterial infections because their phagocytes do not take up bacteria efficiently. Deficiencies in the lytic pathway components (C5–C9) can render patients more susceptible to neisserial infections because the lytic pathway can damage the outer membrane of Gram-negative bacteria such as *Neisseria* spp.

4.2 There is a clear deficiency in C3 and components of the alternative pathway. Components of the classical pathway are on the lower end of normal. At first this looks surprising, because the initial assay for lytic complement required the activity of the classical and lytic pathways. Nevertheless, both the bacterial infections and the lack of total haemolytic complement can be explained by the very low levels of C3. Note that the genes for C3, FB and FI are not genetically linked and therefore we cannot explain this apparent multiple deficiency of alternative pathway components by some multiple gene deletion. The explanation lies in the alternative pathway amplification loop. Because the children lack FI, they cannot break down the alternative pathway C3 convertase C3bBb. Therefore, C3 is continuously activated and binds FB. All the FB is consumed, as is most of the free C3. The genetic deficiency of FI therefore leads to secondary deficiencies in the components of the alternative pathway and this then affects C3 and the function of the classical and lytic pathways.

4.3 The children have a homozygous FI deficiency – both copies of the gene are missing. Replacing FI, either by an infusion of normal serum or by providing pure FI, restores all other components to normal levels and allows the children to clear bacterial infections. Antibiotic prophylaxis will help prevent bacterial infections.

Discussion point: What problem might occur if you inject a protein such as FI into an individual who lacks it due to a genetic deficiency?

5. THE ROLE OF MACROPHAGES IN TOXIC SHOCK SYNDROME

5.1 TNFα, IL-1, IL-6, IL-10.

5.2 Lack of activity, ruffling of fur, respiratory distress, possibly leading to death within 24 hours

5.3 BCG activates macrophages via infection of APCs and induction of IFNγ by NK and CD4$^+$ T cells, which primes macrophages. LPS delivers stimulus via LPS-binding protein, CD4, Toll-like receptors and NF-κB activation to enhance pro-inflammatory cytokine release. TNFα and IL-1, especially, act locally and systemically on vascular endothelium, neutrophils and central nervous centres, causing hypotension and circulatory collapse.

5.4 CD14 knockout mice are extremely resistant to septic shock. Scavenger receptor A knockout mice are more susceptible to septic shock. IFNγ knockout mice are relatively resistant to septic shock.

5.5 CD14 is central to the LPS recognition and signalling pathway. SR-A clears LPS from the circulation to protect the host. IFNγ is needed to prime macrophages.

THE ROLE OF MACROPHAGES IN TH1 AND TH2 RESPONSES

5.6 Macrophage activation involves a complex pattern of altered gene expression, covering a spectrum of activities and not just polar opposites between activation (TH1, IFNγ)

and deactivation (TH2, IL-10). IL-4 and IL-13, TH2 cytokines, use common receptor chains to induce an alternative pathway of macrophage activation involved in humoral immunity and possibly repair (enhanced APC function via MHC class II expression and MRs, as well as other effects on B-cell production of antibody). IFNγ and IL-10 regulate cellular immune effector functions.

5.7 Broaden the range of macrophage markers examined, ultimately by DNA gene chip analysis and look for consistency and reproducibility of similar patterns of altered gene expression by the cytokines above. Analyse macrophage functions in mice with knockouts of cytokines or their receptors.

5.8 Find model antigens (e.g. parasites) that induce TH2 responses in vivo and establish whether these are recognized by APC receptors that enhance IL-4/IL-13 or inhibit IFNγ production by appropriate cells.

6. MHC RESTRICTION

6.1 This is an example of genetic restriction of antigen presentation. The SM/J T cells are primed with antigen on MHC molecules of the SM/J haplotype and will only respond to this combination of antigen/MHC. They cannot recognize antigen being presented by MHC molecules of the Balb/c haplotype.

6.2 MHC molecules are co-dominantly expressed, so the F1 mice have molecules of both the SM/J and the Balb/c haplotype. Therefore, the APCs from the F1 mice are able to stimulate the primed T cells from the SM/J mice by presenting antigen on SM/J haplotype MHC molecules.

6.3 The minimum peptide needed to activate the T cells appears to be 80–94, which is 15 residues long and therefore corresponds to the expected size of antigen peptides that can fit into the MHC class II binding groove. This peptide is included within peptides 80–102, which also stimulate strongly. Peptides 84–98 and 73–88 lack the N- and C-terminals of the antigenic peptide, respectively, and therefore lack some of the anchor residues needed to hold them in the MHC peptide-binding groove.

6.4 The serine is an anchor residue for this peptide. The mutated peptide lacks the anchor residue and as a result cannot be presented by the MHC.

6.5 This peptide will have a stronger binding affinity for the MHC molecule and/or the TCR. Such a peptide is called a super agonist.

7. ANTIGEN PROCESSING AND PRESENTATION

7.1 Live flu virus infects the macrophages and flu virus polypeptides are synthesized in the cytoplasm of the cell. The viral antigens are presented by the internal (MHC class I) pathway as well as the external (MHC class II) pathway. Inactivated virus is taken up by the macrophage, processed and presented via the class II pathway only; because there is no viral protein synthesis, there is no presentation via the MHC class I pathway.

7.2 Macrophages express both MHC class I and class II molecules and can therefore present antigen to either of the clones. Fibroblasts do not generally express MHC class II molecules and one would not expect them to stimulate the MHC class II-restricted clone.

7.3 XCR1 + DCs are able to cross-present exogenous antigen on MHC class I. Therefore, we might expect them to be able to stimulate the MHC class I-restricted clone using inactivated virus that they have taken up.

7.4 Because emetine blocks protein synthesis, no protein fragments are fed into the MHC class I pathway by the proteasomes. Chloroquine prevents phagosome/lysosome fusion and therefore endocytosed virus cannot be broken down into peptides. Consequently, no peptides are available for the MHC class II pathway.

7.5 The MHC class I-restricted T cells express CD8 and the MHC class II-restricted cells express CD4 because CD8 and CD4 are co-receptors for MHC class I and class II molecules, respectively.

8. MECHANISMS OF CYTOTOXICITY

8.1 CTLs and NK cells effect cytotoxicity by inducing apoptosis in their targets. In this assay, targets with fragmented DNA are assumed to be undergoing apoptosis. Note that there is always a low level of DNA fragmentation in the controls that contain no effector cells.

8.2 Tumour line 1 is susceptible to killing by CTLs but less so to killing by NK cells. Tumour line 1 S is susceptible to killing by NK cells but resistant to killing by CTLs. These observations are consistent with Tumour line 1 expressing MHC class I molecules, which are recognized as foreign by CTLs, while Tumour line 1 S is MHC class I negative and thus a target for NK cells.

8.3 NK cells do effect some killing of Tumour line 1, even though it expresses MHC class I. Therefore, the NK cells must be recognizing the tumour cells via activating receptors. Tumour cells often express surface proteins that can activate NK cells via NKG2D; therefore this is a likely candidate. You could test this hypothesis by blocking the interaction of NKG2D with its cellular ligands either using a blocking antibody or soluble NKG2D ligands.

8.4 Blocking interactions with MHC class I prevents CTL killing of Tumour line 1 because it is no longer able to recognize the target cell class I molecules as foreign. In this condition, however, NK cell killing of Tumour line 1 actually increases. This is likely to be because NK cells are now able to recognize the antibody-coated target cells via their Fc receptor, CD16. Note that the addition of anti-class I has no effect on the MHC class I negative Tumour line 1 S.

9. DEVELOPMENT OF THE ANTIBODY RESPONSE

9.1 In a developing immune response to a TD antigen, B cells will switch from IgM production to IgG. Because the antigen is continuously present as a depot, by day 14 the response has the characteristics of a secondary response – IgG antibody titres are climbing rapidly.

9.2 Perhaps the two mice have already been infected by mouse hepatitis virus. By day 5 they are already making a secondary IgG response. This could be a problem in the colony, although all animals housed together would usually become infected. If these mice have been naturally infected, it would be through the gut (unlike the vaccine) and a stronger IgA response would be expected.

9.3 IgA-producing clones tend to be located in the mucosa-associated lymphoid tissues (see Chapter 2) and it is not surprising that no IgA-producing clones were generated from the spleen.

9.4 IgG-producing clones at day 14 are likely to be of higher affinity than IgM producers.

10. THE SPECIFICITY OF ANTIBODIES

10.1 In the presence of the antibodies, mutated variants of the virus are selected that do not bind those antibodies. By detecting which of the virus proteins are mutated, it can be inferred that these are the proteins that would normally bind to the antibody. Neutralizing antibodies against viruses are generally directed against proteins in the capsid of the virus, particularly against the proteins that the virus uses to attach to the surface of its target cell. Antibodies cannot gain access to the inside of the virus; hence neutralizing antibodies do not bind the core protein VP4.

10.2 The antibody VP1-a binds to an epitope that includes two closely spaced residues (91 and 95). This is a continuous epitope and is located on a single external loop of polypeptide. By contrast, the epitope recognized by VP1-b is located in at least two distinct areas of the polypeptide chain (83–85 and 138–139). This is a discontinuous epitope: examination of the VP1 antigen shows that these residues are located on two adjacent areas of β-pleated sheet.

10.3 A mutation of residue 138 does not affect the epitope recognized by antibody VP1-a and it continues to bind with high affinity to the antigen. This confirms that the epitopes recognized by VP1-a and VP1-b are physically separate. The mutant with Gly at position 95 still binds the VP1-a antibody weakly. Glycine is a smaller amino acid than aspartate, which is present in the wild type, and the antibody can still bind to the epitope, although the 'fit' is less good and the affinity of binding is lower. By contrast, lysine (Lys) is a larger residue than aspartate. It protrudes further out into the antibody's binding site and completely disrupts the antigen–antibody bond.

11. IMMUNOLOGICAL TOLERANCE

11.1 **Clonal deletion:** Immature B cells that recognize antigen in the bone marrow can undergo clonal deletion. T cells start rearranging their antigen receptors in the thymus, where they undergo the processes of positive and negative selection. T cells that do not receive survival signals during positive selection and T cells that recognize self antigens with high affinity will undergo apoptosis.

Receptor editing: This is a B-cell specific tolerance mechanism. Immature B cells that recognize antigen in the bone marrow get a second chance: they can continue V(D)J recombination to assemble another, non-self reactive antigen receptor. Only if that fails will they undergo apoptosis. T lymphocytes assemble one receptor that cannot be changed during development.

Anergy: This describes the inability of a lymphocyte to respond to antigenic stimulation. This was first described for B cells but also occurs in T cells. The molecular mechanisms for anergy may differ between the two lymphocyte populations.

Lack of T-cell help: B cells need T-cell help to switch from IgM to other isotypes. Therefore, robust tolerance in the T-cell compartment will also help to ensure B-cell tolerance. T cells depend on co-stimulatory signals from antigen-presenting cells. This could be viewed as somewhat similar to the B cells' dependence on T-cell help.

11.2 Mutations in AIRE have been identified as the cause of the APECED (**a**utoimmune **p**olyendocrinopathy-**c**andidiasis-**e**ctodermal **d**ystrophy) syndrome and mice that lack AIRE have a similar phenotype. AIRE has been shown to direct the ectopic expression of otherwise strictly tissue restricted antigens by medullary thymic epithelial cells (mTECs) in the thymus.

11.3 T cells which have rearranged their TCR in the thymus need to receive survival signals (cytokines) from cortical thymic antigen-presenting cells (APCs). In order to receive these signals, the TCR must be able to recognize self MHC. Only T cells that express TCRs capable of recognizing self-MHC will receive survival signals; the other T cells will undergo apoptosis. T cells recognize only antigen that is complexed with self MHC. Therefore, a T cell that cannot recognize self MHC would be useless. B cells, in contrast, can recognize antigen without the help of APCs. Therefore, B cells do not need to be selected for self MHC recognition.

11.4 Dendritic cells (DCs) in the thymus contribute to thymic selection of the T-cell repertoire. Outside the thymus, DCs are important antigen-presenting cells (APCs) for T cells, in particular for naive T cells. DCs are located in many organs and constantly take up antigen, both self and non-self. Only if the DCs recognize danger signals (PAMPs), via their pattern recognition receptors (PRRs, e.g. TLRs), will they undergo certain maturation steps, including the upregulation of co-stimulatory ligands for T cells, which transform them into powerful APCs. To become activated, effector T cells need to recognize antigens and receive co-stimulatory signals. If a DC presents only antigens but does not provide co-stimulatory signals, the corresponding T cell will become anergic or undergo apoptosis. Self antigens usually do not provide danger signals for the DC. Therefore, the DC will not provide co-stimulatory signals for the T cells and the T cells recognizing self antigen presented by a non-activated DC will become anergic or apoptotic rather than activated.

11.5 These pathogens do not present danger signals to the antigen-presenting cells (APCs) in the tissue. Consequently, the APCs do not take up the pathogen and deliver it to the T-cell zones in the draining lymph nodes. Therefore, an adaptive immune response against such pathogens is not primed.

11.6 Immunological ignorance describes a state in which fully functional T cells are kept away from the antigen, which they recognize in vivo. Anergy describes a state in which lymphocytes do not respond with effector functions upon recognizing antigen. If the TCR transgenic T cells were ignorant in vivo, they would still respond to antigen in vitro, e.g. they would proliferate and produce cytokines. These effector functions can be assayed in vitro. If the TCR transgenic T cells were anergic, they would proliferate very little and fail to produce IL-2 in response to antigen presentation in vitro.

11.7 This is still an open question. The two most likely explanations are (i) the effector cells have become resistant to regulation by Tregs or (ii) the Tregs lack the relevant effector functions necessary to prevent the effector cells from causing damage.

12. REGULATION OF THE IMMUNE RESPONSE

12.1 EAE requires a type 1 response to develop and one possibility is that the T cells of C57BL/6 mice are more inclined than those of BALB/c mice to make TH1 responses.

12.2 You could sort CD4$^+$ T cells from the two strains of mice, culture them under neutral conditions and measure their production of IFNγ and IL-4. You might expect T cells from the type 1 dominant C57BL/6 mice to make more IFNγ, and T cells from the type 2 dominant BALB/c mice to make more IL-4.

12.3 In general, a type 1 response is most effective against intracellular pathogens.

12.4 C57BL/6 mice tend to make a type 1 response, which is highly effective against *Leishmania*, whereas BALB/c mice make a less-effective type 2 response. Therefore, in this disease, BALB/c mice are the more susceptible strain.

12.5 IL-12 promotes a type 1 response; hence we might expect exogenous IL-12 to make the BALB/c mice less susceptible to *Leishmania*.

13. IMMUNE REACTIONS IN THE GUT

Oysters are a food item that is normally tolerated by the body. Eating an infected shellfish causes the antigens in the food to be presented in association with components of the pathogen that can activate PAMP receptors, induce co-stimulatory molecules and break tolerance. Additionally, bacterial toxins may damage the gut epithelium again, enhancing antigen presentation and allowing antigens to access the gut-associated lymphoid tissues more readily. Once tolerance is broken, the TH2-type response, which is characteristic of the gut, will lead to production of antigen-specific IgE antibodies. Consequently, eating another oyster, even a good one, will lead to an allergic reaction to antigen in the food.

14. VIRUS–IMMUNE SYSTEM INTERACTIONS

14.1 The non-neutralizing antibodies may have mediated protection by activating complement to mediate virolysis, virion opsonization for uptake and destruction by macrophages, or destruction of virus-infected cells expressing glycoprotein D on their surface. They may also have mediated protection by mobilizing Fc receptor-expressing effector cells to combat the infection, promoting virion uptake by macrophages, or targeting macrophages or NK cells to lyse virus-infected cells and produce soluble antiviral factors.

14.2 Whether the protective capacity of the non-neutralizing antibodies was dependent on the presence of their Fc region could be evaluated by testing the capacity of the $F(ab')_2$ portion of the antibody to mediate protection. Although the antibodies were not able to neutralize virus in vitro alone, whether they were capable of doing so in the presence of complement, macrophages or NK cells could be assessed. The roles played by complement, macrophages and NK cells in antibody-mediated virus neutralization in vivo could also be explored by depleting mice of complement or these innate subsets just prior to antibody administration and determining whether or not the antibodies were still able to mediate protection in their absence.

14.3 No. Although epitopes derived from all of the HIV proteins can be presented on infected cells and target these cells for T-cell recognition, T cells recognizing epitopes in proteins that are present in cells early after the cell becomes infected are likely to be able to control virus replication most effectively, as these T cells will have a longer window of opportunity to detect and to lyse the infected cell before new virus particles start to be produced from it. Epitopes derived from structural proteins that are present in virions in sufficient quantities for the protein introduced into the cytoplasm as infection occurs to be processed and presented (e.g. the HIV Gag protein) will be displayed on an infected cell most rapidly, followed by epitopes derived from proteins that are synthesized in infected cells relatively early in the viral life cycle (e.g. the HIV Nef protein).

14.4 One way in which this could be achieved is by designing vaccines to induce T-cell responses to epitopes in the most invariant regions of the virus, where any amino acid changes introduced to confer escape from T-cell recognition are likely to have a high cost to viral fitness. It would also be helpful for vaccines to stimulate strong T-cell responses to a large number of different viral epitopes so that the virus will need to acquire multiple mutations to escape from the entire vaccine-induced response.

15. IMMUNOENDOCRINE INTERACTIONS IN THE RESPONSE TO INFECTION

15.1 The immune system cannot be understood in isolation from the rest of mammalian physiology. One of the many effects of stress is increased production of adrenocorticotrophic (ACTH) from the pituitary. This in turn drives increased production of cortisol by the adrenal. The proof is that, in the animal models mentioned, the stressor can be replaced by mimicking the stress-induced levels of cortisol (or the rodent equivalent, corticosterone) with implanted slow-release cortisol pellets. The cortisol downregulates cell-mediated immunity to tuberculosis.

15.2 These observations provide clues to why increased cortisol levels can lead to reduced immunity to tuberculosis. Raised cortisol levels cause APCs to release more IL-10 and less IL-12; hence newly recruited T cells tend to develop a T_H2 cytokine profile. Moreover, cortisol actually synergizes with some functions of T_H2 cytokines and enhances the ability of IL-4 to drive IgE production. It is interesting that BCG vaccination does not lead to protective immunity if the BCG is given to animals bearing cortisol pellets that mimic stress levels of cortisol. Cortisol also reduces the anti-mycobacterial functions of macrophages.

These points emphasize the need for a physiological approach to the understanding of infection. A narrow immunological approach has solved some infections, but global emergencies such as tuberculosis, HIV infection and septic shock may require integrated physiological thinking as well as pure immunology.

16. IMMUNITY TO PROTOZOA AND HELMINTHS

16.1 Protozoa replicate within the host and there is usually a balance between the effectiveness of the immune response and the virulence of the parasite. With certain parasites, the infections may be short-lived and may kill the host, but this may not be a disadvantage to the parasite if it has already been transmitted to a new host. A good example is falciparum malaria, which is potentially fatal, particularly in children in endemic areas who have not developed any immunity but are likely to have been bitten during the course of the infection by mosquitoes, which will ensure further transmission. Helminths, by contrast, do not replicate within the host and are generally long-lived chronic infections. Transmission is by the release of eggs and larvae from an adult parasite, which may be excreted or be taken up by a vector.

16.2 By adopting an intracellular mode of existence, parasites may be able to hide from the immune response. A good example is falciparum malaria, which lives in mature red blood cells. Because this cell type has no nucleus, it cannot express MHC class I molecules on its surface; hence the parasite is invisible to $CD8^+$ cytotoxic T cells. Other parasites live in nucleated cells, which will express class I MHC molecules, but experiments have shown this to be downregulated in cells infected with some parasites. *Toxoplasma gondii* avoids being killed by the macrophage by inhibiting the fusion of the lysosome with the phagosome; *Trypanosoma cruzi* escapes from the phagosome into the cytoplasm of the cell; and *Leishmania* spp. can resist the low pH of the phagolysosomes and are resistant to lysosomal enzymes.

16.3 Extracellular parasites can adopt a number of ways of avoiding immune attack. Parasites may disguise themselves: for example, by undergoing antigenic variation (African trypanosomes) or by adsorbing host molecules or undergoing molecular mimicry of the host (schistosomes). Parasites may hide from the host immune response by becoming cysts (*Entamoeba* spp.) or by living in an immunoprivileged location (*Toxoplasma* in brain). They may resist attack by having a physical barrier (helminths) or by producing enzymes that resist the oxidative burst or disable antibodies. Many parasites are able to modulate the host immune response to their advantage.

17. VACCINATION

17.1 Successful attenuation results in an organism still capable of generating an immune response against the wild-type virulent organism, but no longer capable of causing disease. This is a delicate balance to achieve. In some instances (e.g. hepatitis B and C viruses), the organisms cannot be cultured and attenuation by repeated in vitro passage is impossible.

17.2 There is no reason to believe that a vaccine cannot improve on nature. Many organisms express gene products that interfere with immune responses. Removal of these from the vaccine may allow protective responses to be generated.

17.3 Although smallpox was eliminated because there was no animal reservoir or carrier state, this is also the case for some other microorganisms and it should be possible to eliminate them. For other organisms, elimination will be difficult and maintenance of herd immunity will remain important.

17.4 Vaccines are unlikely to replace antibiotics completely. Microorganisms evolve very rapidly and vaccine production against complex organisms, such as mycobacteria, has proved very difficult. In addition, immunodeficient individuals and the elderly remain at risk even after vaccination.

17.5 BCG clearly has multiple effects. Specific immune responses to BCG antigens can be detected, but cell wall and other components of the bacterium have potent immunomodulatory effects. The efficacy of BCG as a vaccine has been suggested to depend on cross-reactions of BCG with environmental mycobacteria as well as *Mycobacterium tuberculosis* itself.

17.6 Strong immune responses may cause tissue damage in individuals with parasites already present. However, a vaccine that prevented establishment of infection would be unlikely to be damaging.

17.7 Antigens that induce T-cell immunity may be useful vaccine antigens. Molecules that contribute to virulence, such as toxins, may be the best targets for vaccines. Because the genomes of many pathogens have been or are being sequenced, searching homologous gene products may identify potential targets.

18. HYPER-IgM IMMUNODEFICIENCY

18.1 This child presented with bacterial pneumonia, a history of recurrent respiratory tract infections, lymphadenopathy and abnormal immunoglobulin levels, with increased IgM and low IgG and IgA. These features are consistent with a hyper-IgM phenotype. The normal number and distribution of T and B lymphocytes rules out both SCID and congenital agammaglobulinaemia. CD40L deficiency is inherited as an X-linked trait and is characterized by severe infections (including opportunistic infections) and neutropenia. The patient was a female child who did not present with opportunistic infections or neutropenia. This makes the diagnosis of CD40L deficiency very unlikely.

18.2 The association of hyper-IgM phenotype and recurrent lymphadenopathy is typical of AID deficiency, which is inherited as an autosomal trait, affecting both males and females. This is the most likely diagnosis in this patient.

18.3 Antibodies formed to tetanus toxoid immunization are of the IgG class. Because this child is incapable of undergoing isotype switching, she cannot make IgG antibodies. However, antibodies to the blood group substances are predominantly of the IgM isotype, which this child can synthesize.

18.4 The child should be given intravenous immunoglobulin (IVIG) at regular intervals (every 3–4 weeks) to protect her against bacterial infections. As this child is incapable of making IgG, she will need IVIG for life. She may benefit also from prophylactic antibiotics, along with IVIG administration. This treatment should result in a significant reduction of infectious episodes. However, AID deficiency also carries an increased risk of autoimmune manifestations.

19. SECONDARY IMMUNODEFICIENCY

19.1 If untreated, approximately 97% of HIV-positive individuals seroconvert within 3 months of infection. ELISAs for antibodies to gp41, a HIV surface glycoprotein, and p24, a core protein, are most widely used to detect HIV infection. The ELISA is followed by a Western blot to confirm that antibodies are binding to the correct viral protein. A diagnosis can be made on the basis of the ELISA (sensitivity of 99.7% and specificity of 98.5%) and the Western blot, which in combination give a specificity and sensitivity of >99.98%. Tests may also be performed for the presence of the p24 protein, which appears early after infection. Reverse-transcription PCR may be used to amplify and to detect viral nucleic acid. Interpretation of the findings is made in conjunction with other factors including CD4$^+$ T-cell count and the patient's history. However, the combination of ELISA and the Western blot is highly accurate.

19.2 Acute seroconversion causes an infectious mononucleosis-like illness in up to 50% of infected individuals. Common symptoms are fever, lymphadenopathy, pharyngitis, rashes and myalgia. At this point, there is a drop in the $CD4^+$ and $CD8^+$ T-cell counts and a rise in plasma viraemia and p24 antigen concentration. Antibodies to surface glycoproteins g120 and gp41 are produced from approximately 6 weeks after infection and are initially IgM. IgG antibodies of the same specificity follow the IgM response and persist during the latent phase. Viraemia and p24 levels are generally low during this period. Disease progression is heralded by a declining $CD4^+$ lymphocyte count and a rise in plasma viraemia. Clinically, $CD4^+$ T-cell counts are a fair index of progression, although plasma viraemia gives a more accurate measure of disease progression.

20. AUTOIMMUNITY AND AUTOIMMUNE DISEASE

20.1 It is thought that free DNA filtered in the kidney fixes to the glomerular basement membrane and can then be bound by anti-DNA antibodies, which then form an immune complex in situ. Complement is then fixed, resulting in local damage.

20.2 This is a vexed question. Although DNA–anti-DNA complexes are found in tissues, efforts to find these complexes in the serum have failed. In addition, immunizing lupus-prone animals with DNA does not produce clinical lupus. However, introduction of transgenes encoding anti-dsDNA in mice can produce lupus.

20.3 A possible explanation is that the mononuclear–phagocyte system becomes saturated and is therefore unable to clear the soluble complexes, which are thought to be most likely pathogenic. It is also possible that the reduction in the complement receptors on red cells (complement receptor-1, CR1) might predispose to poor clearance of complexes.

20.4 Over 95% of patients with SLE have ANA as the major autoantibody. Antibodies to extractable nuclear antigens are also seen, but much less frequently. Anti-dsDNA antibodies are the most specific to SLE because anti-single-stranded antibodies are found in a variety of other situations, such as other autoimmune disease, a variety of infections and inflammatory conditions.

21. TRANSPLANTATION

21.1 In group 1, there was a large major histocompatibility complex (MHC) mismatch between the two strains and the graft underwent a rapid acute rejection. In group 2, the donor and recipient are identical and therefore there is no immune response against the grafts. Hence there was no rejection and the grafts survived indefinitely.

21.2 In group 3, the grafts survived slightly longer than in group 1. This is probably because the irradiation of the animals suppressed the immune system. The survival in group 4 is very similar to group 3 and the difference is likely to be by chance. Animals treated with the vector to block CD40

(group 5) and CD80 (group 6) showed longer survival, with blockade of CD40 showing greater graft prolongation. Statistical analysis should be performed to see whether these differences are significant but, assuming that they are, this indicates that blocking either CD40 or CD80 can prolong graft survival, presumably by suppressing the immune response against the graft, but they cannot cause indefinite graft survival. However, animals injected with both vectors that block CD40 and CD80 (group 7) show long-term graft survival (>100 days). This suggests that blocking both CD40 and CD80 is more effective than blocking just one of them and that there may be a synergistic interaction between blockades of these co-stimulatory molecules. This might be a result of more complete suppression of the immune response or the induction of some form of tolerance. To determine whether the animals in group 7 are tolerant, it would be necessary to carry out a second transplant of a BALB/c organ into those mice. If that is accepted with no rejection (and control organs are rejected), it would indicate tolerance induction.

21.3 The researchers could look at the phenotype of cells in the graft and blood of the animals in group 7 to see whether they have markers of regulatory cells, such as FoxP3. They could also take cells from those animals and see whether they can suppress the response of other T cells in in vitro assays (such as the mixed lymphocyte reaction). Finally, they could transfer cells from these animals to new (naive) animals and see whether they could help prolong graft survival.

21.4 In any experiment using animals, it is important to use the fewest animals possible, while ensuring that there are enough animals to get a clear result. If you use more animals than you need, you are subjecting too many animals to the experimental procedures. If you use too few animals, you may not be able to get a clear result and you have wasted those animals that you did use. It important for ethical reasons to carry out statistical tests to determine the optimal group size. The experimenters in this case would have used these tests to decide how many animals they needed in each group.

21.5 Immunosuppressive drugs require the patients to take their medication continually, which is inconvenient. More importantly, the drugs can have toxic side effects on patients, which reduce their quality of life and can cause other disease. In addition, patients who are immunosuppressed have a greater risk of developing infections and some cancers. This may be because of a lack of immune surveillance against the cancer cells or failure to control viruses that cause cancer.

21.6 Jane is blood group O and will have antibodies against blood group A. It is likely that if the organ were transplanted into this patient, it would undergo hyperacute rejection. Therefore, under normal circumstances, Jane is not suitable for receiving this kidney. To receive an organ when there are pre-existing antibodies, the recipient must undergo a desensitizing protocol (as discussed in

Chapter 21). While Seema is a more likely recipient, it will still be important to check that she does not have pre-existing antibodies against other molecules expressed on the graft (for example, HLA molecules). The degree of HLA match and the priority of each of the patients on the transplant list will also need to be considered.

22. IMMUNITY TO CANCERS

22.1 For CAR T-cell therapy, the target antigen must be expressed on the cell surface, since CARs do not recognize intracellular antigen presented on MHC class I. Ideally, the target antigen should only be expressed by tumour cells to prevent off-target effects.

22.2 These are all symptoms of a systemic inflammatory response and point to cytokine release syndrome (CRS), which is a well-known side effect of CAR T-cell therapy.

22.3 High serum IL-6 supports the idea that the volunteers are experiencing CRS. It also suggests that it might be possible to treat this side effect using therapies that target IL-6, such as anti-IL-6 antibodies.

22.4 This suggests that the target antigen, mesothelin, may be expressed in the lining of the lungs. In fact, it is expressed at low levels in the mesothelial cells that line the pleura, peritoneum and pericardium.

22.5 It might be possible to reduce the off-target effects by reducing the dose of CAR T cells, although this might also result in a smaller anti-tumour response. It might also be possible to engineer the T cells with an 'off switch': for example, by introducing a suicide gene (such as caspase 9) whose expression in the T cells can be induced by giving the patient a specific drug. The CAR T cells could also be engineered to express an antigen, such as CD20, which would allow them to be depleted using a monoclonal antibody if necessary.

23. SEVERE ANAPHYLACTIC SHOCK

23.1 Traditionally, the term anaphylaxis has been used to describe a systemic clinical syndrome caused by IgE-mediated degranulation of mast cells and basophils. Susceptible individuals exposed to a sensitizing antigen produce specific IgE antibodies, which bind to high-affinity IgE receptors (FcεRI) found on mast cells and basophils. The receptor binds the Fc portion of the antibody, leaving the Fab binding sites available to interact with antigen. The avidity of this Fc binding reaction is high and therefore the dissociation of IgE from the receptors is slow, with a long half-life. On subsequent exposure, the antigen is bound by the IgE-receptor complexes, which causes receptor-mediated activation of the cells with release of preformed and de novo synthesized mediators. Degranulation is rapid and completed within 30 minutes. These mediators, released on a large scale, are responsible for the clinical manifestations of anaphylaxis. The IgE-mediated mechanism of mast cell degranulation has been implicated in the pathogenesis of anaphylaxis triggered by

a variety of agents. These include antibiotics (e.g. penicillins, cephalosporins), foods (e.g. milk, nuts, shellfish), foreign proteins (e.g. insulin, bee venom, latex) and pharmacological agents (e.g. streptokinase, vaccines). Patients who have anaphylaxis might or might not have a history of atopy. Natural exposure to common allergens such as pollen or dust mites is rarely a cause of anaphylaxis. However, when patients who also have asthma develop anaphylaxis resulting from venom, penicillin or food antigens, the reactions are more dangerous because they can include rapid onset of bronchospasm.

Mast cell degranulation can occur by IgE-independent pathways. In these cases, prior exposure is not a prerequisite because specific IgE antibodies are not involved. Three putative mechanisms of anaphylactoid reactions are given below:

- Blood, blood products and immunoglobulins can cause an anaphylactoid reaction. The suggested mechanism is the formation of immune complexes with subsequent complement activation and production of C3a and C5a. Both of these complement components (anaphylatoxins) are capable of degranulating mast cells directly. In addition, both components increase vasopermeability and may induce hypotension.

- Certain therapeutic and diagnostic agents, such as opiates, muscle relaxants and contrast media, are also capable of directly causing mast cell degranulation and anaphylaxis.

- 5%–10% of asthmatic subjects produce a reaction to non-steroidal anti-inflammatory drugs (NSAIDs), such as aspirin or indometacin. Symptoms commonly include bronchospasm, rhinorrhoea and, rarely, vascular collapse. The ability of these agents to cause anaphylaxis appears to correlate with their effectiveness in inhibiting prostaglandin synthesis. The mechanism of this sensitivity is unknown, but increased leukotriene production occurs, which suggests that triggering mast cells is part of the reaction.

23.2 There is a great variation in the timing and nature of anaphylactic symptoms. The onset is usually within seconds or minutes of exposure, although delays of an hour have been reported. The following are common presentations, which may occur singly or in combination:

- cutaneous: erythema, pruritus of hands, feet and abdomen, urticaria, angioedema;
- respiratory: laryngeal oedema causing hoarseness, which may progress to asphyxia, bronchoconstriction causing wheezing, rhinorrhoea;
- cardiovascular: hypotension, arrhythmias, tachycardia, vascular collapse;
- gastrointestinal: cramping abdominal pain, nausea, vomiting, diarrhoea.

The majority of cases of anaphylactic reaction are not fatal. It has been estimated that 1%–2% of penicillin therapy courses are complicated by systemic reactions, but only 10% of these are serious. In the USA, some

400–800 people die annually from penicillin anaphylaxis, with a similar figure for contrast media; 70% of deaths result from respiratory complications (laryngeal oedema and/or bronchospasm) with 25% resulting from cardiovascular dysfunction. Prompt treatment of anaphylaxis is essential because death may occur rapidly. The patient is placed in the recovery position, oxygen is given by mask and 0.5–1.0 mL epinephrine (adrenaline) 1:1000 w/v is injected intramuscularly. This has the effect of increasing the blood pressure, relaxing bronchial smooth muscle and preventing additional mediator release. Intravenous antihistamines (e.g. 10 mg chlorpheniramine) can be useful because histamine can cause vasodilation, cardiac arrhythmias and bronchospasm. Corticosteroids (e.g. 100 mg hydrocortisone) intravenously may help to reduce any late-phase response.

23.3   The first step is to obtain a thorough history of previous adverse reactions. The timing and nature of such reactions should be noted. Skin prick testing with insect venom is a fast and sensitive method of detecting anti-venom IgE. Serum venom-specific IgE are positive in only 80% of those with significant reactions to venom skin prick tests. Immunotherapy is best reserved for those with life-threatening systemic reactions to insect venom. The patient is given increasing subcutaneous dosages and then a monthly maintenance dose of 100 µg. The clinical protection rate is in the order of 98% for both adults and children.

24. BLOOD GROUPS AND HAEMOLYTIC DISEASE OF THE NEWBORN

24.1   Because Mrs Chareston has clearly become sensitized to Rhesus D, it is most likely that her first child is RhD$^+$. The alternative explanation (that she has become sensitized by a blood transfusion) is highly unlikely, because of the routine matching of this blood group when carrying out transfusions.

24.2   HDNB usually becomes more serious with successive pregnancies because the mother has become sensitized to the fetal red cells and successive sensitizations produce progressively stronger responses in the mother and more serious disease in susceptible children.

24.3   Anti-Rhesus D antibodies are given to the mother to clear the fetal RhD$^+$ erythrocytes before they have a chance to sensitize the mother's immune system.

24.4   If the antibodies are given pre-partum, they would cross the placenta and produce or exacerbate HDNB in the fetus.

24.5   Rhesus prophylaxis is not always successful, but in this case there was no treatment after the first pregnancy and Mrs Chareston was already sensitized to RhD. Preventing further responses in an individual who is already sensitized is less likely to succeed because of the nature of secondary immune responses – less antigen is required to trigger the response.

24.6   The most likely explanation is that the child is Rh$^-$. Indeed, this turns out to be the case. An Rh$^-$ child must have received a Rh$^-$ gene from both parents. Assuming that Mr Chareston is the father of the fourth child, we can say that his genotype is RhD$^+$/RhD$^-$ (heterozygote) and that the child received RhD$^-$ genes from both parents.

24.7   Antigens of the ABO blood group are carbohydrates and tend to induce IgM antibodies, which do not undergo affinity maturation or class switching (see Chapter 9). IgM does not cross the placenta (see Chapter 10) and therefore does not produce HDNB.

24.8   The second child was definitely not fathered by Mr Chareston because ABO blood groups are co-dominantly expressed. For a child to have the blood group B, one or both parents must have blood group B. As neither Mr nor Mrs Chareston has this blood group, the B gene must have come from someone else.

25. TYPE III SERUM SICKNESS AFTER FACTOR IX ADMINISTRATION

25.1   This is a classic example of serum sickness induced by a foreign protein factor IX because the boy does not produce it.

25.2   Corticosteroids were prescribed to decrease inflammation and for immunosuppression.

25.3   The likelihood that this type of reaction will develop again is relatively high because a memory response will be produced; T cells and plasma cells will respond more rapidly during re-exposure to the same foreign antigen (i.e. factor IX).

25.4   Short courses of corticosteroids with/without transient immunosuppression.

25.5   In this case, the clinical presentation is associated with an apparent non-inflammatory process (inferred because there is only proteinuria and inflammation has not reduced the glomerular filtration rate). Although the precise pathogenesis is uncertain, it is thought that the administered factor IX gets modified (becomes more positively charged) in the circulation. Because of its charge, it becomes trapped during normal filtration between the negatively charged glomerular basement membrane and glomerular epithelial cells, where it serves as a planted antigen for circulating anti-factor IX antibodies. The Fc regions of local or in situ formed immune complexes activate the classical complement system, whereby C5b–9 causes sublytic injury to the epithelial cells, leading to their detachment. Because these cells normally participate in maintaining the glomerular integrity and limiting protein filtration, this pathological process causes loss of large amounts of protein in the urine. Inflammation is not observed because FcR engagement on circulating inflammatory cells is prevented by the intact basement membrane. Pathologically, there is epithelial cell effacement from the basement membrane, but a conspicuous absence of inflammation. By contrast, in acute serum sickness, when immune deposits form between the endothelium and the basement membrane (or on the basement membrane), the deposited IgG engages FcR on circulating cells and inflammation (with cellular infiltration) is the predominant feature.

25.6 The likelihood that this type of reaction will develop again is relatively high because a memory response will be produced; T cells and plasma cells will respond more rapidly during re-exposure to the same foreign antigen (i.e. factor IX).

25.7 Immunosuppression until the proteinuria resolves to treat the present episode. Because the probability of immunological recall is high, transient immunosuppression with each factor IX therapy is indicated to reduce the production of antibodies to factor IX.

26. A HYPERSENSITIVITY TYPE IV REACTION

26.1 Granulomas are composed of lymphocytes, macrophages and epithelioid cells. The latter develop from macrophages after chronic antigenic stimulation and may fuse to form multinucleate giant cells, typical of granulomas. Cytokines involved in this process include T-cell-derived IFNγ and TNF, both for the activation of macrophages and for the organization of the granuloma.

26.2 Histological examination at the site of a DTH reaction reveals oedema of the dermis with an infiltrate of monocytes and lymphocytes. This resolves over 1–2 weeks. Granulomas do not form at the sites of DTH reactions if a soluble antigen, such as tuberculin, is used. By contrast, in the lymph node a chronic granulomatous response develops as the mycobacteria survive within macrophages, leading to persistent stimulation of T cells and chronic inflammation.

26.3 CD4$^+$ T lymphocytes are the major cells responsible for the recognition of soluble recall antigens and the stimulation of DTH reactions.

26.4 Other infections, such as cat scratch fever caused by *Bartonella henselae*, histoplasmosis and tularaemia, may cause granulomas in lymph nodes. These are diagnosed by the clinical pattern and microbial cultures. Sarcoidosis causes non-caseating granulomas and is diagnosed by clinical features, histology and the absence of an infectious cause. Granulomas may also develop in response to foreign bodies, such as talc and silica, or exposure to beryllium.

26.5 The brother's DTH reaction is evidence of a strong T-cell response to soluble antigens from *M. tuberculosis*. This indicates that he has been infected with *M. tuberculosis* but does not mean that he has active tuberculosis disease at present. Normally he would have investigations to exclude active tuberculosis and, if this is not present, he would be considered for chemoprophylaxis to eradicate the infection and prevent progression to disease in later life.

GLOSSARY

A

Acquired immune deficiency syndrome (AIDS) A progressive immune deficiency caused by infection of CD4$^+$ T cells and mononuclear phagocytes with the human retrovirus HIV.

Activation-induced cytidine deaminase (AID) An enzyme expressed in activated B cells that causes somatic mutation in the immunoglobulin gene locus.

Acute phase proteins Serum proteins whose levels increase during infection or inflammatory reactions.

ADAMs (a disintegrin and metalloprotease) A family of proteases; some members are involved in inflammation, leukocyte migration and remodelling of tissue.

ADCC (antibody-dependent cell-mediated cytotoxicity) A cytotoxic reaction in which Fc-receptor-bearing killer cells recognize target cells via specific antibodies.

Adhesion molecules Cell surface molecules involved in the binding of cells to extracellular matrix or to neighbouring cells, where the principal function is adhesion rather than cell activation (e.g. integrins and selectins).

Adjuvant A substance that non-specifically enhances the immune response to an antigen.

Affinity A measure of the binding strength between an antigenic determinant (epitope) and an antibody-combining site.

Affinity maturation The increase in average antibody affinity frequently seen during a secondary immune response.

AIRE A transcription factor that promotes expression of multiple tissue genes in medullary thymic epithelial cells and is hence involved in T-cell education.

Allelic exclusion This occurs when the use of a gene from the maternal or paternal chromosome in one cell prevents the use of the other. It is seen with antibody and T-cell receptor genes.

Allergen An agent (e.g. pollen, dust, animal dander) that causes IgE-mediated hypersensitivity reactions.

Allergy Usually refers to a type I hypersensitivity reaction.

Allotype The protein of an allele that may be detectable as an antigen by another member of the same species.

Alternative pathway The activation pathways of the complement system involving C3 and factors B, D, P, H and I, which interact in the vicinity of an activator surface to form an alternative pathway C3 convertase.

Amplification loop The alternative complement activation pathway that acts as a positive feedback loop when C3 is split in the presence of an activator surface.

Anaphylatoxins Complement peptides (C3a and C5a) that cause mast cell degranulation and smooth muscle contraction.

Anaphylaxis An antigen-specific immune reaction mediated primarily by IgE that most commonly results in urticaria, vasodilation, and constriction of smooth muscle, including those of the bronchus and gut, and may result in death.

Anergy Failure to make an immune response following stimulation with a potential antigen.

Antagonist peptides Analogues of antigenic peptides that bind to MHC molecules and prevent stimulation of specific clones of T cells.

Antibody A molecule produced by B cells or plasma cells in response to antigen that has the particular property of combining specifically with the antigen that induced its formation.

Antigen A molecule that reacts with antibody and the specific receptors on T and B cells.

Antigen receptors The lymphocyte receptors for antigens, including the T-cell receptor (TCR) and surface immunoglobulin on B cells, which acts as the B-cell's antigen receptor (BCR).

Antigen presentation The process by which certain cells in the body (antigen-presenting cells) express antigen on their cell surface in a form recognizable by lymphocytes.

Antigen processing The conversion of an antigen into a form in which it can be recognized by lymphocytes.

Antigenic determinants See 'epitopes'.

Antigenic peptides Peptide fragments of proteins that bind to MHC molecules and induce T-cell activation.

Antiviral proteins Proteins whose synthesis is induced by interferons. They become activated if the cell is infected by virus and limit viral replication.

APCs (antigen-presenting cells) A variety of cell types that carry antigen in a form that can stimulate lymphocytes.

Apoptosis Programmed cell death that involves nuclear fragmentation and condensation of cytoplasm, plasma membranes and organelles into apoptotic bodies. The process may be induced by internal controls on cell survival (intrinsic pathway) or external signals, such as from tumour necrosis factor (TNF) family molecules (extrinsic pathway).

Arthus reaction Inflammation seen in the skin some hours following injection of antigen. It is a manifestation of a type III hypersensitivity reaction.

Atopy The clinical manifestation of type I hypersensitivity reactions, including eczema, asthma, rhinitis and food allergy.

Autocrine This refers to the ability of a signalling molecule (such as a cytokine) to act on the cell that produced it.

Autoimmunity Immune recognition and reaction against the individual's own tissue.

Avidity The functional combining strength of an antibody with its antigen, which is related to both the affinity of the reaction between the epitopes and paratopes (complementarity determining regions) and the valencies of the antibody and antigen.

B

β₂-Microglobulin A polypeptide that constitutes a component of some membrane proteins, including the class I MHC molecules.

B7–1 (CD80), B7–2 (CD86) Two molecules present on antigen-presenting cells. They ligate CD28 on T cells and act as powerful co-stimulatory signals.

B cells Lymphocytes that develop in the bone marrow in adults and produce antibody. They can be subdivided into two groups, B1 and B2. B1 cells use minimally mutated receptors, which are close to the germline immunoglobulin sequences, whereas B2 cells are the major responding population in conventional immune responses to protein antigens.

B-cell co-receptor complex A group of cell surface molecules consisting of complement receptor type 2 (CD21), CD81 and CD19, which act as a co-stimulatory receptor on mature B cells.

B-cell receptor complex (BCR) B-cell surface immunoglobulin and its associated signalling molecules, CD79a and CD79b.

Basophil A population of polymorphonuclear leukocytes that stain with basic dyes and have important roles in the control of inflammation.

BCG (bacillus Calmette–Guérin) An attenuated strain of *Mycobacterium tuberculosis* used as a vaccine, an adjuvant or a biological response modifier in different circumstances.

Bcl-2 An anti-apoptotic molecule first discovered in activated B cells that had been rescued from apoptosis.

Bim (Bcl2 interacting mediator of cell death) A pro-apoptotic protein that antagonizes Bcl2.

Biozzi mice Lines of mice bi-directionally bred to produce low or high antibody responses to a variety of antigens (originally sheep erythrocytes).

Blood groups Sets of allelically variable molecules expressed on red cells and sometimes on other tissues that may be the target of transfusion reactions.

Bone marrow Spongy tissue found in the centres of bones, which is the primary site of immune cell production.

Bradykinin A vasoactive nonapeptide that is the most important mediator generated by the kinin system.

Bursa of Fabricius A lymphoepithelial organ that is the site of B-cell maturation and is found at the junction of the hindgut and cloaca in birds.

Bystander lysis Complement-mediated lysis of cells in the immediate vicinity of a complement activation site that are not themselves responsible for the activation.

C

C domains The constant domains of antibody and the T-cell receptor. These domains do not contribute to the antigen-binding site and show relatively little variability between receptor molecules.

C genes The gene segments that encode the constant portion of the immunoglobulin heavy and light chains and the α, β, γ and δ chains of the T-cell antigen receptor.

c-Kit (CD117) A receptor for stem cell factor, which is required for the early development of leukocytes and is a cell surface marker for mast cells.

C1–C9 The components of the complement classical and lytic pathways, which are responsible for mediating inflammatory reactions, opsonization of particles and lysis of cell membranes.

C3 convertases The enzyme complexes C3bBb and C4b2a that cleave complement C3.

Capping A process by which cell surface molecules are caused to aggregate (usually using antibody) on the cell membrane.

Carrier An immunogenic molecule or part of a molecule that is recognized by T cells in an antibody response.

Caspases A group of enzymes that are particularly involved in the transduction of signals for apoptosis.

Cathelicidins A group of cytotoxic peptides produced by granulocytes.

CD markers Cell surface molecules of leukocytes and platelets that are distinguishable with monoclonal antibodies and may be used to differentiate different cell populations.

CDRs (complementarity determining regions) The sections of an antibody or T-cell receptor V region responsible for antigen or antigen–MHC molecule binding.

Cell adhesion molecules (CAMs) A group of proteins of the immunoglobulin supergene family involved in intercellular adhesion, including ICAM-1, ICAM-2, ICAM-3, vascular cell adhesion molecule-1 (VCAM-1), mucosal addressin cell adhesion molecule-1 (MAdCAM-1) and platelet endothelial cell adhesion molecule (PECAM).

Central tolerance Tolerance of T cells or B cells induced during their development in the thymus or bone marrow.

Chemokines A large group of cytokines falling into four families, of which the main families are the CC and the CXC group. Chemokines are designated as ligands belonging to a particular family (e.g. CCL2). Many chemokines have older descriptive names: for example, CCL2 is macrophage chemotactic protein-1 (MCP-1). They act on G protein-linked, seventransmembrane pass receptors and have a variety of chemotactic and cell-activating properties.

Chemokinesis Increased random migratory activity of cells.

Chemotaxis Increased directional migration of cells, particularly in response to concentration gradients of certain chemotactic factors.

Ciclosporin (cyclosporine in the USA) A T-cell suppressive drug that is particularly useful in suppression of graft rejection.

Class I/II/III MHC molecules Three major classes of molecule are coded within the MHC. Class I molecules have one MHC-encoded peptide complexed with β₂-microglobulin, class II molecules have two MHC-encoded peptides that are non-covalently associated and class III molecules are other molecules including complement components.

Class I/II restriction The observation that immunologically active cells will co-operate effectively only when they share MHC haplotypes at either the class I or class II loci.

Class switching The process by which an individual B cell can link immunoglobulin heavy chain C genes to its recombined V gene to produce a different class of antibody with the same specificity. This process is also reflected in the overall class switch seen during the maturation of an immune response.

Classical pathway The pathway by which antigen–antibody complexes can activate the complement system, involving components C1, C2 and C4, and generating a classical pathway C3 convertase.

Clonal selection The fundamental basis of lymphocyte activation in which antigen selectively causes activation, division and differentiation only in those cells that express receptors with which it can combine.

CMI (cell-mediated immunity) A term used to refer to immune reactions that are mediated by cells rather than by antibody or other humoral factors.

Collectins A group of large polymeric proteins, including conglutinin and mannan-binding lectin (MBL), that can opsonize microbial pathogens.

Complement A group of serum proteins involved in control of inflammation, activation of phagocytes and lytic attack on cell membranes. The system can be activated by interaction with the antibodies of the immune system (classical pathway).

Complement control protein (CCP) domains (also called short consensus repeats) A domain structure found in many proteins of the complement classical and alternative pathways and in some complement receptors and control proteins.

Complement receptors (CR1–CR4 and C1qR) A set of four cell surface receptors for fragments of complement C3. CR1 and CR2 have numerous complement control protein (CCP) domains and CR3 and CR4 are integrins. C1qR binds C1q.

ConA (concanavalin A) A mitogen for T cells.

Congenic Animals that are genetically constructed to differ at one particular locus.

Conjugate A reagent that is formed by covalently coupling two molecules together, such as fluorescein coupled to an immunoglobulin molecule.

Constant regions The relatively invariant parts of immunoglobulin heavy and light chains and the α, β, γ and δ chains of the T-cell receptor.

Contact hypersensitivity A delayed inflammatory reaction on the skin seen in type IV hypersensitivity.

Corticosteroids A class of steroid hormones that are also used as anti-inflammatory drugs, especially in the context of transplantation and autoimmune disease.

Co-stimulation The signals required for the activation of a lymphocyte, in addition to the antigen-specific signal delivered via their antigen receptors. CD28 is an important co-stimulatory molecule for T cells and CD40 for B cells.

Cross-reaction The sharing of antigenic determinants by two different antigens.

CSFs (colony stimulating factors) A group of cytokines that control the differentiation of haematopoietic stem cells.

CTLs Cytotoxic T lymphocytes: see cytotoxic T cells (Tc).

CTLA-4 (CD152) A downregulatory signalling molecule of T cells that competes with CD28 for ligation by CD80 and CD86 on antigen-presenting cells.

Cytokines A generic term for soluble molecules that mediate interactions between immune cells.

Cytotoxic T cells (Tc) Cells that can kill virally infected targets expressing antigenic peptides presented by MHC class I molecules.

D

D genes Sets of gene segments lying between the V and J genes in the immunoglobulin heavy chain genes and in the T-cell receptor β and δ chain genes, which are recombined with V and J genes during ontogeny.

DAMPs Damage-associated molecular patterns are signatures associated with damaged or apoptotic cells.

Decay accelerating factor (DAF) A cell surface molecule on mammalian cells that limits activation and deposition of complement C3b.

Defensins Defensins are peptides produced by cells of the immune system and epithelial cells that are active against bacteria, fung, and some viruses.

Degranulation Exocytosis of granules from cells such as NK cells, Tc cells, mast cells and basophils.

Dendritic cells A set of cells present in tissues that capture antigens and migrate to the lymph nodes and spleen, where they are particularly active in presenting the processed antigen to T cells. Dendritic cells can be derived from either the lymphoid or mononuclear phagocyte lineages.

DM molecules Molecules related to MHC class II molecules that are required for loading antigenic peptides onto class II molecules.

Domain A region of a peptide with a coherent tertiary structure. Both immunoglobulins and MHC class I and II molecules have immunoglobulin supergene family domains.

DTH (delayed-type hypersensitivity) An older term that includes the four classes of type IV hypersensitivity, mediated by T cells.

E

Education of T cells The process by which developing thymocytes are selected for those that recognize peptides on self MHC molecules, but not for those that recognize self-antigenic peptides.

Effector cells A functional concept, which in context means those lymphocytes or phagocytes that produce an end effect.

Eicosanoids Products of arachidonic acid metabolism, including prostaglandins, leukotrienes and thromboxanes.

Endocytosis Internalization of material by a cell by phagocytosis or pinocytosis.

Endothelium Cells lining blood vessels and lymphatics.

Endotoxin Lipolysaccharide produced by Gram-negative bacteria that activates B cells and macrophages.

Eosinophils A population of polymorphonuclear granulocytes that stain with acidic dyes and are particularly involved in reactions against parasitic worms and in some hypersensitivity reactions.

Eotaxins The older name for a group of chemokines that attract eosinophils.

Epithelioid cells A population of activated mononuclear phagocytes present in granulomatous reactions.

Epitopes The parts of an antigen that contact the antigen-binding sites of an antibody or the T-cell receptor.

Epstein–Barr virus (EBV) Causal agent of Burkitt's lymphoma and infectious mononucleosis that has the ability to transform human B cells into stable cell lines.

F

Fab The part of an antibody molecule that contains the antigen-combining site consisting of a light chain and part of the heavy chain; it is produced by enzymatic digestion.

Factors B, P, D, H and I Components of the alternative complement pathway.

Fas (CD95) A molecule expressed on a variety of cells that acts as a target for ligation by Fas ligand (FasL) on the surface of cytotoxic lymphocytes.

Fc The portion of an antibody that is responsible for binding to antibody receptors on cells and the C1q component of complement.

Fc receptors Surface molecules on a variety of cells that bind to the Fc regions of immunoglobulins. They are antibody class specific and isotype selective.

Ficolins A group of opsonins that recognize carbohydrate PAMPs.

Flow cytometry Analysis of cell populations in suspension according to each individual cell's binding to fluorescently conjugated antibodies.

Fluorescence-activated cell sorter (FACS) An instrument that analyses cells by flow cytometry and then allows them to be sorted into different populations and collected separately.

Follicular dendritic cells (FDCs) Antigen-presenting cells in the B-cell areas of lymphoid tissues that retain stores of antigen.

Formylmethionyl peptides Prokaryotes initiate protein synthesis with f-Met. Peptides such as f-Met-Leu-Phe are highly chemotactic for mononuclear phagocytes and neutrophils.

Foxp3 A transcription factor required for differentiation of regulatory T cells.

Framework segments Sections of antibody V regions that lie between the hypervariable regions.

Freund's adjuvant An emulsion of aqueous antigen in oil. Complete Freund's adjuvant contains killed *Mycobacterium tuberculosis*, whereas incomplete Freund's adjuvant does not.

Frustrated phagocytosis A term to describe the events that occur when a phagocyte attempts to internalize an antigen or antigenic particle but is unable to do so (e.g. because of its size).

G

γδ T cells The minor subset of T cells that express the γδ form of the T-cell receptor.

Galectins A family of proteins that bind carbohydrates and are involved in signalling, cell adhesion and the control of apoptosis during thymic education of T cells.

GALT (gut-associated lymphoid tissue) The accumulation of lymphoid tissue associated with the gastrointestinal tract.

Genetic restriction The term used to describe the observation that lymphocytes and antigen-presenting cells co-operate most effectively when they share particular MHC haplotypes.

Genome The total genetic material contained within the cell.

Genotype The genetic material inherited from parents; not all of it is necessarily expressed in the individual.

Germinal centres Areas of secondary lymphoid tissue in which B-cell differentiation and antibody class switching occur.

Germline The genetic material that is passed down through the gametes before it is modified by somatic recombination or maturation.

Giant cells Large multinucleated cells sometimes seen in granulomatous reactions and thought to result from the fusion of macrophages.

GPI (glycosylphosphatidylinositol)-linkage A way in which proteins become attached to the outer leaflet of the phospholipid bilayer that forms the plasma membrane.

Granulocytes Neutrophils, eosinophils and basophils.

Granulomatous reactions Chronic inflammatory reactions (often a manifestation of type IV hypersensitivity) caused by a failure to clear antigen.

Granzymes Granule-associated enzymes of Tc cells and NK cells, which enter their target cells through perforin pores and induce apoptosis.

GvHD (graft-versus-host disease) A condition caused by allogeneic donor lymphocytes reacting against host tissue in an immunologically compromised recipient.

H

H-2 The mouse major histocompatibility complex.

Haemagglutination Clumping of erythrocytes caused by antibody. This forms the basis of a number of immunoassays and blood group typing.

Haplotype A set of genetic determinants located on a single chromosome.

Hapten A small molecule that can act as an epitope but is incapable by itself of eliciting an antibody response.

Heat shock proteins A group of proteins that are induced in response to cell stress. Many of them act as chaperones for other proteins and some act as DAMPs to induce inflammation.

Helper T cells (TH) A functional subclass of T cells that can help to generate cytotoxic T cells (Tc) and co-operate with B cells in the production of antibody responses. TH cells recognize antigen in association with MHC class II molecules.

HEV (high endothelial venule) An area of venule from which lymphocytes migrate into lymph nodes, Peyer's patches and other encapsulated secondary lymphoid tissues.

Hinge The portion of an immunoglobulin heavy chain between the Fc and Fab regions that permits flexibility within the molecule and allows the two combining sites to operate independently. The hinge region is usually encoded by a separate exon.

Histamine A major vasoactive amine released from mast cell and basophil granules.

Histocompatibility The ability to accept grafts between individuals.

Human immunodeficiency virus (HIV) The causative agent of AIDS.

HLA (human leukocyte antigen) The human major histocompatibility complex.

Homologous restriction factors Complement components that restrict the action of the membrane attack complex on cells of the host.

Humoral Pertaining to the extracellular fluids, including the serum and lymph.

Hybridoma Cell line created in vitro by fusing two different cell types, usually lymphoid cells.

5-Hydroxytryptamine (serotonin) A vasoactive amine present in platelets and a major mediator of inflammation in rodents.

Hypersensitivity An inordinately strong immune response that causes more damage than the antigen or pathogen that induced the response.

Hypervariable region The most variable areas of the V domains of immunoglobulin and T-cell receptor chains. These regions are clustered at the distal portion of the V domain and contribute to the antigen-binding site.

I

ICAM-1 (CD54), ICAM-2 (CD102) and ICAM-3 (CD50) (intercellular adhesion molecules) Cell surface molecules found on a variety of leukocytes and non-haematogenous cells that interact with leukocyte functional antigen-1 (LFA-1, αLβ2-integrin).

Iccosomes Immune complexes in the form of small inclusion bodies found in follicular dendritic cells.

Idiotope A single antigenic determinant on an antibody V region.

Idiotype The antigenic characteristic of the V region of an antibody.

IELs (intraepithelial lymphocytes) A population of lymphocytes defined according to location in which γδ T cells are strongly represented.

Immune complex The product of an antigen–antibody reaction that may also contain components of the complement system.

Immunoblotting (Western blotting) A technique for identifying and characterizing proteins using antibodies.

Immunofluorescence A technique used to identify particular antigens microscopically in tissues or on cells by the binding of a fluorescent antibody conjugate.

Immunogenic Having the ability to evoke B-cell- and/or T-cell-mediated immune reactions.

Immunoglobulins The serum antibodies, including IgG, IgM, IgA, IgE and IgD.

Immunoglobulin supergene family (IgSF) Molecules that have domains homologous to those seen in immunoglobulins, including MHC class I and II molecules, the T-cell receptor, CD2, CD3, CD4, CD8, ICAMs, VCAM and some of the Fc receptors.

Immunological synapse The closely apposed region of the plasma membranes between T cells or NK cells and antigen-presenting or target cells, centred on MHC–peptide complexes interacting with their receptors.

Induced fit A description of the way in which an antigen can alter the normal tertiary structure of the binding site on a receptor following binding, by displacing amino acids.

Inducible nitric oxide synthase (iNOS) An enzyme induced by inflammatory cytokines in macrophages that catalyses the synthesis of nitric oxide (NO).

Inflammasome A multi-protein complex that assembles within a cell in response to PAMPs and that can activate caspase-1. The exact composition depends on the initiating stimulus.

Inflammation A series of reactions that bring cells and molecules of the immune system to sites of infection or damage. This appears as an increase in blood supply, increased vascular permeability and increased trans-endothelial migration of leukocytes.

Innate lymphoid cells (ILCs) Lymphocytes that do not have rearranged antigen receptors. The group includes three subsets of cells (ILC1, ILC2 and ILC3), which are innate equivalents to their T-cell counterparts (TH1, TH2, TH17, respectively), the natural killer cells (NK) and the lymphoid tissue inducer cells (LTi) important in organogenesis of secondary lymphoid tissues.

Integrins A large family of cell surface adhesion molecules, some of which interact with cell adhesion molecules (CAMs), others with complement fragments and others with components of the extracellular matrix.

Interferons (IFNs) A group of molecules involved in signalling between cells of the immune system and in protection against viral infections.

Interleukins (IL-1–IL-36) A group of molecules involved in signalling between cells of the immune system and the tissues.

Isotype Refers to genetic variation within a family of proteins or peptides such that every member of the species will have each isotype of the family represented in its genome (e.g. immunoglobulin classes).

ITAMs (immunoreceptor tyrosine-based activation motifs) and ITIMs (immunoreceptor tyrosine-based inhibitory motifs) These are target sequences for phosphorylation by kinases involved in cell activation or inhibition.

J

JAKs (Janus kinases) A group of enzymes with two catalytic domains. They activate by cross-phosphorylation and are particularly involved in signalling from type I and II cytokine receptors.

J chain A monomorphic polypeptide present in polymeric IgA and IgM and essential to their formation.

J genes Sets of gene segments in the immunoglobulin heavy and light chain genes and in the genes for the chains of the T-cell receptor, which are recombined during lymphocyte ontogeny and contribute to the genes for variable domains.

K

K cells An older term for NK cells. Defined as lymphocytes that are able to destroy their target by antibody-dependent cell-mediated cytotoxicity.

κ (kappa) chains One of the immunoglobulin light chain isotypes.

Karyotype The chromosomal constitution of a cell that may vary between individuals of a single species depending on the presence or absence of particular sex chromosomes or on the incidence of translocations between sections of different chromosomes.

Killer immunoglobulin-like receptors (KIRs) Receptors on NK cells that belong to the Ig superfamily, having either two or three extracellular domains. They may either inhibit or activate cytotoxicity, depending on their intracellular domains.

Kinins A group of vasoactive mediators produced following tissue injury.

Knockout An animal whose endogenous gene for a particular protein has been deleted or mutated to be non-functional.

Kupffer cells Phagocytic cells that line the liver sinusoids.

L

λ (lambda) chains One of the immunoglobulin light chain isotypes.

Langerhans cells Antigen-presenting cells of the skin that emigrate to local lymph nodes to become dendritic cells; they are very active in presenting antigen to T cells.

Large granular lymphocytes (LGLs) A group of morphologically defined lymphocytes containing the majority of NK-cell activity. They have both lymphocyte and monocyte/macrophage markers.

Lectin pathway A pathway of complement activation initiated by mannan-binding lectin (MBL) that intersects the classical pathway.

Leukotrienes Pharmacologically active derivatives of arachidonic acid produced by the 5-lipoxygenase pathway.

LFAs (leukocyte functional antigens) A group of three molecules that mediate intercellular adhesion between leukocytes and other cells in an antigen non-specific fashion. LFA-1 is CD11a/CD18, LFA-2 is CD2 and LFA-3 is CD58.

Ligand A linking (or binding) molecule.

Line A collection of cells produced by continuous growth of a particular cell culture in vitro. Such a cell line will usually contain a number of individual clones.

Linkage The condition where two genes are both present in close proximity on a single chromosome and are usually inherited together.

Linkage disequilibrium A condition where two genes are found together in a population at a greater frequency than that predicted simply by the product of their individual gene frequencies.

LPS (lipopolysaccharide) A product of some Gram-negative bacterial cell walls; a PAMP that activates many cell types and can act as a B-cell mitogen.

Ly antigens A group of cell surface markers found on murine T cells that relate to the differentiation of T-cell subpopulations. Many are now assigned to the CD system.

Lymph nodes Secondary lymphoid organs present throughout the body and connected by lymphatic vessels. They are the major sites of communication for immune cells during an immune response.

Lymphocytes A lineage of immune cells that is the main type of cell found in the lymph. It includes T cells, B cells and innate lymphoid cells (ILCs).

Lymphoid tissue inducer cells (LTi) Cells of the innate lymphoid cell (ILC) family, which initiate the development of secondary lymphoid tissue.

Lymphokines A generic term for molecules other than antibodies that are involved in signalling between cells of the immune system and are produced by lymphocytes (cf. interleukins).

Lymphokine activated killer cells (LAKs) Cytotoxic cells generated ex vivo by stimulation with interleukin 2 (IL-2) and possibly other cytokines.

Lymphotoxins A group of cytokines, related to tumour necrosis factors (TNFs), that act on TNF receptors and mediate inflammatory reactions and leukocyte activation.

Lysosomes Intracellular vesicles containing stored enzymes, adhesion molecules or toxic molecules, depending on the cell type.

Lysozyme An enzyme secreted by mononuclear phagocytes that hydrolyses bonds present in bacterial cell walls.

Lytic pathway The complement pathway effected by components C5–C9 that is responsible for damage to plasma membranes and potentially causes cell lysis.

M

Macrophages are fully differentiated mononuclear phagocytes, located in different tissues. They may be classed as M1 cells, which are pro-inflammatory, or M2 cells, which help maintain tissue integrity.

MALT (mucosa-associated lymphoid tissue) Generic term for lymphoid tissue associated with the gastrointestinal tract, bronchial tree and other mucosal tissues.

Mannose receptor (MR) A lectin-like receptor found on mononuclear phagocytes.

MAMPs Microbe-associated molecular patterns are molecular signatures that originate from bacteria, parasites and fungi and are recognized by the innate immune system.

MAP kinases A group of intracellular enzymes involved in signalling cascades that lead to the activation of transcription factors.

Marginal zone An area surrounding the splenic white pulp that separates the lymphoid areas from the surrounding red pulp.

Mast cells Cells distributed near blood vessels in most tissues. These cells are the major effector cells of immediate type hypersensitivity reactions (type I) and are full of granules containing inflammatory mediators.

Matrix metalloproteases (MMPs) A group of zinc-containing degradative enzymes that can break down components of the extracellular matrix (e.g. collagenase).

MCPs (macrophage chemotactic proteins) Old term for a group of CCL chemokines that attract macrophages.

Membrane attack complex (MAC) The assembled terminal complement components C5b–C9 of the lytic pathway that becomes inserted into cell membranes.

Memory cells Long-lived lymphocytes that have already been primed with their antigen but have not undergone terminal differentiation into effector cells. They react more readily than naive lymphocytes when re-stimulated with the same antigen.

MHC (major histocompatibility complex) A genetic region found in all mammals, the products of which are primarily responsible for the rapid rejection of grafts between individuals and which function in antigen presentation to T cells.

MHC restriction A characteristic of many immune reactions in which cells co-operate most effectively with other cells that share a MHC haplotype.

Microglia Mononuclear phagocytes resident in the brain and spinal cord. Microglial precursors colonize the human central nervous system early in gestation.

MIF (migration inhibition factor) A group of peptides produced by lymphocytes that are capable of inhibiting macrophage migration.

MIIC An endosomal compartment where MHC class II molecules are loaded with antigenic peptides.

MIPs (macrophage inflammatory proteins) The old name for a group of chemokines.

Mitogens Substances that cause cells, particularly lymphocytes, to undergo cell division.

MLR/MLC (mixed lymphocyte reaction/mixed lymphocyte culture) Assay system for T-cell recognition of allogeneic cells in which response is measured by proliferation in the presence of the stimulating cells.

Mononuclear phagocyte system The lineage of fixed and mobile long-lived phagocytic cells, including blood monocytes and tissue macrophages.

Myeloid cells The lineage of bone marrow-derived phagocytes, which includes neutrophils, eosinophils and monocytes.

Myeloma A lymphoma produced from cells of the B-cell lineage that can invade bone.

N

N regions Gene segments present in recombined antigen receptor genes that are not present in the germline DNA.

Neoplasm A synonym for cancerous tissue.

Neutrophils Polymorphonuclear granulocytes, which form the major population of blood leukocytes.

NF-κB A transcription factor that is widely used by different leukocyte populations to signal activation – sometimes called the master switch of the immune system.

NK (natural killer) cells A group of lymphocytes that have the intrinsic ability to recognize and to destroy some virally infected cells and some tumour cells.

NKT cells T cells that express an invariant form of the T-cell receptor and can recognize glycolipid antigens presented by CD1d. They also express some NK-cell receptors.

Nod-like receptors (NLRs) Nucleotide oligomerization domain-like receptors are pattern recognition receptors (PRRs) that sense intracytoplasmic pathogens.

Nucleotide oligomerization domains (NODs) Domains in intracellular receptors for pathogen-associated molecular patterns (PAMPS).

Nude mouse A genetically athymic mouse that lacks a transcription factor, which is also required for hair production.

O

Opsonization A process by which phagocytosis is facilitated by the deposition of opsonins (e.g. antibody and C3b) on the antigen.

P

PAF (platelet activating factor) A factor released by basophils that causes platelets to aggregate.

PALS (peri-arteriolar lymphatic sheath) The accumulations of lymphoid tissue constituting the white pulp of the spleen.

Paneth cells Cells present in the crypts of the small intestine that secrete anti-microbial peptides.

Paracrine The action of a signalling molecule (such as a cytokine) on a cell that is distinct, but that is in close proximity, from the cell that produced it.

Passenger cells Donor leukocytes present in a tissue graft that may sensitize the recipient to the graft.

Patch test Application of antigen to skin on a patch to test for type IV hypersensitivity reactions.

Pathogen An organism that causes disease.

Pathogen-associated molecular patterns (PAMPs) Biological macromolecules produced by microbial pathogens that are recognized by receptors on mononuclear phagocytes and some opsonins in serum and tissue fluids.

Pattern recognition receptors (PRRs) Receptors that recognize pathogen- or damage-associated molecular patterns (PAMPs or DAMPs).

PC (phosphorylcholine) A commonly used hapten that is also found on the surface of a number of microorganisms.

Pentraxins A group of acute-phase pentameric molecules present in serum that recognize PAMPs and opsonize bacteria for phagocytosis.

Perforin A granule-associated molecule of cytotoxic cells, homologous to complement C9. It can form pores on the membrane of a target cell.

Peyer's patches Collections of lymphoid cells in the wall of the gut that form a secondary lymphoid tissue.

PFC (plaque-forming cell) An antibody-producing cell detected in vitro by its ability to lyse antigen-sensitized erythrocytes in the presence of complement.

PHA (phytohaemagglutinin) A mitogen for T cells.

Phagocytosis The process by which cells engulf material and enclose it within a vacuole (phagosome) in the cytoplasm.

Phenotype The expressed characteristics of an individual (cf. genotype).

Plasma cell An antibody-producing B cell that has reached the end of its differentiation pathway.

Plasmin system One of the plasma enzyme systems that generates the fibrinolytic enzyme plasmin and contributes to inflammation and tissue remodelling.

Polymorphs A common acronym for polymorphonuclear leukocytes, including basophils, neutrophils and eosinophils.

Prick test Introduction of minute quantities of antigen into the skin to test for type I hypersensitivity.

Primary lymphoid tissues Lymphoid organs in which lymphocytes complete their initial maturation steps; they include the fetal liver, adult bone marrow and thymus and bursa of Fabricius in birds.

Primary response The immune response (cellular or humoral) following an initial encounter with a particular antigen.

Prime To induce an initial sensitization to antigen.

Privileged tissues/sites In the context of transplantation these are tissues that induce weak immune responses or sites of the body that are partly shielded from graft rejection reactions.

Prostaglandins Pharmacologically active derivatives of arachidonic acid produced by the cyclo-oxygenase pathway. Different prostaglandins are capable of modulating cell mobility and immune responses.

Proteasomes Organelles that degrade cellular proteins tagged for breakdown by ubiquitination.

Protein A and protein G Components of the cell wall of some strains of staphylococci that bind to Fc of most IgG isotypes.

Pseudoalleles Tandem variants of a gene: they do not occupy a homologous position on the chromosome (e.g. C4).

Pseudogenes Genes that have homologous structures to other genes but are incapable of being expressed (e.g. *Jk3* in the mouse).

Pyrogen A microbial product or chemokine that induces fever (e.g. LPS, IL-1).

R

Radioimmunoassay (RIA) A number of different sensitive techniques for measuring antigen or antibody titres using radiolabelled reagents.

RAG-1 and RAG-2 Recombination activating genes required for recombination of V, D and J gene segments during generation of functional antigen receptor genes.

Rapamycin A bacterial product, used as an immunosuppressive agent in transplantation.

Receptor A cell surface molecule that binds specifically to particular extracellular molecules.

Receptor editing A process by which immunoglobulin genes can undergo a secondary recombination event in order to rescue B cells that are producing non-functional or autoreactive antibodies.

Recombination A process by which genetic information is rearranged during meiosis. This process also occurs during the somatic rearrangements of DNA, which occur in the formation of genes encoding antibody molecules and T-cell antigen receptors.

Relative risk A number that expresses how much more likely (>1) or less likely (<1) an individual is to develop a particular disease if they possess a particular genotype.

Respiratory burst Increase in oxidative metabolism of phagocytes following uptake of opsonized particles.

Reticuloendothelial system A diffuse system of phagocytic cells derived from the bone marrow stem cells that are associated with the connective tissue framework of the liver, spleen, lymph nodes and other serous cavities. An old-fashioned term that is rarely used – mononuclear phagocyte system is the preferred term.

RLRs (rig-like receptors) A group of intracellular helicases that can detect dsRNA and act as sensors of viral infection.

ROIs/RNIs (reactive oxygen intermediates/reactive nitrogen intermediates) Bactericidal metabolites produced by phagocytic cells, including hydrogen peroxide, hypohalites and nitric oxide.

S

Scavenger receptors A group of receptors that recognize cell debris and are involved in the phagocytosis of apoptotic cells and some pathogens.

SCID (severe combined immunodeficiency) A group of genetic conditions leading to major deficiencies or absence of both B cells and T cells.

Secondary lymphoid tissue Sites where lymphocytes interact with each other and with non-lymphoid cells to generate an immune response. These include the spleen, lymph nodes and mucosa-associated lymphoid tissue (MALT).

Secondary response The immune response that follows a second or subsequent encounter with a particular antigen.

Secretory component A polypeptide produced by cells of some secretory epithelia that is involved in transporting secreted polymeric IgA across the cell and protecting it from digestion in the gastrointestinal tract.

Selectins Three adhesion molecules – P-selectin (CD62P), E-selectin (CD62E) and L-selectin (CD62L) – involved in slowing leukocytes during their transit through venules.

Serotonin 5-Hydroxytryptamine.

Serotype A variant of a pathogen, identified by its ability to bind a specific antibody.

Siglecs (Sialic acid-binding immunoglobulin-type lectins) A family of adhesion molecules found mostly on leukocytes (e.g. CD22, CD33), with inhibitory functions mediated via ITIMs.

SLE (systemic lupus erythematosus) An autoimmune disease (non-organ specific) of humans usually involving anti-nuclear antibodies.

Somatic hypermutation (SHM) A process occurring during B-cell maturation and affecting the antibody gene region that permits refinement of antibody specificity.

Spleen A major secondary lymphoid organ in the peritoneal cavity next to the stomach.

STATs A group of proteins that form components of transcription factors following activation by kinases.

Stem cell factor (SCF) Also called c-kit ligand or steel factor. A cytokine required for the earliest stages of leukocyte development in bone marrow. The receptor for SCF is CD177 (also known as c-kit).

Superantigens Antigens that stimulate clones of T cells with different antigen specificity but using the same TCR V genes.

Surface plasmon resonance A biophysical phenomenon that can be used to measure the association and binding constants of proteins in solution interacting with bound ligands.

Synergism Co-operative interaction.

Syngeneic Strains of animals produced by repeated inbreeding so that each pair of autosomes within an individual is identical.

T

T cells Lymphocytes that differentiate primarily in the thymus and are central to the control and development of immune responses. The principal subgroups are cytotoxic T cells (Tc) and T-helper cells (TH0, TH1, TH2 and TH17). T cells can also be defined according to their location, e.g. T-follicular helper cells (TFH).

Tregs (regulatory T cells) A functionally defined group of T cells that control (especially) autoimmune reactions and inflammation in the gut and skin.

TAP transporters A group of molecules that transport proteins and peptides between intracellular compartments.

TCR (T-cell receptor). The T-cell antigen receptor consisting of either an αβ dimer or a γδ dimer associated with the CD3 molecular complex.

T-dependent/T-independent antigens T-dependent antigens require immune recognition by both T and B cells to produce an immune response. T-independent antigens can directly stimulate B cells to produce specific antibody.

TGFs (transforming growth factors) A group of cytokines identified by their ability to promote fibroblast growth and tissue regeneration; they are also generally immunosuppressive.

Thoracic duct Drains efferent lymph into the venous system.

Thromboxanes Products of arachidonic acid metabolism, some of which are involved in inflammation.

Thymus A primary lymphoid organ in the thoracic cavity over the heart.

Tissue inhibitors of matrix metalloproteases (TIMPs) A group of proteins released by cells in tissues that limit the activity of matrix metalloproteases.

Tissue typing Determination of an individual's allotypic variants of MHC molecules.

TNF (tumour necrosis factor) A pro-inflammatory cytokine released by activated macrophages that is structurally related to lymphotoxin released by activated T cells.

Tolerance A state of specific immunological unresponsiveness.

Toll-like receptors (TLRs) A group of receptors, mostly located on the plasma membrane, that recognize PAMPs and transduce signals for inflammation.

Tonsils Paired lymphoid organs in the throat that form part of the mucosa-associated lymphoid tissue (MALT).

Transformation Morphological changes in a lymphocyte associated with the onset of division. Also used to denote the change to the autonomously dividing state of a cancer cell.

Transgenic animal An animal in which one or more new genes have been incorporated. These are often placed under specific promoters so that they are expressed only in particular tissues for limited periods.

V

V domains The N-terminal domains of antibody heavy and light chains and the α, β, γ and δ chains of the T-cell receptor that form the antigen or antigen/MHC binding site.

Vaccination A general term for immunization against infectious disease, originally derived from immunization against smallpox, which uses the vaccinia virus.

Vasoactive amines Products such as histamine and 5-hydroxytryptamine (serotonin) released by basophils, mast cells and platelets that act on the endothelium and smooth muscle of the local vasculature.

Veiled cells Cells of the dendritic cell lineage as seen in afferent lymph. They may be derived from Langerhans cells or other dendritic cell types.

VLA-1–VLA-6 (very late antigens) The set of integrins that share a common β1 chain (CD29).

W

Waldeyer's ring The secondary lymphoid tissues of the nasopharynx that includes the tonsils and adenoids.

Western blotting A technique for identifying and characterizing proteins using antibodies; synonymous with immunoblotting.

White pulp The lymphoid component of spleen consisting of peri-arteriolar sheaths of lymphocytes and antigen-presenting cells.

X

Xenogeneic Refers to interspecies antigenic differences.

INDEX

Note: Page numbers followed by *f* indicate figures, *t* indicate tables, and *b* indicate boxes.